ANIMAL
MICROBIOLOGY

ANIMAL MICROBIOLOGY

VOLUME 2

Rickettsias and Viruses

A. BUXTON

Ph.D. F.R.C.V.S. F.R.S.E.
Professor of Veterinary Pathology,
Royal (Dick) School of Veterinary Studies, University of Edinburgh

and

G. FRASER

B.Sc. Ph.D. M.R.C.V.S.
Senior Lecturer in Veterinary Microbiology,
Royal (Dick) School of Veterinary Studies, University of Edinburgh

BLACKWELL SCIENTIFIC PUBLICATIONS

OXFORD LONDON EDINBURGH MELBOURNE

© BLACKWELL SCIENTIFIC PUBLICATIONS LTD. 1977

Osney Mead, Oxford
8 John Street, London WC1
9 Forrest Road, Edinburgh
P.O. Box 9, North Balwyn, Victoria, Australia

First published 1977

British Library Cataloguing in Publication Data
Buxton, A.
    Animal microbiology.
    Vol. 2: Rickettsias and virology.
    1. Micro-organisms, Pathogenic
    I. Title II. Fraser, G.
    591.2'3   QR175

    ISBN 0 632 00941 1

Distributed in the United States of America by
J. B. Lippincott Company, Philadelphia,
and in Canada by
J. B. Lippincott Company of Canada Ltd., Toronto

*Typesetting by Dai Nippon Printing Co., Hong Kong, and
Printed and bound by T. & A. Constable Limited, Edinburgh*

(handwritten annotations: (215) 574 4200 — New edit. info — 1-800-638 3030 — out of print — (212) 593 7213)

Contents

(Detailed contents are found at the start of each chapter)

VOLUME 2

VOLUME 1

Preface

Our purpose in writing this book has been to collect together information on animal micro-biology required both by undergraduates studying for their primary veterinary degrees and by veterinarians undertaking postgraduate courses. We also hope that the book will be of use to veterinary surgeons in different walks of professional life as well as being of interest to medical microbiologists and others requiring information on this subject. To cater for these various interests we have included discussions on the epidemiology, pathogenesis, clinical features, diagnosis, control, public health and other aspects of infectious diseases as well as on purely microbiological matters. We hope that the tables of contents at the beginning of each chapter, the textual headings and lists of further reading, together with the general index, will enable the reader to locate easily any required information.

In order to present the subject in a manner equally acceptable to all readers, we have supported the text with a selection of coloured photographs and drawings as well as mono-chromes illustrating the appearance of microbiology as seen in a diagnostic laboratory. For the benefit of postgraduate students, and particularly those in tropical and subtropical countries, we have tried to maintain a balance between our discussions on microbial diseases of animals occurring in warmer climates and those in more temperate zones. Consequent upon the recent expansion of fish farming throughout the world and as a result of the increasing importance of controlling and preventing diseases of fish, a chapter has been devoted to this specialist subject.

During the prolonged gestation period of this book we have become increasingly aware of the difficulties that can beset two authors when trying to ensure that a text covering such a wide canvas as animal microbiology is up-to-date in all its facets, while simultaneously avoiding undergraduate indigestion arising from the inclusion of too much detailed infor-mation in particular areas. It is inevitable in a first edition of a book of this size that some errors and omissions will have occurred and we hope that readers will call our attention to any shortcomings. While the preparation of the whole book has been the concern of both of us, the senior author has dealt in particular with the introductory chapters, bacteriology and the appendices and the junior author has been responsible for the sections on mycotic, rickettsial and viral infections.

During the writing and correction of the text we have received advice and encouragement from many people, and we should like to mention in particular Dr. G. H. K. Lawson for information on *Campylobacter*, Dr. W. J. Penhale on Immunology and Dr. J. E. Phillips on *Actinobacillus*. We are especially grateful to Dr. W. B. Martin for reading the whole of the manuscript on Virology and for making many valuable suggestions and corrections.

It is a special pleasure to acknowledge the apparently inexhaustible patience and skill of Mr. R. C. James, who was responsible for photographing most of the colour plates used in this book. We also hope that we have done justice to those who have contributed illustrative material and we accord our thanks to Mr. I. S. Beattie, Mr. K. W. Head and Mr. A. C. Rowland for allowing us to include some of their coloured transparencies of pathological lesions in the section on Bacteriology. Recognition of colleagues, research students and correspondents who have kindly provided us with many of the illustrations in the chapters dealing with Mycology and Virology is recorded in the captions of the relevant plates. To all those and to others, too numerous to mention individually, who have helped in many ways, large and small, we offer our sincere thanks.

It is a pleasure to record the untiring assistance we have received from Miss M. Millar, who has not only typed the entire manuscript but has also helped in numerous other ways towards the completion of the final text.

Finally, our grateful thanks are due to our publisher, in particular Mr. Per Saugman, who invited us to write the book, and Mr. Nigel Palmer for his constant advice in matters relating to production.

A. Buxton
G. Fraser

Edinburgh, April 1977

VOLUME II

CHAPTER 36

THE RICKETTSIAS

The Rickettsias

The unicellular microorganisms can be arranged in order of decreasing size and complexity, viz: protozoa, yeasts and certain fungi, bacteria, mycoplasmas, rickettsiae and chlamydiae. Members belonging to these last two groups resemble bacteria in some ways and viruses in others, and are not immediately identifiable as either. They are generally smaller than bacteria but larger than viruses (300–500 nm), and most species are obligate intracellular parasites.

Most workers are now agreed that *Rickettsia* and *Chlamydia* (the psittacosis-lymphogranuloma venereum agents), have properties more closely related to bacteria than to viruses in that: (1) they contain both DNA and RNA, (2) multiplication is by binary fission or budding, and (3) particles possess bacterial cell wall constituents and certain growth enzyme systems which render them susceptible to some antibiotics. Thus, rickettsiae and chlamydiae are probably very small bacteria which have developed an ultra-parasitic mode of life.

The general properties of these organisms are compared with those of bacteria, mycoplasmas and viruses in Table 36.1.

THE RICKETTSIAE

Rickettsiae constitute a relatively small but important group of obligate, intracellular microorganisms that mostly occur naturally in the tissues of arthropods and are transmissible to man and animals in which they may cause disease. The name rickettsia was assigned to these organisms in memory of Dr H. T. Ricketts who died of typhus accidentally contracted while studying the disease.

Classification

Organisms of the order *Rickettsiales* may be classified into three families based on their morphology, serology, mode of transmission and whether they occur in the cytoplasm or nucleus of the cells they infect (Fig. 36.1). All are small, rod-shaped or coccoid and often pleomorphic microorganisms that are usually obligate intracellular parasites and grow only in living tissues. The one exception to this general rule is *R. quintana*, the causative agent of trench fever, which grows extracellularly in the louse

TABLE 36.1. Biological relationships of microorganisms.

	Bacteria	Mycoplasmas	Rickettsiae	Chlamydiae	Viruses
Visible by light microscopy	+	+	+	+	−†
Size (nm)	c. > 1000	Variable	c.300	c.300	< 300
Nucleic acids	DNA+RNA	DNA+RNA	DNA+RNA	DNA+RNA	Either DNA or RNA
Muramic acid	+	—	+	+	—
Ribosomes and other organelles	+	+	+	+	—
Growth in non-living media	+	+	—	—	—
Intracellular replication	—*	+	+	+	+
Mode of replication	Binary fission	Binary fission & budding	Binary fission	Binary fission & budding	Synthesis of viral NA and viral proteins
Eclipse phase	—	—	—	—(?)	+
Sensitivity to antibiotics	+	+	+	+	—
Sensitivity to interferon	—	—	—	+	+

* Some will replicate intracellularly, e.g. *Mycobacterium tuberculosis*
† Some are just visible, e.g. vaccinia.

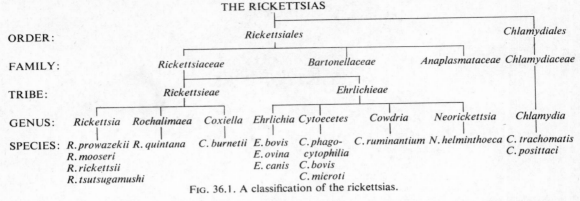

FIG. 36.1. A classification of the rickettsias.

gut and has been cultivated successfully on modified blood agar. Most but not all species of rickettsiae are transmitted by arthropod vectors and many cause diseases in man and animals.

Members of the family *Rickettsiaceae* usually inhabit the gut cells of the arthropods which transmit the microorganisms to other susceptible hosts, and those that affect mammals parasitize the cells of the vascular endothelium or other tissue cells. The properties of *Chlamydiaceae* are so similar to those of *Rickettsiaceae* that many authors prefer to classify them with rickettsiae even though they have no arthropod vectors. In contrast, members of the families *Bartonellaceae* and *Anaplasmataceae* primarily parasitize mammalian erythrocytes and may be transmitted by arthropod vectors. (Table 36.2).

The *Rickettsiaceae* may be divided into two tribes, the *Rickettsieae*, which are adapted to arthropods and cause disease in mammals, and the *Ehrlichieae*, some of which are adapted to arthropods and are pathogenic for mammals but not for man.

The *Rickettsieae* consist of three important genera, each of which contains pathogenic species that cause diseases of man and animals. Members of the genus *Rickettsia* are transmitted by lice, fleas, ticks or mites and include several important species, e.g. *R. prowazekii* of epidemic typhus, *R. mooseri* of endemic typhus or murine typhus, *R. tsutsugamushi* of scrub typhus, *R. conorii* of Mediterranean fever, and *R. rickettsii* of Rocky Mountain spotted fever. The genus *Coxiella* includes the important species *C. burnetii*, of Q fever, which is not dependent on arthropod transmission and does not produce a typhus-like rash on the skin of the patient. The third genus, *Rochalimaea*, includes *R. quintana* of trench fever.

The tribe *Ehrlichieae* includes four genera, viz. *Ehrlichia*, which are lymphocytic parasites associated with 'rickettsiosis' of cattle (*E. bovis*), sheep (*E. ovina*) and dogs (*E. canis*); *Cytoecetes*, which are present in the granular leucocytes and monocytes

in cases of tick-borne fever in sheep (*C. phagocytophilia*) and cattle (*C. bovis*), and in a disease of voles (*C. microti*); *Cowdria*, which form characteristic clusters in the cytoplasm of vascular endothelial cells in heartwater fever of ruminants (*C. ruminantium*); and, *Neorickettsia*, occurring as short rods, crescents or rings in the cytoplasm of reticuloendothelial cells of mammals and in the tissues of fluke vectors of salmon disease of dogs (*N. helminthoeca*) (Table 36.3).

General properties

Rickettsiae are mostly obligate intracellular parasites having properties that are intermediate between those of bacteria and viruses. They are usually smaller than bacteria and their size ranges from 0·3 to 2·0 μm in length by 0·3–0·5 μm in width. Most species are highly pleomorphic and their shape may vary from coccoid, ellipsoid or coccobacillary to rod-shaped and, occasionally, filamentous forms. They are Gram-negative and mostly stain poorly with watery solutions of aniline dyes. The most satisfactory methods for staining them are Giemsa, Leishman, Castaneda and Macchiavello; some, e.g. *R. prowazekii* and *C. burnetii* retain basic fuchsin but others, e.g. *C. ruminantium* and *C. phagocytophilia* do not. Electron micrographs show that the individual organism is surrounded by a plasma membrane and a rigid cell wall which is chemically and structurally very similar to that of *E. coli*. The cytoplasmic material is granular in appearance and contains irregular, filamentous bodies which are believed to constitute the nucleus.

Rickettsiae resemble bacteria in that they are composed of protein, neutral fat, phospholipids and carbohydrates and the cell wall contains aminoacids, polysaccharide and muramic acid. Unlike viruses which contain either DNA or RNA, but never both, the nucleic acid of rickettsiae consists of relatively constant amounts of DNA and variable quantities of RNA, which is usually about

TABLE 36.2. Some diseases associated with members of the families *Bartonellaceae* and *Anaplasmataceae*.

Organism	Host	Transmission	Natural disease	Activated by splenectomy	Remarks
BARTONELLACEAE (Four genera)					
Bartonella bacilliformis	Man	Sand fly (Phlebotomus)	(1) Oroya fever – anaemia (2) Verruga peruana – granulomatous skin disorder		Grows in non-living media
Haemobartonella muris	Rodents	Louse (*Polyplax spinulosum*)	Not primary pathogen		May grow slowly in non-living media
H. bovis	Cattle	?Insect vector	Not primary pathogen	Yes	
H. canis	Dogs	Not known	Severe anaemia, or none	Yes	
H. felis	Cats	?Insect vector	Fever and anaemia	?	
Grahamella spp.	Rodents	Not known	Not primary pathogen	?	
Eperythrozoa suis	Pigs	?Ectoparasites, e.g. lice	Icteroanaemia	?	not cultivated
E. parva	Pigs	?Ectoparasites	Not primary pathogen	Yes	
E. wenyoni	Cattle	?Ectoparasites	Not primary pathogen	Yes	
E. ovis	Sheep, goats	?Ectoparasites	Haemolytic anaemia	Yes	
E. felis	Cats	?	Anaemia or none	?	
E. coccoides	Laboratory mice	?	Not primary pathogen	Yes	
ANAPLASMATACEAE					
Anaplasma marginale	Cattle	Ticks (7 genera) (Biting flies – 19 species)	'Gall-sickness' – may be severe icteroanaemia	Yes	Widely distributed in the tropics and sub-tropics.
A. centrale	Cattle	Various arthropods	Mild anaemia		
A. ovis	Sheep, goats	Various arthropods	Mild anaemia		

TABLE 36.3.   Some diseases caused by members of the family *Rickettsiaceae*.

Species	Disease	Geographical distribution	Host	Transmission	Straus Reaction	Weil-Felix Reaction
RICKETTSIA						
R. prowazekii	Epidemic typhus	Worldwide	Man	Body louse. Infected louse faeces into broken skin	—	OX-19
R. mooseri (R. typhi)	Endemic (murine) typhus	Worldwide	Rats, mice (man)	Flea. Infected flea faeces into broken skin	+	OX-19
R. tsutsugamushi	Scrub typhus	Asia, Far East.	Wild rodents (man)	Mite. Bite of trombiculid mite	—	OX-K
R. rickettsii	Rocky Mountain spotted fever	America	Wild rodents, dogs (man)	Tick. Bite of wood tick or dog tick (*Dermacentor* spp.)	+	OX-19, OX-2
COXIELLA						
C. burnetii	Q fever	Worldwide	Small animals, cattle, sheep, goats, man	Inhalation of dried infective material from placentas, discharges, etc. ?Ingestion, ?Tick bite or faeces	Rarely	—
EHRLICHIA						
E. canis	'Rickettsiosis' (dog typhus)	Africa, India.	Dogs	Tick. Bite of *Rhipicephalus sanguineus*	—	?OX-19, OX-K
CYTOECETES						
C. phagocytophilia	Tick-borne fever	Europe.	Sheep, cattle	Tick. Bite of *Ixodes ricinus*	—	—
C. bovis						
COWDRIA						
C. ruminantium	Heartwater	Africa, south of the Sahara.	Sheep, goats, cattle	Tick. Bite of *Amblyoma* spp.	—	—
NEORICKETTSIA						
N. helminthoeca	Salmon poisoning	N.W. Pacific seaboard	Dogs, foxes	Ingestion of raw fish containing fluke cercaria infected with neorickettsia. No arthropod transmission	—	—

three times that of DNA. Although rickettsiae possess their own enzyme systems which enable them to oxidise intermediate metabolites like pyruvate and succinate, they depend on living susceptible host cells for essential metabolic reactions and cannot, therefore, be cultivated in artificial media.

Most species of rickettsiae can survive only briefly outside the living cell and are quickly inactivated by chemical disinfection, drying, heat and other adverse environmental conditions, and their growth is inhibited by broad-spectrum antibiotics, e.g. tetracyclines. Recent isolates of rickettsiae are inactivated within a few hours at room temperature but may be preserved in 50 per cent glycerol-saline at 4°C or by freeze-drying emulsions of infected tissues suspended in sterile skimmed milk, serum albumen or other suitable stabilizer.

Pathogenicity

Most species of rickettsiae have a predilection for vascular endothelium and stimulate the cells lining the small capillaries to swell and divide. Hyperplasia of the endothelial cells, localised thrombus formation and the release of erythrocytes into the surrounding tissues give rise to some of the more prominent clinical manifestations of rickettsial infections such as petechial rash and stupor. Other rickettsia-like organisms, e.g. *Ehrlichia* spp. and *Cytoecetes* spp. mostly parasitize granular leucocytes and monocytes.

Cultivation

Most rickettsiae can be propagated in a wide range of laboratory animals, in the yolk sacs of embryonated hens' eggs and in various cell culture systems. Growth may occur in different parts of the host cell; members of the typhus group usually parasitize the cytoplasm while those of the spotted fever group are mostly to be found in the nucleus. So far, only one member of the *Rickettsiaceae*, *R. quintana*, which causes trench fever, has been shown to grow on cell-free media; all other species require living susceptible cells and grow best when the cell metabolism is depressed. Thus, their rate of multiplication in chicken embryos is enhanced when the temperature of incubation is reduced to 32°C. In many cases, enhanced growth is also obtained in the presence of sulphonamides.

A few species of rickettsiae are capable of producing lethal toxins. For example, if large numbers of *R. mooseri* or *R. prowazekii* are inoculated intravenously or intraperitoneally into mice, the animals usually die within 2–8 hours due to the direct effects of the toxins. It is significant that these toxins are not neutralized by antisera prepared against the rickettsial cell wall and that they cannot be separated from the intact living organism. Further evidence suggests that they are heat labile and are detoxified by formaldehyde. It is also interesting to note that yolk sac suspensions of *R. mooseri* and *R. prowazekii* can haemolyse sheep and rabbit red blood cells, *in vitro*, but have no effect on those of human origin.

Ecology

Rickettsial infections vary enormously in severity, from symptomless, mild and self-limiting illnesses to some of the most fulminating diseases known; and most are transmitted through the bite of infected lice, fleas, mites or ticks or by their infected faeces through broken skin.

The role of arthropods in the transmission of rickettsial infections is well illustrated in the case of epidemic typhus of man. The causative agent, *R. prowazekii*, is spread from man-to-man by the bite of the human body louse (*Pediculus corporis*) which acquires the infection when it bites either a patient suffering from typhus or a latent carrier in whom the organism has persisted for many months or years. When rickettsiae in the blood-meal reach the insect's gut they invade the epithelial cells and multiply therein. In due course the cells swell and rupture, releasing enormous quantities of organisms into the intestinal contents. The louse contaminates the skin with its infected faeces and the organisms are probably introduced into the human host through abrasions caused by scratching rather than by actual lousebites.

In contrast to epidemic typhus, the spotted fever group of diseases represent accidental infections in man following the bite of infected ticks. Several species of tick, e.g. wood ticks and dog ticks are the principal vectors. Some may carry the organism in all stages of their development but it is the adult tick that is mainly responsible for transmitting the infection to humans. In many cases the rickettsiae are maintained in various mammalian reservoir hosts.

A number of important rickettsial infections of domesticated animals are also transmitted by tick bite, e.g. *C. ruminantium* of heartwater by the bont tick, *Amblyoma hebraeum*, and *C. phagocytophilia* of tick-borne fever by *Ixodes ricinus*. On the other hand, although *C. burnetii* of Q fever is often conveyed from animal to animal by tick-bite, man usually acquires the infection by inhaling infected dust from straw and bedding soiled by animals or from fomites, placentae and uterine discharges and, perhaps, by drinking infected milk.

Diagnosis

The isolation of a known strain of rickettsia from a typically affected individual probably constitutes the best evidence that the organism is the cause of the disease but technical difficulties limit the usefulness of the method, especially in human medicine. In many rickettsial infections of domesticated animals a tentative diagnosis can usually be made by demonstrating the rickettsial bodies in stained blood or tissue smears, e.g. within the granular leucocytes in tick-borne fever (Plate 36.1b), the endothelial cells of the capillaries in heartwater (Plate 36.1c) and in the uterine discharges and placentae of cattle and sheep infected with Q fever (Plate 36.1a, facing p. 388).

For confirmatory diagnosis a number of serological tests are available. These include the Weil-Felix agglutination reaction with Proteus OX antigens for certain human infections, specific agglutination tests, complement-fixation tests which can detect antibodies to both group and type specific antigens, neutralization tests performed in guinea-pigs or yolk sacs of developing chicken embryos, and fluorescent antibody staining.

Biological methods for the isolation and identification of rickettsiae are also available but, as the identification procedures are not always easy and many are extremely hazardous to perform, these should never be attempted except by highly trained personnel in suitably equipped laboratories.

Whole blood, emulsified blood clot or tissue suspensions are inoculated intraperitoneally into male guinea-pigs. Rectal temperatures are taken twice daily and, if the animals fail to show signs of clinical illness such as fever, scrotal swelling (Straus reaction), emaciation or death, serum samples should be obtained by cardiac puncture and examined for the presence of specific antibodies. At autopsy, carcases should be examined for macroscopic lesions such as swellings or other changes in the spleen, liver and other tissues. Impression smears of the viscera are stained and examined for the presence of rickettsiae and tissues may be passaged to other male guinea-pigs.

It is emphasised that the Straus reaction is not produced by all species of rickettsiae. Characteristic scrotal lesions, due to inflammatory changes in the *tunica vaginalis*, are generally found in guinea-pigs infected with Rocky Mountain spotted fever (*R. rickettsii*), Fièvre boutonneuse (*R. conorii*), South African tick-bite fever (*R. rickettsii var. pijperi*), Rickettsial pox (*R. akari*) and endemic typhus (*R. mooseri* or *R. typhi*) but not by epidemic typhus (*R. prowazekii*), scrub typhus (*R. tsutsugamushi*) and only very occasionally by Q fever (*C. burnetii*).

Antigenicity
Each species of rickettsia possesses its own antigens which stimulate the production of homologous antibodies. The presence of these antigens can be demonstrated by various serological tests including agglutination, serum neutralization, complement-

fixation and immunofluorescence. All species except *C. burnetii* also possess a soluble group antigen which is probably derived from the mucoid envelope of the organism and is released when shaken with ether.

Antibodies formed in the course of typhus fever and certain other rickettsial infections have been found to react, fortuitously, with the polysaccharide somatic antigens of certain non-motile O variants of *Proteus*, the so-called OX strains. This is because these rickettsiae contain an alkali-stable carbohydrate hapten, identical to a somatic constituent of these particular proteus bacilli which are readily agglutinated by sera from convalescent cases of typhus. This agglutination test is usually referred to as the Weil-Felix reaction which forms the basis of a simple and safe diagnostic procedure since it does not require the use of dangerous rickettsial antigens. Three strains are used: *Proteus* OX-2, OX-19 and OX-K, and the agglutination reactions to all three help to differentiate the important human rickettsial diseases. The agglutinins tend to disappear a few months after recovery and thus a positive Weil-Felix reaction is a useful indication of a recent infection. On the other hand, complement-fixing antibodies persist for much longer periods and provide evidence of past infection.

Treatment
Chloramphenicol, erythromycin and especially tetracyclines are effective in treating many rickettsial diseases. Unfortunately, however, they are rickettsistatic rather than rickettsicidal and do not always cure the body of organisms but rather suppress their growth. Since recovery largely depends on immunity, the course of treatment should continue for several days after the temperature has returned to normal. It should also be noted that if antibiotics are given early in the disease before immunity has developed, relapses may occur unless a second course of treatment is given about a week after the original treatment was stopped. Sulphonamides enhance the growth of many strains of rickettsiae and are generally contra-indicated.

It is of interest that rickettsiae can survive in recovered patients for many months or years and in Brill's disease, which is a recrudescence of an old epidemic typhus infection due to *R. prowazekii*, the organisms can persist for as long as 20 years in the tissues without the patient showing symptoms of the illness.

Control
In rickettsial diseases, control is often best achieved by breaking the infection chain, by treatment with antibiotics and by immunization if suitable vaccines are available.

Q fever

Synonyms Abattoir fever, Query fever, Burnet's rickettsiosis.

Definition

An infectious but usually symptomless condition of cattle, sheep, goats and other animals that is transmissible to humans in whom it causes an acute, and sometimes serious illness characterised by sudden onset, severe headache, high fever and, frequently, an interstitial 'atypical' pneumonia.

History

Q fever was first recognised as a 'local' disease among slaughterhouse workers in Brisbane, Australia, in 1933. The original name, 'abattoir fever' was changed to 'query fever' until 1937 when the causative agent was isolated and identified as belonging to the genus *Rickettsia*. In 1939 the name of *Rickettsia burnetii* was proposed for this organism but this has now been changed to *Coxiella burnetii*. In 1940 it was shown that several species of wild-living animals carried *Rickettsia* and probably formed the natural reservoir of infection in Australia. In the same year it was found that ticks belonging to the genera *Ixodes, Ornithodorus* and *Rhipicephalus* could become infected from carrier animals and shed the agent in their faeces or transmit it by tick-bite. In America during the late 1930s, it was shown that an agent isolated in Montana from the tick *Dermacentor andersoni* was identical with *C. burnetii* and that an earlier isolation made in 1926 was probably of the same organism. Although a serious epidemic of Q fever occurred among laboratory workers at Bethesda, U.S.A., in 1940, it was only during the later years of the second world war, when numerous outbreaks of a febrile pulmonary disease occurred in German and Allied troops stationed in Italy and the Balkan countries, that Q fever was recognised as a serious health problem in human and veterinary medicine.

The disease was first reported in the U.K. at the end of 1945 and a serological survey carried out in 1956 showed that about 3 per cent of healthy blood donors gave positive reactions.

Distribution

At first, Q fever was thought to be confined to Australia but the results of both cultural and serological surveys have shown that infection occurs extensively in many countries and is probably worldwide in its distribution.

Hosts affected

C. burnetii is widely distributed in nature and has been isolated from a variety of ticks and from many animal species, both wild and domesticated, including cattle, sheep, goats, horses, camels, pigs, dogs, bandicoots and birds. Although the organism rarely produces clinical illness in animals several species, including domesticated cattle and sheep, are important reservoirs of infection for man.

Aetiology

C. burnetii occurs within the cytoplasm of infected cells as large masses (20–30μm in diameter) of tightly packed organisms. Each organism occurs as a very short rod or as a tiny paired coccus with a bipolar appearance: some of the particles may be as large as medium-sized bacteria, while others are so small (0.3×0.15 μm) that they will pass membrane filters with an average pore diameter of 0·4 μm. They are weakly Gram-negative but stain Gram-positive when alcoholic iodine is used as a mordant. They stain readily with Romanowsky stains, appearing reddish-blue or purple with Giemsa and bright red with Macchiavello or the modified Ziehl-Neelsen (Brucella differential) method. In this respect they closely resemble both *Brucella abortus* and the agent of enzootic abortion of ewes, and their presence in ruptured cells in stained smears of uterine discharges or fetal membranes may cause confusion in diagnosis. Best results are probably obtained by staining *Coxiella* with auramine and examining the smear under the fluorescence microscope.

Although *C. burnetii* possesses many of the morphological and cultural characters of rickettsiae and does not grow in non-living media, it is unusually stable outside the host cell. It resists dessication or putrefaction and remains viable for prolonged periods at room temperature in excreta, secretions, water and milk, and in tissues suspended in 50 per cent glycerol–saline. It is relatively resistant to many physical and chemical bactericidal agents and to heat, and is capable of withstanding a temperature of 70°C for several minutes. Heating of infected raw milk at 143°F for 30 minutes is not sufficient to destroy all viable organisms but the 'flash' method of pasteurization, at 162°F for 15 seconds, is highly efficient. It is emphasised, that *C. burnetii* may remain virulent for days or weeks in milk, cream, butter and cheese. Tick faeces have been shown to retain infectivity for up to 586 days and infected dried blood for 186 days. *C. burnetii* resists merthiolate at 1:1000, hypochlorite solutions containing 100 mg/litre of active chlorine and phenol at 1 per cent. for 24 hours, but is inactivated by 2 per cent formalin, 1 per cent lysol, 5 per cent H_2O_2 and ethyl ether. Lyophilised yolk sacs and tissue suspensions retain their infectivity for years.

Cultivation

C. burnetii is an obligate intracellular parasite that cannot be grown in non-living media. In the labora tory it is readily propagated by the intraperitoneal inoculation of guinea-pigs, rabbits, hamsters and mice, and less easily in the yolk-sacs of 6–8-day old embryonated· hens' eggs incubated at 35°C. Experimentally infected animals usually develop a fever after 5–28 days but male animals rarely show a typical Straus reaction (orchitis). In chick embryos, the infection is confined to the yolk-sac and does not spread to other tissues. Infected yolk sacs are commonly used for the preparation of antigens for complement-fixation and agglutination tests but they are dangerous to handle and frequently cause infection of laboratory workers by inhalation. The agent can also be grown in cell cultures, producing colonies of organisms in the cytoplasm of the infected cell, but often without destructive cytopathic changes of the monolayer. Growth is improved after 14 days of incubation when the metabolic level of the host cell system is reduced.

Pathogenicity

Apart from an occasional report that *C. burnetii* has been found in association with bronchopneumonia in sheep and goats, and with abortions in sheep, goats and cattle, there is little evidence that it is responsible for any specific disease in domesticated animals. Indeed, most workers are of the opinion that Q fever infections of animals produce an astonishing lack of clinical signs. In naturally and artificially acquired infections of sheep and cattle there is a marked predilection for the mammae and placenta and, as a result, heavily infected uterine discharges and fetal membranes are probably the main sources of infection for other animals and for veterinarians, abattoir workers, farmers and others engaged in agriculture. Infection in chronically affected cows and goats resides in the udder and the agent may persist in the tissues for many months or years or be excreted in the milk over very long periods.

In man, on the other hand, Q fever causes a sudden onset of illness following an incubation period of between 14–28 days. The clinical picture is similar to that of influenza and is characterised by a sharp rise in temperature, a severe headache and photophobia, accompanied by symptoms of fever and chills; but there is no rash nor local lesion of the skin as in other rickettsial infections. Primary 'atypical' pneumonia is not uncommon and there may be some involvement of the central nervous system. During the febrile stage of the illness *C. burnetii* is present in the blood stream and may be excreted in the urine and sputum, and even in the milk, but inter-human spread is rare. The course of the disease is usually short but it may vary from a few days to several months. Although the mortality rate is low, recovered patients may require a prolonged period of convalescence, but subsequent immunity is fairly solid. Convalescence from Q fever is usually uneventful but chronic infections may occur and cases have been described at autopsy in which there is endocarditis, with vegetations on the heart valves containing rickettsiae. In man, and especially in children, the disease can also run a symptomless course which is only detectable by serological examinations.

Ecology

The most likely source of infection in the original cases of Q fever among abattoir workers in Queensland was an animal reservoir in bandicoots from which two species of tick were infected. It is believed that cattle acquired the infection from ticks and that the slaughtermen became infected by inhaling the organisms from contaminated hides. Despite the fact that many different varieties of ticks can carry the organism and spread it by contaminated faeces or tick-bites, it is now believed that they play only a minor role in the epidemiology of Q fever. There can be no doubt that *C. burnetii* is now firmly established among domestic animals and that animal-to-animal infection occurs readily by direct contact, without the necessity for intermediate vectors. In fact, the introduction of a single infected animal into a herd results in the rapid dissemination of infection among all the cattle; and several surveys have shown that in some areas as many as 50 per cent of cattle may become infected within a period of 6 months.

In man, infection by inhalation is undoubtedly the commonest route by which *C. burnetii* enters the body. In rural areas large numbers of organisms reach the external environment by means of infected uterine discharges, after-births, milk and other secretions and excretions. Much of this material becomes dried on exposure to air and sunlight and the tiny infectious particles, which are among the most resistant of the non-sporogenic organisms, become suspended in the air and may be transported for considerable distances before being inhaled by susceptible humans. Hay, straw, bedding and clothing contaminated by carrier sheep and cattle also remain infective for many weeks or months, and in Italy during the Second World War a number of severe outbreaks of pneumonia occurred among servicemen sleeping on straw palliases contaminated with *C. burnetii*.

It has also been suggested that dogs, especially sheepdogs, become infected by eating contaminated placentas and consequently spread the organisms over great distances via their infected faeces. Furthermore, in a recent epidemic in Germany it was found that dogs acquired infected ticks from fields grazed by cattle and subsequently carried the infection to a number of neighbouring farms.

Man may also become infected by the oral route and it has frequently been shown that milk samples from cows, sheep and goats contain rickettsiae and that the organisms can survive for considerable periods in cream, butter, cheese and other milk by-products. A survey conducted in the U.K. in 1952 showed that 7 per cent, 2 per cent and 1 per cent of the milk from farms in England, Wales and Scotland, respectively, were contaminated with *C. burnetii*. In an American survey carried out in an area where only 5 per cent of the community consumed raw milk, it was shown that 32 per cent of 300 people who had contracted Q fever were habitual drinkers of unprocessed milk. In an outbreak in England 41 per cent of cases were thought to have resulted from the patients drinking raw milk. While there is known to be a real risk of man contracting Q fever from animals, it is remarkable that the disease does not appear to occur in certain agricultural countries such as New Zealand and Scandinavia. Birds may also play a part in spreading *C. burnetii* and several cases of Q fever have been reported in human patients associated with pigeons.

Diagnosis

Laboratory diagnosis of Q fever includes the demonstration of the organisms in stained smears and the isolation and identification of *C. burnetii* by the inoculation of laboratory animals and chick embryos with blood and sputum from human sources, and with uterine discharges, placental material or other secretions and excretions from animal sources.

The direct microscopical examination of stained smears of pathological material from human patients has only limited application but the method is of value in veterinary medicine. The presence of large masses of red-coloured spherical or cocco-bacillary particles in preparations stained by Macchiavello or modified Ziehl-Neelsen methods is strong presumptive evidence of Q fever infection provided the organisms are not mistaken for *Brucella abortus* or psittacosis agents (Plate 36.1a, facing p. 388).

The isolation of *C. burnetii* by the intraperitoneal inoculation of guinea-pigs, rabbits, mice and hamsters or by the yolk sac route in embryonated hens' eggs has been described earlier (p. 366).

A confirmatory diagnosis may be obtained by serological methods including complement-fixation, agglutination and allergic tests.

Serology

Serological tests have confirmed the individuality of *C. burnetii* and there are no cross-reactions with other species of *Rickettsia* or with antigens of the PLGV group of organisms (*Chlamydia*).

Complement-fixation is the most widely used serological test for the diagnosis of Q fever in man and animals, and is generally carried out with antigens prepared from infected yolk sacs. In human patients, complement-fixing antibodies are present in from 60–100 per cent of cases after 2–3 weeks. The maximum reaction occurs after 1–2 months and then slowly declines, but sometimes high titres persist for many months. In cattle and sheep the complement-fixation test remains positive for shorter periods than in man. The test is also useful for detecting *C. burnetii* antibodies in the whey of infected milk.

Newly isolated strains of *C. burnetii* are characteristically in Phase I and react only with antibodies in late convalescent sera, but after repeated passages in eggs the organism converts to Phase II which reacts with antibodies in early convalescent-phase sera. This host-controlled variation resembles the S–R change in bacteria.

An agglutination test can also be used for the diagnosis of Q fever and was, in fact, the first serological test employed in the study of this disease. There are many techniques for performing this reaction but the same antigen that is used for the complement-fixation test may also be used for the agglutination test. For the microslide method a dilution ten times greater than that used for the macrotube agglutination method is desirable. The test is not so widely used as that of complement-fixation, largely on account of the difficulties of standardising the technique and because of the variable results that may arise. Specific agglutinins do not usually appear before the 10th day and up to a month may pass before all the animals react. An opsonic test may also be used, but the technique is complex and some workers are doubtful as to its specificity.

Allergic tests may be employed in animals for the diagnosis of Q fever. These include an intrapalpebral reaction which has proved useful in cattle, horses and sheep, and an intradermal test which has given good results in experimentally infected guinea-pigs. In the intrapalpebral tests the animal is inoculated with killed *Coxiella* antigen intracutaneously into the lower eyelid. In a positive reaction an intense swelling of the eyelid develops in 3–4 days and the animal becomes acutely febrile. Unfortunately, the allergic response develops later than either the complement-fixation or agglutination reaction and is not suitable, therefore, for early diagnosis of infection. Moreover, the allergic response may lead to the development of antibodies in the animals tested and these may subsequently interfere with agglutination tests carried out at a later date. Its use in uninfected animals does not lead to false results in later complement-fixation tests.

Other serological methods include neutralization, antiglobulin sensitization and conglutinating complement absorption tests, all of which are of value in experimental studies but not for the diagnosis of disease under natural conditions.

Treatment
Antibiotic therapy is of very limited value for the treatment of animal infections, and attempts to eradicate *C. burnetii* from the milk of cows by intramammary and intravenous injections of tetracyclines have proved unsuccessful. It is of interest that cortisone administered to experimentally infected guinea-pigs is said to bring about a more rapid recovery.

In the medical field there is some evidence that chloramphenicol, tetracycline and lincomycin are active against *C. burnetii*. Unfortunately, this activity is bacteriostatic rather than bactericidal, and in several cases illness has recurred despite prolonged courses of treatment.

Control
Ether-extracted yolk sac vaccines and live attenuated vaccines have been used to protect laboratory workers, livestock attendants and abattoir workers against Q fever, but with varying degrees of success. Many of the preparations produce severe reactions including sterile abscess formation.

The use of inactivated yolk sac vaccines in cattle produces some immunity and may lead to a reduction in the incidence of infection in dairy herds, but unfortunately the method is not practicable on a large scale.

Raw milk is a likely source of infection and should be sterilized by the 'flash' method of pasteurization.

In infected herds every precaution should be taken to remove and destroy placentas, straw, bedding and other materials soiled by excretions and secretions. Contaminated utensils and vehicles used for animal transport should be thoroughly cleansed and disinfected.

THE EHRLICHIAE

Ehrlichieae, the second tribe of the family *Rickettsiaceae* consists of at least four genera, *Ehrlichia*, *Cytoecetes*, *Cowdria* and *Neorickettsia*. In contrast to rickettsiae, the ehrlichia group of organisms occur mostly in circulating monocytes and are pathogenic for animals but not for man. The genus *Ehrlichia* includes three species, *E. canis* which causes an important 'rickettsiosis' of dogs, and two other very similar species, *E. bovis* and *E. ovina*, which are associated with mild illnesses in ruminants.

About ten years after these three species were first described in 1935–37, organisms were observed in monocytes and occasionally lymphocytes of pigeons,

and in monocytes and endothelial cells of pigs. It is possible that these latter two species will be included in the genus when more information becomes available.

Rickettsiosis of dogs

Synonyms
Canine rickettsiosis. Canine typhus. Nairobi bleeding disease.

Definition
An infectious, febrile, tick-borne disease of dogs. The severity of the clinical symptoms is greatly enhanced by concurrent infections with *Babesia*, *Leishmania* and *Bartonella*. Acute illness is characterised by hyperplasia of the lymph nodes, nasal and ocular discharges, emaciation and death.

History and Distribution
A virulent rickettsial infection of dogs was first described in Algeria in 1935 and in Kenya in 1937. The causative agent was identified in 1938 and the name *Rickettsia canis* was changed in 1945 to *Ehrlichia canis*. In subsequent years canine rickettsiosis has been reported from other parts of Africa including South Africa, Nigeria, Uganda, Zaire and the Sudan. It occurs along the Mediterranean littoral and may also be present in Iran, India, Sri Lanka and the U.S.A. Thus, canine rickettsiosis has a very wide distribution and it seems likely that the occurrence of the causative organism corresponds fairly closely with that of *E. bovis* and *E. ovina*.

Hosts affected
The natural disease affects both wild and domestic dogs, and symptomless infections can be produced in jackals and Macaca monkeys.

Aetiology
Ehrlichiae are present in the circulating blood of affected dogs and examination of stained blood films shows that they occur almost exclusively in the cytoplasm of the monocytes. There are a number of reports that they may occasionally parasitize neutrophils, histiocytes and endothelial cells of the meningeal vessels.

In most cases the organisms are found as clusters or colonies within the cytoplasm of infected cells. These colonies may be small and contain only a few deeply staining granules or they may be large, consisting of aggregates of amorphous particles which tend to fill the cytoplasm and indent the nucleus. The number of colonies in a cell is usually between one and 8 but may vary from one to as many as 20 or even 40. The individual particles are pleomorphic, spherical or cocco-bacillary bodies which vary in size from 0·2–0·3 μm to larger particles measuring from 0·5 μm up to 1·5 μm. By Giemsa's method the small particles stain a deep purple colour whereas the larger 'initial-bodies' usually appear slate-grey or light blue.

E. canis has not been propagated in chicken embryos or cell cultures and all attempts at filtration have proved negative. They are fragile organisms and do not remain viable in defibrinated blood at room temperature for longer than 48 hours.

Pathogenicity

In natural cases of canine rickettsiosis the incubation period is about 6–21 days compared with 3–15 days in experimental infections. This is followed by a sharp rise in temperature up to 106°F (41°C) which usually persists for about a week. During the early febrile stage there is a marked increase in the number of monocytes in the circulating blood and eosinophils may disappear almost completely. Organisms seldom appear before the fourth day of the febrile reaction. In recovered animals *E. canis* may persist for many weeks or months and give rise to a state of premunition.

Many cases of canine rickettsiosis are symptomless and may pass unnoticed but others are quite dramatic in appearance, particularly if the patients are concurrently infected with *Babesia, Leishmania* or *Bartonella*, which are believed to enhance the virulence of *E. canis*. In these circumstances most dogs suffering from 'rickettsiosis' show injected mucous membranes, especially of the lips and gums, a purulent discharge from the eyes and nose, gastritis, intermittent vomiting, progressive emaciation and paraplegia. The breath becomes foetid and a characteristic purple or dark brown discolouration develops on the gums and teeth. In the majority of cases there is marked hyperplasia of the lymph nodes and careful palpation of the abdomen reveals enlargement of the spleen. In a few instances skin lesions are seen in the form of shallow, red erosions up to 2 cm in diameter which may become pustular as the disease progresses. Cases occurring in dogs in West Africa are characterised by marked nervous symptoms in the form of convulsions, hysteria, encephalitis and paralysis.

The mortality rate in acute canine rickettsiosis is usually very high and most dogs succumb to the disease within 10–15 days although others may show a more protracted illness lasting for several weeks.

Pathology

At autopsy, the most consistent macroscopical lesions are oedema of the hind limbs, pulmonary oedema, petechial haemorrhages of the lungs, hydrothorax, gastroenteritis, hyperplasia of the lymph nodes and *tumor splenis* with prominent malpighian corpuscles. In addition, there is usually evidence of subendocardial haemorrhages, petechiation of the gastro-intestinal tract, skin erosions, ulceration of the buccal mucosa and congestion of the liver.

In mild cases of *E. canis* infection the only abnormality may be enlargement of the spleen. The same holds good for *E. ovina* and *E. bovis* infections except that hydropericardium may be present in cattle.

Ecology

Ticks have been incriminated as vectors of the *Ehrlichia* group of organisms and there is general agreement that the dog tick, *Rhipicephalus sanguineus*, is the usual vector of *E. canis*. The agent is transmitted from adult females through the eggs to their progeny and all three stages of the tick may be infectious.

Little is known about possible vectors of *E. bovis* and *E. ovina* but there is evidence that the former may be transmitted by a species of *Hyaloma* and the latter by *R. bursa*.

Diagnosis

In endemic areas, where the dog tick, *R. sanguineus*, is known to occur, the clinical symptoms and post-mortem findings in acute forms of the illness are usually characteristic. A confirmatory diagnosis is obtained by the demonstration of rickettsia-like bodies in blood films stained by Giemsa. *Ehrlichia* species are mostly confined to the cytoplasm of monocytes and do not stain by Castaneda's method. Clean slides must be used and it is also recommended that only the first drop of blood that emerges from a prick-incision on the edge of the ear should be taken. The disease must not be confused with canine babesiosis or other possible concurrent infections.

It is interesting to note that a slight rise of titre against *Proteus* OX-19 and OX-K may develop during the course of canine rickettsiosis.

Treatment

Ehrlichiae are sensitive to certain antibiotics and the administration of tetracyclines early in the disease may have beneficial effects although they do not prevent the development of a carrier state. Four daily doses of 25 mg/kg of aureomycin or terramycin are given orally, or 10 mg/kg on two successive days by the intravenous route.

Control

The only satisfactory method of controlling canine rickettsiosis is by the eradication of ticks from kennels and from the dogs themselves. If dogs are kept well nourished and diseases such as canine babesiosis are treated adequately, most cases of *E. canis* infection are of the mild or symptomless variety and seldom require to be treated.

Tick-borne fever

Synonym
Sjodogg (Nor.).

Definition
Tick-borne fever is an infectious, non-contagious, febrile disease occurring in sheep, and occasionally in cattle, on tick infested pastures: uncomplicated cases usually recover.

History and Distribution
This disease was for many years confused with louping-ill of sheep since both are tick-borne and have the same seasonal incidence and geographical distribution in Scotland. However, in 1932 it was shown that the two diseases can be clearly distinguished on clinical, histological and immunological grounds and that their causal agents are borne by the same arthropod vector, *Ixodes ricinus*. The rickettsia-like nature of the infective organism of tick-borne fever and its distribution in the cytoplasm of granular leucocytes and monocytes was first reported in 1939. It is now known that tick-borne fever is present in tick-infested regions of Scotland, England and Wales and that sporadic cases occur in other parts of Europe including Norway, Finland, the Netherlands and Yugoslavia. It was first recognised as a mild infection of cattle in England in 1950.

Aetiology
The causative agent of tick-borne fever is an obligate intracellular parasite which shows many of the properties of a rickettsia. Some believe that it should be incorporated either in the genus *Ehrlichia*, i.e. parasites of the circulating leucocytes, or in the genus *Cytoecetes* because it is a parasite of phagocytes. However, others consider that it shows too many differences to warrant inclusion in either. It is interesting to note that workers at the Moredun Research Institute, Edinburgh, where the disease was first described, have assigned the organism to the genus *Cytoecetes* with the specific epithet *phagocytophilia* for sheep strains and *bovis* for cattle strains.

The causative agents of tick-borne fever in sheep and cattle can readily be demonstrated in blood smears taken during the acute phase of the illness. With Romanowsky stains the organisms appear in the neutrophils, eosinophils, basophils or monocytes as highly pleomorphic, intracytoplasmic bodies varying in colour from pale blue or slate grey to deep blue or lilac. Using Macchiavello's stain or

the modified Ziehl-Neelsen (Brucella differential) staining method, the basic fuchsin is not retained and the particles stain faintly with the malachite green or methylene blue counter stain. This is in marked contrast to rickettsiae which retain the carbol fuchsin stain and appear as bright red particles within the cytoplasm of the affected cells.

Although a life-cycle for tick-borne fever organisms has not been established, examination of stained blood films from infected sheep clearly shows the presence of various developmental forms in the cytoplasm of granular leucocytes and monocytes (Plate 36.1b, facing p. 388). They do not invade the nucleus. The organisms may occur singly or in clusters and are usually in the form of: (1) small, spherical granules measuring about 0·3–0·5 μm in diameter, (2) larger, round or oval bodies up to 2·5 μm in diameter many of which seem to be breaking up into irregular clusters or an orderly circular pattern, and (3) large, round or oval morulae (or plaques), 2·5–3·5 μm in diameter, composed of small particles only, large particles only or a mixture of both. At the height of the febrile reaction, occasional cells packed with tiny particles may be seen. Some appear to be developing in the morulae but the majority are freelying in the cytoplasm. These minute particles probably represent the infectious elementary bodies that are released by lysis of the affected cell.

Cultivation
The organism is an obligate intracellular parasite and does not grow on artificial media, in developing chicken embryos or in cell cultures of various animal tissues.

Experimental transmission of the sheep agent is readily achieved by inoculating infected blood intravenously into susceptible sheep or goats. There are reports that sheep and cattle strains produce a mild, febrile reaction in adult cattle. Infected, citrated sheep blood may retain its infectivity for 13 days at 4°C. This suggests that the parasite is less fragile than that of bovine petechial fever or heartwater. Attempts to infect many different species of laboratory animal have generally been unsuccessful but sheep strains have been adapted and will grow well in splenectomized guinea-pigs.

Pathogenicity
Following infection from tick-bites and invasion of phagocytes by the causative organisms, the affected animal may show clinical signs that are typical of the disease. The course of the infection is characterised by an incubation period of varying length, usually ranging between 4–8 days, followed by a febrile phase of approximately 10 days' duration. The sharp rise of temperature (40–42°C) is associated with

the presence of the parasite in polymorphs and with a marked increase in the neutrophil count. During this stage of the illness the affected animals quickly lose condition and pregnant ewes and cows may abort. The mortality rate is low and uncomplicated cases generally recover. The plateau-type of febrile reaction usually terminates with a gradual fluctuating decline in temperature which lasts from 6–22 days. The subsiding temperature is accompanied by rapid disappearance of the organism from the circulating blood and a progressive but pronounced neutropenia. Although the parasites are rarely seen in blood films after the neutropenic phase, experimental transmission studies have shown that the blood from recovered sheep remains infective for considerable periods, up to 2 years, after an acute attack of the disease. Moreover, an occasional sheep may show a spontaneous relapse and the parasites reappear in the blood during the febrile phase of the illness.

Affected lambs rarely show clinical symptoms of the disease but the neutropenia is believed to predispose the animal to various other disease conditions including tick pyaemia and pneumonia. There is also evidence that the severity of louping-ill is enhanced in sheep concurrently infected with tick-borne fever and that the encephalitic symptoms of louping-ill are commoner in sheep that are immune to tick-borne fever.

In cattle, tick-borne fever usually runs a mild course and clinical symptoms are mostly confined to animals that have recently arrived from tick-free areas. The febrile phase of the illness may result in a pronounced drop in milk yield which may remain subnormal for the rest of the lactation, and non-infected pregnant heifers may abort soon after being introduced into hill areas where the disease is endemic.

There are no characteristic lesions in affected sheep and cattle although a number of workers have observed enlargement of the spleen.

Ecology
The infection is transmitted to susceptible sheep, cattle, goats and deer by the tick *Ixodes ricinus*. The great majority of ticks on an infected pasture carry the causative organism and, while transovarian infection from one generation to the next does not take place, ticks that become infected in the larval or nymphal stage are capable of transmitting the infection during a subsequent stage of their development.

Diagnosis
Tick-borne fever is usually a mild or symptomless infection and many uncomplicated cases may pass undetected. The presence of the disease is usually diagnosed by the demonstration of characteristic particles of the organism in the granular leucocytes and monocytes in Giemsa-stained blood films obtained during the early febrile stage of the illness. A confirmatory diagnosis can be obtained by inoculating susceptible sheep intravenously with freshly drawn blood from reacting animals. Alternatively, splenectomised guinea-pigs may be used.

Immunity
Animals recovered from natural infections of tick-borne fever develop varying degrees of protection against subsequent attacks of the disease. Since the causative agent persists in the tissues for many months and the sera do not contain demonstrable antibodies, the recovered animals are said to be in a state of 'premunition'. Cattle strains have low infectivity for sheep and *vice versa*. Moreover, cattle strains do not protect sheep against reinfection with sheep strains.

Treatment
Terramycin and other broad-spectrum antibiotics curtail the febrile phase of the illness, but there is a tendency for the organisms to reappear and for symptoms to recur. For this reason the use of antibiotics is of little practical value.

Control
There are no adequate measures for the control of tick-borne fever other than complete eradication of the vector. This is impracticable because incomplete destruction of the tick population might result in the development of a more severe form of the disease in many adult animals which escaped infection as lambs.

Bovine petechial fever

Synonyms
Bovine infectious petechial fever, transmissible petechial fever, Ondiri disease, Nairobi quarantine disease.

Definition
An infectious, non-contagious disease of cattle which is characterized by fever, oedema of the conjunctiva, petechiae of the mucous membranes and, in severe cases, sudden collapse and death.

Hosts affected
The natural disease occurs only in cattle of more than 6 months of age, and most cases have been observed in adult animals of exogenous breeds. Transmission experiments in sheep, goats and dogs elicit a slight febrile response with no other symptoms.

History and Distribution

Bovine petechial fever, better known locally as Ondiri disease, was first reported in 1933 among dairy cattle on a Kikuyu farm but there is some evidence that the disease has been known since 1929 as Nairobi quarantine disease.

Clinical illness is usually restricted to only one or two animals in a herd and most cases occur in the highland regions at altitudes above 1500 m (5000 ft) where cattle have access to indigenous forest or thick scrub. The disease may occur at any time of the year but is most commonly seen during the drier periods especially when short spells of rain follow bright, sunny weather.

Although outbreaks have occurred in most parts of the Highlands, the disease appears to be restricted to Kenya and has not been reported from adjacent territories or any other country.

Aetiology

Bovine petechial fever is probably caused by a rickettsia-like organism having properties similar to those of *Ehrlichia* (*Rickettsia*) *phagocytophilia* of tick-borne fever. It is suspected that wild ruminants act as reservoirs of the infection and that a species of tick is the vector.

In blood films stained by Giemsa the organisms are to be found in the neutrophils, large lymphocytes (monocytes) and eosinophils while in spleen smears they normally occur in the lymphocytes or, occasionally, as free-lying forms. The organisms occur singly or in colonies of between 3–8 μm in diameter. The individual particles are highly pleomorphic and vary in size from small elementary bodies of about 1·3 μm to larger initial bodies of about 2 μm in diameter. They may be spherical, oval, cocco-bacillary or rod-shaped, and usually stain from pale blue or slate grey to dark blue or purple. In blood films the colonies may consist of masses of tightly packed aggregates or the particles may be well separated and often lie around the periphery of the colony. The interspaces are unstained and the colony may have the appearance of a 'broken dinner-plate'.

Blood from reacting animals retains its infectivity for 9 days at 4°C but for only 48 hours at 37°C. Spleen tissue remains infective for at least 6 months at —60°C. The organism is said to be resistant to *in vitro* contact with penicillin, chloramphenicol and streptomycin but sensitive to oxytetracycline.

Cultivation

Infection can be transmitted artificially to cattle, sheep and goats with blood, spleen or lymph node material obtained from affected cattle. For serial passage, large volumes of heparinized blood (e.g. 300 ml for cattle or 20 ml for sheep and goats) is administered by the intravenous route. Approxi-mately 50 per cent of adult susceptible cattle infected in this way recover from the clinical illness. The agent is mostly associated with the leucocyte fraction of the blood which is infectious from the first day of the thermal reaction until about 4 days after the clinical symptoms have disappeared. The disease does not appear to be contagious.

The causative agent of bovine petechial fever has not been grown in horses, rats, mice or guinea-pigs but there are reports that dogs and rabbits may react to artificial infection. All attempts to cultivate the organism in embryonated hens' eggs and in ruminant cell cultures of testis or kidney have proved unsuccessful, and subsequent inoculation of these cell cultures into susceptible adult cattle failed to elicit a clinical response.

Pathogenicity

The incubation period following artificial infection of cattle with blood is usually 7–14 days. Infected animals may show high fever and, in lactating cows, there is a sharp drop in milk yield. In most cases the temperature remains elevated for a day or two and then returns slowly to normal. On the second day of the clinical illness small petechial haemorrhages appear on the gums, under the tongue, and on the conjunctiva and mucosa of the vulva and vagina. The petechiae may persist for 1–10 days. In some cases there is an offensive blood-stained diarrhoea and severely affected animals show a characteristic, unilateral, 'poached-egg eye' appearance. These eye changes consist of swelling and eversion of the conjunctival sac with accumulations of blood in the lower part of the aqueous humor.

The mortality rate may be high, particularly in high-grade mature cattle of exogenous breeds, and pregnant cows that survive usually abort. In other cases, e.g. young animals reared on farms known to be infected, the clinical picture is usually mild and may pass unnoticed.

Pathology

The post-mortem findings are characterized by widespread submucous and subserosal haemorrhages, lymphoid hyperplasia and oedema. Petechiae are present in the mouth and may extend to the larynx and pharynx while the trachea may show ecchymoses throughout its length. A constant finding is the presence of extensive haemorrhage on the inner and outer surfaces of the heart. Sheet haemorrhages are found on the epicardial and endocardial surfaces, particularly on the left side, and ecchymoses appear below the serous covering of the fat around the coronary vessels.

Petechial haemorrhages may occur in the adrenals, urinary bladder, peri-renal fat and throughout the whole length of the intestines, and in many cases are to be found scattered in almost any tissue of the body. Oedema of the subcutaneous and intra-muscular tissues is frequently present and in most per-acute cases lung oedema is marked and appears to be the immediate cause of death.

Ecology

The mode of natural transmission of bovine petechial fever is unknown but, in view of its sporadic, non-contagious nature together with the fact that it is confined to high-altitude forest or scrub areas, it is presumed that a tick or other blood-sucking arthropod vector is responsible. The arthropods that are most commonly found on naturally infected cattle include *Rhipicephalus hurti, R. kochi* and a number of unnamed species of *Ixodes*. All are three-host-ticks but, so far, none has been proved to be the vector of bovine petechial fever.

The causative agent has very limited powers of survival outside the living animal and the fact that it persists for many months in enzootic areas in the absence of clinical disease suggests that wild ruminants or other animals may act as reservoir hosts.

Immunity

Cattle bred on farms with a history of the disease are believed to acquire some degree of resistance to the infection but all attempts to demonstrate cir-culating antibodies in reacting and recovered animals have been unsuccessful. Most cattle re-covered from experimental infections resist challenge inoculations for at least 2 years, while in others, the duration of immunity might be less than one year. There is no cross-immunity between bovine petechial fever and heartwater.

Diagnosis

In enzootic areas, typical cases of bovine petechial fever are usually diagnosed by the history, geogra-phical location, clinical signs and post-mortem lesions of the suspected case. Where doubt exists, the diagnosis should be confirmed by the demons-tration of the rickettsia-like organisms in stained blood films taken early in the course of the disease or in spleen smears obtained at autopsy. If the animal dies or is killed, smears should be prepared as soon as possible since the organisms rapidly lose their staining affinity after death of the host. Unfortunately, it is not possible to demonstrate the agent in every blood film taken from an affected animal, particularly from cattle showing severe clinical symptoms, because at this stage of the illness, the leucocytes tend to be immature and difficult to identify.

If facilities for transmission experiments are available, whole blood collected at the beginning of the febrile reaction should be preserved in citrate solution and dispatched to the laboratory on ice, by the quickest means available.

Differential diagnosis

There are a number of disease conditions which must be excluded before a case of bovine petechial fever can be confirmed. These include, anthrax, *Trypanosoma vivax* infection, *Theileria lawrenci* infection (corridor disease), heartwater, Rift Valley fever, East Coast fever and the septicaemic form of pasteurellosis.

Treatment and control

There are no satisfactory methods of treatment and control. Although tetracyclines are effective in experimentally infected cattle when administered during the incubation period or at the onset of clinical symptoms, they are of little value in field cases where the disease is usually too far advanced when diagnosed.

The only effective control measure in enzootic areas is to ensure that cattle are not grazed on infected paddocks and that the bush is cleared as far as possible to discourage natural reservoir hosts and possible vectors of the disease.

No vaccines are available for the control of bovine petechial fever. However, because animals born and bred on infected farms are often resistant to the infection it has been suggested that a method of immunization based on that used to protect cattle against heartwater might prove effective (*vide infra*).

Heartwater

Synonyms

Veld poisoning. Dronkgalsiekte (Afrikaans). Peri-cardité exudative infectieuse (Fr.). Herzwasser (Ger.). Hidrocarditis infectiosa (Sp.).

Definition

An infectious, non-contagious, tick-borne disease of sheep, goats and cattle characterized by fever and nervous symptoms. Hydropericardium is the com-monest lesion in small ruminants but is not always present in cattle.

History and distribution

Heartwater was first reported among sheep in South Africa in 1838. In subsequent years it was described in goats and cattle, and has been recorded in West African territories south of the Sahara, the Sudan, Eritrea, Ethiopia as well as in many parts of East, Central and South Africa, and in the neighbouring island of Madagascar. Regions with a very low rainfall and/or cold climate are believed to be free from the disease.

In 1900, heartwater was recognised as a specific disease entity of ruminants and, in the following year, it was proved that the bont tick, *Amblyoma hebraeum* was an important vector of the infection. In 1926, Cowdry clearly demonstrated the aetiological significance of an organism which he named *Rickettsia ruminantium*, and which was renamed *Cowdria ruminantium* in 1953.

Hosts affected

The clinical disease occurs naturally in sheep, goats and cattle but wild-living ruminants including blesbuck, springbuck and black wildebeest may acquire symptomless infections. Mature animals are generally more susceptible than young animals and lambs, and calves up to the age of 3 weeks usually possess a high degree of resistance.

Aetiology

C. ruminantium is a small (0·2–0·8 μm in diameter) pleomorphic, obligate, intracellular parasite that is confined to the endothelial cells of the mammalian host. They stain poorly, are Gram-negative and appear as slate-blue, dark blue or reddish-purple particles when stained with Giemsa. Stained 'brain-crush' smears or intima smears prepared from the jugular vein show colonies within the vascular endothelial cells (Plate 36.1c, facing p. 388). These colonies range from 2–15 μm in size and generally consist of masses of spherical or pleomorphic particles. The shape of the individual granule varies from spherical, cocco-bacillary and bacillary to horse-shoe and ring forms. The organism contains RNA and DNA and is susceptible to various antibiotics including oxy- and chlortetracycline. *C. ruminantium* is remarkably fragile and usually does not survive in infected defibrinated blood for more than 24 hours at room temperature. However, infected blood and spleen emulsions stored at −80°C remain viable for periods of up to 2 years. The organism appears to be firmly attached to the red blood cells and cannot readily be removed by repeated washings in buffered saline. It is seldom present in the plasma and does not pass Berkefeld W or Seitz filters.

Cultivation

C. ruminantium does not grow in non-living laboratory media and there is, as yet, no evidence that it can be cultivated in embryonated hens' eggs or in cell cultures of different animal tissues.

Sheep, goats and cattle can readily be infected by artificial inoculation and high concentrations of the organism can be found in the blood from about the 4th day of fever until the death of the animal. In recovered animals, the agent may persist for a variable period, and times of 60–105 days have been reported in sheep. The ferret is believed to be the only laboratory animal that is susceptible to the infection and it can be used to maintain the organism by serial passage.

C. ruminantium will survive in mice for periods of up to 90 days following the intraperitoneal injection of infective blood, spleen and brain suspensions, but it does not multiply in this host. Serial alternating passages between sheep and mice do not result in adaptation of the agent to mice.

Pathogenicity

The incubation period of heartwater varies considerably but in experimentally infected animals it is usually about 12 days in sheep and goats, and between 12 and 18 days in cattle. Following natural transmission by tick-bite a period of 14–28 days generally elapses before the development of clinical symptoms. In natural infections the organisms are conveyed from the site of the tick-bite by the circulating blood to various tissues and are demonstrable in stained blood films about 24 hours after the initial temperature rise. Fever (40–42°C) usually persists throughout much of the illness but the temperature drops rapidly as death approaches. Multiplication of the organism within the endothelial cells lining the blood vessels gives rise to a toxin which increases the permeability of the capillary walls and causes oedema of the lungs and hydropericardium.

In the peracute form of the disease, death may supervene within 48 hours and before clinical symptoms have appeared, but in the less acute forms there is pyrexia, followed by nervous symptoms and paroxysmal convulsions. When marked nervous signs develop recovery is rare. The mortality rate varies from 50–90 per cent depending on the strain of organism, the locality of the outbreak, the season of the year and the breed and age of the affected animals. In the sub-acute form the course of the disease is longer, recoveries are more frequent, nervous symptoms are less pronounced but a severe diarrhoea may develop. The signs of involvement include protrusion of the tongue, frequent chewing movements and twitching of the eyelids. The affected animal usually walks in circles with a high-stepping, unsteady gait or stands with its legs apart and head held low. In the mild form of the disease the clinical signs are so slight, or even inapparent, that the disease is seldom diagnosed, and most animals recover.

Pathology

Lesions of heartwater vary greatly according to the duration and severity of the disease but in typical cases the most outstanding features are hydrothorax, hydropericardium and ascites. Oedema of the lungs and hydrothorax of varying degree are regular lesions, and hydropericardium is usually present in sheep and goats but not in cattle. The amount of fluid in the pericardial sac is considerable but is generally proportionately less in cattle than in sheep. The heart muscle is dull in appearance and may show evidence of cloudy swelling, fatty degeneration and small subepicardial and subendocardial haemorrhages. The lymph nodes are generally enlarged and congested, the liver is engorged and there is almost invariably *tumour splenis* which is especially marked in cattle. Although the brain may be congested and moist in appearance there are usually no outstanding features in the central nervous system.

Ecology
It is generally agreed that heartwater of sheep, goats and cattle is now confined to regions where the environmental conditions are favourable for the development and survival of the tick vector. The proven vectors include several species of the genus *Amblyoma* including *A. hebraeum*, *A. variegatum*, *A. pomposum* and *A. gemma*. The tick acquires infection during the larval or nymphal stage when it feeds on an infected animal, and transmits the disease during a subsequent stage in its development. Transovarial infection from one generation to the next does not take place and other reservoirs of infection are possible. Ticks feeding on non-susceptible animals do not free themselves of the infection. Thus, if they acquire the infection as larvae they can maintain the agent for a period of more than 3 years.

Indigenous breeds of cattle in endemic areas, Persian sheep, Africander sheep, indigenous antelopes and some other wild-living ruminants may develop inapparent infections and act as reservoir hosts, thereby maintaining the infection in the tick population and perpetuating the disease in the locality.

Diagnosis
In endemic areas, a provisional diagnosis of heartwater can usually be made on the basis of the history, geographical locality, clinical symptoms and lesions at autopsy. However, a confirmatory diagnosis depends upon the demonstration of colonies of *C. ruminantium* within the cytoplasm of the vascular endothelial cells. Specimens taken 2–4 days after the onset of fever generally give the best results, but organisms may also be found comparatively easily in fresh intima smears prepared from the jugular vein or other large blood vessels of an animal that has died from the disease. They can also be identified readily in 'crush' smears made from the cerebral cortex, hippocampus or spinal cord. The smears are fixed in alcohol and stained with Giemsa. *C. ruminantium* is a remarkably fragile parasite and quickly dies if infected blood or other tissues are not rapidly inoculated into other animals, e.g. sheep, or stored at —80°C. Mice inoculated intraperitoneally with suspected material at field autopsies may be used as a means of transporting the organism to the laboratory where it can be injected into susceptible ruminants 14–21 days after inoculation of the mice. In South Africa the material is inoculated into heartwater-susceptible but bluetongue-immune sheep. The incubation period of bluetongue is about 5 days whereas in heartwater fever it is around 11 days. It should be noted that heartwater does not occur in the absence of the vector so the finding of bont ticks on the suspected animal may be of significance.

Differential Diagnosis
Heartwater fever must be differentiated from tetanus, strychnine poisoning, hypomagnesaemia and other conditions causing nervous involvement.

Infectious conditions which must be eliminated include anthrax, piroplasmosis, anaplasmosis, East Coast fever, listeriosis, louping-ill, scrapie and rabies.

Treatment
Chlortetracycline or oxytetracycline administered by the intravenous route is extremely effective for treating heartwater provided the course of treatment is carried out in the earliest stages of the disease. The use of arsenical and antimony compounds is said to stimulate the multiplication of *C. ruminantium* and is contra-indicated in the treatment of heartwater.

Immunity
In recovered animals, *C. ruminantium* persists for periods of up to 3 months and healthy ticks may acquire the infection during this time. The presence of the persisting organism induces a temporary state of premunition which is usually followed by a period of solid, sterile immunity which may be as short as 6 months or as long as 5 years. As the period of immunity declines, animals in endemic areas may become reinfected with symptomless infection, although the blood remains infective to ticks.

Control
Heartwater fever is confined to areas where the tick vector occurs, thus eradication of *Amblyoma* ticks would eliminate the disease. In infected areas dipping and hand-dressing of all domestic stock should be carried out at regular intervals of not more than 5 days, and the introduction of tick infested stock into clean areas must be avoided.

The fact that calves and lambs of up to 4 weeks and 7 days of age, respectively, possess a marked resistance to heartwater provides a practical and comparatively safe and effective means of immunization. Young animals inoculated as soon as possible after birth with *C. ruminantium* in the form of infected blood from a reacting animal develop a durable immunity. In heavily infected areas the possible loss of a few young calves through the use of live vaccines is preferred to heavier losses in older calves from natural infection. Adult cattle may also be immunized by this method provided the resulting symptoms are carefully controlled with antibiotics which should be given at the onset of fever and every 12 hours, thereafter, until the temperature subsides.

Salmon poisoning in dogs

Synonym
Salmon disease of dogs.

Definition
An acute, often fatal, infectious, non-contagious febrile disease of dogs, characterised by severe depression, extreme thirst and frequent vomiting.

Hosts affected
Dogs are the commonest natural host but the disease has also been reported in foxes. Coyotes are susceptible to experimental infection.

History and distribution
The disease has been recognised for many years along the seaboard of the Northwest Pacific. Its association with the ingestion of raw fish parasitized by metacircariae of the fluke *Nanophyetus (Troglotrema) salmincola* was first reported in 1924. The presence of intra-cytoplasmic bodies in the reticuloendothelial cells of affected animals, suggesting that the causative organism was a type of rickettsia, was reported in 1947.

There can be no doubt that the disease is limited to areas where dogs, foxes and coyotes have access to fish infested with the metacircariae of *Nanophyetus salmincola*. The parasites have been found in trout in freshwater streams of Oregon, California and Idaho, and in salmon along the coastline of Alaska and as far south as San Francisco in California. In some areas of the Pacific coast, salmon poisoning is considered to be one of the three most important infectious diseases of dogs.

Aetiology
Clusters of small (c.300 nm) coccoid or pleomorphic organisms occurring in the form of short rods or crescents are present in the tissues of the fluke vectors. In dogs and other *Canidae* affected with the disease they are frequently to be found in stained smears of the large reticuloendothelial cells of the lymph nodes, intestinal lymphoid follicles, tonsils,

thymus and spleen and are sometimes seen in macrophages of the circulating blood, lungs and liver. The organisms are Gram-negative but stain dark blue or purple by Giemsa and red with Macchiavello's stain. In some cells stained by Macchiavello, larger pale-blue particles resembling the LCL bodies of psittacosis are seen.

The causative agent of salmon poisoning is an obligate intracellular organism which has many of the morphological and tinctorial properties of rickettsiae. However, since it is not immediately identifiable as a member of the *Rickettsiaceae* or *Chlamydiaceae* and is independent of arthropod transmission, it is generally classified in the genus *Neorickettsia* with the specific epithet *helminthoeca*.

Pathogenicity
The incubation period following ingestion of raw parasitized fish is usually about 5–7 days but, according to some workers, the onset of symptoms may be delayed for 62 days. The course of the natural disease is very rapid and the onset of infection is characterized by a sudden rise in temperature which reaches a peak of between 104–107°F. This period of fever continues for 3–7 days and then declines for 6–8 days, followed by hypothermia and death. Early clinical signs include anorexia, weakness, loss of weight, deep depression, vomiting, diarrhoea and extreme thirst. A number of animals may show serous nasal discharge and conjunctivitis. The mortality rate in untreated cases is usually above 90 per cent.

Pathology
The principal macroscopic lesions include hyperplasia of carcase and visceral lymph nodes, sometimes with petechiae or necrosis. The tonsils, thymus and spleen may also be enlarged. Many affected animals show haemorrhagic enteritis. Large numbers of flukes and fluke eggs may be present in the intestinal contents.

Ecology
Salmon poisoning of dogs is caused by *Neorickettsia helminthoeca* and is one of the first examples of a rickettsial disease of animals that is transmitted by a trematode. The fluke vector, *Nanophyetus salmincola* has a three host life cycle involving dogs, snails and fish; and the following method of transmission has been suggested. Infected metacircariae encysted in the musculature of fish belonging to the family *Salmonidae* are ingested by dogs and the ova passed by adult flukes in the dogs' intestines. These ova develop miracidia which infect the snail *Goniobasis plicifera var. silicula*. Cercariae develop and pass from the snail and infect suscepti-

ble species of fish which are eaten raw by dogs, foxes and other carnivores.

Diagnosis

In endemic areas the clinical symptoms are usually characteristic of the disease. Additional evidence is obtained by examining the patient's faeces for the presence of the fluke eggs and by demonstrating the rickettsia-like bodies in stained smears of fluid aspirated from the swollen mandibular lymph nodes. The organisms stain well with Romanowsky stains and are found diffusely arranged or in tight clusters within the cytoplasm of infected cells. The bodies have also been seen in Giemsa-stained 'buffy-coat' smears from sedimented blood.

Treatment

Early treatment with sulphonamides or broad spectrum antibiotics given parenterally or orally may alleviate the condition and, in some cases, effect a cure. Streptomycin is ineffective. In salmon poisoning of dogs the treatment should include fluid replacement therapy and measures to control the diarrhoea.

Control

Although recovered dogs are probably solidly immune there are no vaccines available. In some endemic areas young dogs are deliberately infected and then treated with antibiotics early in the disease.

THE CHLAMYDIAE

Members of the family *Chlamydiaceae* are in many ways so different from true viruses that most workers now believe they should be considered as bacteria and classified with the rickettsias (Order *Chlamydiales*) although they have no true vectors.

Unfortunately, the adoption of a linguistically simple and taxonomically reasonable name for these agents has presented considerable difficulties. In this chapter the generic term *Chlamydia* will be used in preference to *Miyagawanella* or *Bedsonia*, but they will also be referred to as members of the psittacosis-lymphogranuloma venereum group or, simply, as PLV-agents.

Chlamydia can be divided into two species viz. *C. trachomatis* and *C. psittaci*. The former comprises the causative agents of two diseases confined to man, namely trachoma and inclusion conjunctivitis, which are sometimes called the TRIC agents. The second species contains a large number of agents which may be conveniently classified on the basis of their natural host range into avian, human, and other-mammalian strains.

Properties of the agents

Chlamydiae are relatively large Gram-negative organisms which multiply only in living cells and are not dependent on arthropod transmission. They stain readily with basophilic dyes and take Castaneda and Macchiavello stains in the same way as rickettsiae. The various species of *Chlamydia* are indistinguishable morphologically and are large enough to be clearly visible in the light microscope. Suspensions of *Chlamydia* under the electron microscope contain two main types of particle. The first is the elementary body which measures about 300 nm in diameter and appears as a dense electron-opaque, central nucleoid separated from an outer membrane of three distinct layers by a wide clear zone. The second is the initial body which is larger (700–1200 nm) and has no central core. The elementary body is the highly infective extracellular form while the initial body represents the intracellular replicating form of the organism.

Several members agglutinate mouse and hamster red blood cells, but not those of human or avian origin. The haemagglutinins are soluble and group specific but are produced irregularly and in low titres. The reaction occurs at 37°C and 22°C but not at 4°C, and the optimum pH is about 7·0. The haemagglutinin consists of lecithin and nucleoprotein and does not react with receptor areas for myxoviruses.

Multiplication of *Chlamydia* is inhibited when the host cells are treated with adequate concentrations of penicillin, chloramphenicol, tetracyclines or erythromycin. Most chlamydiae are susceptible to sulphonamides but the psittacosis agents are generally resistant. Streptomycin is not inhibitory and can be added to suspensions of the organisms to combat bacterial contamination.

Chlamydiae are rapidly inactivated by heat and they lose their infectivity completely after 10 minutes at 60°C and when stored in glycerol. They maintain their viability for years at —70°C. although much of their infectivity may be lost during the process of freeze-drying. Lipids are abundant and all species of the organism are inactivated by ether within 30 minutes.

PLV-agents contain both DNA and RNA. In the small, infective particles (elementary bodies) the DNA is mostly concentrated in the electron-dense central core, while in the large particles (initial bodies) it is distributed irregularly throughout the cytoplasm. The large particles contain four times as much RNA as DNA whereas the elementary bodies contain about equal amounts of RNA and DNA, much of the RNA being situated in the outer protective coat. Fluorescence microscopy after acridine orange staining supports the suggestion that RNA is present in the developing forms as well as DNA (Plate 36.2c, facing p. 388a).

Organisms of sub-group A, viz. trachoma, inclusion conjunctivitis, lymphogranuloma-venereum and mouse pneumonitis have compact intracytoplasmic inclusions with a glycogen matrix that is detectable by staining with iodine; and are inhibited by sodium sulphadiazine. Other chlamydiae including psittacosis, ornithosis, feline pneumonitis and bovine encephalomyelitis do not produce glycogen or show susceptibility to sulphadiazine and are classified as sub-group B. An additional differentiating feature between members of the two sub-groups is the greater susceptibility of sub-group A chlamydiae to D-cycloserine.

Comparison with viruses

Discussion about the true nature of the psittacosis-lymphogranuloma venereum group of organisms continues, and a good deal of evidence is accumulating to show that the group lies somewhere between the Gram-negative bacteria on the one hand and the viruses on the other. Although they are obligate intracellular parasites, chlamydiae differ from viruses in the following important respects:

(1) Purified preparations of *Chlamydia* contain both RNA and DNA, whereas viruses contain only one nucleic acid.

(2) They mostly possess cell walls containing muramic acid which is usually present in bacteria and rickettsiae but not in viruses.

(3) They possess ribosomes but viruses do not.

(4) They have their own metabolic enzymes and are sensitive to several antibiotics.

(5) During the developmental cycle at least one form of particle multiplies by binary fission; viruses do not.

Cultivation

Chlamydiae can be grown readily in the yolk sacs of 6–8-day old chicken embryos, and this was the only means of cultivating members of the trachoma sub-group until the recent introduction of irradiated cells provided a more sensitive alternative. All other species have a wide host range and can be propagated by the inoculation of mice, embryonated eggs or various cell culture systems (Plate 36.2b, facing p. 388a).

The growth cycle of *Chlamydia* has been studied in all of these systems and most workers believe that infection is usually initiated by a tiny, highly specialised particle (elementary body) which is able to survive the brief extracellular journey from one cell to another. It is emphasised that the elementary particle is incapable of multiplying in the cell in which it is formed and must undergo a long internal reorganization into a large initial body before multiplication can begin in the cell which it invades.

Growth cycle (Fig. 36.2)

Large numbers of elementary bodies measuring about 0·2–0·3 µm in diameter are adsorbed on to the surface of a susceptible host cell, but only a few gain entry and these quickly cease to be demonstrable. Once inside the cell's cytoplasm the elementary bodies go through a characteristic sequence of chemical and morphological changes. During the lag phase which lasts about 1–10 hours, the particles undergo an internal reorganization and change from small, spherical structures into larger, less deeply staining 'initial bodies' measuring about 0·5–0·7 µm in diameter. From about 15–20 hours after infection the number of initial bodies increases rapidly without obvious division, and they aggregate in clusters in an homogeneous fluid-like matrix which appears to digest the surrounding cytoplasm to form a vacuolar structure or vesicle. This phase of development is followed by a stage of rapid multiplication when the large bodies appear to break down into smaller bodies with dense centres, either from a single large particle by budding or by division in several planes to form four or five small particles of equal size. Towards the end of the multiplication cycle, the cytoplasm of the host cell may be packed with particles of both types, but the nucleus is not affected and the cell may continue to grow and divide. The larger particles stain pale blue with Macchiavello's method and are not infectious whereas the more numerous tiny spherical particles which constitute the new population of elementary bodies stain bright red and are highly infectious. The particles are ultimately released by lysis of the infected cell.

Antigenicity

The antigens of *Chlamydia* fall into two main categories, viz. a heat-stable complement-fixing antigen which is common to the group, and a heat-labile species-specific antigen. The former is closely associated with the cell wall. The latter which is usually associated with the inner part of the elementary particle, is toxic for mice and identified by neutralization tests. It is of interest that the lethal toxin is not separable from the elementary particles and kills mice when injected intravenously.

Although most members of the genus *Chlamydia* can be differentiated antigenically, and in their pathogenicity for different species of animals, there is an urgent need for a more satisfactory method of classification in order to determine which of the strains should be elevated to specific rank. For example, the word ornithosis is frequently used as a synonym for psittacosis in non-psittacine birds or for the disease in man acquired from them. Recent evidence suggests that the agent of ornithosis can now be distinguished from that of psittacosis

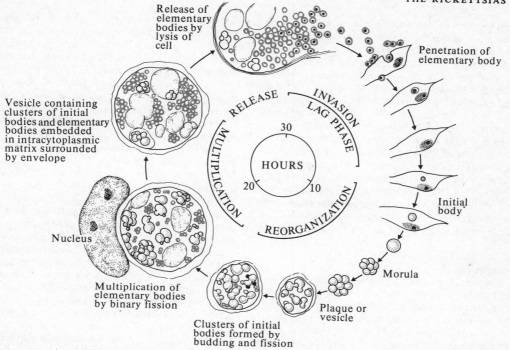

Release of elementary bodies by lysis of cell

Penetration of elementary body

Vesicle containing clusters of initial bodies and elementary bodies embedded in intracytoplasmic matrix surrounded by envelope

RELEASE

INVASION LAG PHASE

MULTIPLICATION

REORGANIZATION

30

HOURS

20   10

Initial body

Nucleus

Morula

Multiplication of elementary bodies by binary fission

Plaque or vesicle

Clusters of initial bodies formed by budding and fission

FIG. 36.2 Multiplication cycle of the agent of enzootic abortion of ewes.

not only by its pathogenicity for certain laboratory animals but also by the fact that it may possess a type specific antigen.

Pathogenicity

There are a number of well-recognised human diseases that are due to *Chlamydia*, e.g. trachoma, inclusion conjunctivitis, lymphogranuloma venereum and psittacosis. In the veterinary field, psittacosis and ornithosis are primarily diseases of birds but man occasionally acquires infection from them. In addition, PLV-agents are probably responsible for a number of diverse pathological processes in a wide range of animals including sheep, cattle, goats, cats, mice, hamsters and guinea-pigs. The more important of these conditions are enzootic abortion of ewes, catarrhal pneumonias of sheep and goats, respiratory disorders of calves, sporadic encephalitis of calves, late abortions of calves, gastrointestinal disorders of cows, pneumonia and fibrinous pericarditis of swine, stiffness, lameness and polyarthritis of lambs, meningopneumonitis of mice and pneumonitis of cats.

Psittacosis and ornithosis

Synonyms

Psittacosis or parrot disease. Papageien Krankheit und Geflügelornithose (Ger.).

Definition

Psittacosis is essentially a disease observed in or derived from parrots, budgerigars and other psittacine birds whereas ornithosis is an almost identical disease originating in pigeons, domestic poultry, turkeys, ducks, sea-birds and other non-psittacine species. The diseases, whether affecting birds, animals or humans, are all caused by members of the family *Chlamydiaceae*

History

It had long been known that parrots suffered from an infectious disease to which man was highly susceptible and the terms psittacosis and parrot disease were used on account of its psittacine origin. The condition was probably first recognised as a distinct clinical entity in 1879 during an outbreak of severe pneumonia in a household in Switzerland in which three of the seven cases proved fatal. During the next 20 years further outbreaks were described in France (1892), Italy (1894 and 1897) and Germany (1898). The first outbreak in the USA occurred in 1917 following an importation of Amazonian parrots. The largest known epidemic was in 1929–30 when 143 deaths were reported in some 750–800 human cases of psittacosis in Europe and America. This extensive outbreak involved twelve countries, including the UK, and was attributed to a consignment of infected parrots imported from South America.

In 1930 workers in Britain, the U.S.A. and Germany showed independently that a filterable agent was responsible for both the human and avian types of infection and that it could be demonstrated by the inoculation of mice. In the same year, Levinthal, Coles and Lillie demonstrated tiny coccal bodies in stained smears of infective material. These were later proved to be the causal agent and are sometimes referred to as the LCL bodies of psittacosis.

In 1932–34 the developmental cycle of the psitta-cosis agent was clearly defined by Bedson and, subsequently, many workers have suggested that the term Bedsonia should be adopted as the group designation in his memory. However, following recent recommendations of an international committee the generic term *Chlamydia* (Gr. *chlamys*, a 'cloak') is now widely used for all the agents in the group.

Hosts affected
The disease occurs mostly in psittacine birds and man, but latent and clinical infections may also occur naturally in fulmars, petrels and certain other sea-birds, pigeons, pheasants, domestic fowls, geese, ducks and turkeys, as well as in sheep, goats, cattle, pigs, cats and many other species of domestic and laboratory animals.

Distribution
The infection is enzootic among wild parrots and other psittacine birds in Australia, New Zealand, South America and, possibly, in parts of Africa and Asia. It is also prevalent in breeding establishments in France, North Africa, Argentina and, probably, in many other countries where large aviaries are maintained. The presence of latent ornithosis infections among ducklings, turkeys and poultry in large commercial breeding farms in the U.S.A. and Europe constitutes a serious occupational health hazard for people working in poultry-processing plants and other branches of the poultry industry. From time to time spectacular outbreaks in turkeys cause serious economic losses.

Aetiology
All members of the genus *Chlamydia* differ to some extent antigenically and in their pathogenicity for birds and mammals; otherwise they resemble each other closely and pass through similar developmental cycles. None of the species has been shown to divide and grow outside living susceptible host cells.

The general characters of the psittacosis organisms are similar to those of other members of the group, and have been described previously.

Cultivation
The host range of *Chlamydia* is extensive and natural infection occurs in many species of mammals and birds. According to a report published in 1964, spontaneous infection has been recorded in 127 avian species. It is generally believed that man acts only as an occasional host.

The agent can readily be grown in mice, guinea-pigs and some other species of laboratory animals. Parrot and certain turkey strains produce fatal infections in mice when inoculated intraperitoneally, whereas pigeon strains rarely produce clinical symptoms of the disease. However, both types produce a fatal infection if introduced intracerebrally or give rise to pneumonia when instilled intranasally.

All types of *Chlamydia* proliferate in embryonated hens' eggs, particularly in the yolk sac. This simple, direct route is the method of choice for producing large quantities of uncontaminated infectious material. The chick embryo usually dies after 3–8 days of incubation and smears of the infected yolk sac reveal large numbers of organisms. The agent can also be grown on the chorioallantoic membrane and generally produces small, greyish lesions which may start to heal by the third day when the infection will have generalised.

Most members of the psittacosis group have been adapted to grow on a wide range of cell culture systems. Secondary monolayer cultures and continuous cell lines derived from a variety of avian and mammalian sources can be used but, since large numbers of organisms are usually required to initiate infection, it is doubtful if cell culture techniques will supplant yolk sac inoculation for primary isolations. Evidence of propagation of the agent is provided by the appearance of characterisitic 'vesicles', containing both large and small particles, and infectivity titrations can readily be performed by counting the number of cells showing these inclusions. High titres are obtained but regular serial passages of the agent in cell culture may prove difficult. Most strains of *Chlamydia* do not produce cytopathic effects and the infection may proceed until almost 100 per cent of cells are affected. A few strains of trachoma and inclusion conjunctivitis (TRIC agents) are characterised by their ability to lyse human fibroblasts in cell culture.

Pathogenicity
In the natural psittacine and non-psittacine hosts, the disease is commonly latent except when birds are shipped abroad, and particularly when they are kept intensively under conditions of bad husbandry. Outbreaks of clinical disease are especially prevalent during the breeding season when nestlings become infected. Affected birds appear sleepy, refuse to eat, have fits of shivering and are disinclined to perch. In large aviaries the characteristic chattering noises

of a healthy colony are noticeably absent. Sick birds may show ruffled plumage, nasal discharge, watery-green diarrhoea with pasting of the feathers around the vent, and marked wasting of the pectoral muscles. The mortality rate is often high with large numbers of birds dying suddenly after a short illness.

In pigeons, the symptoms of ornithosis are not always characteristic. Infected squabs are usually undersized and weak, and diarrhoea is common. Adult pigeons, especially racing birds, may suffer from an acute respiratory form of the disease. In epizootics among turkeys, affected birds are feverish, disinclined to move and show acute respiratory distress.

Human infections may be subclinical, mild or severe. After an incubation period of about 7–14 days the resultant illness is pneumonic in type and, in untreated cases, may be severe with a 20 per cent mortality. Fortunately, however, the illness is usually mild and resembles an attack of influenza with fever, severe headache and chest pains associated with a patchy pneumonia involving the bases of the lungs.

Infections of laboratory workers are not uncommon.

Pathology
At autopsy, the main macroscopical lesions in psittacine birds consist of wasting of the pectoral muscles, focal liver necroses, enlargement of the spleen, purulent, serous or fibrinous pericarditis, fibropurulent thickening of the air-sacs with adhesions to the sternum, mucous plugs in the nasal passages, enteritis and, on occasion, a well marked erythematous rash on the skin over the body and legs. It is emphasised that visibly healthy, well-nourished psittacines with chronic infections may show only enlarged spleens at post-mortem examination. Adult pigeons dying from a relapsing latent infection show enlarged, congested livers with pin-head necrotic lesions, but the spleens are not so enlarged as in psittacine species.

Ecology
Transmission of the infectious agent occurs during close contact of birds with one another and the disease is probably acquired by inhaling dust from feathers contaminated with dried infectious excreta. The disease is endemic in wild birds of the parrot family, and captured psittacines from South America and Australia may constitute an important public health hazard. Carrier birds may excrete the agent in their droppings for long periods and disseminate the organisms widely to other birds and man. Despite the prevalence of ornithosis in pigeons, the incidence of human clinical infections arising from contact with pigeons is generally low, but clinical and inapparent infections among pigeon fanciers are not unusual. Although bird-to-bird transmission of psittacosis is common, interhuman infections are rare.

Diagnosis
Confirmation of psittacosis or ornithosis may be difficult in the living bird because the symptoms often resemble those of other avian diseases. Usually, only a tentative diagnosis is possible, based on the clinical findings and a known history of close contact with other infected birds. In some of the larger avian species acute and convalescent blood samples can be examined by complement-fixation tests for a four-fold or greater rise in antibody titres. In human patients complement-fixation with group antigen is probably the most useful diagnostic test. The antigen used is the agent of enzootic abortion of ewes grown in the yolk sac of chick embryos. Acute and convalescent phase sera are examined and the demonstration of a four-fold or greater rise of antibody level is diagnostic when correlated with the clinical history. The single observation of a titre of group complement-fixing antibody at levels of 1/128 or 1/256, usually indicates recent infection. Antibodies usually develop within 10 days but the use of antibiotics may delay their development for 20–40 days or suppress it altogether.

In avian species the diagnosis is mostly based on the post-mortem findings, the demonstration of organisms in stained tissue smears and the isolation and identification of the causative agent.

Great care must be taken in handling dead birds and in performing post-mortem examinations because psittacosis is highly contagious and dangerous to man. As a routine, all avian carcases should be dipped in a suitable disinfectant to inactivate the agent and minimise the risk of scattering and inhaling small particles of dried, infected excreta adhering to the down and feathers around the cloaca of diseased birds. Laboratory workers should wear protective clothing, disposable gloves, face masks and goggles during all manipulations. After careful consideration of the history, clinical signs and post-mortem findings, smears are prepared from the air sac membranes and from the pericadium if exudate is present, as well as from the liver and spleen. The smears are stained by Giemsa or, preferably, by the modified Macchiavello or Brucella differential techniques and examined under the high-power oil immersion lens. When the Brucella differential stain is used, the elementary bodies of psittacosis appear as minute (300–450 nm) red spheres against a pale-blue background. Small or large clusters will be seen within the cells, but for the most part, the elementary particles are lying free due to damage to the cells when the smear is being prepared.

For isolation of the organism, mouse or egg inoculation is used. The suspect material is ground thoroughly in sterile nutrient broth (pH 7·2–7·6) to make a 10–20 per cent emulsion. If it is likely to be heavily contaminated, the emulsified tissue is treated by light centrifugation (c. 3000 rev/min for 5 minutes) or coarse filtration through sand and paper filters and passed through membrane filters of average pore diameter 1·0 μm. Alternatively, since so much of the agent is lost through filtration, certain antibiotic solutions, e.g. streptomycin and tyrothricin, may be added to the tissue suspension in appropriate concentrations up to a maximum of 2000 μg/ml. The use of penicillin and other antibiotics is contra-indicated. The prepared suspensions are then either instilled intranasally (0·03–0·05 ml) or injected intracerebrally (0·03 ml) or intraperitoneally (0·5 ml) into small groups of mice. Most strains of psittacosis agent will produce fatal infections in mice by one or other of these procedures. Smears prepared from pneumonic lungs, enlarged spleens or other affected tissues abound with organisms.

From recent observations of ornithosis of turkeys and pigeons and in surveys of wild birds in Australia, it is becoming increasingly evident that the pathogenicity of *Chlamydia* may be so low that the mouse alone cannot be regarded as a suitable indicator host for non-psittacine infections. However, chick embryos are particularly susceptible and it is recommended that egg inoculation should be used con-

serum neutralization or, if species identification is required, by toxin-antitoxin neutralization tests in mice.

Indirect complement-fixation test

The complement-fixation test is a useful and reliable means of diagnosing psittacosis in man and animals. Unfortunately, however, certain birds infected with psittacosis or ornithosis produce antibodies which do not combine with guinea-pig complement in the presence of homologous antigens, and their sera cannot, therefore, be used in the direct complement-fixation test. It should be noted that heated sera in decreasing order of their ability to fix complement are those from mammals, psittacine birds, older pigeons, turkeys, pheasants and chickens. Therefore, the antibody levels are detected by an indirect complement-fixation test, using the direct reaction as an indicator. In this technique a standard serum, i.e. specific CF indicator antibody, is added to the test serum-antigen mixture. If the antigen combines with the antibody of the **test** serum, no antigen remains to combine with the antibody of the **standard** serum. Since there is insufficient antigen left to combine with the standard serum, the complement will not be fixed and the red blood cells will lyse. The last tube, or the highest dilution of the test serum which shows lysis, is the indirect complement-fixing titre of the serum. In its simplest form the reaction can be represented as shown in Fig. 36.3.

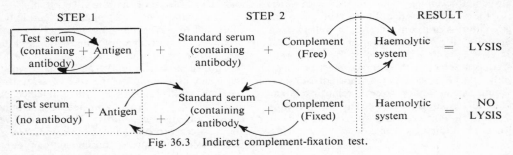

Fig. 36.3   Indirect complement-fixation test.

currently with mouse inoculation for the isolation of *Chlamydia* from non-psittacine and animal sources. The suspected tissue suspension is injected in 0·25 ml amounts directly into the yolk sac of 6–8-day old embryonated hens' eggs. The eggs are candled daily and non-specific deaths occurring within the first 48 hours are discarded. Infected embryos usually die in 3–8 days after inoculation. Stained impression smears prepared from the yolk sac, which has been carefully washed in sterile saline until free from yolk, show an abundance of elementary particles. Large quantities of the organims can be obtained by further passages in eggs and their identity confirmed by complement-fixation, fluorescent antibody staining,

Treatment

The agent of psittacosis is susceptible to many antibiotics including penicillin, aureomycin and terramycin. It is not sensitive to streptomycin, and most strains are unaffected by sulphonamides. Tetracyclines are highly effective in human infections and bring about marked improvement in acute cases of the disease. The best results are obtained with doses of 1–2 g administered daily until several days after the temperature has returned to normal.

Tetracyclines are also effective in treating sick birds provided they are injected intramuscularly with doses of 100 mg/kg or orally with over 200 mg/kg/day for 7–10 days. Latent avian infections have been successfully eradicated when the daily intake in medicated feed has exceeded 100 mg/kg/day and has been maintained for 30 days.

Control

After an outbreak of disease, carcases, droppings and litter should be carefully collected and burned, the cages thoroughly cleansed and sterilized and the premises generally cleaned. Sick birds respond promptly to antibiotic therapy, especially to aureomycin and terramycin, and there may be some justification for permitting rare or valuable birds to be treated provided the course of treatment is adequate. In some countries the infection is controlled in intensively-reared poultry, ducklings and turkeys by the application of routine but intensive and prolonged chemotherapy under careful supervision.

Some authorities consider that all consignments of imported psittacine birds should be held in quarantine for 30 days and examined for evidence of clinical disease. Also, that a proportion of each shipment should be tested for antibodies and that some be sacrificed and examined for the organism. Recent evidence suggests that this procedure is ineffective and that there is almost a ten-fold increase in the incidence of psittacosis by the end of the quarantine period. It is now proposed that all imported psittacines should be given medicated feed for a period of 45 days before and during shipment from abroad. Upon arrival, the birds will be housed under sanitary conditions, isolated from untreated birds and will continue to receive the same antibiotic feed until they are sold to the public.

There are no practical vaccines available against psittacosis, but laboratory workers have successfully vaccinated themselves by giving large doses of live organisms subcutaneously.

Chlamydial infections in other hosts

In 1937, some seven years after the first report that laboratory mice were highly susceptible to artificially induced infections with parrot strains of psittacosis, it was discovered that many colonies of clinically normal mice were latently infected with PLV-agents. Until then, psittacosis was widely regarded as being a disease of parrots or other psittacine birds only, and that man was an incidental host. Soon afterwards, the natural host range was extended to fulmars, petrels, pigeons and other non-psittacine birds and to various laboratory animals including guinea-pigs and hamsters. The first accounts of the isolation of PLV-agents from natural infections of non-laboratory mammals were reported from America; the first, in 1944, from an acute respiratory, distemper-like disease in cats called feline pneu-

monitis and the second, in 1949, from cases of meningitis in opossums.

By 1950, it became increasingly clear that members of the psittacosis lymphogranuloma group of organisms are responsible for a large number of diverse overt and inapparent infections in man and animals. Investigations carried out in many parts of the world during the last 40 years have shown that PLV-agents can infect no fewer than 130 species of birds, belonging to 12 orders, and that an ever-growing number of animals are also susceptible. Among mammals, naturally occurring infections with *Chlamydia* have been identified in primates, ungulates, carnivores, rodents and marsupials.

A report from Scotland, in 1950, of the causal organism of enzootic abortion of ewes was the first definitive account of a PLV-infection in farm animals. This was followed during the next 3 years, by reports from America of PLV-agents causing enteritis in calves, pneumonitis in sheep, encephalomyelitis in cattle, and from Japan of pneumonitis in goats. In subsequent years (1955–60) psittacosis-like organisms were isolated from cases of pneumonitis in cattle, epizootic bovine abortion, keratoconjunctivitis in sheep and, following an earlier preliminary report, from arthritis, pericarditis and peritonitis of pigs. Since then, PLV-agents have been isolated from the faeces of inapparently infected ruminants and carnivores, and associated with abortions in goats, conjunctivitis in pigs and cats and as the causative agent of polyarthritis of sheep and cattle. A report that psittacosis organisms can cause pneumonitis in dogs awaits confirmation.

Enzootic abortion of ewes

Synonyms

Virus abortion of sheep. Ovine virus abortion. Pararickettsial abortion. Psittacosis-lymphogranu-coma abortion. 'Kebbing'.

Definition

A placentitis of young ewes, characterized by abortion and premature lambing as a result of chlamydial infection.

History and distribution

Although flockmasters are usually reluctant to disclose the fact that their flocks are affected, there is good evidence that the disease has been experienced as an annual occurrence on farms of south-east Scotland for at least a hundred years. On one farm alone, its existence has been recorded for over 50 years.

Very little was known about the aetiology of the disease until 1950 when the causative agent was first isolated and identified as being a member of the psittacosis-lymphogranuloma group of organisms. Since that time, enzootic abortion of ewes has been recorded in England and much of continental Europe, including France, Germany, Hungary, Rumania, Bulgaria, Italy, Turkey and Cyprus. It was first reported in New Zealand in 1952 and in the U.S.A. in 1958.

An inactivated egg-adapted vaccine was introduced in 1959 and has greatly reduced the incidence of ewe abortions in endemic areas.

Hosts affected
The disease is almost entirely confined to gimmers and adult ewes; it also causes abortions in goats. Rams do not appear to undergo natural infections. Artificial intranasal infection of mice results in pneumonitis and death, and an acute disease has been produced in experimentally infected monkeys.

Aetiology
The causative agent occurs in considerable numbers in the placentae and uterine discharges of aborting sheep. It is indistinguishable in size, morphology and staining avidity from other members of the psittacosis family and shares the group-specific, heat-stable, complement-fixing antigen of *Chlamydia*. The specific antigen is labile and less readily demonstrable compared with some other chlamydiae. It is believed to be the only mammalian species to produce a good endotoxin.

The agent of enzootic abortion of ewes grows to very high titres in the yolk sac of developing hens' eggs and generally causes a fatal infection of the embryos after 3–8 days' incubation.

Mice infected by the intranasal route invariably develop pneumonia and die, but guinea-pigs and most other laboratory animals inoculated subcutaneously, intraperitoneally or intracerebrally usually remain healthy. Experimentally infected cows and gravid rabbits may abort.

The agent can be propagated on a very wide range of avian and animal cell culture systems and undergoes the normal psittacosis-type of life cycle with the formation of large intracytoplasmic vesicles containing both large and small developmental forms. Cellular degeneration is uncommon and infected monolayer cultures may remain intact for several weeks without replenishing the maintenance medium. The different morphological forms of the agent are clearly visible under dark-ground illumination and by Giemsa, modified Macchiavello, acridine orange or immunofluorescence staining.

The agent is susceptible to sulphathiazole, penicillin, aureomycin and terramycin but is insensitive to streptomycin and para-aminobenzoic acid.

Pathogenicity
The incidence of enzootic abortion varies considerably but it may be as high as 25 per cent in first and second lamb ewes. Most cases of abortion or premature lambing occur late in the gestation period from about 2–3 weeks before 'term', but some may occur 3 or 4 weeks earlier. Although the majority of lambs are delivered dead, normal vigorous lambs may be born even when the placenta is heavily infected, and it is not unusual for one of a pair of twins to be affected while the other is normal. Infected ewes show little or no ill-effects unless the placenta is retained or the lambs have been found dead *in utero*. In these circumstances the ewes may rapidly lose condition and some may die from secondary bacterial infections. Ewes which have aborted produce a pink, creamy discharge from the vulva for some time after lambing but sterility is not a common sequel to the infection.

Pathology
The most characteristic feature of enzootic abortion of ewes is the appearance of the fetal membranes. The affected placentae show various stages of necrosis of the cotyledons and chorion, and the colour of the cotyledons varies from dark red or pink to a dull clay-like colour, instead of the purple appearance of the normal tissue. The chorion presents irregular areas of thickening due to oedema, but more often the tissue is tough, crumpled and leather-like. In contrast, the uterine mucosa and uterine cotyledons show no macroscopic abnormalities.

Ecology
Most workers consider that lambs become infected by the ingestion of large numbers of organisms either at the time of birth, shortly thereafter or as adults. The agent has little affinity for tissues other than the placenta and may remain dormant in the clinically normal, non-pregnant animal until the onset of gestation. Infected placentae contain considerable numbers of organisms and are mainly responsible for contaminating lambing pens and pastures, and for spreading the infection to other members of the flock. Ewes that acquire the infection while pregnant may not abort or deliver weakly lambs until the subsequent pregnancy.

The infection is usually introduced into clean flocks through the agency of 'bought-in', latently infected ewes and gimmers, or when ewes from an abortion-free district have been introduced in the autumn before service into a known infected flock. In either case, abortions do not occur in the originally non-infected ewes at the first lambing after the mixing of the two groups, even though the incidence of abortion amongst the originally infected ewes may have been high at that lambing.

Parenteral inoculation of the agent into healthy sheep causes a sharp rise in temperature (40–42°C within 24–36 hours) which persists for 2–3 days. Pregnant animals will abort in about 5 weeks but are usually free from demonstrable infection at the next pregnancy; and will resist further challenge. Less consistent results are obtained if suspensions of the organism are administered by the oral route when the time required to produce abortion is at least 7 weeks.

Chlamydial infections constitute a distinct hazard to animal economy but only two clinical cases have been reported in man where the causative agent was a strain derived from an animal host. Both were acquired in the laboratory and one was due to the agent of enzootic abortion of ewes.

Diagnosis

The appearance of the placental lesions is fairly characteristic of the disease but a tentative diagnosis should always be confirmed by demonstrating the psittacosis-like organisms in the affected fetal membranes and uterine discharges. In the absence of these tissues, swabs taken from the moist woollen coats of newly aborted fetuses may suffice but it is stressed that, in contrast to *Brucella abortus* infections, the causative organisms are not present in the fetal stomach contents.

Smears stained by the modified Macchiavello or Brucella differential method and examined under the oil-immersion lens show the organisms as tiny, spherical, bright red particles about 250–450 nm in size. (Plate 36.2a, facing p. 388a). Careful examination will reveal the larger, granular 'initial bodies' as blue-staining structures against the paler blue background of the smear. These do not occur in tissue smears of rickettsial infections and, to the experienced observer, their presence will prove helpful in distinguishing between the agents of enzootic abortion and Q fever in the placentae and discharges of sheep. The minute elementary particles are also clearly visible in infected tissues if examined microscopically under dark-field illumination.

Complement-fixing antibodies are usually present in the sera of infected and vaccinated sheep and a direct complement-fixation test performed on acute and convalescent phase sera taken between 2 weeks and 4 months after abortion is a useful method of confirming or refuting a diagnosis. Wherever possible, serum samples should be collected from several sheep in a flock. In infected animals, the paired sera should show a four-fold or greater rise in antibody levels.

The presence of serum neutralizing antibodies can be demonstrated by the intranasal inoculation of mice, using infected yolk sac emulsions as the antigen. The serum-antigen mixtures are instilled intranasally in 0·25–0·3 ml amounts and will cause fatal infections in 3–5 days if antibodies are absent. In infected ewes, neutralizing antibodies appear later than complement-fixing antibodies, but persist longer. Serological methods including complement-fixation, serum-neutralization and fluorescent-antibody staining, are useful for identifying organisms isolated from field material by the usual mouse and egg inoculation methods. Large quantities of agent can readily be obtained by further passages in embryonated eggs.

Although the agent of enzootic abortion grows well in a variety of secondary and established cell cultures, large inocula are required to initiate infection and the method is not suitable, therefore, for primary isolation.

Treatment

Various chemotherapeutic substances including sulphonamides and antibiotics have been used for the treatment of individual cases. Encouraging results have been obtained with chloromycetin, aureomycin and terramycin. Penicillin is less effective although it has inhibitory properties *in vitro*.

Control

Ewes that have aborted once usually develop an effective resistance to re-infection and do not abort a second time. But ewe-lambs from immune mothers are not protected against infection and may abort at the first pregnancy.

A satisfactory vaccine has been produced from infected yolk sac tissues inactivated with formalin and precipitated with a water-in-oil emulsion of alum. If young sheep are vaccinated before mating the subsequent immunity persists for at least 30 months and significantly reduces the incidence of abortion in subsequent lambing seasons.

Every effort should be made to prevent dissemination of the causative agent from ewes at lambing time. Ewes showing clinical signs of infection should be isolated, while young lambs and breeding ewes should always be kept apart around lambing time. Infected placentae must be collected and destroyed. They should not be left in places that are accessible to sheepdogs or foxes.

Feline pneumonitis

Feline pneumonitis variously known as cat distemper, cat influenza or nasal catarrh is a highly infectious debilitating disease caused by a member of the psittacosis group of organisms. The illness, which lasts about a month, is characterized by anorexia, sneezing, snuffling and coughing and the presence of a heavy mucopurulent discharge which tends to block the eyes and nasal passages. Many of the affected cats develop a chronic infection of the upper and lower respiratory tract, and, although pneumonia may not be evident clinically, post-mortem examination shows that the anterior lobes of the lungs are consolidated and have a grey appearance.

The disease is highly contagious and spreads directly to other cats by the respiratory route. The incubation period in natural infections is from 6–10 days. During the early period of the illness the causal agent can be recovered from the liver and spleen and, in experimentally infected cats, from the lungs and oculonasal secretions. The typical clinical disease can readily be reproduced by the intranasal inoculation of susceptible kittens; other routes are not effective. Mice, hamsters and young guinea-pigs inoculated intranasally develop fatal pneumonia but older guinea-pigs and rabbits undergo non-fatal infections. Infected mice do not transmit the agent to other mice. The feline pneumonitis agent forms a potent endotoxin which kills intravenously injected mice in 12–24 hours.

The mortality rate is generally very low and recovered cats are able to carry the PLV-agent for long periods, thereby maintaining the chain of infection without the need for another host. The feline pneumonitis agent is also responsible for an unusual form of keratoconjunctivitis in cats. Reports suggesting that it is a source of human infection have not been confirmed.

The characters of the causative agent are similar to those of other members of the PLV-group. However, it is inactivated not only by ether but also by sodium dodecyl-sulphate and quickly dies out at 37°C: the half-life at 37°C being 90 minutes. It survives for 24 hours between pH 6·5 and 7·5 at 0°C and is stable at –70°C. It agglutinates mouse red blood cells at 20°C but the haemagglutinin, which is separable from the elementary particle, is said to be unstable at 50°C. The agent grows well in the yolk sac of fertile hens' eggs and kills the chick embryos after 2–3 days. It can also be propagated in various cell culture systems, producing characteristic psittacosis-like developmental forms.

Affected kittens respond well to treatment with tetracyclines but penicillin, which is active *in vitro*, does not eliminate the infection completely.

Polyarthritis of lambs and calves

Polyarthritis or stiff-lamb disease is due to invasion of the joints of lambs by a member of the psittacosis group of organisms. The disease has been observed in many parts of the U.S.A. and usually occurs during the summer and autumn months of the year, mostly in lambs from 3–8 months of age.

Affected animals are febrile and walk with a stiff, stilted gait. Movement is characterized by extreme carpal flexion with the weight being borne on the carpal joints. The mortality rate is low and seldom exceeds 1–2 per cent, but a few animals become permanently lame.

The causative organisms are found in the cytoplasm of the synovial cells and monocytes, and are clearly visible in smears of joint fluids stained by Giemsa. Macchiavello's stain gives irregular results. The agent can readily be isolated from the joint fluids by the inoculation of yolk sacs of embryonated hens' eggs. It can also be recovered from various other tissues including the brain, blood, spleen, liver, kidney and lymph nodes. The widespread distribution of the agent in the affected carcase is indicative of a generalised infection.

Little is known about the epidemiology of stiff-lamb disease but some workers believe that the causative organism is a strain of *Chlamydia* normally inhabiting the alimentary tract of sheep.

A polyarthritis syndrome associated with PLV-agents has also been reported in young calves, usually between 1–3 weeks of age. The disease is characterized by pyrexia, anorexia, mild diarrhoea and disinclination to walk. The gait is stiff, due to gross enlargement of the joints, and the tendons are painful when handled. The mortality rate is high and death usually occurs 2–10 days after the onset of clinical symptoms.

At autopsy, the synovial sacs are distended with a greyish-yellow, turbid fluid and the membranes often show petechiae. The liver and spleen are enlarged and the lymph nodes are swollen and oedematous.

The causative agent is present in the affected joints and various visceral organs but is more difficult to isolate than that of stiff-lamb disease. Antibiotic therapy has little effect on the course of the illness.

Bovine encephalomyelitis

Bovine encephalomyelitis, sometimes called sporadic bovine encephalomyelitis (SBE) or Buss disease, was first described in the midwestern United States as a disease of calves and was shown in 1953 to be caused by a member of the psittacosis-lymphogranuloma venereum group of organisms. The disease, which occurs only in cattle, is characterized by sudden onset of fever, anorexia, weakness, depression and paralysis. Many of the animals salivate freely, show a nasal discharge and cough, and the breathing becomes rapid and laboured. Occasionally there is diarrhoea and the faeces are apt to be watery and blue-grey in colour. The clinical symptoms may be mild and most animals make an uneventful recovery but in others, nervous symptoms may appear. Within about a week badly affected calves have difficulty in walking due to stiffness of the gait and knuckling of the fetlocks and they stagger in circles and frequently fall. Finally, paralysis sets in and at least 50 per cent of calves with established symptoms die. The incidence of the disease is probably affected by the age of exposed animals and the degree of herd immunity. In endemic areas, adult cattle are seldom affected with the acute clinical form of the disease which usually causes a mortality rate considerably lower than that in calves less than 6 months of age.

At autopsy, a common finding is the presence of a fibrinous net enveloping the omentum and covering the surfaces of the liver and spleen. In many cases there is also a yellow, watery fluid in the pleural, pericardial and peritoneal cavities.

The disease has been observed in Canada, Germany, Australia, South Africa and in many parts of the U.S.A. Little is known about its incidence or mode of transmission since many of the infections are inapparent and the clinical disease is of a sporadic nature. Calves can be readily infected by the intracerebral or subcutaneous routes. The incubation period varies from 4–27 days and the visceral lesions commonly encountered in field cases of the disease are reproduced more readily than the nervous ones.

It is generally agreed that the causative agent of sporadic bovine encephalomyelitis is a member of the PLV-group of organisms. Its properties are very similar to those of other members of the group and characteristic intracytoplasmic elementary bodies can be seen in stained smears prepared from the exudates overlying the spleen and mesencephalon. The agent grows readily in the yolk sacs of fertile hens' eggs and retains its infectivity for long periods at $-70°C$ or when stored in 50 per cent glycerol-saline at 4°C. It is sensitive to ether and chloroform, and is heat labile. Complete inactivation of the agent occurs within 15 minutes at 62°C or within 30 minutes at 56°C. There is no evidence that it produces an haemagglutinin.

Although the agent causes fatal infection in chick embryos within 5–10 days, it differs from other chlamydiae in that it is usually non-pathogenic for Swiss mice. Nevertheless, when given intraperitoneally to guinea-pigs it often causes death in 4–5 days with fibrinous peritonitis. Cotton rats and hamsters are susceptible and show fever, encephalitis, paralysis and death when inoculated by the intracerebral route. Domestic rabbits are not susceptible. Rhesus monkeys inoculated intracerebrally and intraperitoneally are infected and show fever and encephalitis. The accidental infection of a laboratory worker has been confirmed.

Although the agent is sensitive to sulphonamides and antibiotics including penicillin and the tetracyclines, there is no clear evidence that clinically affected animals respond satisfactorily to antibiotic therapy. There are no effective vaccines against the disease.

Further reading

Rickettsiae

BABUDIERI B. (1959) Q fever: a zoonosis. *Advances in Veterinary Science*, **5**, 81.

CARMICHAEL J. AND FIENNES R.N.T.-W. (1942) Rickettsia infection of dogs. *Veterinary Record*, **54**, 3.

CORDY D.R. AND GORHAM J.R. (1950) The pathology and etiology of Salmon disease in the dog and fox. *American Journal of Pathology*, **26** (2), 617.

DANSKIN D. AND BURDIN M.L. (1963) Bovine petechial fever. *Veterinary Record*, **75**, 391.

EWING, S.A. (1969) Canine Ehrlichiosis. *Advances in Veterinary Science and Comparative Medicine*, **13**, 331.

FARRELL R.K., OTT R.L. AND GORHAM J.R. (1955) The clinical laboratory diagnosis of salmon poisoning. *Journal of the American Veterinary Medical Association*, **127**, 241.

FOGGIE A. (1951) Studies on the infectious agent of tick-borne fever in sheep. *Journal of Pathology and Bacteriology*, **63**, 1.

GORDON W.S., BROWNLEE A., WILSON D.R. AND MACLEOD J. (1932) Tick-borne fever. A hitherto undescribed disease of sheep. *Journal of Comparative Pathology and Therapeutics*, **45**, 301.

HAIG D.A. (1955) Tickborne rickettsioses in South Africa. *Advances in Veterinary Science*, **2**, 307.

HAIG D.A. AND DANSKIN D. (1962) The aetiology of bovine petechial fever (Ondiri disease). *Research in Veterinary Science*, **3**, 129.

HUDSON J.R. (1950) The recognition of tick-borne fever as a disease of cattle. *British Veterinary Journal*, **106**, 3.

KITAO, T., FARRELL, R.K. AND FUKUDA, T. (1973) Differentiation of salmon poisoning disease and Elokomin fluke fever: fluorescent antibody studies with *Rickettsia sennetsu*. *American Journal of Veterinary Research*, **34**, 927.

KRAUSS, H., DAVIES, F.G., ODEGAARD, O. A. AND COOPER, J.E. (1972) The morphology of the causal agent of Bovine Petechial Fever [Ondiri Disease]. *Journal of Comparative Pathology*, **82**, 241.

MALHERBE W.D. (1948) The diagnosis and treatment of rickettsiosis in dogs. *Journal of the South African Veterinary Medical Association*, **19**, 135.

NYINDO, M.B.A., RISTIC, M., HUXSOLL, D.L. AND SMITH, A.R. (1971) Tropical canine pancytopenia: *in vitro* cultivation of the causative agent — *Ehrlichia canis*. *American Journal of Veterinary Research*, **32**, 1651.

PHILIP C.B., HADLOW W.J. AND HUGHES L.E. (1954) Studies on salmon poisoning disease of canines. I. The rickettsial relationships and pathogenicity of *Neorickettsia helminthoeca*. *Experimental Parasitology*, **3**, 336.

PURCHASE H.S. (1945) A simple and rapid method for demonstrating *Rickettsia ruminantium* (Cowdry) in heartwater brains. *Veterinary Record*, **57**, 413.

RISTIC, M., HUXSOLL, D.L., WEISIGER, R.M., HILDEBRANDT, P.K. AND NYINDO, M.B.A. (1972) Serological diagnosis of tropical canine pancytopenia by indirect immunofluorescence. *Infection and Immunity*, **6**, 226.

SLAVIN G. (1952) Q fever. The domestic animal as a source of infection for man. *Veterinary Record*, **64**, 743.

STOKER M.G.P. (1949) Serological evidence of Q fever in Great Britain. *Lancet*, **1**. 178.

WEITZ W.O., ALEXANDER R.A. AND ADELAAR T.F. (1947) Studies on immunity in heartwater. *Onderstepoort J.*, **21** (2), 243.

Chlamydiae

BAKER J.A. (1944) A virus causing pneumonia in cats and producing elementary bodies. *Journal of Experimental Medicine*, **79**, 159.

McEWEN A.D., LITTLEJOHN A.I. AND FOGGIE A. (1951) Enzootic abortion in ewes. Some aspects of infection and resistance. *Veterinary Record*, **63**, 489.

MENDLOWSKI B. AND SEGRE D (1960) Polyarthritis in sheep. I. Description of the disease and experimental transmission. *American Journal of Veterinary Research*, **21**, 68.

MENGES R.W., HARSHFIELD G.S. AND WENNER H.A. (1953) Sporadic bovine encephalomyelitis. *American Journal of Hygiene*, **57**, 1.

MEYER K.F. (1953) Psittacosis group. *Annals of the New York Academy of Science*, **56**, 545.

MEYER K.F. AND EDDIE B. (1964) Psittacosis-lymphogranuloma venereum group (Bedsonia infections). In '*Diagnostic Procedures for Viral and Rickettsial Diseases*', 3rd Edition, Ed. E.H. Lennette and N.J. Schmidt, pp. 603–639. New York: American Public Health Association, Inc.

MEYER K.F. (1965) Ornithosis. In '*Diseases of Poultry*', 5th Edition, Ed. H.E. Biester and L.H. Schwarte, pp. 675–770. Ames, Iowa:

PARKER H.D., HAWKINS W.W. AND BRENNER E. (1966) Epizootiologic studies of bovine virus abortion. *American Journal of Veterinary Research*, **27**, 869.

STAMP J.T., McEWEN A.D., WATT J.A.A. AND NISBET D.I. (1950) Enzootic abortion in ewes. Transmission of the disease. *Veterinary Record*, **62**, 251.

STORZ, J. AND PAGE, L.A. (1971) Taxonomy of the chlamydiae: reasons for classifying organisms of the genus Chlamydia, family Chlamydiaceae, in a separate order, Chlamydiales ord. nov. *International Journal of Systematic Bacteriology*, **21**, 332.

STORZ J., SHUPE J.L., JAMES L.F. AND SMART R.A. (1963) Polyarthritis of sheep in the intermountain region caused by a psittacosis-lymphogranuloma agent. *American Journal of Veterinary Research*, **24**, 1201.

STORZ J., SMART R.A., MARRIOTT M.E. AND DAVIS R.V. (1966) Polyarthritis of calves: isolation of psittacosis agents from affected joints. *American Journal of Veterinary Research*, **27**, 633.

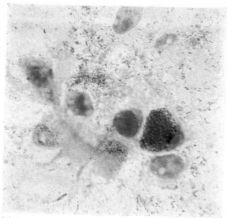

36.1a

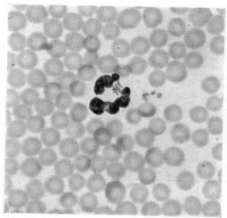

36.1b

36.1c

36.1a A smear from the placenta of a sheep heavily infected with *Coxiella burnetii* of Q fever. The rickettsiae are seen as intracellular masses of red-coloured coccobacilli. Brucella differential stain, × 650.

36.1b A blood film from a sheep affected with tick-borne fever. The infective agents are seen as a cluster of small, spherical bodies within the cytoplasm of a polymorphonuclear leucocyte. Leishman stain, × 1000.

36.1c A crush preparation from the brain of a sheep found suffering from heartwater fever. The organisms (*Cowdria ruminantium*) are seen forming large clusters in the endothelial cells lining the brain capillaries. Giemsa stain, × 1030.

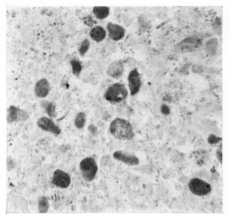

36.2a

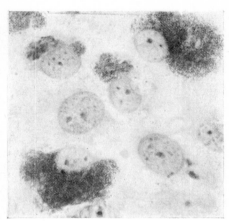

36.2b

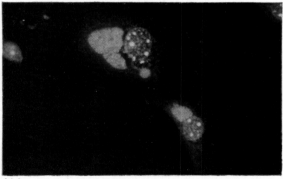

36.2c

36.2a A smear from the placenta of a sheep infected with the agent of enzootic abortion of ewes. The organisms (*Chlamydia*) are seen as masses of tiny red particles within the cytoplasm of the infected cells. In some areas the cells have ruptured and the organisms are escaping. Brucella differential stain, × 645.

36.2b A monolayer of sheep kidney cells 7 days after inoculation with the psittacosis agent (*Chlamydia psittaci*). Notice the presence of a few large blue-staining particles and numerous tiny red-coloured elementary bodies within the cytoplasm of the infected cells. Brucella differential stain, × 645.

36.2c Sheep kidney cells 5 days after inoculation with *Chlamydia*. The monolayer culture was stained with acridine orange and photographed in the ultraviolet light microscope. The presence of orange-red fluorescence indicates that the intracytoplasmic plaques of organisms contain RNA. The nuclei are never infected, × 500.

VIROLOGY

CHAPTER 37

FUNDAMENTAL CHARACTERS OF VIRUSES

Fundamental characters of viruses

In the early days of virology, the presence of a virus could only be detected by its filterability and by its ability to infect susceptible animals. Thus, it was soon discovered that most viruses were extremely minute microorganisms which were not recognizable in the optical microscope and could not be cultivated in non-living media.

Since filterability was the main character that distinguished viruses from fungi, yeasts, bacteria and protozoa, the term 'filterable virus' was commonly used to distinguish them from other microorganisms. However, this term is no longer regarded as a unique feature of viruses because certain species of bacteria are smaller than the largest viruses and modern filters can be produced that are fine enough to retain even the smallest virus particles.

For many years the majority of viruses remained 'ultramicroscopic' and only the largest species, the poxviruses, could be recognised as minute amorphous granules under the ordinary light microscope. From 1940 onwards the introduction of improved techniques in electron microscopy revolutionized the study of viral morphology and, in due course, most of the common viruses had been observed and photographed. Then, in 1959, the method of negative staining greatly enlarged our knowledge of viral ultrastructure, and the term 'ultramicroscopic viruses' became meaningless.

Virology is a new and important field of science which comprises the study of both the infecting microorganism and its host. In general terms, the subject is divided into four main divisions:

(1) the viruses of man and animals (animal viruses),

(2) the bacterial viruses (bacteriophages),

(3) the viruses of insects and worms (insect viruses) and

(4) the viruses of plants (plant viruses).

Viruses are very simple structures and the mature virus particle (virion) consists of a central core of nucleic acid surrounded by a protective coat of protein. They vary greatly in size ranging from the poxvirus, which at 300×200 nm is about the size of the elementary body of *Chlamydia*, down to the picornavirus, e.g. foot-and-mouth disease virus which, at 20–28 nm in diameter, is little more than the size of a large protein molecule. The size and shape of the main virus groups, compared with a bacterial cell (*E. coli*), are shown diagrammatically in Fig. 37.1.

Definition

Viruses are small, obligate intracellular 'parasites' which can replicate only in living susceptible cells. They differ fundamentally from other classes of microorganisms in that:

(1) The mature virus particle consists essentially of a central core of nucleic acid, the genetic material, enclosed within a protein-rich outer coat which protects the viral genome (complete set of genes) from adverse environmental conditions and assists the penetration of the virus into its host cell.

(2) The genome nucleic acid is either DNA or RNA and is either single-stranded or double-stranded. (But see also Chapt. 46. page 586)

(3) Viruses have no metabolic activity of their own and lack enzyme systems and other constituents fundamental for independent growth and multiplication.

(4) They do not possess ribosomes, nor transfer RNA and enzymes required for synthesis of nucleic acids and proteins, but the viral genome can divert the metabolism of the infected host cell from the manufacture of normal cellular constituents towards the synthesis of viral components and the assembly of new progeny virus.

(5) Viruses are unable to grow or to undergo binary fission as are other microorganisms, and are reproduced solely from their nucleic acid by a complicated process of biosynthesis.

(6) They are metabolically inert and, consequently, are not susceptible to antibiotics or other agents that act against the metabolic pathways of microorganisms.

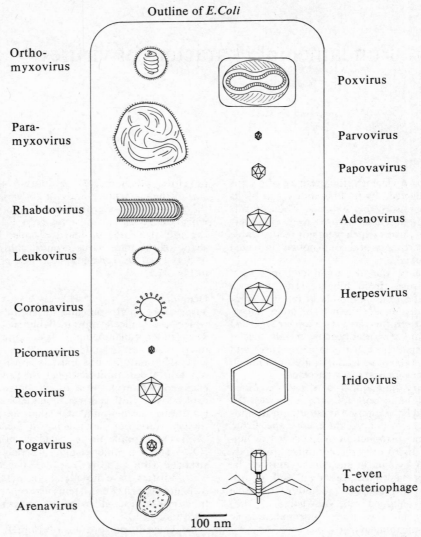

FIG. 37.1. Size and shape of the main virus groups compared with a bacterial cell (*E. coli*).

(7) Most species are sensitive to interferons.

(8) Some are capable of inducing latent infections by the integration of their nucleic acid with the DNA of the host cell.

Despite these unusual features, most workers are agreed that viruses behave like microorganisms and should be considered as living entities; but others believe that they are not organisms (e.g. they may contain RNA and not DNA as the repository of their genetic information) and are non-living. The debate as to whether viruses are living or non-living stems from the discoveries that certain viruses, e.g.

tobacco mosaic virus and poliovirus, can be crystallized and that the viral nucleic acid of others can enter susceptible host cells and replicate therein. Although the argument is now little more than one of semantics, interest has been revived by recent reports that purified RNA or DNA can be induced to multiply *in vitro*, albeit in the presence of essential precursors and enzymes.

Physical methods of studying viruses

Unit of mass

The unit of mass is the **dalton;** one dalton being the

mass of one hydrogen atom which is equal to 1.67×10^{-24} g. The molecular weight of the nucleic acid component of a virus is expressed in daltons and is obtained by disrupting highly purified viral suspensions with phenol or by treatment with detergents such as sodium deoxycholate or by proteolytic enzymes. The intact nucleic acid liberated from the virion by these procedures is then sedimented in an analytical centrifuge and its molecular weight estimated.

The molecular weight of the nucleic acid of most RNA viruses is between 2×10^6 and 4×10^6 but in the case of double-stranded RNA viruses, e.g. reovirus, the molecular weight is five times greater, approximately 15×10^6. On the other hand, most DNA viruses have nucleic acids with a much higher and more variable molecular weight than the RNA viruses, e.g. vaccinia has a DNA molecule of 160×10^6 and herpes DNA has a molecular weight of $50–90 \times 10^6$ daltons.

Units of length

Viruses, because of their small size, are usually measured in millimicrons ($m\mu$) but recent adoption of the MKS system (metres, kilograms and seconds) has introduced alternative methods of measurement. Thus, the micron (μ) is now termed a micrometer (μm) and the millimicron is called a nanometer (nm), which is equal to 10^{-6} millimetres (mm). The Angström unit (Å or AU) is used by some workers for recording the size of very small structures such as virus capsomeres or for scale bars on optical micrographs. The relationship between these units of length is shown as follows:

```
1 metre (m)     = 1000 millimetres (mm)
1 millimetre    = 1000 micrometres (μm)
1 micrometre    = 1000 nanometres (nm)
1 nanometre     = 10 Angström units (Å or AU).
```

Purification of virus

Before attempting to define the physical and chemical characteristics of a virus, the virus particles must be purified in such a way that the suspension contains as little host cell constituents as possible. In cell culture systems relatively small amounts of virus are present in the fluid phase of the culture, and most of the infectious and non-infectious particles are attached to cellular debris having similar physical and chemical properties. As a general rule virions with helical symmetry are more difficult to purify because their protective envelope contains lipids derived from the host cell whereas cubical viruses with no envelope are easier to purify. Thus, the first step in obtaining concentrated purified virus preparations involves the release of the infectious virions by disrupting the host-cell membranes. This is usually achieved by breaking down the infected tissue cells in a homogenizer, with detergent or enzyme treatment, by disrupting the cells with ultrasonic vibration or by alternately freezing and thawing the cell suspension. The material may then be clarified by filtration through various types of bacteriological filters followed by secondary filtration through fritted glass or cellulose membrane filters of suitable average pore diameter (APD). Alternatively, the cellular constituents can be pelleted by slow speed centrifugation and the suspended virus particles concentrated by alternate cycles of low and high speed centrifugation; thereby providing a preparation that is suitable for purification.

Methods of purification include a) differential centrifugation which is useful for most viruses whose particles are appreciably different in size from the cellular constituents, b) density gradient centrifugation where sucrose gradients ensure finer separation of particles with slightly different sedimentation properties and c) equilibrium sedimentation in caesium columns which separates the particles according to their buoyant density. Because viruses are basically protein macromolecules, those techniques that are commonly used for the 'salting-out' of proteins from solution are sometimes employed for viral purification. Precipitation with $(NH_4)_2SO_4$ or alcohols can be done provided enough material is available and the virus is not inactivated in the process. Virus particles can also be separated from contaminating materials by using fluorocarbons or other organic solvents to remove large quantities of host cell material selectively. This procedure is especially useful for removing lipid material and denatured host protein.

In the case of haemagglutinating viruses suspensions of healthy red blood cells can be used to remove the virus particles by adsorption. The virions are then eluted from the erythrocytes at higher temperatures of incubation, e.g. 37°C, or following treatment with receptor destroying enzyme (RDE). Adsorption on to ion exchange compounds such as diethylaminoethyl cellulose (DEAE-cellulose) followed by selective elution at certain pH values or salt concentrations have also been used as a means of purifying viruses.

Determination of particle size

Many procedures are available for determining the size of virus particles. These range from filtration through filters of graded porosity and sedimentation of the particles by centrifugal force, to the most frequently used and generally most accurate method of direct observation under the electron microscope.

Filtration

Originally, viruses were measured by their capacity to pass through earthenware filters and many different types have been used for this purpose. Since the pore diameter of filters depends on the proportion of materials used in their manufacture, various grades of earthenware candles were produced of which the Chamberland candle of unglazed porcelain and the Berkefeld filters of diatomaceous earth (kieselguhr) proved most effective. The coarser grades of the Chamberland filters are similar in porosity to the Berkefeld types but the finer grades of Chamberland candles pass only certain viruses of extreme minuteness such as the virus of foot-and-mouth disease. The use of earthenware candles has now largely been replaced by a method of filtration through collodion or cellulose acetate membranes of graded pore sizes. One of the advantages of these membrane filters is that by careful arrangement of the conditions of manufacture it is possible to produce membranes of nearly uniform pore size, in contrast to Seitz and some other types of asbestos pad filters (Appendix 2, Vol. 1). Membrane filters are non-toxic to cells in culture, they do not alter the pH of the medium and they do not adsorb large quantities of virus particles during filtration.

When a purified virus suspension is passed through a series of membrane filters of known APD, the approximate size of the virions can be estimated from the average APD of the two membranes, one of which allows the virus to pass freely while the other retains it completely. By this method the limiting pore diameter multiplied by 0·64 gives the diameter of the virus particle. Inevitably this is an approximation and does not take into account variations in shape or in particle size which may vary considerably. Although filtration methods have no high degree of precision in virus measurements and have been largely replaced by newer techniques, e.g. electron microscopy, they are still of value in measuring very small particles contained in material contaminated with so much host-cell protein that other methods cannot be used.

Centrifugation
Another procedure which can be used for determining the size of viruses is that of high speed centrifugation. The method depends upon the fact that the rate of sedimentation of a suspended particle is dependent upon its size, its density and the viscosity of the suspending fluid. The relationship between the particles' size and rate of sedimentation follows Stoke's Law and holds good even when forces many times greater than gravity (g) are applied to a virus preparation in a fast-moving centrifuge. In modern ultracentrifuges, forces of more than 100 000g may be used to drive the particles to the foot of the tube. Thus, from values for the density and viscosity of the medium, the distance from the axis of rotation

and the speed of the rotor, the diameter of the particle can be calculated.

The following methods can be used:

Density gradient centrifugation. Particles are suspended in a liquid column whose density is distributed in a continuous gradient. Two procedures are available.

(1) *Rate zonal centrifugation* in a sucrose gradient separates particles with different sedimentation constants on the basis of particle size, shape and density. The density gradient prevents diffusion in the tube during centrifugation. At the end of a 'run' the zones can be sampled by collecting fractions through a small hole punctured in the bottom of the centrifuge tube.

(2) *Equilibrium density centrifugation* involves suspension of particles in a solution of a high-density salt such as caesium chloride. Centrifugation separates the particles according to their buoyant density and is used to separate viruses of different types from each other and from cellular debris. After prolonged centrifugation the solution forms a stable density gradient and the particles collect at the level where the density of the medium equals their own, and ultimately form a band.

Chromatography and electrophoresis
Additional methods used to separate virus particles according to the electrostatic charge on their surfaces include column chromatography and electrophoresis. In chromatography, the virus is allowed to filter through a gel in a column under appropriate ionic conditions; gels of different pore sizes are available. The cellular material is washed out and then the virus particles are eluted with a solution of different ionic strength which competitively adsorbs to the gel.

In electrophoresis, the particles are separated according to the number and distribution of charges on their surfaces and the speed of migration of the particles in the electron field is measured. The method, which is primarily intended for purifying and identifying proteins, is also useful for characterization of viruses.

Microscopy
The earliest microscopical observations on the morphology of viruses appear to have been made in 1887 by Buist who accurately described minute particles in stained smears of vaccinial material. Similar observations were made in 1904 by Borrel who noted minute coccal bodies in stained smears of fowlpox lesions and concluded that they were the virus particles. In later years convincing photographs of poxviruses were obtained by increasing the resolving power of the ordinary light microscope by using the shorter wave of ultraviolet

light, the limit of resolution falling from 200 to 80 nm, in combination with quartz lenses and a special dark-ground condenser. Despite these refinements, visible light microscopy is not generally suitable for observing the vast majority of viruses since the particles will not be resolved adequately and, if attempts are made to do so, the image rapidly becomes blurred and indistinct.

Until comparatively recently, most viruses have remained 'ultra-microscopic' and studies of their morphology were largely confined to poxviruses, rickettsiae and psittacosis-like organisms: the discrete particles or rods being referred to as 'elementary bodies'.

In recent years improvements in the electron microscope and the development of new techniques suitable for the study of viruses have undoubtedly provided a most useful and accurate method of estimating virus size and structure by simple direct observation and measurement.

The most successful of the various types of electron microscopes is the high-power transmission electron microscope which, as its name implies, is intended solely for the examination of thin specimens by transmitted electrons. In many respects it is an electronic counterpart of the standard light microscope, the principal differences being due to the type of illumination used, the electromagnetic lens system and the degree of resolution obtainable.

In most modern electron microscopes the actual source of electrons is a pure tungsten filament (the electron gun) which, when heated electrically to incandescence, emits a stream of electrons. The beam is accelerated by a potential difference in the range 30–100 kV and the electrons, moving at such high velocities, travel through the microscope at uniform speed and possess an extremely short wavelength of the order of 0·04 Å (0·004 nm). Glass is very opaque to electron beams and, therefore, the lens system consists essentially of a number of magnetic coils which control the magnetic fields through which the electrons pass. After passing the first or 'condenser' lens system, the electrons are deflected by the specimen and the image is enlarged some 200 times by the second or 'objective' lens system. The image is finally enlarged a further 500 times and projected by the 'ocular' or 'projector' lens system on to a fluorescent screen where it can be viewed at magnifications of 100 000 times or greater. The image may also be photographically recorded and then magnified to give a picture with a total magnification of about 1 million. Although the electron microscope has exceptionally good resolving power the efficiency of the lens system does not match that of optical lenses and the resolution of the instrument is only about 200–300 times better than that of the best light microscope. The penetrating power of the electron microscope is very poor also and, for this

reason, only very small objects or ultra-thin sections of tissues can be examined. Moreover, the specimens must be mounted on thin films of high transparency to electrons and, because they are extremely fragile, these are supported by a small copper supporting mesh or perforated disc. Another serious disadvantage of the electron microscope in virological studies is due to the fact that the passage of electron beams can only be achieved in a vacuum so that wet specimens, e.g. virus suspensions, cannot be introduced into the microscope and examined in their natural state.

To overcome these difficulties and to enable virus suspensions to be examined in greater detail a number of techniques have been devised to enhance the contrast and to improve the quality of the electron micrographs. These include metal shadowing or shadow casting and positive staining or negative staining methods.

Metal shadowing

In metal shadowing, heavy metals such as chromium, gold and platinum or palladium alloys are evaporated from an electrically heated filament in a vacuum. The source of the evaporating metal is so arranged that the metal atoms are directed at an oblique angle to the grid containing the specimen. The atoms of metal travel in almost parallel straight lines and, on striking the specimen at an oblique angle, pile up on the near side of the virus particle, casting a shadow beyond it. Because the metal atoms are more opaque to the electron beam a three-dimensional effect is produced and this enables the size of the virus to be calculated provided the angle of incidence of the metal atoms is known. Accurate measurement is also made possible by including in the virus suspensions a number of small latex particles of known diameter, e.g. 250 nm.

Since 1946, the method of shadow casting has provided useful but limited information about the shape of virus particles. For example, the majority of poxviruses were found to be brick-shaped, myxoviruses appeared to be highly pleomorphic with filamentous as well as spherical bodies, tobacco mosaic virus was in the form of a slender, rigid rod, and bacterial viruses were tadpole-shaped with a spherical or polyhedral head joined to a large cylindrical tail. Despite its obvious limitations, the shadow-casting technique was used to show that the virion of *Tipula* iridescent virus, which attacks the larvae of the common crane fly or daddy-long-legs, is in the form of an icosahedron with twenty equilateral triangular faces. This interesting observation was discovered quite simply by double shadowing a frozen-dried particle of the virus by means of two metal sources positioned some 60° apart and comparing the appearance of the two shadows in the electron microscope with that produced by a cardboard model of an icosahedron shadowed by two light-sources and orientated so that one apex of the hexagonal contour pointed directly towards each light source. In both cases one of the shadows was five-sided and blunt-ended while the other had four sides and a pointed end.

Negative staining

Recent improvements in electron microscopes, and especially in the methods of preparing and staining specimens, have made it possible to resolve fine differences in the basic morphology of viruses. The most notable advance in our knowledge of viral ultrastructure occurred in 1959 when negative staining techniques were first applied to the electron microscopy of viruses. The method is extremely simple to perform and consists essentially of mixing suspensions of virus particles with a salt solution which is highly opaque to electrons, usually sodium phosphotungstate. The mixture is then spread in a thin layer on a carbon-coated membrane, dried in air, transferred to the electron microscope and examined through the fluorescent screen. Because the surface contours and depressions of the virus particle attract the tungstate solution, fine details of the external surface of the virion are revealed as electron-lucent areas on an opaque background. In these early experiments the resulting electron micrographs showed a degree of fine detail not previously possible and allowed resolution of structure which, in some instances, had been predicted earlier by theoretical considerations and X-ray diffraction studies.

The first animal viruses examined by negative staining or negative contrast techniques were adenoviruses and herpesviruses, and in both cases a regularly arranged subunit structure was discovered. The method also revealed that the protein coat of the virion is composed of a large number of morphological units, termed capsomeres, and that two main kinds of symmetry exist, cubical, (e.g. adenovirus) and helical, (e.g. Newcastle disease virus.)

Positive staining

The electron density of virus particles can be greatly increased by staining them with chemicals with an affinity for protein molecules, usually osmium tetroxide or potassium phosphotungstate. The stain tends to obliterate the fine detail of particulate material and is generally unsuitable for studies of viral ultrastructure, but it is invaluable for increasing the contrast of ultra-thin sections of infected tissues or cell cultures. Uranyl acetate, on the other hand, is sometimes useful in positive staining of virus suspensions since it stains the nucleic acid of the particle as well as its protein component.

A specialised form of positive staining is used to show that antibodies conjugated to an electron-opaque molecule, such as ferritin, stain the proteins for which they have specificity.

Thin sectioning

A considerable amount of information on viral replication and cytopathology has been obtained in recent years by studying ultra-thin sections of infected material. Tissues, cells or pellets of centrifuged virus are fixed, dehydrated and embedded in a plastic such as methyl methacrylate. Thin sections are cut with an ultratome equipped with a plate glass or diamond knife, mounted on specimen grids and examined in the electron microscope. Sections of infected cells are especially valuable for ascertaining the distribution of virus particles within the cells and for studying viral development.

It is emphasised that the size of a virion will appear greatest in shadowed preparations which usually enhance the contrast at the periphery of the particles. It will be smaller in negatively stained specimens because the stain penetrates the surface contours of the virion, and even smaller in ultra-thin sections of infected cells since the method of cutting the preparations often disrupts the virion. Furthermore, the size of the particle is probably artificially small in all electron micrographs since drying causes considerable shrinkage of the specimens.

Freeze-etching

Attempts are now being made to overcome the disadvantages of fixation and dehydration which causes structural changes in the specimens, by the method known as freeze-etching. In this technique the specimen is supercooled in a drop of water to form a solid block of ice and is placed in an evaporating unit under liquid nitrogen. The nitrogen is removed briefly to produce a sublimation or etching of the iceblock, thereby exposing the surface of the specimen which is then shadowed. The fixation of carbon–platinum replicas of fractured surfaces of the material enables the investigator to observe the ultrastructure of the specimen as it appears in the living condition.

X-ray diffraction

Purified preparations of virus particles that form either crystals (e.g. poliovirus) or paracrystals (e.g. tobacco mosaic virus), lend themselves to structural analysis by means of X-ray diffraction. For X-ray diffraction analysis, a beam of X-rays is directed at a preparation, e.g. a crystal of purified virus, and produces a characteristic diffraction pattern which is recorded on a photographic plate. If the atoms are aligned in an orderly or crystalline pattern then the X-rays will be diffracted in an orderly manner, and from the angle of scattering the atomic arrangement can be deduced. In experienced hands this gives a pattern of a three-dimensional picture of the molecular arrangement of the virus.

The technique was first used to provide evidence that a virion is not an amorphous object and that the protein molecules of the viral coat, the capsid, are regularly assembled around the central nucleic acid molecule in a symmetrical arrangement. These observations were dramatically confirmed when negative staining techniques were first applied to studies of viral ultrastructure.

The chemical composition of viruses

The chemical composition of a virus was first determined by Schlesinger in 1933 who showed that a bacterial virus consisted essentially of protein and deoxyribonucleic acid (DNA). This was followed in 1935 by Stanley's report on the isolation and crystallization of the virus of tobacco mosaic (TMV) which consisted of protein and ribonucleic acid (RNA). Since then, biochemists have studied the chemistry of many other viruses and it is now accepted that all viruses, be they from plants, insects, bacteria or animals, contain only one type of nucleic acid, ribonucleic acid or deoxyribonucleic acid, plus a protective coat of protein. In addition, some viruses may contain lipids, carbohydrates and certain other minor constituents but none contains the growth enzyme systems required for synthesis of nucleic acids and proteins. Although it would be a simple matter to define the constituents of any one virus in terms of carbon, nitrogen, phosphorus, etc., the result would be very much the same as the elementary composition of an average bacterial culture and would show nothing beyond the fact that virus particles are not very dissimilar in their chemical composition from other microorganisms.

The observation that purified crystals of tobacco mosaic virus contained about 95 per cent protein, overshadowed for many years the all important role of the 5 per cent nucleic acid component until it was discovered, in 1952, that it was DNA which infected the bacterial cell during phage replication and initiated the synthesis of progeny virus; whereas most of the protein component of the virus particle remained outside the host cell and played no further part in the infection. Thus, it was clearly shown that it was the nucleic acid component that was responsible for carrying the genetic information of the virus.

The importance of viral nucleic acid in the replicative cycle was further emphasized 4 years later when it was discovered that chemically degraded preparations of tobacco mosaic virus consisting only of RNA were infectious and that the RNA molecule, in the absence of its protein covering, was capable of carrying all the genetical information the host cell required to manufacture new virus. Furthermore, the exposed nucleic acid was stable only for very short periods and was less infective than the normally protected nucleic acid of the intact virion.

As well as having a protective role, the protein coat has surface properties that enable the intact virus to reach and penetrate the susceptible host cell. Also, it is the protein components which alone, or together with other macromolecules, provide the principal antigenic determinants of the virus particle.

Plant viruses contain only RNA and most of them have only one species of structural protein. Bacterial and animal viruses, on the other hand, may contain either DNA or RNA, and many have a few or several different kinds of protein molecules.

The proportions of nucleic acid to protein in the intact virion vary considerably with different viruses. For example, the DNA content of a typical bacteriophage (e.g. the T_2 phage of E. coli) is about 40 per cent of its dried weight compared with that of a DNA animal virus, (e.g. vaccinia) which is only about 6 per cent. The differences are not so great in the case of most RNA viruses and, although a three-fold variation between viruses has been described, the majority of single-stranded RNA viruses contain about the same amount of nucleic acid. The overall chemical composition of the larger animal viruses tends to be more complex and in influenza virus there is, in addition to protein, RNA (1 per cent.), polysaccharides (4–6 per cent), phospholipids (11 per cent), and cholesterol (6 per cent).

Many viruses contain significant amounts of lipids in their structure and in the surrounding envelope, if present. In the case of myxoviruses, whose component parts are assembled at the periphery of the host cell, the envelope materials react with antisera prepared against uninfected cells indicating, therefore, that some of the lipoprotein of the envelope is derived from the host cell. The lipid nature of the envelope enables the virion to be readily disintegrated by organic solvents such as ether, and the susceptibility of these 'lipoviruses' to the action of 20 per cent ethyl–ether is particularly useful in methods of classification. Lipid, when present, varies from about 5 per cent for some poxviruses to 50 per cent for togaviruses.

Myxoviruses and many other animal viruses contain small amounts of carbohydrates in addition to that of their pentose sugars but muramic acid, which is a characteristic component of bacterial cells, rickettsiae and chlamydiae (PLGV agents), is not present in viruses.

Structure of nucleic acids

Genes are composed of a number of long-chain molecules (polymers) called nucleic acids, and the genetic information of all cells (animal, plant and bacterial) and of many viruses is stored in double-stranded DNA. In other viruses, however, it is in the form of single-stranded DNA (phage ØX174), single-stranded RNA (myxoviruses) or, occasionally, double-stranded RNA (reoviruses).

The manner in which this information is passed from the genes is not fully understood but it has been suggested that, following unmasking of the viral nucleic acid within the cell, the viral genome is incorporated with that of the cell as provirus (e.g. bacteriophages) and then replicates with the DNA of the cell to produce infectious progeny virus. A more likely alternative so far as animal viruses are concerned, is that the viral genome replicates independently of the cellular DNA to produce new virus. This is supported by the fact that the production of cellular enzymes is usually halted abruptly following infection and the cell then proceeds to

cytosine and uracil (Fig. 37.2). Thus, DNA differs from RNA in that it contains thymine instead of uracil and its pentose sugar, deoxyribose, lacks one OH (hydroxyl) group compared with ribose, as in RNA (Fig. 37.3). Adenine and guanine are purines whereas cytosine, uracil and thymine are pyrimidines.

The many thousands of adjacent molecules are linked together by phosphate bonds between the $3'$ OH of the ribose (or deoxyribose) of one nucleotide and the $5'$ OH of its neighbour (Fig. 37.4). It has been estimated that there are about 40 000 nucleotides in some viral RNAs, over 500 000 nucleotides in certain DNA viruses and that the bacterial genome is a single DNA molecule with chains of about 10^7 nucleotides.

Following upon the classical theories of the structure of DNA by Watson and Crick, it is now known that the DNA molecule normally consists of

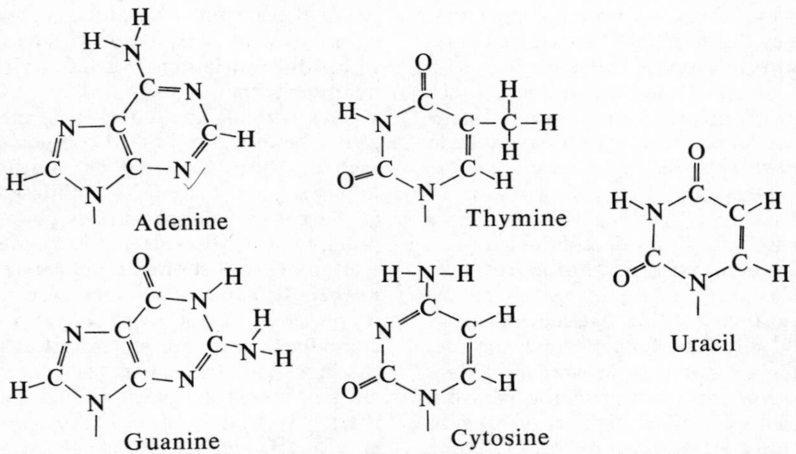

FIG. 37.2. The four bases (adenine, thymine, guanine & cytosine) of DNA. In RNA, uracil replaces thymine.

produce only those enzymes that are necessary for the manufacture of virus particles.

The nucleic acid chain is composed of a string of basic units called nucleotides, each of which is the result of condensation of three components. These are: (1) a nitrogenous base consisting essentially of a ring compound containing nitrogen and carbon, (2) a molecule of a 5-carbon pentose sugar which is either ribose (in RNA) or deoxyribose (in DNA), and (3) a molecule of phosphoric acid residue which links the base to the pentose sugar.

There are four kinds of nucleotides depending on which of the four major nucleic acid bases is contained in each nucleotide. In the DNA molecule the four bases are guanine, adenine, cytosine and thymine, whereas in RNA they are guanine, adenine,

two complementary strands of polynucleotides running in opposite directions (Fig. 37.5). Unlike most threads they are not twisted around one another but are wound together around an imaginary core to form a double spiral or, as it is usually called, a double helix (Fig. 37.6). The ends of a DNA strand can be distinguished by the fact that one has a free $5'$ phosphate while the other has a free $3'$ phosphate. Moreover, the two strands in the DNA molecule are always arranged in such a way that one of them lies in a $5 \rightarrow 3$ direction whereas the other runs $3 \rightarrow 5$ in the opposite direction, thereby forming an antiparallel double helix. Thus, enzyme reactions passing along one of the DNA threads moves either in a $3 \rightarrow 5$ or $5 \rightarrow 3$ direction. The long chemical threads of the double helix are held

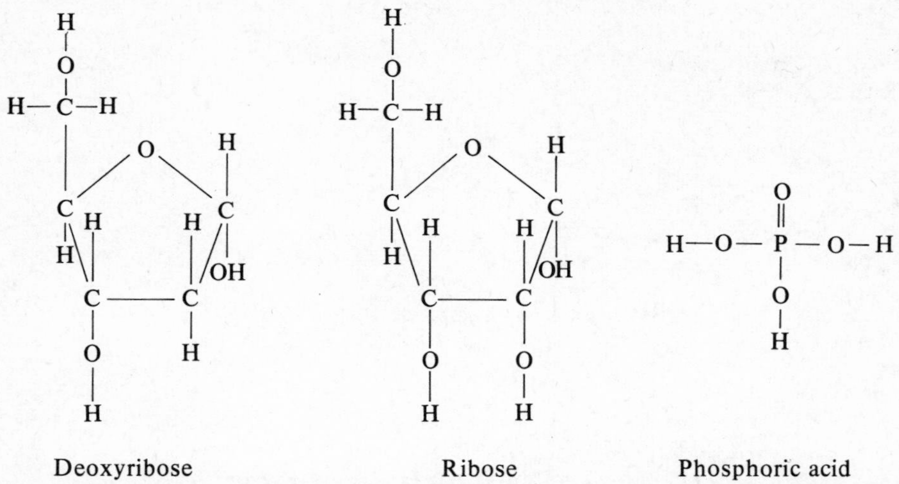

Deoxyribose   Ribose   Phosphoric acid

FIG. 37.3. In DNA, deoxyribose and phosphoric acid form chains to which the bases attach. In RNA, ribose replaces deoxyribose.

together by a regular system of hydrogen bonds linking the bases (guanine to cytosine and adenine to thymine) of pairs of opposite nucleotides. It should be noted, however, that the complementary base pairs adenine and thymine share two hydrogen bonds, while guanine and cytosine share three hydrogen bonds. In the double-stranded DNA molecule the number of guanine units always equals the number of cytosine units, and adenine always equals thymine. Thus, each strand of the double helix bears the molecular component of the other and wherever a thymine is present in one chain then an adenine exists opposite to it in the other chain; similarly guanine is always paired with cytosine. The same relationships apply to double-stranded RNA except that uracil occurs in place of thymine. In virus studies, the ratio of each pair of bases, that is $(A+T)/(G+C)$ may vary from one virus group to another; and is an important feature in virus characterization.

Molecules of RNA generally consist of a single strand of nucleotides that may be folded back on itself so that the bases from one region of the strand join up with the complementary bases from a different region: but there is also evidence that 2 helical strands interwoven in the fashion of the DNA molecule may occasionally occur.

Replication of DNA

The Watson-Crick model of DNA reproduction, called 'semi-conservative', suggests that each strand (i.e. half molecule) of the double helix serves as a template for the manufacture of a new strand. Replication probably occurs by the unravelling of the two original (parent) strands which is followed by the synthesis of a complementary new (daughter) strand — by means of free adenine attaching to an exposed thymine base and guanine to cytosine, on each of the two parent strands, resulting in the formation of two double-stranded molecules. Thus, after one cycle of DNA replication each of the two strands of the double helix is converted into a hybrid molecule, half old (parent) and half new (daughter) (Fig. 37.7).

The replication of linear DNA molecules is thought to begin at one end and is completed at the opposite end. On the other hand, replication in circular molecules begins at some point on its circumference, probably with either adenine or guanine depending on the specific start signal in the DNA template, and proceeds in one direction around the ring until two rings are formed. Each ring consists of one old and one new polynucleotide strand. Synthesis ends upon reaching stop signals, which like start signals, are specific nucleotide sequences (vide infra).

The enzyme requirements for DNA synthesis are not well understood but it is known that although protein synthesis is necessary for initiating replication, it is not required to maintain the process once it has started. In the case of DNA, the replicative form is probably a two-stranded intermediate, each strand of which contains matching amounts of the complementary base pairs, adenine–thymine and guanine–cytosine. It is also possible that this double-stranded replicative form may serve as a template from which many copies of the single-stranded form are peeled off.

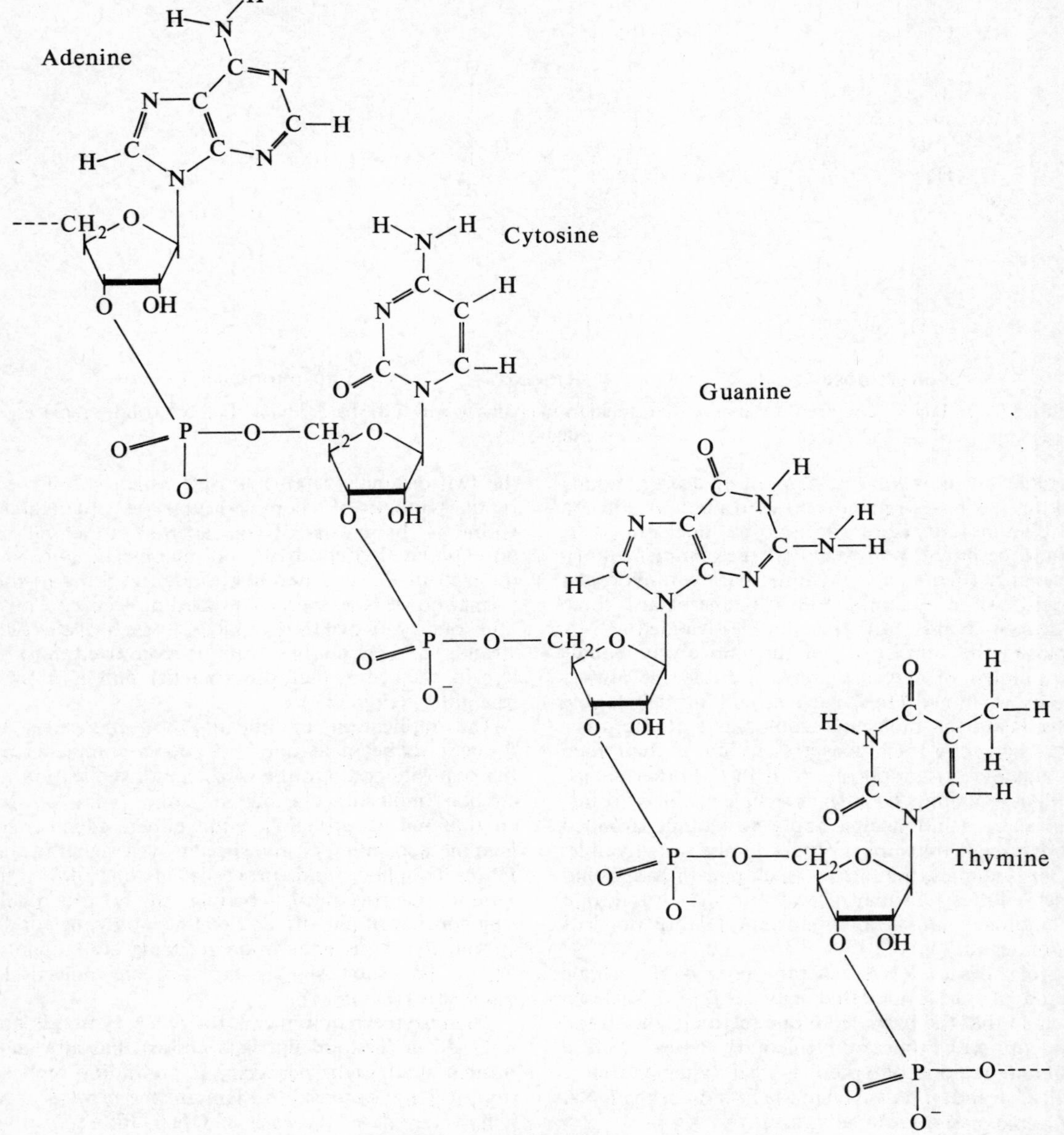

FIG. 37.4. Fragment of chain of deoxyribonucleic acid.

Replication of RNA

The replication of RNA is, in many ways, very similar to that of DNA since it probably occurs by a stepwise extension of the molecule, whereby one unit at a time is attached to the end of the strand.

The mechanisms by which the appropriate bases are inserted in their correct position in the growing nucleotide backbone of RNA are also very similar to those of DNA. In DNA replication, the double strand produces its own information as to the correct

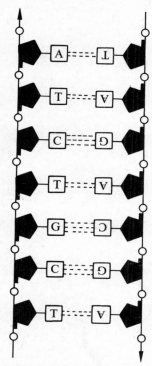

FIG. 37.5. DNA molecule shown in the form of a straight ladder, consisting of a long double chain of nucleotides—(deoxyribose sugar ⬠, attached base ☐ , and phosphate group –O–). Hydrogen bonds (broken lines) link pairs of complementary bases (A + T/C + G) to form the double chain.

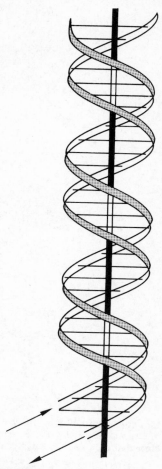

FIG. 37.6. The double helix, showing the arrangement of the anti-parallel strands.

sequence of insertion of its bases whereas in RNA this information is provided by one of the strands of the DNA molecule. In other words, DNA provides its own template whereas RNA must utilise a DNA template. The process illustrated in Fig. 37.7 shows how DNA, by using the base sequence of the old (parental) strands as a guide, forms two double-stranded DNA molecules, each with one old and one new strand. This type of DNA replication, termed semi-conservative, is carried out by an enzyme known as DNA-dependent DNA polymerase. In RNA replication, the base sequence of one DNA strand provides the template for the insertion of the bases in the correct position along the growing chain. In this case adenine is paired with uracil instead of thymine. The enzyme responsible for RNA synthesis is a DNA-dependent RNA polymerase. Where double-stranded RNA is required, the single-stranded RNA molecule which is formed first, usually bends back on itself so that the bases from one region of the strand join up with

the complementary bases from a different region; but without extending over the whole length of the RNA molecule.

Since many viruses contain only one molecule of nucleic acid, the molecular weight is an indication of the amount of information coded in its nucleic acid.

Structure and synthesis of protein

Proteins are large molecules composed of long chains called polypeptides which are assembled from about twenty common kinds of amino acids. Typical amino acids carry an amino ($-NH_2$) and a carboxylic ($-COOH$) group that make the peptide bonds that form the backbone of the polypeptide chains. All amino acids have a common structure except for the attached R-group which represents a side chain that distinguishes one amino acid from another (Fig. 37.8).

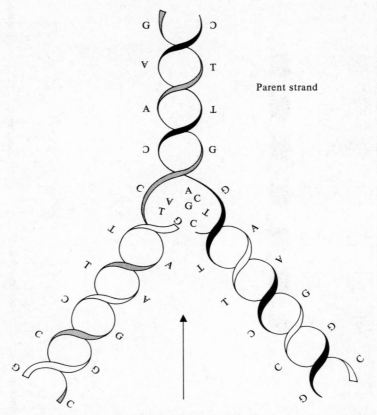

FIG. 37.7. Biosynthesis of DNA. As the vertical double (parental) strand unwinds, synthesis proceeds upwards along the two arms which serve as templates for the synthesis of complementary (daughter) strands. Note that each double daughter strand consists of one new (white) and one old (black) strand.

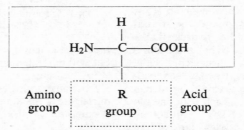

FIG. 37.8. Structure of a typical amino acid.

In the smaller viruses there is probably no other constituent except nucleic acid and protein; the protein being a polypeptide chain of at least 145 amino acids. The structure of any one protein is determined by the sequence of the amino acids in the chains that constitute the protein molecule.

For protein synthesis, the four bases guanine (G), adenine (A), cytosine (C) and uracil (U) code for the twenty major amino acids required to form the protein molecule. It is obvious, however, that the four individual bases cannot determine the order of insertion of at least twenty amino acids into the growing polypeptide chain, but it is now accepted that a sequence of at least three bases (the so-called 'triplets' or RNA 'codons') is the minimum number of nucleotides needed for each amino acid.

If the shortest code-group that represents one particular amino acid is a triplet, this would permit the possibility of 4 × 4 × 4 or 64 different nucleotide combinations. Recent observations have largely confirmed the accuracy of this assumption and not only has the pattern of the genetic code been established, but a catalogue of three-letter code words for the different amino acids has now been devised; with the proviso that most amino acids can be coded for by more than one triplet. In fact, no fewer than sixty-one of the sixty-four available triplets can code for the insertion of individual amino

Synthesis of viral proteins

During the course of virus infection, a variety of proteins are formed as a result of the information contained in the viral genome. These include not only the new proteins (enzymes) that enable the viral nucleic acid to replicate, but also the structural proteins that are incorporated into the new virus particles and assembled to form the capsid. However, not all viral proteins take part in the formation of the capsid and some viruses (e.g. myxoviruses) also

TABLE 37.1. Specification of amino acids by RNA triplets (codons).

2nd base	U	C	A	G	
1st base					3rd base
	Phenylalanine	Serine	Tyrosine	Cysteine	U
U	Phenylalanine	Serine	Tyrosine	Cysteine	C
	Leucine	Serine	*(STOP)	(STOP)	A
	Leucine	Serine	(STOP)	Tryptophan	G
	Leucine	Proline	Histidine	Arginine	U
C	Leucine	Proline	Histidine	Arginine	C
	Leucine	Proline	Glutamine	Arginine	A
	Leucine	Proline	Glutamine	Arginine	G
	Isoleucine	Threonine	Asparagine	Serine	U
A	Isoleucine	Threonine	Asparagine	Serine	C
	Isoleucine	Threonine	Lysine	Arginine	A
	Methionine	Threonine	Lysine	Arginine	G
	Valine	Alanine	Aspartic acid	Glycine	U
G	Valine	Alanine	Aspartic acid	Glycine	C
	Valine	Alanine	Glutamic acid	Glycine	A
	Valine	Alanine	Glutamic acid	Glycine	G

*(STOP) = 'chain termination' (see text).

acids during protein synthesis while the remaining three [UAA, UAG and UGA], which do not code for amino acids, are possibly useful as 'punctuations' for signalling the starting and ending of sequences in a given polypeptide chain. Since most amino acids can be coded for by more than one triplet the genetic code is said to be 'degenerate'. The full list of triplets assigned to each of the twenty amino acids (Table 37.1) shows that three of the amino acids can be specified by any of six different triplets, e.g. leucine by UUA, UUG, CUU, CUC, CUA and CUG. Five amino acids each have four triplets, one has three, nine have two, while two, methionine (AUG) and tryptophan (UGG), are specified by a single triplet only.

The information coding for each protein is carried by a single gene. Viruses may contain upwards of several hundred genes, bacteria about 1000 and a human cell may contain about a million. The human genes are not assembled in one long chain but are divided amongst at least forty-six DNA molecules — the forty-six human chromosomes.

contain haemagglutinins and neuraminidase. In addition, members of the myxovirus, herpesvirus and togavirus groups possess a well-defined lipoprotein envelope.

Protein synthesis is carried out by the small intracellular particles called ribosomes which contain protein as well as RNA — the so-called **ribosomal RNA** (rRNA). The DNA is not directly involved in the synthesis of protein, instead the genetic information of the DNA is first transferred to RNA molecules. The RNA molecules, in turn, serve as the primary templates that order the amino acid sequences in protein synthesis. The template RNA, which acts as the essential intermediary in this process, carries the genetic message from the DNA molecules to the cellular sites of protein synthesis (ribosomes) and is termed **messenger RNA** (mRNA). The transfer of genetic information from DNA to this template is called 'transcription'. When RNA is being formed on the DNA template through the action of the enzyme DNA-dependent RNA polymerase, uracil is taken up on the RNA chain wherever adenine appears at the complementary site on the DNA chain (Fig. 37.9). After the strand of mRNA leaves the nucleus it attaches itself to the cytoplasmic ribosomes where its message (in the form of sequences of bases) is read, and on which it directs the synthesis of amino acids — the building blocks for protein. Most mRNA molecules are long enough to embrace five or more ribosomes. The transfer of information from mRNA to protein involves a change from a 'language' with four letters (the nucleotides) to one with twenty letters (the amino acids), and is called 'translation'. The amino acids are transported, in turn, to their proper position in the protein chain by means of yet another form of RNA called **transfer RNA** (tRNA).

Architecture of viral particles

Viruses are unique in that they are small obligatory intracellular parasites that do not grow on synthetic media and do not multiply by binary fission. They have only one kind of nucleic acid in their genome, RNA or DNA, which may in either case be single-stranded or double-stranded. The complete virus

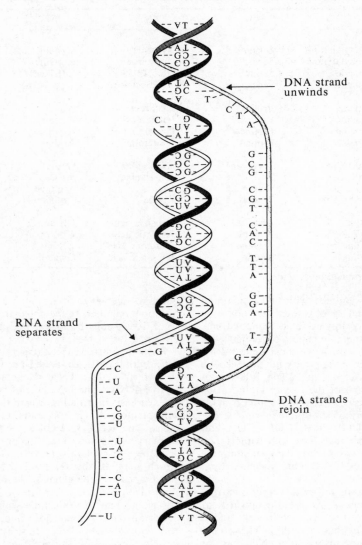

FIG. 37.9. Messenger RNA (mRNA) transcription. The new mRNA thread is a complementary copy of one of the DNA strands, with uracil (U) replacing thymine (T).

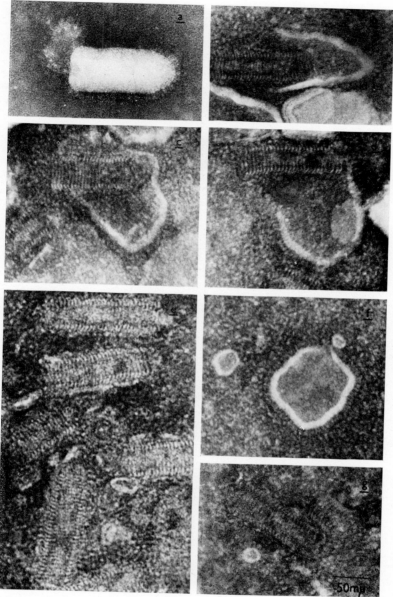

37.1 Uncoating of rhabdovirus (vesicular stomatitis virus) with Tween-ether, showing the internal regular coil of ribonucleoprotein. Bar represents 50 nm. (Courtesy of Dr F. Brown and Mr C. J. Smale.)

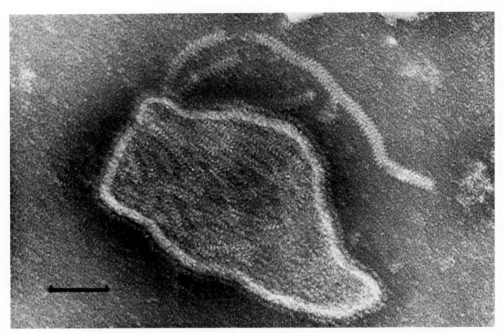

37.2 Electron micrograph of a Newcastle disease virus particle negatively stained with phosphotungstic acid. Notice the 'herring-bone' structure of the nucleocapsid strands, one of which can be seen escaping through a small break in the envelope of the virion. The fringe of evenly spaced 'spikes' lining the surface of the envelope is also visible. Bar represents 100 nm.

particle, or virion, can be regarded as consisting of a central core of genetic material, the nucleic acid, surrounded by a protective outer covering of protein. Some virions may also contain lipids and carbohydrates but all lack the enzyme systems and other constituents that are essential for growth and multiplication.

Viruses range in size between the largest molecules and the smaller bacteria, and ultracentrifugation and electron microscopic studies suggest that the greatest dimensions lie between 18 and 300 nm. Thus, the largest viruses, (e.g. poxviruses) are similar in size to the rickettsia–chlamydia group of organisms and are just visible with the ordinary light microscope, whilst the smallest viruses (e.g. adeno-satellite viruses and the coliphage ØX174) measuring about 20 nm are only slightly larger than the molecule of haemoglobin.

The size of virus particles was first estimated by filtration through Elford collodion membranes and, more recently, by the much more accurate methods of ultracentrifugation and electron microscopy. Electron microscopy has the additional advantage that it provides information about the shape of the virion and, in many instances, about the structure of the virus particle itself, especially when negative staining methods are used.

Structural features of viruses

In 1956, Crick and Watson postulated that the simplest form of a virion would be represented by nucleic acid protected by protein in the form of identical repeating subunits packed in a regular arrangement. Experimental support for this hypothesis was provided by X-ray crystallography studies which showed the presence of repetitive features in the structure of those viruses that can be crystallised. The findings also suggested that the subunits of a virus particle would be arranged symmetrically and that the symmetry would be one of two types, helical or cubic (isometric). Shortly afterwards, the application of negative staining techniques in electron microscopy not only confirmed the subunit theory of viruses but showed pictorially that viruses once thought to be spherical were, in fact, of cubic symmetry and particles described as rod - shaped had helically arranged subunits.

Chemical analysis and X-ray diffraction studies together with the high resolution provided by the negative staining method have revealed that one of the simplest forms of virus, that of tobacco mosaic virus, is a long, hollow, rigid rod-shaped structure composed of a single spiral of RNA surrounded by regular closely-packed protein subunits called capsomeres. The rod has a diameter of about 18 nm, and its minimal infective length is about 300 nm. The RNA strand lies in a groove between the protein

structural units of which there are about seventeen on each turn of the spiral. The rows of protein monomers (capsomeres) make up the protein coat (capsid) which closely surrounds the nucleic acid to form the nucleocapsid. Thus, the tobacco mosaic virus consists of a hollow cylinder surrounded by a spiral structure and, since its nucleocapsid is not invested by an outer coat or envelope, it is described as a naked virion showing helical (spiral) symmetry

Apart from tobacco mosaic virus there are other RNA viruses with helical symmetry and some are enveloped. The group of enveloped RNA helical viruses, or compound helical RNA viruses as they are sometimes termed, includes several important animal pathogens such as fowl plague, Newcastle disease, distemper, rinderpest, vesicular stomatitis and rabies viruses. The envelope of compound helical RNA viruses usually contains lipids, carbohydrates and antigenically specific proteins some of which have enzymic activity. The main components of the envelope are of viral origin but some normal host components may also be incorporated in its structure since the envelope is frequently formed from the cell surface. The membranous envelope is not rigid and the virion may show a regular or highly pleomorphic outline. Changes in osmolarity during the drying of specimens for electron microscopy frequently produce changes in the envelope and cause it to assume a bizarre tadpole-like shape. Within the envelope of most species of compound helical RNA viruses lies the hollow nucleocapsid which is flexible, unlike the rigid rods of tobacco mosaic virus, and forms a tight regular coil, (e.g. rhabdoviruses) (Plate 37.1 facing page 402) or a loose irregular pattern as in paramyxoviruses. Electron micrographs of disrupted compound helical RNA viruses frequently show strands of nucleocapsids lying outwith the envelope. Direct measurement of these 'herring-bone' structures is of value since the diameter of the nucleocapsid of members of the orthomyxovirus group, e.g. fowl plague virus, is about 9 nm compared with that of 12–14 nm for metamyxoviruses (e.g. respiratory syncytial virus) and 18 nm for Newcastle disease virus and other paramyxoviruses viruses (Plate 37.2, facing p. 403).

In myxoviruses and certain other animal viruses, the membranous envelope is covered with numerous spikes clearly visible with negative staining as a row of projections 10 nm long and about 8 nm apart. In many instances, the envelope contains two biologically active fractions responsible for the haemagglutinating and neuraminidase activities of the virus. The haemagglutinins of myxoviruses appear as triangular prisms forming a fringe of projections on the surface of the envelope, whereas the neuraminidase components are mallet or mushroom shaped and are mostly located between the haemagglutinin spikes. Very little is known about the molecular organisation of the envelope and, until recently, there was little evidence that it conformed to the requirements of a virus structure with identical repeating subunits. However, electron micrographs of the envelope of fowl plague and influenza C viruses have revealed an arrangement of hexagonal subunits each one of which is surrounded by either five or six others. If this finding is confirmed it would suggest that at least some orthomyxoviruses have two components; first the nucleic acid which has helically arranged protein around it and, second, the envelope (or what is really a capsid) consisting of protein units arranged as hexamers or pentamers. It would also mean a change in terminology from cubic and helical viruses to cubic and pleomorphic viruses.

Many RNA and DNA animal viruses do not possess helical symmetry and these include most of the species that were previously known as the 'spherical viruses'. Early studies with a method of metal shadowing from two angles showed that preparations of *Tipula* iridescent virus or adenoviruses produced two types of shadow that could only be caused by a particle having a hexagonal outline with 20 equilateral triangular faces, i.e. an icosahedron.

Since then, many other hexagonal viruses have been studied and, because of the similarity of their morphology, have been described as 'cubic viruses' or viruses with cubic symmetry. The more recent application of negative staining to virus particles has revealed other details of their structure due to the ability of the phosphotungstic acid to penetrate even the finest contours of their surface. Many viruses appear to be faceted and each facet forms an equilateral triangle consisting of a regular arrangement of protein subunits or capsomeres. There are generally 20 equilateral triangular faces and a particle is, therefore, an icosahedron. In adenoviruses, each side of an equilateral face consists of six hollow spheres (capsomeres) linked to each other by divalent bonds. A model of an icosahedron having a side of six subunits can be built from 252 polystyrene spheres to give the appearance of a typical adenovirus (Plate 55.1c, facing p. 726). The majority of the protein subunits of the adenovirus virion, the 240 capsomeres, are termed hexons because each is surrounded by six adjacent capsomeres. The remaining 12 capsomeres are called pentons since they have only five neighbouring subunits. Electron micrographs of mature adenovirus virions taken at high resolving powers have shown that there are 12 additional smaller subunits one of which is attached by a thin straight fibre to each of the 12 pentons which are located at each corner of the icosahedron. Herpesviruses have a similar morphology to that of adenoviruses except that they are usually enveloped and their capsomeres have a distinctly hollow core and are hexagonal or pentagonal in outline. (Plate 37.3, facing p. 430).

The total number of capsomeres in any virion can be calculated from the formula $10 (N-1)^2+2$, where N is the number of capsomeres on one edge of any facet. Thus, a herpesvirus which has only five capsomeres along each axis has 162 capsomeres in all; while reoviruses with only four capsomeres along each face have 92 capsomeres. The bacteriophage, ØX174, with only two capsomeres along the side of each triangle has only 12 capsomeres in all but there are, nevertheless, 20 facets and its symmetry is still that of an icosahedron. The triangular facets of the icosahedron can be subdivided further into a number of smaller equilateral triangles. Thus, viruses showing icosahedral symmetry can be grouped according to the triangulation number or T-value; and the total number of capsomeres expressed by the simple formula $10T+2$. For example, the T-value for a herpesvirus is 16, therefore the capsid consists of $10 \times 16+2=162$ capsomers, and adenovirus with a T-value of 25 has 252 capsomeres.

As we have seen, the capsids of viruses with cubic symmetry generally consist of clusters of morphological units called capsomeres. The capsomeres, in turn, are composed of chemical subunits called structural units. Because of this, it has been suggested recently, that the helical ribonucleoprotein of the myxovirus is a misnomer and that the protein units should be termed 'structure units' and not capsomeres because they appear to be the chemical subunits of the virus.

One type of cubic symmetry, as shown by the icosahedron, is termed 5:3:2 because there are five-fold, three-fold and two-fold axes of symmetry, drawn through its centre. Axes through the corners are five-fold axes of rotational symmetry because every time the icosahedron is rotated around this axis, by one-fifth of a turn, it gives rise to an identical figure. The three-fold axes of symmetry are located in the centre of each triangular face while the two-fold axes are situated in the middle of any one edge of a triangle (Fig. 37.10).

Viruses showing cubic symmetry may or may not be enclosed in a protective membranous envelope. Electron micrographs of herpesvirus preparations frequently show enveloped and non-enveloped virions. Usually the envelope contains only a single virion but occasionally two or three particles may be present. Both mature and immature particles can occur, the latter being identified by their dark 'empty' central core (procapsids) due to the accumulation of the PTA stain in the absence of the DNA material. Adenoviruses and many other icosahedral viruses do not possess an envelope.

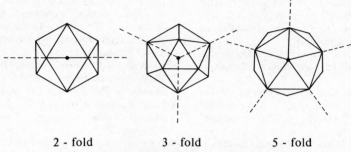

2 - fold   3 - fold   5 - fold

FIG. 37.10. Axes of symmetry for a regular icosahedron.

Reovirus capsids are naked icosahedrons consisting of 92 prismatic hollow capsomeres. In a few instances, an inner protein coat may be observed lying between the outer capsid and the central core of RNA. Togaviruses, on the other hand, possess a closely adherent outer envelope covered with fine projections and an inner capsid which appears to have icosahedral symmetry and surface capsomeres.

Most animal viruses show either helical symmetry or cubic symmetry but poxviruses are exceptional and their ultrastructure appears to be complex. Some poxviruses are brick-shaped (Plate 37.4a, facing p. 431), while others are ovoid and the DNA is contained in a nucleoid, shaped like a biconcave disc, and is surrounded by one or more membranes. Negative staining shows that the virion contains a surface layer of hollow tube-like fibrils which may give the particles a striated appearance. In some species of poxviruses, e.g. 'orf', the thread appears to be continuous and is arranged in a criss-cross or figure-of-eight pattern across the surface of the virion giving it the characteristic 'ball of wool' appearance (Plate 37.4b, facing p. 431).

The architecture of bacterial viruses is more complex and sophisticated than any of the viruses so far considered. The large bacteriophages, e.g. the even-numbered coliphages, which consist of a polygonal head and cylindrical tail, are said to have binal symmetry since they show both icosahedral and helical symmetry within the same virion. A further account of the structure of bacterial viruses is given in Chapter 39.

Details of the ultrastructure of animal viruses are of some importance since they form a useful part of most modern methods of classifying the viruses.

Further reading

BURNET F.M. AND STANLEY W.N. (1959). *The Viruses*: Vol. 1, *General virology*; Vol. 3, *Animal viruses*. London: Academic Press.

CRAMER R. (1964) Purification of animal viruses. In, *Techniques in Experimental Virology*, Ed. R.J.C. Harris, p. 146. London: Academic Press.

CRICK F.H.C. (1954) The structure of the hereditary material. *Scientific American*, **191**, 54.

CRICK F.H.C. (1962) The genetic code. *Scientific American*, **207**, 67.

DOANE F.W., ANDERSON N., ZBITNEW A. AND RHODES A.J. (1969) Application of electron microscopy to the diagnosis of virus infections. *Canadian Medical Association Journal*, **100**, 1043.

FINCH J.T. AND HOLMES K.C. (1967) Structural studies of viruses. In, *Methods in Virology*, Eds. K. Maramorosch and H. Koprowski, Vol. 3, p. 351. New York: Academic Press.

GAREN A. (1968) Sense and nonsense in the genetic code. *Science*, **160**, 149.

HAYNES R.H. AND HANAWALT P.C. (1968) *The Molecular Basis of Life: an introduction to molecular biology*. Folkestone: W.H. Freeman.

HORNE R.W. (1961) In, *Techniques for Electron Microscopy*, Ed. D. Kay, p. 150. Oxford: Blackwell Scientific Publications.

HORNE R.W. (1963) The structure of viruses. *Scientific American*, **208**, 48.

HORNE R.W. (1967) Electron microscopy of isolated virus particles and their components. In, *Methods in Virology*, Ed. K. Maramorosch and H. Koprowski, Vol. 3, p. 521. New York: Academic Press.

HORNE R.W. AND WILDY P. (1963) Virus structure revealed by negative staining. *Advances in Virus Research*, **10**, 101.

HSIUNG G.D. (1965) Use of ultracentrifugation for animal virus grouping. *Bacteriological Reviews*, **29**, 477.

KNIGHT C.A. (1954) The chemical constitution of viruses. *Advances in Virus Research*, **2**, 153.

LWOFF A. (1957) The concept of virus. *Journal of General Microbiology*, **17**, 239.

MERCER E.H. AND BIRBECK M.S.C. (1966) *Electron Microscopy: A Handbook for Biologists*, 2nd Edition. Oxford: Blackwell Scientific Publications.

The Nature of Viruses (1957) Ciba Foundation Symposium. London: Churchill.

NUNN R.E. (1970) *Electron Microscopy: Microtomy, staining and specialized techniques*. London: Butterworth.

PARSONS D.F. (1964) Electron microscopy of viruses in cells and tissues. In, *Techniques in Experimental Virology*, Ed. R.J.C. Harris, p. 381. London: Academic Press.

RICHMOND M.H. (1971) I. Macromolecules in micro-organisms, p. 11. II. Biosynthesis in micro-organisms, p. 37. In, *Micro-organisms — function, form and environment*, Eds. L.E. Hawker and A.H. Linton. London: Edward Arnold.

SMITH W., GRAY E.W. AND MACKAY J.M.K. (1968) A sandwich-embedding technique for monolayers of cells cultured on araldite. *Journal of Microscopy*, **89**, 359.

SPRADBROW P.B. AND FRANCIS D. (1969) Electron microscopy as an aid to the rapid identification of animal viruses. *Veterinary Record*, **84**, 244.

VALENTINE R.C. (1961) Contrast enhancement in the electron microscopy of viruses. *Advances in Virus Research*, **8**, 287.

WATERSON A.P. (1964) Ultrastructural studies. In, *Techniques in Experimental Virology*, Ed. R.J.C. Harris, p. 359. London: Academic Press.

WILDY P. AND HORNE R.W. (1963) Structure of animal virus particles. *Progress in Medical Virology*, **5**, 1.

WILDY P. AND WATSON D.H. (1962) Electron microscopic studies on the architecture of animal viruses. *Cold Spring Harbour Symposia on Quantitative Biology*, **27**, 25.

WILLIAMS R.C. AND WYCKOFF R.W.G. (1946) Applications of metallic shadow-casting to microscopy. *Journal of Applied Physiology*, **17**, 23.

CHAPTER 38

THE CLASSIFICATION OF ANIMAL VIRUSES

Since this text went to press, the International Committee on the Taxonomy of Viruses (ICTV) has published a listing of officially approved and common names of virus groups (Fenner, F., 1976, *J. gen. Virol.*, **31**, 463). For the convenience of the reader, a summary of the current position regarding viral families and genera is given below:

Approved family and generic names	Names used in the present text
Family: Orthomyxoviridae	Orthomyxovirus group
Genus: Influenzavirus (influenza types A and B virus)	Influenza A and B viruses
Probable genus: (no name approved) Influenza type C virus	Influenza C virus
Family: Paramyxoviridae	Paramyxovirus group
Genera: Paramyxovirus (Newcastle disease virus group)	Paramyxovirus
Morbillivirus (measles virus group)	Pseudomyxovirus
Pneumovirus (respiratory syncytial virus group)	Metamyxovirus
Family: Rhabdoviridae	Rabiesvirus group
Genera: Vesiculovirus (vesicular stomatitis virus group)	Vesicular stomatitis virus group
Lyssavirus (rabies virus group)	Rabies virus group
Probable genera: (no names approved)	
Exemplified by sigma and ephemeral fever viruses	other rabiesviruses
Family: Coronaviridae	Coronavirus group
Genus: Coronavirus (may be subdivided later)	Coronavirus
Family: Retroviridae	Leukovirus group
Subfamilies: Oncovirinae (RNA tumour virus group)	Leukovirus (oncornavirus)
Spumavirinae (foamy agents)	unclassified RNA viruses
Lentivirinae (visna and related agents)	Slow virus group
Family: Picornaviridae	Picornavirus group
Genera: Enterovirus	Enterovirus
Rhinovirus	Rhinovirus
Possible genus: Calicivirus	Calicivirus
Family: Reoviridae	Diplornavirus group
Genera: Reovirus	Reovirus
Orbivirus	Orbivirus
Probable genus: (no name approved)	Rotavirus (Duovirus)
Family: Togaviridae	Togavirus group
	Arthropod-borne togaviruses
Genera: Alphavirus (group A arboviruses)	Alphavirus
Flavivirus (group B arboviruses)	Flavivirus
	Non-arthropod-borne togaviruses
Pestivirus (hog cholera and related viruses)	Swine fever virus group
Rubivirus (rubella virus)	Rubella virus group
Family: Bunyaviridae (formerly Bunyamwera Supergroup)	Bunyamwera supergroup of viruses
Genus: Bunyavirus	group C arboviruses and others
Family: Arenaviridae	Arenavirus group
Genus: Arenavirus	Arenavirus
Family: Poxviridae	Poxvirus group
Genera: Orthopoxvirus (vaccinia and related viruses)	Orthopoxvirus
Avipoxvirus (fowlpox and related viruses)	Avipoxvirus
Capripoxvirus (sheep pox and related viruses)	Capripoxvirus
Leporipoxvirus (myxoma and related viruses)	Leporipoxvirus
Parapoxvirus (milkers' node and related viruses)	Parapoxvirus
	Molluscovirus
Entomopoxvirus (poxviruses of insects)	Entomopoxvirus
Family: Parvoviridae	Parvovirus (picodnavirus) group
Genera: Parvovirus	Parvovirus (sub-group A)
Densovirus (viruses of insects)	
Other genus: (no name approved)	
Adeno-associated virus group	Parvovirus (sub-group B)
Family: Papovaviridae	Papovavirus group
Genera: Papillomavirus	Papovavirus-A (papillomavirus)
Polyomavirus	Papovavirus-B (polyomavirus)
Family: Adenoviridae	Adenovirus group
Genera: Mastadenovirus (adenoviruses of mammals)	Adenovirus
Aviadenovirus (adenoviruses of birds)	
Family: Herpetoviridae	Herpesvirus group
Genus: Herpesvirus (herpes simplex and related viruses)	Herpesvirus sub-group A
Probable genera: (no names approved)	Herpesvirus sub-group B and others
Family: Iridoviridae	Iridovirus group
Genus: Iridovirus (iridescent viruses of insects)	Iridovirus
Other probable genera: African swine fever virus and other cytoplasmic icosahedral DNA viruses of vertebrates may belong to the same family but not to the genus *Iridovirus*	

The classification of animal viruses

The early systems proposed for the classification of animal viruses were based on their tissue specificity, host susceptibility or on the clinical and pathological changes they produced; but all have proved unsuitable for a variety of reasons. Attempts to introduce a classification based on the Linnean binomial nomenclature, as used for bacteria, have also been abandoned but some Latinised names whereby each generic name is followed by the suffix 'virus' are still in common usage, e.g. *Poxvirus variolae* (smallpox virus), and *Herpesvirus suis* (Aujeszky's disease virus).

At the present time, most of the viruses isolated from vertebrates have been separated into some fifteen or sixteen major groups and a number of subgroups according to their physical and chemical properties, and this has proved most useful. The names given to these groups are: Orthomyxovirus, Paramyxovirus and Pseudomyxovirus, Rhabdovirus, Coronavirus, Leukovirus (Oncornavirus), Picornavirus, Diplornavirus (Reovirus and Orbivirus), Togavirus, Arenavirus, Poxvirus, Parvovirus (Picodnavirus), Papovavirus, Adenovirus, Herpesvirus and Iridovirus. The following are the principal features of these viruses.

Properties of the major groups of RNA viruses

Orthomyxovirus (Gr. *myxa*, slime, mucus).
Orthomyxoviruses derive their name from the affinity they possess for the mucus and other mucoprotein substances present in the respiratory tract and elsewhere. Members of the group are medium-sized, ether-sensitive, acid labile, single-stranded RNA viruses (80–120 nm in diameter) having helical symmetry and an envelope surrounding the nucleocapsid. The virion matures at or near the margin of the cell membrane and the surface of the virus particle is invested with numerous short, sharp-pointed projections. Most contain haemagglutinin and neuraminidase and are capable of haemadsorb-

ing red blood cells. They possess a type or subgroup antigen associated with the nucleocapsid.

Paramyxovirus
Members of the paramyxovirus group are morphologically similar to but slightly larger (100–250 nm) than the orthomyxoviruses. The diameter of the ribonucleoprotein helix (nucleocapsid) is 18 nm compared with 6–9 nm for orthomyxoviruses while the molecular weight of its RNA is at least twice as great (4–8×10^6 daltons compared with 1.5–6×10^6 daltons). Unlike the orthomyxoviruses, the paramyxoviruses are resistant to the action of actinomycin D. They may also produce a soluble haemolysin, are more active in cell cultures and frequently produce intracytoplasmic inclusions and, sometimes, multiple intranuclear bodies. Genetic recombination does not occur with paramyxoviruses and nuclear involvement is not a feature of their multiplication.

Pseudomyxovirus
These large compound helical RNA viruses include the antigenically related measles-rinderpest-distemper triad of viruses. They are structurally similar to the myxoviruses and paramyxoviruses but differ from them in that they do not possess the enzyme neuraminidase. Some of these viruses (e.g. measles) haemagglutinate red blood cells while others do not.

Rhabdovirus (Gr. *rhabdos*, rod).
These are also enveloped helical single-stranded RNA viruses but their morphology is sufficiently distinctive to merit their inclusion in a separate group. The type species is vesicular stomatitis virus. The virions which are formed by budding at plasma or cytoplasmic membranes are characteristically bullet-shaped or bacilliform and measure about 60×225 nm but the length is very variable. There are numerous surface projections and some members haemagglutinate red blood cells. There is no common group antigen but antigenic relationships exist between some members.

Coronavirus

Avian infectious bronchitis virus, murine hepatitis virus, haemagglutinating encephalomyelitis virus of swine, transmissible gastroenteritis virus of swine and certain human respiratory viruses have a fringe of widely spaced pear-shaped bulbous projections resembling a crown, hence the suggested name of this 'new' group of ether-sensitive, single-stranded RNA viruses. The symmetry of coronaviruses has not been determined but may be helical. The virions are spherical in shape and measure 80–160 nm in diameter. Avian infectious bronchitis virus is antigenically different from the other members of the group and it possesses a haemagglutinin. Growth of coronaviruses takes place in the cytoplasm and maturation is by budding into cytoplasmic vesicles.

Leukovirus (Oncornavirus)

This term refers to leukaemia viruses of avian, murine, feline and other animal species but does not include human leukaemia since a causal agent has not yet been identified in the disease in man. Most members are spherical or enveloped single-stranded RNA viruses, about 50–100 nm in diameter, and some at least show helical symmetry. They are ether-sensitive, heat and acid labile and sensitive to actinomycin D. The molecule of RNA is approximately 1.3×10^7 daltons. Leukoviruses mature by budding from cytoplasmic membranes.

Picornavirus

These are very small (18–40 nm) spherical ether-resistant single-stranded viruses showing icosahedral symmetry. The group name, Picornavirus, is derived from **Pico** which means 'very small' and **RNA** indicates the nucleic acid composition. It includes three major subgroups:

(1) the enteroviruses, e.g. poliomyelitis, Coxsackie, Teschen/Talfan and, possibly, swine vesicular disease viruses,

(2) the many types of rhinoviruses causing human colds, and a number of unassigned members including the viruses of foot-and-mouth disease and infectious avian encephalomyelitis (epidemic tremor), and

(3) the caliciviruses which include vesicular exanthema virus of swine. The virions are non-enveloped and the capsid is composed of either 60 or 180 identical protein subunits (triangulation numbers T1 and T3, respectively.). In contrast to other picornaviruses, members of the enterovirus group are acid resistant. Acid lability varies with the species and molar $MgCl_2$ protects many but not all picornaviruses against inactivation by heat. There is no group antigen. Virus synthesis and maturation occur in the cytoplasm with occasional formation of crystalline arrays of particles.

Diplornavirus

This new group of double-stranded RNA viruses includes two genera, Reovirus and Orbivirus. The name reovirus was derived from 'Respiratory Enteric Orphan' since the viruses occur widely in the respiratory and enteric tracts of man and animals. They are small, (60–75 nm in diameter), non-enveloped, ether- and acid-resistant cubic viruses. The capsid is generally twin-layered with 92 or 180 hollow capsomeres on the outer shell. The nucleic acid core of RNA is unusual in that it is composed of double-stranded molecules with the high total molecular weight of $10–15 \times 10^6$ daltons. Multiplication is intracytoplasmic with the formation of characteristic perinuclear inclusions, sometimes containing virus particles in crystalline arrays.

Orbiviruses are also cubic, double-stranded RNA viruses with icosahedral symmetry, but the capsid is single-layered having only 32 capsomeres, although some particles may show a diffuse outer layer composed of 92 capsomeres. The mature virion has a diameter of 54–64 nm. Orbiviruses resist lipid solvents and, unlike reoviruses, are markedly labile at pH 3.0.

A third morphologically distinct genus has recently been described, and has provisionally been named Rotavirus.

Togavirus (L. toga, cloak).

The group of **AR**thropod-**BO**rne viruses (arboviruses), recently designated togaviruses (*Family Togaviridae*), contains over 150 members most of which multiply in some arthropod host (e.g. insects, mites or ticks). They are small spherical enveloped viruses, (40–60 nm, sometimes larger), with a high but single-stranded RNA content. Little is known of their structure but, from the present limited knowledge, most of the virions show cubic symmetry while others may be helical. The molecular weight is $3–4 \times 10^6$ daltons. They are all ether-sensitive and acid-labile and most have an haemagglutinin which agglutinates the erythrocytes of newly-hatched chicks or geese. Haemagglutinating strains show radially arranged spikes passing through the envelope, whereas those devoid of haemagglutinating activity have a smooth surface to their envelope. Two genera have been proposed: the subgroup A or alphaviruses which are insensitive to trypsin and the subgroup B or flaviviruses which are sensitive to trypsin. Non-arthropod-borne togaviruses (e.g. swine fever) have also been described.

Arenavirus (L. arenosus, sandy)

Members of the recently formed arenavirus group are round, oval or pleomorphic virions, 50–150 nm in diameter. The surrounding envelope contains closely packed surface projections while the interior of the capsid appears unstructured and contains a number of electron-dense granules 20–30 nm in diameter. The virus particle probably contains RNA, but its strandedness and molecular weight have not yet been determined. It is ether-sensitive, grows in the cytoplasm of the host cell and matures by budding from the marginal membranes. All strains of arenavirus, e.g. lymphocytic choriomeningitis virus (LCM), share a group specific antigen.

Properties of the major groups of DNA viruses

Poxvirus

Poxviruses are large (170 × 300 nm), double-stranded DNA viruses that replicate wholly within the cytoplasm of the cell and produce well-defined eosinophilic cytoplasmic inclusions. The capsid symmetry is complex but most virions are brick-shaped or ovoid, and possess a central core, lateral bodies and outer envelope. Characteristic surface patterns are seen in negatively stained preparations and some particles, e.g. orf, show a definite crossed helical pattern. Although the nucleocapsid is enveloped, most members are resistant to ether but a few, e.g. the Neethling strain of lumpy skin disease, are partly or highly ether-sensitive. The molecular weight of poxvirus DNA is unusually high, being about $150–160 \times 10^6$ daltons. All members exhibit non-genetic reactivation and most can recombine genetically. There is a common group antigen.

Characteristically, poxviruses infect epithelial cells in which they produce papules, vesicles and pustules (pock formation).

Parvovirus (Picodnavirus)

The parvovirus or picodnavirus group consists of very small (pico), naked, cubic DNA viruses. Most members, e.g. feline panleukopenia virus have single-stranded DNA but in others such as adeno-associated (satellite) viruses the single strands are complementary and come together *in vitro* to form a double strand. It is interesting to note that the associated or adeno-satellite virus are defective and require an adeno 'helper-virus' to replicate. The capsid of the parvovirus is small (18–24 nm), shows icosahedral symmetry and has 32 capsomeres of about 2–4 nm in diameter. Multiplication takes place within the nucleus of the host cell.

Papovavirus

Members of the papovavirus group include the papilloma-polyoma and vacuolating viruses. They are naked, cubic, ether-resistant and acid-stable DNA viruses. They are characterised by having their DNA molecules in circular form with a molecular weight of $3·2–5·0 \times 10^6$. The capsid is between 40–55 nm in diameter and is made up of 72 (or 42) capsomeres in a skew arrangement. Some members, e.g. polyoma and SV40, have oncogenic properties especially in species other than their normal habitat, and some haemagglutinate. Multiplication and assembly occur in the nucleus. There is no common group antigen.

Adenovirus

The name of this group was first given to previously unidentified viruses isolated from a latent infection of the adenoid tissues of man. They are medium-sized (70–90 nm), naked, ether- and acid-resistant, cubic, double-stranded DNA viruses (molecular weight $20–25 \times 10^6$). The capsid contains 252 capsomeres, each 7 nm in diameter, of which 240 are hexons and 12 are pentons. Each penton base carries a thin, fibre-like structure with a small terminal 'knob'. Most adenoviruses possess a common group specific (hexon) antigen as well as type specific (penton and fibre) antigens. Mammalian strains have a common group antigen. Several members haemagglutinate red blood cells and some have oncogenic properties under certain experimental conditions. All adenoviruses multiply and mature within the nucleus but the process is inefficient and only 10 per cent of the viral DNA and protein is incorporated into virions. The rest remains unassembled and produces intranuclear inclusions.

Herpesvirus (Gr. *herpes*, to creep).

These are all ether-sensitive and acid-labile, double-stranded, DNA viruses (molecular weight $50–100 \times 10^6$). The capsid has cubic symmetry with 162 prismatic hollow capsomeres (150 are hexagonal and 12 are pentagonal). The nucleocapsid is formed within the nucleus where it produces typical Cowdry type A inclusions and acquires an envelope as it buds through the membrane to the perinuclear space. The enveloped virion measures between 150–200 nm in diameter but smaller (100–110 nm), naked virions are also frequently present. In some cases, e.g. Aujeszky's disease virus, active herpesvirus is readily released from infected cells whilst in others, e.g. Marek's disease virus, the virus is strongly cell-associated. After primary infection some herpesviruses can persist in a latent form for the lifespan of the host. There is no common group antigen.

Iridovirus

The type species of the recently proposed Iridovirus group is *Tipula* iridescent virus, and some possible members include lymphocystis virus of fish and African swine fever virus.

The icosahedral virion is 130 nm in diameter and the capsid shell consists of about 812 protein subunits; but others with as many as 1500 capsomeres have been described. The virus particle contains a single molecule of double-stranded DNA having a molecular weight of about 130×10^6 daltons. Although the type species and other members of the group appear to be devoid of lipids some possible members are believed to have a lipid-containing envelope.

A comprehensive list of viruses belonging to the major groups of RNA and DNA viruses is given in Table 38.1.

Because of the rapid advances in knowledge of virus properties any system of virus classification is subject to continuous modification. A simple scheme which is probably acceptable at the present time is outlined in Tables 38.2 and 3, and is based on such characteristics as the nature of the viral nucleic acid, the type of capsid symmetry, the presence or absence of a membrane or envelope, the number and shape of the capsomeres, the size of the virus particle, its acid stability and ether susceptibility. Unfortunately, there is insufficient information about the properties of other viruses causing diseases of domestic animals to justify their inclusion in this present system of classification.

Some diseases of animals, birds and fish caused by or frequently associated with viruses, rickettsiae or chlamydiae are shown in Tables 38·4–10.

TABLE 38.1. Members of the major groups of viruses.

RNA-CONTAINING VIRUSES

ORTHOMYXOVIRUS GROUP
Influenza virus A
Human influenza virus A (AO), A1, A2 (Asian)
Swine influenza virus
Equine influenza virus (Equi-1, Equi-2)
Avian influenza virus
Fowl plague virus (Classical; and England/63)
Tern virus (and Smith/Scotland/59 virus)
Virus N (Dinter)
Duck influenza virus (Duck/England; Duck/Czechoslovakia)
Influenza virus B (B, B1, B2, B3 Taiwan)
Influenza virus C

METAMYXOVIRUS GROUP (proposed)
Respiratory syncytial virus (RSV)
Pneumonia virus of mice (PVM)

PARAMYXOVIRUS GROUP
Newcastle disease virus (NDV)
Mumps virus
Yucaipa virus of chicks
Turkey virus, Canada/58
Parainfluenza type 1 (Sendai, Haemadsorption virus-2 (HA2), or Haemagglutinating virus of Japan (HVJ))
Parainfluenza type 2 (Croup-associated (CA) virus, avian strain, simian SV5, etc.)
Parainfluenza type 3 (Haemadsorption virus-l; bovine SF4)
Parainfluenza type 4 (2 subtypes)
Parainfluenza types 5–7 (SV 41)

PSEUDOMYXOVIRUS GROUP (unofficial)
Measles virus
Rinderpest virus
Distemper virus

RHABDOVIRUS GROUP
(a) Vesicular stomatitis and other bullet-shaped viruses
Vesicular stomatitis virus (Indiana; New Jersey)
Cocal virus of fruit flies
Flanders and Hart-Park viruses of mosquitoes and birds
Kern canyon virus of bats
Egtved virus (rainbow trout haemorrhagic septicaemia)
Sigma virus of fruit flies
Lagos bat virus
Mount Elgon bat virus

(?) Bovine ephemeral fever virus
(?) Marburg monkey virus
Infectious haematopoietic necrosis (IHN)
Spring viraemia of carp (SVC)
(b) Rabies virus

CORONAVIRUS GROUP (CORONAVIRIDAE)
Avian infectious bronchitis virus (IBV)
Human coronavirus (HCV)
Murine hepatitis virus (MHV)
Transmissible gastroenteritis virus of swine (TGEV)
Haemagglutinating encephalomyelitis virus of swine (HEV)
Rat coronavirus (RCV)
Sialodacryoadenitis virus of rats (SDAV)
Turkey bluecomb disease virus (TBDV)
Neonatal calf diarrhoea coronavirus (NCDCV)

LEUKOVIRUS GROUP

Subgroup A (Avian types)
Rous sarcoma virus (3 subgroups)
Rous-associated viruses (RAV types 1–6)
'Resistance inducing factors' (RIF-1, 2)
Avian leukosis virus strain RPL 12
Fujinami sarcoma viruses
Fujinami-associated virus (FAV1)
Avian leukosis virus, visceral (2 or more subgroups)
Avian leukosis virus, erythroblastic
Avian leukosis virus, myeloblastic
Osteopetrosis virus

Subgroup B (Murine types).
Leukaemia viruses (of Gross; Friend; Graffi; Moloney; Rauscher and others)
Sarcoma viruses (of Harvey; Moloney)

Subgroup C (Feline types)
Feline leukaemia virus (of Jarrett; Rickard; Kawakami)
Feline sarcoma virus

Subgroup D
Bittner's mouse mammary tumour virus (MTV)
Mouse nodule-inducing virus

Others
Bovine, canine, cavian and (??) human leukaemia viruses.

Candidate members
Visna-maedi viruses of sheep
Progressive pneumonia and Zwoegerziekte viruses of sheep
Bovine syncytial virus
Foamy agent.

PICORNAVIRUS GROUP

Enterovirus
Poliovirus (Types 1 Brunhilde; 2 Lansing; 3 Leon)
Coxsackie virus A (Types 1–23, 24)
Coxsackie virus B (Types 1–6)
Swine vesicular disease virus
Echo viruses (Types 1–9, 11–27, 29–34)
Simian enteroviruses (SV2 and many other SV types)
Bovine enteroviruses (2 subgroups; 63 or more serotypes)
Feline enteroviruses (2 or more serotypes)
Avian enteroviruses (15 or more serotypes)
Porcine enteroviruses (30 or more serotypes)
    e.g. Teschen disease group
        Subtype 1 Konratice; Bozen; Reporyje
        Subtype 2 Talfan; Tyrol
Murine encephalomyocarditis virus (EMC) e.g. Col-Sk, MM and Mengo strains
Avian encephalomyelitis virus (AEV)
Murine encephalomyelitis virus (T.O., F.A., GD VII and MHG)
Duck hepatitis virus
(?) Acute bee paralysis virus

Rhinovirus
Human rhinoviruses (100 or more types)
Equine rhinoviruses (Types 1 and 2)
Bovine rhinoviruses (3 serologically related strains)
Foot-and-mouth disease virus (7 serotypes; 65 or more subtypes)
            O (11 subtypes)
            A (32 subtypes)
            C (5 subtypes)
    SAT –1 (7 subtypes)
    SAT –2 (3 subtypes)
    SAT –3 (4 subtypes)
    Asia –1 (3 subtypes)

Calicivirus
  Vesicular exanthema virus (13 serotypes)
  Feline picornavirus (several serotypes)

DIPLORNAVIRUS GROUP (REOVIRIDAE)

Viruses from man, horses, cattle, sheep, pigs, kangaroos, birds, mice and other vertebrate hosts
Viruses from invertebrate, bacterial, plant and fungal hosts

Genus reovirus
  Serotypes 1, 2 and 3 (ubiquitous in vertebrates)
  Avian reoviruses (5 serotypes)

Genus rotavirus (proposed)
  acute gastroenteritis virus of children
  acute diarrhoea virus of newborn calves

Genus orbivirus (proposed)
  Bluetongue virus of ruminants (12 serotypes)
  Epizootic haemorrhagic disease virus of deer
  African horsesickness virus (9 serotypes)
  Colorado tick fever virus of man
  Epizootic mouse diarrhoea virus
  Infectious pancreatic necrosis virus (IPNV) of trout
  (?) Equine encephalosis virus
Many candidate members including:
  Blue-comb virus of poultry
  Gumboro disease virus of poultry (Infectious bursal agent)

TOGAVIRUS GROUP

Arthropod-borne togaviruses
  Alphavirus (Arbovirus group A)
    Eastern equine encephalitis virus
    Western equine encephalitis virus
    Venezuelan equine encephalitis virus
    Semliki forest virus
    Sindbis virus
    O'Nyong-nyong virus
    15 other named viruses
  Flavivirus (Arbovirus group B)
    Yellow fever virus
    Dengue viruses (4 types)
    St. Louis group of viruses
      St. Louis encephalitis virus
      Japanese B encephalitis virus
      Murray valley encephalitis virus
      West Nile fever virus
      Ilheus virus
    Tick-borne encephalitis group of viruses
      Russian spring-summer encephalitis virus
      Far-Eastern encephalitis virus
      Central European encephalitis virus
      Omsk haemorrhagic fever (2 types)
      Langat virus
      Powassan virus
      Louping ill virus
      Kyasanur Forest disease virus
      2 or more named viruses
    Other flaviviruses
      Wesselsbron virus
      Spondweni virus
      Israel turkey meningoencephalitis virus
      14 other named viruses

Bunyamwera supergroup (?Hylovirus)
Includes arbovirus group C and two other mosquito-borne arbovirus groups; together with 5 other smaller groups. Numerous named members have been assigned to these groups.

Unassigned arboviruses (? togaviruses)
   Rift valley fever virus
   Nairobi sheep disease virus
   and others

Non-arthropod-borne (nonarbo-) *togaviruses*
   (?) Rubella (german measles) virus of man
   Equine arteritis virus
   Bovine viral diarrhoea-mucosal disease virus
   (?) Border disease virus of lambs
   Swine fever (hog cholera) virus
   Lactic dehydrogenase (LDH) virus of mice

ARENAVIRUS GROUP
Lymphocytic choriomengitis (LCM) virus and at least 10 other named members.
? Lassa fever virus

DNA-CONTAINING VIRUSES

POXVIRUS GROUP (POXVIRIDAE)

Subgroup 1 Orthopoxvirus
   Vaccinia virus
   Variola major (smallpox) virus
   Variola minor (alastrim) virus
   Cowpox virus
   Monkeypox virus
   Rabbitpox virus
   Mousepox (ectromelia) virus

Subgroup 2 Parapoxvirus
   Orf (contagious pustular dermatitis) virus
   Bovine papular stomatitis/dermatitis virus
   Milker's nodule (paravaccinia) virus

Subgroup 3 Avipoxvirus
   Fowlpox virus
   Pigeon pox virus
   Canary pox virus
   Starling pox virus
   Turkey pox virus
   Sparrow pox virus
   Junco pox virus

Subgroup 4 Leporipoxvirus
   California myxoma virus
   Myxoma (myxomatosis) virus of rabbits
   Rabbit fibroma (Shope) virus
   Squirrel fibroma virus
   Hare fibroma virus

Subgroup 5 Capripoxvirus
   Sheep pox virus
   Goat pox virus
   Lumpy skin disease (Neethling) virus
   ? Swine pox virus
   ? Horse pox virus
   ? Camel pox virus
   ? Buffalo pox virus
   ? Rhinoceros pox virus

Subgroup 6 Unclassified
Molluscum contagiosum virus of man
Yaba monkey tumour virus

PARVOVIRUS GROUP (Picodnavirus)

Subgroup A
Kilham's latent rat virus
Other rodent viruses (e.g. H, H1, H3, X14)
Minute virus of mice
Minute virus of dogs
Porcine parvovirus
Bovine picodnavirus
Bacteriophages øX174 and S13

Subgroup B
Adeno-associated (satellite) viruses (4 types)

Possible members
Avian parvovirus
Feline panleucopaenia virus
Mink enteritis virus
Haemorrhagic encephalopathy virus of rats
HADEN virus of cattle
Other animal parvoviruses

PAPOVAVIRUS GROUP (PAPOVAVIRIDAE)

Genus Papovavirus A
Type 1 Human papilloma (wart virus)
Type 2 Shope rabbit papilloma virus
Type 3 Bovine papilloma virus
Type 4 Canine papilloma virus
Type 5 Hamster papilloma virus
Probably other viruses causing papillomas of horses, sheep, goats, monkeys and other species.

Genus Papovavirus B
Type 1 Polyoma virus
Type 2 Simian vacuolating virus (SV40)
Type 3 Murine K-papovavirus
Type 4 Rabbit kidney vacuolating virus (RKV)
Type 5 BK virus from human urine after renal transplantation
Type 6 JC virus from progressive multifocal leucoencephalopathy patients.

ADENOVIRUS GROUP

Human adenoviruses (32 serotypes)
Simian adenoviruses (20 or more serotypes)
Bovine adenoviruses (possibly 9 or more serotypes)
Porcine adenoviruses (3 or more serotypes)
Murine adenoviruses
Other mammalian adenoviruses, e.g. of sheep, horse, opossum
Kennel cough adenovirus
Infectious canine hepatitis (Rubarth) virus
Avian adenoviruses (GAL; CELO)
Quail bronchitis virus

HERPESVIRUS GROUP

Subgroup A
Herpes simplex virus (human) (2 or more serotypes)
B virus (Old world monkey)
M (Marmoset) virus (New world monkey)
Pseudorabies (Aujeszky's disease) virus

Equine rhinopneumonitis (mare abortion) virus (Equine virus type-1)
Equine LK herpesvirus type-2
Equine herpesvirus type-3
Infectious bovine rhinotracheitis virus (Infectious pustular vulvovaginitis virus)
Infectious bovine keratoconjunctivitis virus
Canine herpesvirus
Bovine ulcerative mammillitis (Allerton) virus
Calf tracheitis virus
Feline rhinotracheitis virus
Avian infectious laryngotracheitis virus (ILT)
Avian herpesviruses affecting pigeons, owls, parrots and cormorants.
Virus III of rabbits (*Herpesvirus cuniculi*)

Subgroup B
Varicella (varicella/zoster) virus of chickenpox/shingles
Cytomegaloviruses (mostly host-specific, affecting man and many other mammalian species), e.g. Cytomegalic inclusion disease of man
Porcine inclusion body rhinitis virus
Liverpool vervet monkey virus
Salivary gland virus of guinea-pigs and mice

Other members
Malignant catarrhal fever virus of ruminants
Viruses associated with renal carcinoma of leopard frog (Lucké)
Epstein-Barr (EB) virus of Burkitt lymphoma and infectious mononucleosis
Marek's disease (fowl paralysis) virus
Jaagsiekte (sheep pulmonary adenomatosis) virus
Duck plague virus (Duck virus enteritis)
Mouse thymic virus
Snake herpesvirus
? Foal kidney virus
? Australian coital exanthema of horses
? Fish pox or hyperplastic epidermal disease

IRIDOVIRUS GROUP
Tipula iridescent virus of crane fly
Possible members include:
Gecko virus
Amphibian cytoplasmic viruses
Lymphocystis virus of fish
African swine fever virus

VIRUSES NOT YET ADEQUATELY STUDIED

Viruses of man
Rubella (German measles) (? Nonarbo togavirus)
Infectious hepatitis virus
Serum hepatitis virus
Multiple sclerosis (? viral aetiology)
Kuru (Slow or CHINA virus)
Marburg virus (? Rhabdovirus)

Viruses of ungulates
Peste de petits ruminants (? Pseudomyxovirus)
Borna disease (horses, cattle and sheep) (Unclassified RNA)
Near East equine encephalomyelitis
Nigerian equine encephalitis
Equine infectious anaemia (Swamp fever) Unclassified RNA)
Scrapie of sheep and goats (Slow ? virus)
Ephemeral fever of cattle (? Rhabdovirus)
Sweating sickness of cattle (? viral aetiology)
Bovine syncytial virus (? leukovirus)
Grass sickness of horses (? viral aetiology)
Picodna virus of swine (Cartwright's 59e/63 strain)
Border disease of lambs (? Nonarbo-togavirus)

Viruses of other vertebrates
    Mink encephalopathy (? slow virus)
    Plasmacytosis of mink (Aleutian disease) (Slow virus)
    Gumboro disease virus (? orbivirus plus satellite virus)
    Blue-comb disease (? orbivirus)
    Turkey hepatitis
    Simian foamy virus (? leukovirus)
    Various simian viruses
    Feline syncytial virus (? leukovirus)
    Feline infectious peritonitis agent (? RNA virus)
    Guinea-pig paralysis agent.

TABLE 38.2 A classification of the major groups of RNA viruses

Capsid symmetry	Capsid naked or enveloped	Reaction to Ether	Reaction to Acid	Number of capsomeres	Diameter (nm) of Helix	Diameter (nm) of Virion	Morphology	
	Naked					15–30 × 300		
Helical	Enveloped	Sensitive	Labile		6–9	80–120		1
					12–15	100–200 >		
					18	100–250 >		
					18	100–200		2
					18	70 × 180 or longer		3
					?	80–160		4
					?	50–100		5
Cubic	Naked	Resistant	Stable	60 or 180 i.e.		(18)–30		6
			Labile	60 × 1 or 60 × 3 subunits		20–30		
			Labile at low pH			35–40		7
		Resistant	Stable	92 (180)		60–75		8
			?	92 (180)		60–66		
			Very labile	32 (92)		(53)–68–(80)		10
Mostly cubic	Mostly enveloped	Sensitive	Labile	32		30–90		
						45–55		
						45–75		
						60–75–(100)		1
						27–70–(100)		
Not known	Enveloped	Sensitive	Labile	?		50–150		1

Special features	Virus group		Representative members
ø Mol. wt. 2.1×10^6	All known naked helical RNA viruses are plant viruses		Tobacco mosaic (TMV) Potato 'X'
Mol. wt. 2.5×10^6 Sensitive to actinomycin D	ORTHOMYXOVIRUS	1	Influenza viruses: human, porcine, equine and avian (e.g. fowl plague)
Mol. wt. $4-8 \times 10^6$	*METAMYXOVIRUS	2	Pneumonia virus of mice Respiratory syncytial virus
Mol. wt. 7.0×10^6 Insensitive to actinomycin D Haemolysins	PARAMYXOVIRUS	2	Newcastle disease Mumps Parainfluenza types 1–4
Lack neuraminidase	*PSEUDOMYXOVIRUS	2	Measles/rinderpest/distemper
Bullet-shaped or bacilliform or conical Mol. wt. $2-5 \times 10^6$	RHABDOVIRUS	3	Vesicular stomatitis Rabies ? Marburg disease ? Bovine ephemeral fever
Corona of pear-shaped projections Mol. wt. not known	CORONAVIRUS	4	Avian infectious bronchitis TGE of swine HEV of swine Mouse hepatitis
Mol. wt. $10-13 \times 10^6$ Reverse transcriptase activity Sensitive to actinomycin D Symmetry not fully established A, B and C-type particles	LEUKOVIRUS Subgroup A (avian types) Subgroup B (murine types) Subgroup C (feline types) Subgroup D Others	5	Avian leukosis Rous sarcoma Leukaemia viruses (e.g. Gross) Sarcoma viruses (e.g. Harvey) Leukaemia and sarcoma Bittner mouse mammary tumour ? Visna-maedi complex ? Bovine syncytial virus
Mol. wt. 2.5×10^6 Stabilized by 1M $MgCl_2$	PICORNAVIRUS ENTEROVIRUS	6	Poliomyelitis, Coxsackie Swine vesicular disease ECHO, Teschen group Duck hepatitis
Mol. wt. $2.4-2.8 \times 10^6$	RHINOVIRUS	6	Human, equine, bovine strains Foot-and-mouth disease
Mol. wt. 2.0×10^6 Cup-shaped capsomeres	CALICIVIRUS	7	Vesicular exanthema Feline 'picornaviruses'
Double-stranded RNA Mol. wt. $10-15 \times 10^6$ Two distinct coats One distinct coat	*DIPLORNAVIRUS REOVIRUS *ROTAVIRUS *ORBIVIRUS	8 9 10	Many human and animal types Acute calf diarrhoea Bluetongue African horsesickness
Mol. wt. $3-4 \times 10^6$ Insensitive to trypsin Sensitive to trypsin Mostly non-haemagglutinating	TOGAVIRUS Arthropod-borne Alphavirus Flavivirus Bunyamwera Unassigned Non-arthropod-borne	11	Equine encephalitides Yellow fever, louping-ill Ilesha, Batai Rift Valley fever Nairobi sheep disease Mucosal disease Swine fever
Mol. wt. 3.2×10^6	ARENAVIRUS	12	Lymphocytic choriomeningitis

ø= Molecular weight of nucleic acid   *= Proposed names

TABLE 38.3. A classification of the major groups of DNA viruses

Capsid symmetry	Capsid naked or enveloped	Reaction to Ether	Reaction to Acid	Number of Capsomeres	Diameter of virion (nm)	Morphology	
Complex	Enveloped (with complex coats)	Most are ether resistant	Labile	—	170–250 × 300–325		13
							14
				(12) or 32	18–24		15
	Naked	Resistant	Stable	72	40–55		16
				252	70–90		17
Cubic	Enveloped	Sensitive	Labile	162	150–200 (enveloped) or 100–110 (naked)		18
	Mostly naked	Mostly resistant	?	about 1500	130		19

Special features	Virus group		Representative members
Mol. wt. of poxvirus DNA (all groups) = $150-160 \times 10^6$	POXVIRUS 1. ORTHOPOXVIRUS	13	Variola (smallpox), vaccinia Cowpox, rabbitpox Mousepox (ectromelia)
Group 2 No growth on eggs 'ball of wool' morphology	2. PARAPOXVIRUS	14	Orf (CPD) Bovine papular stomatitis Milker's nodule
	3. AVIPOXVIRUS 4. LEPORIPOXVIRUS		Fowlpox, pigeon pox Myxomavirus of rabbits Shope's rabbit fibroma
Group 5 Some are ether sensitive	5. CAPRIPOXVIRUS		Sheeppox, goatpox Lumpy skin disease (Neethling)
Group 6 No growth on eggs	6. (?MOLLUSCOVIRUS)		Molluscum contagiosum
Single-stranded DNA Mol. wt. $1 \cdot 2 - 1 \cdot 8 \times 10^6$	PARVOVIRUS (PICODNAVIRUS)	15	Kilham latent rat virus Feline panleukopenia virus Mink enteritis virus Minute virus of mice Other animal parvoviruses Adeno-associated viruses
DNA molecules in circular form Mol. wt. $3 \cdot 2 - 5 \cdot 0 \times 10^6$	PAPOVAVIRUS PAPILLOMAVIRUS POLYOMAVIRUS	16	Human wart & animal papillomas e.g. Shope's rabbit papilloma Polyomavirus Simian vacuolating virus (SV40) Murine K virus
Mol. wt. $20-25 \times 10^6$	ADENOVIRUS	17	Infectious canine hepatitis Multiple human & animal types Avian GAL, CELO Quail bronchitis virus
Mol. wt. $50-100 \times 10^6$ *Subgroup A* Virus readily released from infected cells	HERPESVIRUS Subgroup A	18	*Herpes simplex* virus *Herpesvirus simiae* (B virus) Pseudorabies (Aujeszky's) virus Infectious laryngotracheitis and other avian herpesviruses Equine rhinopneumonitis Infect. bovine rhinotracheitis Bovine mammillitis (Allerton) Canine herpesvirus
Subgroup B virus strongly cell associated	Subgroup B		Varicella/zoster Cytomegaloviruses of man and animals Marek's disease of poultry Burkitt's lymphoma (EB virus)
Mol. wt. c. 130×10^6 Some possible members have a lipid-containing envelope, e.g. ASF	IRIDOVIRUS	19	*Tipula* iridescent virus ? African swine fever (ASF) ? Lymphocystis virus of fish

TABLE 38.4. Rickettsial, chlamydial and viral diseases of vertebrate animals

Species of Host	Name of disease	Major group of organisms causing or frequently associated with the clinical condition
Cattle	Bovine encephalomyelitis and certain other syndromes	*Chlamydia pecoris* and other PLGV agents
	Heartwater	*Cowdria ruminantium*
	Ondiri disease (or Bovine petechial fever)	?*Ehrlichia spp.*
	*Q-fever	*Coxiella burnetii*
	Tick-borne fever	*Cytoecetes bovis*
	Bluetongue	Diplornavirus (Orbivirus)
	Borna disease	Unclassified RNA virus
	Bovine leukaemia	Leukovirus
	Bovine ulcerative mammillitis	Herpesvirus
	Bovine papular stomatitis	Poxvirus
	Calf diarrhoea, acute	Diplornavirus (Rotavirus)
	Calf diarrhoea, neonatal	Coronavirus
	Calf tracheitis	Herpesvirus
	Coital vesicular exanthema (or Infectious pustular vulvovaginitis)	Herpesvirus
	*Cowpox	Poxvirus
	Encephalomyocarditis	Picornavirus
	Ephemeral fever	?Rhabdovirus
	*Foot-and-mouth disease	Rhinovirus (Picornavirus)
	Inapparent infections	Bovine syncytial virus (? Leukovirus) HADEN virus (? parvovirus)
	Infectious bovine keratoconjunctivitis	Herpesvirus (some forms associated with PLGV)
	Infectious bovine rhinotracheitis	Herpesvirus
	Infertility	Parainfluenza (Paramyxovirus) Enterovirus (ECBO) (Picornavirus)
	*Louping-ill	Flavivirus (Togavirus)
	Lumpy skin disease (Allerton)	Herpesvirus
	Lumpy skin disease (Neethling)	Poxvirus
	Malignant catarrhal fever	Herpesvirus
	*Milker's node (paravaccinia)	Poxvirus
	Mucosal disease complex (Virus diarrhoea of cattle) (Pneumo-enteritis of calves)	Unclassified RNA (?nonarbo togavirus)
	?*Pseudorabies (Aujeszky)	Herpesvirus
	*Rabies	Rhabdovirus
	Respiratory infections	PLGV, paramyxovirus, reovirus, rhinovirus, adenovirus, herpesvirus
	*Rift Valley fever	Togavirus (?Hylovirus)
	Rinderpest	Pseudomyxovirus
	Transit fever (Shipping fever)	Myxovirus (Parainfluenza)
	*Vesicular stomatitis	Rhabdovirus
	Warts	Papillomavirus (Papovavirus)
	*Wesselsbron	Flavivirus (Togavirus)

* = transmissible to man

TABLE 38.5.   Rickettsial, chlamydial and viral diseases of vertebrate animals

Species of Host	Name of Disease	Major group of organisms causing or frequently associated with the clinical condition
Sheep Goats	?*Enzootic abortion of ewes	*Chlamydia* (PLGV)
	Heartwater	*Cowdria ruminantium*
	Pneumonitis, polyarthritis (stiff-lamb disease)	*Chlamydia species*
	*Q-fever	*Coxiella burnetii*
	Tick-borne fever	*Cytoecetes phagocytophilia*
	Balano-prosthitis	Unclassified
	Bluetongue	Diplornavirus (Orbivirus)
	Border disease of lambs	? Nonarbo-togavirus
	Borna disease	Unclassified RNA virus
	*Contagious pustular dermatitis (or Orf)	Poxvirus
	*Foot-and-mouth disease	Rhinovirus (Picornavirus)
	Goat papillomatosis	Papillomavirus (Papovavirus)
	?*Goatpox	Poxvirus
	*Louping-ill	Flavivirus (Togavirus)
	Malignant catarrhal fever	Herpesvirus
	Nairobi sheep disease	?Togavirus (Unclassified arbovirus)
	Pneumonia	Parainfluenza, adenovirus, reovirus, rhinovirus, Chlamydia
	Progressive preumonia	(see Visna-maedi)
	?*Pseudorabies (Aujeszky)	Herpesvirus
	*Rabies	Rhabdovirus
	*Rift Valley fever	Togavirus (?Hylovirus)
	†Rinderpest	Pseudomyxovirus
	*Russian Spring-Summer encephalitis	Flavivirus (Togavirus)
	Sheeppox	Poxvirus
	Visna-Maedi complex	Unclassified 'slow' virus (? Leukovirus)
	*Wesselsbron	Flavivirus (Togavirus)
	Pulmonary adenomatosis (Jaagsiekte)	?Virus (?Herpesvirus)
	Rida	?Virus (?"slow" virus)
	Scrapie	?Virus (?"slow" virus)
	Zwoegerziekte	(see Visna-maedi)

*transmissible to man.
†including peste des petits ruminants.

TABLE 38.6. Rickettsial, chlamydial and viral diseases of vertebrate animals

Species of Host	Name of Disease	Major group of organisms causing or frequently associated with the clinical condition
Horses	African horse sickness	Diplornavirus (Reovirus) (Orbivirus)
	Australian coital exanthema	Herpesvirus
	Borna disease	Unclassified RNA virus
	Coital exanthema	Unclassified (?Herpesvirus)
	*Eastern, Western and Venezuelan encephalitis	Alphavirus (Togavirus)
	?*Equine infectious anaemia (or Swamp fever)	Unclassified, ?RNA virus
	Equine influenza	Orthomyxovirus
	Equine papillomatosis	Papovavirus
	Foal kidney virus	Herpesvirus (inapparent infection)
	*Horsepox	Poxvirus or another unclassified poxvirus
	Infectious equine arteritis (or Infectious arteritis or Pink-eye)	Unclassified, RNA virus (? nonarbo togavirus)
	Infectious rhino-pneumonitis (or Equine abortion or Mare abortion)	Herpesvirus
	*Japanese B. encephalitis	Flavivirus (Togavirus)
	Nigerian horse "staggers"	Unclassified
	Periodic ophthalmia	Paramyxovirus
	Pharyngitis of horses	Rhinovirus (Picornavirus)
	*Rabies	Rhabdovirus
	*Vesicular stomatitis	Rhabdovirus
	*Wesselsbron	Flavivirus (Togavirus)
	Hepatitis in horses (Equine serum hepatitis)	?Virus
	Virus diarrhoea	Unclassified

*transmissible to man.

TABLE 38.7. Rickettsial, chlamydial and viral diseases of vertebrate animals

Species of Host	Name of Disease	Major group of organisms causing or frequently associated with the clinical condition
Swine	African swine fever	?Iridovirus
	Encephalitis and pneumonia	?Cytomegalovirus (Herpesvirus)
	*Foot-and-mouth disease	Rhinovirus (Picornavirus)
	Genital papilloma	Papillomavirus (Papovavirus)
	Inclusion body rhinitis and Atrophic rhinitis	Cytomegalovirus (Herpesvirus)
	*Japanese encephalitis	Flavivirus (Togavirus)
	Pig encephalomyelitis	Coronavirus
	Pig leukaemia	Leukovirus
	Porcine encephalomyelitis (Teschen or Talfan disease)	Enterovirus (Picornavirus)
	?*Pseudorabies (Aujeszky's disease)	Herpesvirus
	*Rabies	Rhabdovirus
	Rinderpest	Pseudomyxovirus
	Swine fever (Hog cholera)	Unclassified, RNA virus (nonarbo togavirus?)
	Swine influenza	Orthomyxovirus
	Swine pox	Poxvirus and other unclassified poxviruses
	*Swine vesicular disease	Enterovirus (Picornavirus)
	Transmissible gastroenteritis (TGE)	Coronavirus
	Vesicular exanthema	Calicivirus (Picornavirus)
	*Vesicular stomatitis	Rhabdovirus
	Viral enteritis	Adenoviruses, reoviruses and enteroviruses (T80, V13, etc.)
	Vomiting and wasting disease	Coronavirus (HEV)
	*Wesselsbron	Flavivirus (Togavirus)

*transmissible to man.

TABLE 38.8. Rickettsial, chlamydial and viral diseases of vertebrate animals

Species of Host	Name of Disease	Major group of organisms causing or frequently associated with the clinical condition
Dogs	Rickettsiosis (Dog typhus)	*Ehrlichia canis*
	Salmon poisoning in dogs	Neorickettsia (*N. helminthoeca*)
	Canine laryngotracheitis	Unclassified (?Adenovirus)
	Contagious rhino-tonsillitis	Unclassified (?Adenovirus)
	Contagious venereal dog sarcoma	?Viral origin
	Distemper	Pseudomyxovirus
	Fading puppy syndrome	Herpesvirus
	Infectious canine hepatitis (Rubarth's disease)	Adenovirus
	*Louping-ill	Flavivirus (Togavirus)
	*Lymphocytic choriomeningitis infection	Arenavirus
	"Minute-virus" infection of dogs	Parvovirus
	Papilloma and oral papilloma	Papillomavirus (Papovavirus)
	?*Pseudorabies (Aujeszky)	Herpesvirus
	*Rabies	Rhabdovirus
Cats	Feline conjunctivitis	?Picornavirus
	Feline pneumonitis	*Chlamydia* (PLGV)
	Feline panleucopenia	Parvovirus
	Feline leukaemia	Leukovirus
	Feline rhinoconjunctivitis	?Picornavirus (?Calicivirus)
	Feline infectious peritonitis	?Parvovirus
	Feline stomatitis	?Picornavirus
	Feline viral rhinotracheitis	Herpesvirus
	*Rabies	Rhabdovirus
	Inapparent infection	KCD (Kitten-cell-degenerating virus)

*transmissible to man.

TABLE 38.9. Rickettsial, chlamydial and viral diseases of vertebrate animals

Species of Host	Name of Disease	Major group of organisms causing or frequently associated with the clinical condition
Birds	*Psittacosis and ornithosis	*Chlamydia psittaci*
		Chlamydia ornithosis
	Avian encephalomyelitis (or Epidemic tremor)	Enterovirus (Picornavirus)
	Avian leucosis — sarcoma complex	Leukovirus
	Blue-comb disease	?Diplornavirus (? Orbivirus)
	Cormorant virus disease	Herpesvirus
	Duck hepatitis	Enterovirus (Picornavirus)
	Duck influenza (sinusitis)	Orthomyxovirus
	Duck plague (duck enteritis)	Herpesvirus
	Fowl plague	Orthomyxovirus
	Fowlpox (pigeon pox, canary pox, turkey pox, etc.)	Poxvirus
	Gumboro disease	?Diplornavirus
	Hepatitis of turkeys	Unclassified (?enterovirus)
	Inclusion disease of owls	Herpesvirus
	Inclusion disease of pigeons	Herpesvirus
	Infectious avian nephrosis	See Gumboro disease
	Infectious bronchitis	Coronavirus
	Infectious bursal disease	See Gumboro disease
	Infectious laryngotracheitis	Herpesvirus
	Israel turkey encephalitis	Flavivirus (Togavirus)
	*Japanese B. encephalitis	Flavivirus (Togavirus)
	Marek's disease	Herpesvirus
	*Murray Valley encephalitis	Flavivirus (Togavirus)
	*Newcastle disease	Paramyxovirus
	Pacheco's disease of parrots	Herpesvirus
	Puffinosis	Unclassified
	Quail bronchitis virus	Adenovirus
	*Rabies	Rhabdovirus
	*St. Louis encephalitis	Flavivirus (Togavirus)
	Tern virus influenza	Orthomyxovirus
	Turkey bluecomb disease	Coronavirus
	Turkey virus infection	See Marek's disease
	Virus 'N' (Dinter) influenza	Orthomyxovirus
	*West Nile encephalitis	Flavivirus (Togavirus)
	Yucaipa virus disease	Paramyxovirus
	None or uncertain	CELO virus (Adenovirus)
		GAL virus (Adenovirus)
		Numerous enteroviruses (avian orphans)

*transmissible to man.

TABLE 38.10. Viral diseases of fish.

Name of disease	Syndrome caused	Virus group
Carp erythrodermatitis [CE] or subacute/ chronic carp dropsy	Inflammation, haemorrhage, necrosis and ulceration of the skin.	Unclassified virus
'Cauliflower' disease of eels	Chronic fibro-epithelial tumours around mouth and head especially of adult females.	?Virus
Contagious stomatitis	Eosinophilic cytoplasmic inclusions. Skin lesions and stomatitis.	Unclassified virus
Fish pox or hyperplastic epidermal disease	Proliferative cutaneous lesions with nuclear and cytoplasmic inclusions. Low mortality.	?Herpesvirus
Infectious pancreatic necrosis in trout [IPN].	Cork-screw type of swimming. Pancreatic necrosis. Cytoplasmic inclusions. High mortality in spontaneous outbreaks.	? Orbivirus
Kidney tumour agent	Kidney tumours, later with metastasis.	Unclassified virus
Lymphocystis of European perch	Cutaneous tumour masses. Cells contain cytoplasmic inclusions. Low mortality.	?Iridovirus
Oregon Sockeye salmon disease or infectious haematopoetic necrosis [IHN]	Haemorrhagic and eroded areas at base of fins. Visceral petechiae. High mortality in young salmon.	Rhabdovirus
Sacramento River Chinook salmon disease or infectious haematopoetic necrosis [IHN]	Skin darkens, haemorrhagic areas behind head. High mortality.	Rhabdovirus
Spring viraemia of carp [SVC]	Pallor of gills, enteritis, peritonitis, oedema and visceral petechiae. High mortality.	Rhabdovirus
Ulcerative dermal necrosis [UDN]	Progressive cytolytic necrosis of skin of head, fins and body.	?Virus
Viral haemorrhagic septicaemia [VHS] or Egtved virus of European trout & other fish	Haemorrhagic septicaemia. Kidney swelling and liver degeneration. High mortality in rainbow trout.	Rhabdovirus
Walleye sarcoma	Cutaneous sarcomata	Unclassified virus
Other neoplastic diseases	—	Unclassified viruses

Further reading

ALMEIDA J.D. (1963) A classification of virus particles based on morphology. *Canadian Medical Association Journal*, **89**, 787.

ANDREWES C.H. (1965) Viruses and Noah's Ark. *Bacteriological Reviews*, **29**, 1.

ANDREWES C.H. (1968) Methods of virus classification, In, *Methods in Virology*, Vol. 4, eds. K. Maramorosch and H. Koprowski, p. 593. New York: Academic Press.

ANDREWES C.H. AND PEREIRA H.G. (1972) *Viruses of Vertebrates*, 3rd Edition. London: Baillière, Tindall.

DALTON A.J. AND HAGUENAU F. (1973) *Ultrastructure of animal viruses and bacteriophages: An atlas*, London: Academic Press.

HUCK R.A. (1964) The classification of viruses. *Veterinary Bulletin*, **34**, 239.

LWOFF A. AND TOURNIER P. (1971) Remarks on the classification of viruses. In, *Comparative Virology*, eds. K. Maramorosch and E. Kurstak, p. 2. London: Academic Press.

MELNICK J.L. (1974) Classification and nomenclature of viruses, 1974. *Progress in Medical Virology*, **17**, 290.

MELNICK J.L. AND McCOMBS R.M. (1966) Classification and nomenclature of animal viruses. *Progress in Medical Virology*, **8**, 400.

WILDY P. (1971) Classification and nomenclature of viruses. In, *Monographs in Virology*, Vol. 5, ed. J.L. Melnick, p. 1. Basle: Karger.

WILDY P., GINSBERG H.S., BRANDES J. AND MAURIN J. (1967) Virus classification, nomenclature and the International Committee on the Nomenclature of Viruses. *Progress in Medical Virology*, **9**, 476.

WILNER B.I. (1969) *A Classification of the Major Groups of Human and Other Animal Viruses*, 4th Edition. Minneapolis: Burgess.

CHAPTER 39

VIRUS-CELL RELATIONSHIPS

Virus-cell relationships

Replication of animal viruses

The developmental cycle
The clinical signs and the tissue reactions in virus diseases are the result, directly or indirectly, of the virus–host interactions. Thus, some knowledge of the mechanisms by which viruses gain entry into the cell and multiply therein is essential before the pathogenesis of virus infections can be fully understood.

Replication of most animal viruses involves a dual process in which the viral protein and nucleic acid are synthesized separately and then assembled into the infectious particle. This is usually followed by release of mature virions into the extracellular environment.

The cycle of development of animal viruses may be described in five separate stages, as follows.

(1) Attachment (adsorption) of the virus to a susceptible cell.

(2) Penetration or engulfment, and uncoating of the virion.

(3) Virus multiplication and the synthesis of new viral components.

(4) Assembly and maturation of the newly-formed virus.

(5) Release of progeny virions from the cell.

The mode of infection of plant, bacterial and animal cells differs because of the nature of their cell walls. Plant cells have rigid cell walls of cellulose, and it appears that plant viruses can only enter into the cell following injury or bruising. Bacterial cell walls are generally less rigid and the nucleic acid of most bacterial viruses, which is usually DNA, is introduced into the cytoplasm of the cell by means of an injection mechanism, resembling the action of a hypodermic syringe. Most animal cells have no rigid cell walls and, consequently, infection with animal viruses is readily achieved, usually with engulfment of the entire virus particle.

Virions are wholly inert in the extracellular state, and they are incapable of multiplication except within the cytoplasm or nucleus of living susceptible cells. Also, they lack the physico-chemical properties and energy components that are essential for the many complex biosynthetic steps associated with viral replication, and which can only be provided by the living cell.

Attachment or adsorption
The first stage of infection is attachment (adsorption) of the virus particle on to the surface of the susceptible host cell. The process, which is probably due to electrostatic attraction between charged groups on the virus surface and a complementary pattern on the cell membrane, is greatly influenced by changes of pH in the medium and occurs optimally in the presence of calcium and magnesium ions. The initial attachment rate is independent of temperature except in so far as Brownian movement is increased at higher temperatures and the likelihood of collision between virus and cell is thereby increased. However, collision does not always result in attachment, even with relatively high concentrations of virus. In most instances, adsorption largely depends on an affinity between the attachment sites on the virus and certain specialized areas on the plasma membrane termed 'receptors'. Sometimes, these specific receptor sites for a given virus are present only on cells of certain species. For example, poliovirus grows readily in cells of primate origin but will not attach to non-primate cells. In other cases, there is no evidence of specificity and some viruses (e.g. toga- and pox-viruses) will adhere to and infect cells from a variety of animal sources. In poliovirus, the virus attachment sites are lipoproteins but in myxoviruses they are mucoproteins similar to the red blood cell receptors involved in haemagglutination. The receptor areas are readily destroyed by receptor-destroying enzyme so that the virus cannot adhere to enzyme-treated cells.

Penetration, engulfment and uncoating of the virion
Most bacterial viruses inject their nucleic acid

through the cell walls, which probably have an increased permeability due to enzymatic digestion, and the viral nucleic acid is released from its protein coat at or near the surface of the cell. With most animal viruses, however, adsorption of the intact virion on to the surface of the host cell is followed in a remarkably short time by a process of active engulfment (pinocytosis) by the closely adherent cell membrane. Engulfment is akin to phagocytosis but, unlike adsorption, is temperature-dependent.

There is, as yet, little information available on the means by which the viral genome is unmasked once the virus enters the cell, but some viruses (e.g. influenza virus) appear to be uncoated at the cell surface, thereby releasing the viral nucleocapsid directly into the cytoplasm. On the other hand, the initial steps in the uncoating of viruses with more than one envelope, and the removal of the capsids from non-enveloped virions, probably occurs in the 'phagocytic' cytoplasmic vacuoles by means of lysosomal enzymes which enter the vacuoles soon after they are formed. In vaccinia virus infections, the partially uncoated nucleic acid core passes from the phagocytic vacuole into the cytoplasm. At this stage, a virus-coded DNA-dependent RNA polymerase contained in the virion transcribes mRNA from the viral DNA by a process involving base-pairing, whereby the genetic information contained in the viral DNA is used to order a complementary sequence of bases in an RNA chain. The newly formed mRNA is, in turn, translated on host cell ribosomes to produce the enzymes necessary to complete the second stage uncoating with the release of the viral nucleic acid. It should be noted that other DNA viruses do not contain a DNA-dependent RNA polymerase within the virion and probably rely, therefore, on a host cell polymerase for the production of mRNA before new viral enzymes can be made.

Virus multiplication and the synthesis of new viral components

Soon after the infectious particle has successfully penetrated the host cell, there follows a short period of development, the eclipse phase, when the virus cannot readily be recovered in the infectious form. With some viruses, the eclipse phase can be divided into two parts: the 'eclipse period' which represents the interval between uncoating of the viral nucleic acid and the presence of new virions within the cell, and the 'latent period' which extends until the first appearance of infectious extracellular virus. The duration of the eclipse phase varies considerably with different viruses. For example, in the case of T_2 bacteriophage of *E. coli* it lasts only 15–20 minutes whereas in most animal virus infections (e.g.

adenovirus and papovavirus) the period is much longer and may extend to 12–15 hours.

Although the mechanisms involved in the multiplication of DNA and RNA viruses differ in a number of important respects, the eclipse phase can be considered, in general terms, as a series of sequential biosynthetic steps leading to assembly, maturation and release of infectious progeny virions.

During the early eclipse period the physical state of the virus is greatly altered and in some instances (e.g. picornaviruses) the virion is broken down into its protein and nucleic acid components within 15 minutes of the initiation of infection.

The eclipse phase is a period of intense metabolic activity during which the unmasked viral genome directs the cell to replicate new viral nucleic acids and to synthesise new viral proteins. The precise mechanism by which this information is passed from the various genes is not fully understood but in experiments with many different kinds of viruses it has clearly been shown that a new virus-specified substance promptly appears which inhibits the synthesis of the host-cell DNA. Thereafter, the infected cell proceeds to manufacture only those enzymes that are necessary for the formation of new viral components. In most DNA viruses, the steps involved in the production of new virions include:

(1) transcription of mRNA from specific sequences of bases on the parental viral DNA,

(2) migration of this virus-induced mRNA to the ribosomes in the cytoplasm where it is translated into virus-coded enzymes and other 'early proteins', which initiate and maintain the synthesis of new viral nucleic acid,

(3) replication of the viral DNA,

(4) further transcription of mRNA from both progeny and parental DNA,

(5) translation of these 'late mRNA's' into 'late proteins' which include most of the structural proteins for the new virions. The 'late proteins' also regulate the production of additional early enzymes.

(6) assembly of progeny virions, and

(7) release of mature virus from the cell.

The nucleic acid of deoxyriboviruses is replicated in the cell nucleus but the DNA of poxviruses and the RNA of riboviruses are mostly produced in the cytoplasm.

Unlike deoxyriboviruses, the multiplication of riboviruses presents a number of unusual features, not only because they must utilise RNA, rather than DNA, as their genetic material but also because the RNA of many members of the group is in the single-stranded form. At the present time, most workers in this field are of the opinion that replication of single-stranded RNA takes place by a method of 'base-pairing' which leads to the formation of a 'replicative

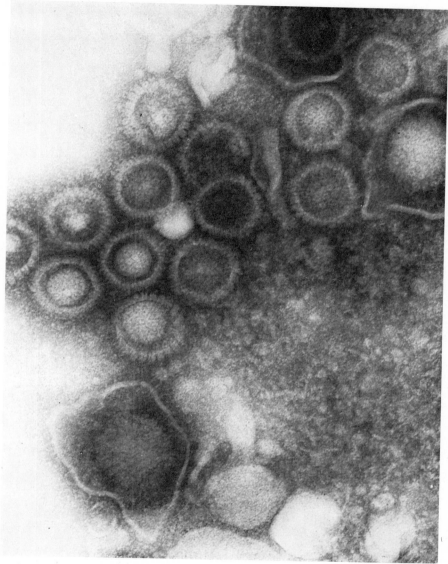

37.3 A group of enveloped and non-enveloped particles of Aujesky's disease herpesvirus, showing the regular arrangement of the hexagonal and pentagonal prisms forming the capsid. Notice the longitudinal hollow core of the capsomeres
on the surface of the naked virions, × 160 000. (Courtesy of Dr Sakkubai Ramachandran.)

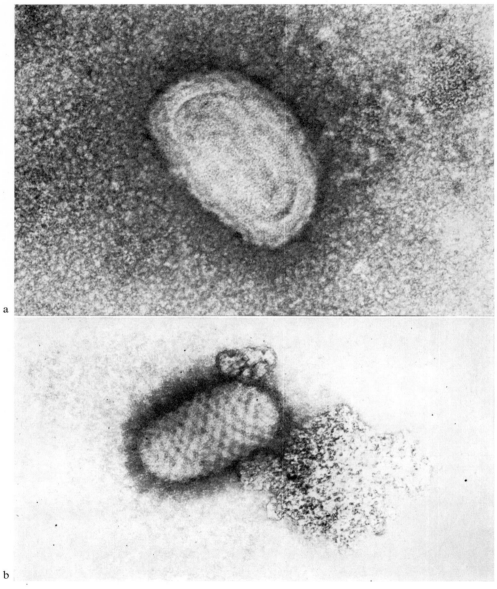

37.4a Vaccinia virus embedded in phosphotungstic acid. The virion is brick-shaped and is surrounded by a thick outer envelope, ×160 000.

37.4b Mature particle of Orf virus negatively stained with phosphotungstic acid, showing the characteristic woven pattern of threads due to the apparent criss-crossing of the surface tubules on the front and back faces of the virion, ×120 000.

intermediate'. As a result, new 'positive' strands are assembled from the 'negative' complementary strands. In the case of the small RNA-containing viruses (picornavirus and togavirus) the single-stranded 'positive' component of both parental and progeny viral RNA is used as mRNA in the process of translation into viral protein. In other words, the nucleic acid of small RNA viruses is infectious, *per se*. Whether similar mechanisms are involved in the replication of large RNA viruses (e.g. myxoviruses) is not yet clear. But recent evidence suggests that some riboviruses, including Newcastle disease virus, are 'negative strand' viruses, in which case the viral RNA must first be transcribed before it is translated; and this is accomplished by a virion-associated enzyme, RNA-dependent RNA polymerase. In reoviruses and other double-stranded riboviruses, the viral RNA is probably transcribed into mRNA by an RNA-dependent RNA polymerase (RNA synthetase) in a manner analogous to that for double-stranded DNA viruses.

Further details of the growth cycles of representative DNA- and RNA-containing viruses are included at the end of this chapter.

Assembly and maturation

After the viral proteins and nucleic acids have been independently synthesised they are assembled at different sites in the host cell, depending on the type of virus involved. This may be in the nucleus (herpesvirus and adenovirus), within the cytoplasm (poxvirus and picornavirus) on the membranes lining intracytoplasmic vacuoles (rhabdovirus) or at the cell surface (myxovirus). After assembly, new virus particles are formed by a process which is generally called virus maturation. In some instances, however, the newly formed viral proteins and nucleic acids do not combine normally but give rise to incomplete or defective virus, or occasionally, to an abortive infection. With ortho- and para-myxoviruses, productive and non-productive types of persistent infections may result.

Once nucleic acid and protein synthesis is initiated assembly of the capsid protein takes place around the nucleic acid molecules. With small riboviruses (e.g. picornavirus), the virions appear in the cytoplasm about 6–8 hours post-infection. In the large RNA-containing viruses such as rhabdoviruses and myxoviruses, the outer envelopes are completed and added to the virion after the proteins have been assembled, by a process of budding of the intracellular or plasma membranes. Thus, the envelope of these 'membrane-forming' viruses frequently contains virus-specified proteins as well as small amounts of host cell-derived proteins, although its lipid constituents are mainly derived from lipids normally present in the cell membrane.

Release of progeny virions from the cell

Comparatively little is known about the mechanisms of viral release from infected animal cells. Since the sites of assembly and maturation differ widely among the various groups of viruses it is reasonable to suppose that the mechanisms of release will also differ. Thus herpesviruses, which replicate in the cell nucleus, are likely to undergo a different cycle of maturation and release and will have a longer way to travel to reach the extracellular fluids than small RNA viruses which multiply only within the cytoplasm, or myxoviruses which mature by budding on the plasma membrane.

Following assembly and maturation, the progeny of the infecting virus usually leaves the cell about one hour after maturation is completed, but the amount of new virus liberated is very variable and, in cell cultures, is independent of the type of cytopathic effect produced. Many RNA viruses are released in about the same quantity in which they are formed but others (e.g. reoviruses) are released rather poorly. Some picornaviruses are freed promptly and continuously while others, such as poliovirus, escape by bursts from individual cells. Most DNA viruses are also released rather poorly and, as in adenovirus infections, as much as 90 per cent or even 99·9 per cent may be retained within the infected cells. Herpesviruses generally acquire a second coat as they enter the cytoplasm through the lamellae of the nuclear membrane, but are also capable of passing to contiguous cells by direct cell-to-cell transfer rather than by the more normal extracellular route. This method of direct cell-to-cell transfer is of interest since it probably enables the virus to spread within the animal body even in the presence of substantial amounts of neutralizing antibody which cannot reach the virus in its intracellular location. This may also account for the latent or chronic type of virus infection that can persist in apparently healthy animals for many months or even years following an acute infection. Viruses which mature and are released by budding from the cell surface are readily accessible to the neutralizing effects of circulating antibodies but those that are completely enveloped in host-cell components are relatively non-antigenic and may not be neutralized by specific antiviral sera.

The growth cycles of the major groups of animal viruses

Multiplication of animal viruses involves three fundamental processes. The first is the method whereby the viral nucleic acid is replicated, the second is the means by which the viral nucleic acid molecules can initiate synthesis of structural proteins, and the third is the mechanism by which the new viral components are assembled into complete virus particles.

The production of several novel enzymes is usually necessary for the replication of viral nucleic acid; and these are the virus-coded or virus-specified enzymes in contrast to the existing cellular enzymes of the normal host-cell. These new enzymes are not only responsible for uncoating the virus particles soon after they enter into the cell, but are also required for synthesis of viral proteins and assembly of the component parts of the progeny virus.

One of the most fundamental differences between cellular and viral nucleic acids lies in the fact that cellular RNA is incapable of self-replication and its synthesis is entirely dependent on the DNA of the cell. Viral RNA, on the other hand, is capable of independent replication whether in the double-or single-stranded form. Deoxyriboviruses are unusual in that they have a virus-specified RNA during one phase of their growth cycle, so that both types of nucleic acid are present during one, albeit brief, stage of their development, whereas most riboviruses can utilise only one nucleic acid — their own RNA. A remarkable feature of the multiplication cycle of RNA tumour viruses is the presence of a novel viral enzyme, RNA-directed DNA polymerase ('reverse transcriptase') which reverses the flow of information from RNA to DNA.

Multiplication of deoxyriboviruses

Poxviruses

The growth and development of vaccinia and other members of the poxvirus group have been intensively studied by electron microscopic, biochemical and immunofluorescence techniques. Soon after the virus enters the host cell, the virions are engulfed in phagocytic intracytoplasmic vacuoles where the outer layer of the protein coat is rapidly removed by means of pre-existing cellular enzymes. This results in degradation of the outer membrane and lateral bodies, and the release of the viral nucleoprotein core into the cytoplasm. The second uncoating step involving degradation of the nucleoprotein and liberation of the viral DNA is more complex, and is not yet fully understood.

It has been suggested that liberation of the viral nucleic acid is rapidly followed by release of a heat-labile 'inducer protein' which is transferred to the nucleus where it de-represses the synthesis of a new protein coded in the cellular DNA. This new protein returns to the cytoplasm where it codes for an additional uncoating protein on the ribosomes which then unmasks the 'naked' DNA. On the other hand, recent observations with vaccinia virus have shown that the virion carries within its core a viral-coded DNA-dependent RNA polymerase which transcribes on RNA from the viral DNA while the DNA

is still within the core structure of the virion. After the mRNA has been transcribed, it is released into the cytoplasm where it is associated with the ribosomes and is translated to synthesise new enzymes necessary to complete the unmasking process. The released viral DNA, which may be present at more than one site in the cytoplasm, is now concerned with the replication of new viral DNA as well as assembly of the viral proteins which have already been synthesized in the polyribosomes under the influence of viral mRNA. The mRNA's for certain other 'early enzymes', including thymidine kinase, DNA polymerase and deoxyribonucleases, become available for translation into protein only after the unmasking process of the viral DNA has been completed. Thymidine kinase is associated with certain essential steps in the incorporation of thymine into DNA but after several hours its production ceases abruptly due, it is believed, to the formation of a virus-specified repressor substance in the cell that is produced only after viral DNA replication has commenced. The synthesis of viral DNA begins in the cytoplasm 1–2 hours after infection, and replication of the double-stranded molecules under the stimulus of a virus-coded DNA polymerase continues to about the fifth or sixth hour when immature virions first appear in the cytoplasm; followed within 2 hours by mature infectious virus.

Little is known about the maturation process of poxviruses except that mature particles (developmental bodies) appear as hollow spheres embedded in a dense cytoplasmic matrix, the so-called 'viroplasm', at the several 'factory sites' in the cytoplasm. In many instances the dense cytoplasmic masses constitute inclusion bodies. In time, the hollow spheres become filled with an homogeneous material and condense into smaller ovoid mature virions each with a pair of large lateral bodies, an electron-opaque central dumbbell-shaped nucleoid covered by two thin membranes and surrounded by protein, and all encased within a thick double-layered outer membrane.

The assembly of pox-virions is not an efficient process since over half the new viral DNA and protein fails to become incorporated into complete progeny particles. Moreover, coding errors sometimes lead to the formation of 'empty' virions and other aberrant forms which are usually non-infectious. Most of the mature virus particles remain cell-associated until the death and disruption of the cell. Release of virus is not inevitable and large aggregates of complete virions may remain in the cell debris even after lysis has occurred.

Herpesviruses

Cubic DNA viruses of the herpesvirus and adenovirus groups present a somewhat different pattern of replication to that of the poxviruses since their maturation takes place in the cell nucleus, although some of their viral products are synthesised in the cytoplasm.

Herpesviruses are adsorbed and transferred to the interior of the cell in a membrane-bound vesicle. Most of the virions lying within the vesicles are enveloped because enveloped capsids attach more readily to the cell than non-enveloped forms, and are engulfed more efficiently. In electron micrographs of infected cells the envelopes of many virions lying within phagocytic cytoplasmic vacuoles appear to have become detached wholly or partially from their nucleocapsids and several non-enveloped forms may be found lying freely in the cytoplasm near the nucleus. This process of uncoating, which is probably due to enzymes already present in the cell, permits the viral DNA-protein complex to escape and enter the nucleus where replication begins. By this stage in the developmental cycle, synthesis of cellular DNA has ceased and there is a marked increase in the activity of certain virus-coded 'early enzymes' including thymidine kinase and DNA polymerase. Following entry of the DNA-protein complex into the nucleus, the viral DNA becomes dissociated from the protein and is transcribed within six hours after infection. The product, virus-specific mRNA, is then transported into the cytoplasm where it enters into free and membrane-bound polyribosomes, and directs the synthesis of new structural and non-structural viral proteins. Most of the proteins specified by the virus migrate to the nucleus where several of the non-structural proteins are involved in the production of viral nucleic acids. The structural proteins entering the nucleus aggregate with the newly synthesized viral nucleic acid to form a capsid near the nuclear membrane. The process of assembly is not efficient and the amount of viral nucleic acid and protein produced is usually greatly in excess over what is eventually incorporated into the mature virion. Indeed, in the case of some herpesviruses, the structural components form aberrant aggregates resembling micro-tubules in both the nucleus and cytoplasm. Shortly after they are assembled, nucleocapsids surrounded by an amorphous material are enveloped by the inner lamella of the nuclear membrane as they bud through the membrane to the perinuclear space. In some herpesvirus infections, however, envelopment seems to occur not only at the nuclear membrane but also at the Golgi apparatus, the endoplasmic reticulum and even at the plasma membrane. Information is lacking on the mechanisms whereby the enveloped virus particles make their way from the space between the inner and outer lamellae of the nuclear membrane to the external environment, but recent evidence suggests that the endoplasmic reticulum forms a network of branched tubules along which the virions pass to the surface of the cell. An alternative hypothesis that portions of the endoplasmic reticulum containing herpesviruses break off, form vesicles and transport the mature virions to the extracellular fluids, is probably misleading since recent reports show that these cytoplasmic vacuoles are not closed and merely represent cross-sections of the highly convoluted and branched tubules. Under these circumstances it is unlikely that the enveloped progeny nucleocapsids are transported across the cytoplasm and released by a process of 'reverse phagocytosis', as was previously supposed. Rather it is now suggested that the tubules provide a pathway for egress of the virus from the site of development in the nucleus to the extracellular fluid; thereby preventing uncoating of the new virion by the lysosomal nucleases in the cytoplasmic vacuoles, and its subsequent destruction. Whether this method of release of herpesviruses along the tubules is a property shared with all DNA viruses which multiply in the nucleus is not yet known, but similar tubules connecting the perinuclear space with the extra-cellular fluid have been described in cells infected with SV4O and adenoviruses.

Not all types of cell are disrupted by herpesviruses, and in certain cases progeny virus may be extruded from infected cells by evagination of the cellular membrane, thereby acquiring an additional envelope. Conversely, in some cell systems the cells may disrupt before the normal method of release can occur so that a number of naked nucleocapsids are freed into the supernatant fluid of the culture. Direct intercellular transmission of virus is a not uncommon feature of *Herpes simplex* and other typical members of the group. It should also be noted that the development of herpesviruses is generally associated with the formation of large acidophilic intranuclear inclusions of Cowdry type A. Early in their development the inclusions stain Feulgen positive, indicating the presence of DNA but, at the time of virus release, most of the DNA has disappeared from the nucleus.

Adenoviruses

These non-enveloped icosahedral DNA viruses are assembled and mature in the nucleus although most of their proteins are synthesized in the cytoplasm. The virus is adsorbed to the host-cell, transferred to the interior in a membrane-bound vesicle and uncoated probably within the nucleus by means of pre-existing cellular enzymes. The growth cycle is slower and the 'latent phase' much longer than with herpesviruses. Synthesis of viral coat protein begins at about 10 hours and maturation occurs between 13 and 28 hours post-infection. The oncogenic adenoviruses have an even longer latent period and a much more prolonged developmental cycle than other adenoviruses. Only about 20 per cent of the new viral DNA and 6 per cent of the protein is incorporated into the virions. The formation of intranuclear inclusion bodies is characteristic of all adenovirus infections and most serological types give rise to large crystalline arrays of virions in the nucleus. Mature progeny virus is released from the nucleus either by disruption of the nuclear membrane or by the formation of large nuclear protrusions filled with virions which subsequently detach from the nucleus to form membrane-enclosed viral crystals in the cytoplasm.

Summary
The various biosynthetic steps involved in the replication of DNA viruses can be summarised as follows:

(1) Attachment, penetration and transfer of the virus to the site of replication, followed by uncoating by existing cellular enzymes, and release of viral DNA either within or in the vicinity of the nucleus.

(2) Early transcription of mRNA from specific base sequences of the parental viral DNA.

(3) Attachment of the viral mRNA to the cytoplasmic polyribosomes.

(4) Translation of this mRNA into virus-coded enzymes including thymidine kinase and DNA polymerase, and other 'early' proteins.

(5) Replication of viral DNA by means of a virus-coded DNA polymerase.

(6) Second wave of transcription of mRNA from parental and progeny DNA.

(7) Translation of these late mRNA's into viral capsid proteins and more enzymes.

(8) Assembly of the viral DNA with structural (capsid) and other proteins to form new mature virions.

(9) Release of virus particles with or without cell lysis.

Multiplication of riboviruses
As we have seen, double-stranded DNA viruses replicate according to the classical Watson–Crick pattern, that is by means of 'base-pair copying'. The DNA viral genome does so by transcription of the parental viral DNA to viral mRNA which then directs the synthesis of virus-specified enzymes and other early proteins upon the polyribosomes situated in the cytoplasm of the host cell. To replicate in this way the nucleic acid of RNA viruses would have to be in the double-stranded form which, in the great majority of cases, it is not. However, since newly formed viral RNA in cells infected with a typical ribovirus is resistant to the action of ribonuclease it seems likely that the newly synthesized viral RNA is, in fact, in the double-stranded form. Thus, the single-stranded RNA of the infecting virus is probably converted to a double-stranded molecule ('replicative form') by the synthesis of a complementary strand on the incoming viral strand, during the first stage in the cycle of development. The next stage would include the production of many copies of the viral genome by means of the complementary strand in the 'replicative form'. The precise mechanisms of viral RNA multiplication are still not fully understood, but a system that has been proposed for the replication of single-stranded DNA may apply equally to single-stranded RNA. According to this so-called 'rolling-circle hypothesis', the incoming strand assumes a circular form on which a complementary circular chain is made. From this circular molecule, a long chain consisting of many copies of the parental strand can be unfolded or 'rolled off'. If this new chain is then severed by specific enzymic action at appropriate points along its length, then many copies of the viral genome are produced. On the other hand it has been clearly shown with certain riboviruses that inhibitors of DNA synthesis and blockage of DNA transcription by actinomycin D have little effect on the replication of small RNA viruses (e.g. poliovirus) and it seems that the RNA of these particular viruses has the capacity to serve as its own mRNA and thereby direct its own duplication.

In most RNA virus infections, the viral mRNA is translated to produce a number of new virus-coded enzymes, one of which is called RNA-dependent RNA polymerase to distinguish it from the existing DNA-dependent RNA polymerase of the uninfected cell. The presence of this novel viral RNA polymerase is essential first for synthesizing the complementary strand and second for producing the multiple copies of the viral genome. The synthesis of viral protein occurs in the same way as for host cell protein, but it is emphasised that a host cell enzyme cannot be used for RNA production as none is known which could make mRNA on an RNA template. This enzyme must, therefore, be virus-coded and either carried into the cell in the virion or synthesised early in the growth cycle by direct translation of the infecting RNA strands. In fact, there are many instances when both mechanisms obtain.

Following its entry into a susceptible host cell, the viral RNA is transcribed by a polymerase or transcriptase enzyme which gives rise to several types of virus-specified mRNA that attach to the ribosomes in the cytoplasm. The mRNA is then translated, with the participation of transfer RNA (tRNA) and produces early and late proteins including replicase and other enzymes, as well as envelope, capsid and other structural proteins. The replicase combines with the parental viral RNA to produce new viral RNA which becomes incorporated into a nucleoprotein capsid, protecting the progeny viral RNA genome.

Picornaviruses

The growth cycles of the small, naked, nonlipid-containing, icosahedral, single-stranded RNA-containing polioviruses have been studied in detail and there is general agreement that all of the biosynthetic steps necessary for the production of new mature virus are independent of the host DNA and occur in the host-cell cytoplasm. The sequence of events is probably the same with enteroviruses, foot-and-mouth disease virus and other members of the family as a whole, since all are of a simple structure with only a few kinds of protein.

The intact virions of poliovirus attach to the surfaces of primate cells in culture through species-specific cell receptor sites, but they do not do so on cell strains of non-primate origin. On the other hand, isolated viral RNA will, in the absence of the protein component of the virus, adsorb to and infect primate cells as well as non-primate cells of rabbit, guinea-pig or chicken and may, in fact, complete one cycle of infection. Only a single cycle of infection is possible on non-primate cells because the progeny virus particles are produced complete with protein coats and only primate cells are capable of supporting them. It is also of interest that cell cultures growing in fluids containing the enzyme ribonuclease can be successfully infected with intact virus, but not with isolated RNA which is not protected against the destructive action of the enzyme. This would suggest that following infection the viral RNA is released within the cell rather than at the cell surface.

Following attachment, intact virions are taken into the cell by pinocytosis, which is quickly followed by the process of uncoating of the viral RNA. It seems likely that in poliovirus, as well as in some other small single-stranded RNA virus infections, the viral RNA becomes attached to the ribosomes where it serves as its own mRNA for direct translation into viral protein. Translation of mRNA during the first 30 minutes after infection is responsible for the synthesis of at least one new virus-coded enzyme, i.e. an RNA-dependent RNA polymerase (RNA synthetase or replicase) which is required to catalyse the replication of viral RNA. This new RNA polymerase is also associated with the formation of a new double stranded protein molecule called the 'replicative intermediate', together with a number of inhibitors that switch off both cellular RNA and protein synthesis by preventing the transcription and translation of host mRNA.

Little is known about the precise method of replication of poliovirus RNA but in the first stage of development the RNA polymerase is considered to bind with the parental (positive) strand which then serves as a template for the transcription of a complementary (negative) strand. The negative strand can, in turn, act as a template for the asymetrical synthesis of other positive strands, identical to the parental RNA, and so on. Single-stranded viral RNA molecules are synthesized from the replicative intermediate in the region of the cytoplasmic polysomes during the first 3 hours of infection. At the same time, viral protein is also in the process of being laid-down by both parental and progeny RNA, acting as mRNA.

The first stage in the construction of the virion involves the assembly of the protein subunits (capsomeres) which condense to form empty protein shells called procapsids. Subsequently, the viral nucleic acid is incorporated into the procapsid, forming the mature virion. The virus particles are usually retained in the cell for some time but are rapidly released when the cell undergoes lysis.

Myxoviruses

Members of the myxovirus group are single-stranded RNA viruses that are much larger than picornaviruses and most other species of riboviruses. They show helical symmetry and are surrounded by an envelope with a high lipid content. They also possess three major antigens, the nucleoprotein antigen of the inner helix, and the haemagglutinin and neuraminidase both of which are contained in the outer envelope.

Unlike other RNA viruses, most members of the myxovirus group do not 'shut down' the synthesis of cellular RNA and protein, but seem to prefer that some degree of cellular activity should continue for the first few hours of the viral replicative cycle. Thus, in myxovirus infections the synthesis of new viral components appears to be superimposed on that of the cell.

In any consideration of the developmental cycles of myxoviruses it is customary to divide them into two groups: those having a stage of synthesis in the nucleus, (e.g. influenza, fowl plague and other orthomyxoviruses), and those that are considered by some workers, but not by others, to multiply exclusively within the cytoplasm of the cell, (e.g. Newcastle disease, mumps and other paramyxoviruses). In all cases, however, the mechanisms of adsorption and entry into the susceptible host-cells are very similar.

Orthomyxoviruses

Infection is initiated by the interaction between the viral surface glycoproteins and the mucopolysaccharide receptor sites on the surface of the host-cell, thereby enabling the virus to attach itself. After the virions become entwined in long mucoprotein chains coating the cell membrane they approach the surface of the cell and are rapidly taken into the cytoplasm by a process of active engulfment (pinocytosis) akin to phagocytosis. The engulfed virions are frequently found enclosed within phagocytic cytoplasmic vacuoles where the first steps in the uncoating process take place. These initial stages in the developmental cycle may not apply to all myxoviruses, however, and recent observations indicate that influenza virus particles may fuse with the cellular membrane during attachment, thereby releasing the viral nucleoprotein directly into the cytoplasm.

As soon as the virion has been liberated from its outer membrane, a transcriptase enzyme present in the unmasked single-stranded viral genome codes for mRNA which, in turn, induces the formation of several types of 'early' and 'late' proteins including the enzymes replicase and transcriptase, before replication of viral RNA takes place. Most of the mRNA associated with the polyribosomes in cells infected with orthomyxoviruses appears to be in the form of short strands of base sequences that are complementary to the parental RNA molecule. In this respect they resemble the discontinuities found in the genetic material of reovirus and other double-stranded riboviruses. But, whether the viral genome of the single-stranded orthomyxovirus consists of discrete segments each capable of being transcribed into mRNA is not yet known.

Immunofluorescence and other serological studies on myxoviruses of the influenza type, suggest that both the viral RNA and the helical ribonucleoprotein component, which is the soluble 'S' or 'g' complement-fixing antigen, are formed within the nucleus and that the latter unites immediately with the viral RNA since nearly all the new RNA in the nucleus is present as ribonucleoprotein. Fluorescent antibody staining methods also show that influenza ribonucleoprotein is present in the nucleus about three hours after infection, and appears in increasing amounts in the cytoplasm from about the fifth hour onwards. The haemagglutinin protein or 'V' antigen is first seen in the perinuclear area of the cytoplasm four hours post-infection; but, an hour or two later, both the envelope and spike (haemagglutinin plus neuraminidase) proteins accumulate on the outer plasma membrane of the cell where they form discrete patches. The sites of synthesis of the viral neuraminidase have not been definitely established but it first appears with the haemagglutinin antigen at the periphery of the cell.

Assembly is completed when the strands of new viral nucleoprotein migrate and become aligned with the surface of the cell and are extruded through the plasma membrane, or into the cytoplasmic vacuoles. All myxoviruses are enclosed in a lipoprotein envelope, the lipids of which vary in amount with the different species of virus. Much of the lipid material is of cellular origin but some of the phospholipids are different from those of the cell, since budding only occurs when the nucleocapsid makes contact with the plasma membrane in which some viral components have already been incorporated. Release of complete infectious virus by the process known as budding occurs over many hours, often without lysis of the infected cells. There is evidence that viral neuraminidase may play an important role in the release process since the extrusion of new intact virus may be inhibited by antibody to neuraminidase. It is emphasised that myxovirus particles are rarely seen within the cytoplasm of infected cells, due to the fact that the processes of assembly and maturation mostly occur at the surface of the cell.

Paramyxoviruses

The sequence of events in the developmental cycle of Newcastle disease virus and other paramyxoviruses is very similar to that described for orthomyxoviruses, but with one or two important differences.

The main point of disagreement concerns the sites of assembly of the different components of the virus. Most workers consider that the various components of paramyxoviruses, including viral RNA, are synthesized exclusively in the cytoplasm and that the different biosynthetic steps take place later than with orthomyxoviruses. If it is confirmed that the nucleic acid of orthomyxoviruses, but not paramyxoviruses, is synthesized in the nucleus it is reasonable to suppose that its viral RNA differs from that of paramyxoviruses by having a DNA-dependent step in its replication.

Summary

Present knowledge regarding the multiplication of large and small single-stranded riboviruses can be summarized as follows.

(1) Attachment of the virus to the surface of the susceptible host-cell.

(2) Penetration of the virus by phagocytic engulfment (pinocytosis) following invagination of the modified plasma membrane; or digestion of cell surface mucoprotein by viral neuraminidase enabling the intact viral genome to enter the cell.

(3) Uncoating of cubic virions (or ribonucleoprotein helices) and unmasking of viral RNA by lysosomal nucleases in phagocytic cytoplasmic vacuoles.

(4) Single-stranded RNA of small ribovirus genome attaches to ribosomes where it serves as

its own mRNA for direct translation into viral proteins.

(5) Translation of viral mRNA into novel enzymes including RNA-dependent RNA polymerase (RNA synthetase or replicase) required to catalyse the replication of viral RNA.

(6) RNA polymerase responsible for:

(a) production of inhibitors of cellular RNA and protein synthesis (most riboviruses), and

(b) the formation of a 'replicative intermediate'.

(7) Replicative intermediate of small riboviruses serves as a double-stranded template for transcription of parental (positive) and complementary (negative) RNA strands.

(8) New viral RNA incorporated in structural viral protein,

(a) to form helical nucleocapsids, or

(b) to convert procapsids into complete cubic virions

(9) Release of cubic virions by cell lysis and of helical viruses by budding of the plasma membrane.

Reoviruses

Reoviruses differ from other riboviruses in that they are composed of structural units of double-stranded RNA. As such, the viral RNA is incapable of acting as its own mRNA, as occurs with most of the small species of single-stranded riboviruses.

When the double-stranded RNA is removed from the purified virions it invariably fragments in a reproducible manner. Recent investigations have shown that the reovirus-genome consists of ten discrete segments within the virion and each of the segments is transcribed independently from end to end and from one strand only, into mRNAs. The mRNAs in reovirus-infected cells correspond exactly in length to the ten double-stranded viral RNA parental molecules since each is transcribed exclusively from that segment of double-stranded viral RNA of corresponding size. A limited number of segments of parental RNA code for early viral function and these can be transcribed in the absence of protein synthesis, probably by a virion-associated polymerase. Seven of the ten segments of reovirus-genome are coded for viral capsid polypeptides and the function of at least one of the remaining three segments is possibly the synthesis of viral RNA polymerase. Whether or not the segments are linked, or how they are bonded inside the virus core has not yet been determined.

Reoviruses have a prolonged growth cycle and a tendency to accumulate within the cell. They multiply exclusively within the cytoplasm and progeny virus particles are frequently found in close association with the centrioles and spindle fibres which are involved in cell mitosis. Later, as virus multiplication proceeds, extensive crystalline arrays of newly formed virions are found in large cytoplasmic 'factory' areas. The virus particles usually remain cell-associated until cell lysis occurs.

Leukoviruses

Unlike DNA viruses which transmit information from DNA to RNA and thence to protein, most RNA viruses replicate directly into new copies of RNA and translate this information into new viral proteins. In contrast to this 'normal' method of information-transfer from DNA to RNA, or RNA to RNA, it has become apparent during the past few years that a reverse flow of information from RNA to DNA might be possible, and recent evidence suggests that this may occur during the multiplication of all oncogenic RNA viruses as well as feline and simian foamy viruses and visna virus of sheep. The mechanism by which this unusual activity takes place is explained by the recent discovery of a DNA polymerase capable of using the viral RNA as a template for DNA synthesis. The enzyme, which copies the sequence of the bases in the RNA viral genome to produce a DNA strand which can then be replicated and finally inserted into the host cell chromosome, has been named RNA-directed DNA polymerase or 'reverse transcriptase'.

Unlike many other viruses which destroy the cells they infect, chicken cells infected with leukoviruses, e.g. Rous sarcoma virus, may not only survive but also be transformed into malignant cells and continue to divide and produce mature infective virions. On the other hand, rat cells infected with Rous sarcoma virus are also transformed and continue to divide but do not produce the virus even though the viral genome persists in the host cells. However, the defective virus can be rescued from the persistently infected cells if they are fused by co-cultivation with normal chicken cells. The manner in which the viral genome of RNA oncogenic viruses persists in a non-infectious form (provirus) in the host cell chromosome is analogous to the formation of prophage in lysogenic bacterial cells.

All RNA tumour viruses grow in the cytoplasm, but not the nucleus, of the susceptible host cell. In productive infections, the virions are assembled and emerge along the margins of membranes lining the cell and its cytoplasmic vacuoles. In general, the mature virus particles are released slowly by a process of budding, often without dramatic impairment of the host cell's viability.

Bacteriophages

A new era was opened in microbiology when Twort in 1915, reported on the presence of curious transparent areas in a culture of staphylococcus in which no cocci could be found. The phenomenon could be reproduced in successive cultures by subcultivation from one of the affected areas, and high dilutions of bacteria-free filtrates from fluid cultures induced the effect in fresh growths of staphylococci. Two years later, D'Hérelle observed that filtrates of a culture obtained from the faeces of a patient suffering from bacillary diarrhoea were able, when added in small quantities to a young culture of dysentery bacilli, to destroy the developing organisms. Although D'Hérelle postulated that the lytic factor was an invisible living microorganism parasitic for bacteria, several years passed before it was realised that bacteriophages are, in fact, viruses that infect bacteria.

When susceptible bacteria are spread on the surface of a dry agar plate and a phage-containing filtrate is inoculated at one point on the surface, the lytic activity of the phage will be indicated after 12–24 hours of incubation by a large clear area, devoid of bacteria, at the point of inoculation. The phage-bacterial cell interaction is highly specific and the destruction of bacteria by these 'virulent' bacteriophages is widely used for the identification of many bacterial species. This method of 'phage-typing' is more sensitive than conventional serology for the recognition of strains within some bacterial species, and has proved invaluable in epidemiological investigations especially of enteric and staphylococcal infections.

Properties of the virus

Much of our knowledge concerning the properties and growth characters of animal viruses, and many of the recent advances in vertebrate virology, stem from earlier detailed studies of bacterial viruses. Because they are capable of multiplying in simple bacterial cultures and are easy to maintain, bacteriophages provide a convenient model for studies of such biological phenomena as viral structure, reproduction, genetics, pathogenesis and infectivity.

Morphology

Bacteriophages are undoubtedly viruses and, by definition, they contain a nucleic acid core surrounded by a coat of protein. The nucleic acid, which represents the genetic material of the virus usually consists of either double- or single-stranded DNA, but small single-stranded RNA viruses have recently been discovered. The protein coat varies considerably in shape and size but most resemble a tadpole or spermatozoan with a spherical, oval or hexagonal head and, usually, a tail with a central hollow axis (Plate 39.1a, facing p. 444b).

Although phages were invisible under the microscopes available to Twort and D'Hérelle, today the more sophisticated methods of shadow-casting and negative-staining by electron microscopy reveal that bacterial viruses exist in five fundamentally different forms.

Group A phage is the most complex type and consists of a head and a long, thick rigid tail with a contractile sheath and terminal tail fibres (Fig. 39.1). The head is a bipyramidal hexagonal prism or a prolate icosahedron (i.e. a twenty-sided object with an extended middle section). All members of the group contain double stranded DNA (2-DNA) and are represented by the T-even (T2, 4, 6) series of coliphages.

Group B phage is similar to the first and contains 2-DNA but lacks a contractile sheath and its tail is flexible. The tail may be long as in T5 or short as in T3. The heads of T3 and T7 phages are octahedral.

Group C is the tailless 1-DNA phage with a relatively large spherical capsomere at each apex of the icosahedron, e.g. the small coliphage ØX174.

Group D phage is similar to group C phage except that the apical sub-units are very small or absent. Its nucleic acid core consists of single-stranded RNA (1-RNA) e.g. R17.

Group E includes the long, flexible filamentous phage, without the head or structural features of the typical phage. The single-stranded nucleic acid component (1-DNA) is thought to be intertwined with the coat protein rather than forming a characteristic head.

Bacterial viruses, like animal viruses, possess two types of symmetry, cubical (polyhedral) and helical (rod-shaped). Tailed bacteriophages differ from animal viruses, however, in that they have 'binal' symmetry with heads that are cubic and tails that are helical. The size of the head and tail varies with the species of virus: T-even phages are morphologically identical having heads of about 95×65 nm and tails of 100 nm in length and 25 nm in width, with a knob or cluster of fibres at the tip. The tail has a sheath surrounded by a network of fine fibres attached to a baseplate at the distal end and a thin disc or collar adjacent to the head. Following attachment to the host cell, the fibres become detached from the collar and extend outwards and downwards from the base plate, firmly anchoring the phage to the cell surface. On adsorption, the sheath contracts to about half its length by rearrangement of its morphological subunits. The main morphological features of a T-even phage, firstly in the intact state as released after lysis of an infected bacterial cell, and secondly in the 'triggered' state attached to the surface of the cell, are shown diagrammatically in Fig. 39.2.

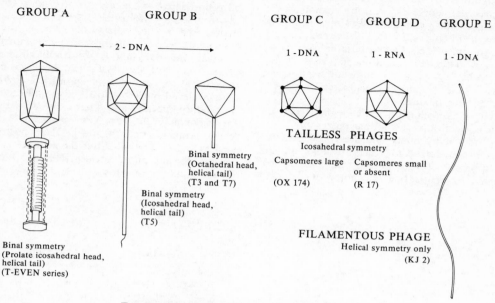

FIG. 39.1. Symmetry of Group A–E bacteriophages.

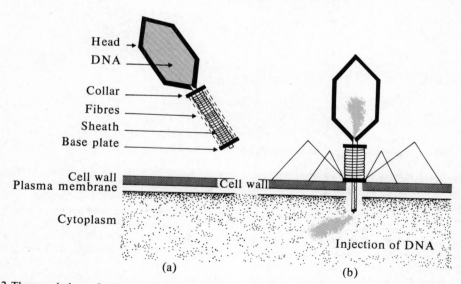

FIG. 39.2. The morphology of a T-even bacteriophage. (a) intact (before attachment), (b) triggered (after attachment).

The T-odd series shows marked differences in size. For instance, T5 has a regular hexagonal head 65 nm in diameter with a tail 170 nm long and 10 nm wide, whereas the identical T3 and T7 phages have heads 47 nm wide and short stubby tails 15 × 10 nm protruding from one corner of the hexagon. Group C (ØX174) and Group D (S13) viruses have no tail,

measure about 60 nm across and resemble small icosahedral animal viruses, with 12–92 surface capsomeres.

Phage replication

The most common source of bacteriophage is the natural host habitat. For example, coliphages pathogenic for *Escherichia coli* can best be isolated from intestinal contents, manure, sewage and contaminated water supplies. Most phages can be readily isolated and cultivated in young actively growing cultures of sensitive bacteria in broth or on digest agar plates. In liquid media, lysis of the bacterial cells may cause a cloudy culture to clear, whereas on agar clear foci or plaques of dead cells are visible to the unaided eye.

The phage reproduction cycle begins when an uninfected genetically susceptible bacterium is exposed to free, active phage and the tip of the virus tail becomes attached to receptor areas on the surface of the cell. This first phase, called **adsorption**, is followed by **penetration** and entry of the viral

After the stage of penetration and entry, there is an **eclipse phase**, when no infective phage particles can be isolated from the host cell. During this period, the injected, chemically inert viral nucleic acid which carries all the hereditary information necessary for the synthesis of progeny virus quickly takes control of the host's metabolic machinery, directing it to synthesize phage nucleic acid rather than bacterial nucleic acid. It also causes the cell to produce enzymes and other substances required for manufacturing new viral particles including 'early proteins' such as new DNA polymerase, kinases and synthetase. After the eclipse phase and towards the end of the **latent period** which accounts for about half of the growth cycle, the newly formed

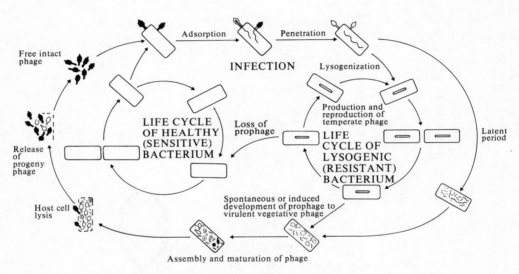

FIG. 39.3. Bacteriophage-host life cycle.

nucleic acid into the cytoplasm of the cell; the process being facilitated by the action of a lysosome-like enzyme incorporated in the tail which increases the permeability of the outer cell membrane or actively digests it. In most instances, the sheath of the tail contracts and the nucleic acid inside the head is injected along the hollow central axis of the tail through the cell wall and cytoplasmic membrane into the cytoplasm of the host cell. With the exception of Group D phages in which the entire filamentous particle may enter the bacterium, the empty protein coat remains outside the cell and is not engulfed by pinocytosis as occurs with many animal viruses. If sufficient phages are adsorbed on to a single cell, leakage through the damaged wall may be so severe that the bacterium is immediately lysed; the phenomenon being termed 'lysis from without'.

viral nucleic acids become irreversibly combined with a protein coat and, as a result, several hundred new vegetative phages are formed. This stage is called **assembly and maturation**. From this point onwards, progeny virus particles are produced at a linear rate until the cell lyses and the phages are **released** to attack further cells. It is generally believed that lysis occurs as a result of osmotic pressure after the cell wall has been weakened by a lytic enzyme produced during the process of viral synthesis. The exception is the filamentous group E phage in which mature viral particles are extruded through the cell wall without destroying the host. The length of the reproduction cycle varies with different species of phages but usually occupies 20–60 minutes. The number of progeny virus particles liberated from an infected bacterium is known as the 'burst size' and is characteristic for each phage strain.

Lysogeny

The entry of phage into sensitive bacterial cells is not invariably followed by a lytic or vegetative cycle of development. In certain circumstances many phages do not undergo the normal lytic cycle and, instead, the phage genome becomes integrated in the bacterial genome and in many respects continues to behave as a bacterial gene. In this situation the DNA of the phage, or prophage as it is now called, is incorporated in the bacterial chromosome with which it multiplies in harmony and persists in a stable non-infectious form. The infected bacterial cell which is termed lysogenic, continues to metabolize and reproduce normally, the viral nucleic acid being transmitted to each daughter cell through all successive generations. However, after an indeterminate number of cell divisions, and in circumstances not well understood, the viral genome becomes detached from the bacterial chromosome, by the process called induction, and enters a lytic cycle leading to the death of its host. Bacteria persistently infected with 'latent' prophage are resistant to super-infection by virulent phages of the same (homologous) type which they are carrying, but heterologous phages can still infect and lyse carrier bacteria. In some instances, it may be possible to induce the prophage of lysogenic bacterial cells into mature virulent phage following treatment of the carrier bacterial cells with certain chemical substances (e.g. mitomycin C) or by ultraviolet irradiation. The phenomenon is analagous to the rescue of defective virus from tissue cells transformed by oncogenic animal viruses. It is interesting to note that spores which develop from lysogenic spore-forming bacteria, e.g. *Bacillus megaterium* will contain prophage which, while it is within the spore, becomes as resistant to adverse environmental factors as the spore itself.

Phages which multiply by the lytic cycle are named 'virulent' while those capable of reduction to prophage are termed 'temperate'.

Transduction

There is a striking similarity between the phenomenon of lysogeny and latent or inapparent infection by animal viruses, but more remarkable is the fact that temperate phages are capable of transmitting genetic material from the cell which they have previously parasitized to another sensitive cell. Through this process of 'transduction', bacteria may become resistant to antibiotics or acquire a variety of new, permanent characteristics. For instance, non-toxic strains of diphtheria bacilli may acquire the ability to produce toxins when they become infected by prophages derived from toxin-forming strains, and, in the same way, new somatic antigens may be acquired by certain strains of *Salmonella*.

It is emphasised, however, that any gene can be transducted, but the incorporation of a new gene into a receptor cell is invariably accompanied by the loss of one of its own genes. (See Vol. 1, p. 24).

Bacteriocins

In 1925, it was discovered that filtrates of a strain of *E. coli* inhibited the growth of another strain of the same species and, subsequently, that the inhibitory substance, termed colicin, was lethal to the organism. Since then, more than twenty colicins have been recognised and similar antibiotic-like substances have been isolated from a variety of Gram-positive and Gram-negative organisms. These have been named according to the species of the donor host, e.g. pyocin from *Pseudomonas aeruginosa* and megacin from *Bacillus megaterium*, but the group as a whole are termed bacteriocins. Although bacteriocins are naturally host specific and usually act only against closely related organisms, some have a much wider spectrum of activity that includes genera other than that of the producer species.

Bacteriocins differ from antibiotics in that they are proteins and have a narrower antimicrobial spectrum. On the other hand, they have a good deal in common with bacteriophages and some types are identical to phages except that they are able to kill the cell but lack the ability to multiply within it. Like phages they act by adsorption of specific receptor sites on the host's cell wall but differ from phages by the fact that they are degraded by trypsin whereas phages are resistant to trypsin.

There are probably two types of bacteriocins, one consisting of phage-like particles or phage components such as head or tail, whereas the other is much smaller, invisible under the electron microscope and is probably a component of the cell wall of the producer organism. Large bacteriocins are thermolabile and are generally inactivated at 80°C or below, whereas small bacteriocins are thermostable and withstand boiling for several minutes. In some bacteriocins the DNA of the head is not injected into the susceptible host cell despite the fact that the particle has a contractile tail; the lethal effect being produced by the protein alone. Other forms have an empty head whilst a third type consists of the headless tail of a contractile phage. It is not known how one molecule of nonreplicating bacteriocin can exert its markedly bactericidal effects.

Because of the specificity of their action and the fact that producer strains are resistant to their own bacteriocin, some of them, e.g. colicins and pyocins have proved useful for 'typing' of enterobacteriaceae. (See Vol. 1, p. 96.)

Episomes

Plasmids, or episomes, are lengths of DNA existing

either in the cytoplasm or attached to the chromosomes of the bacterial cell. They replicate in synchrony with the bacterial chromosomes and are thus perpetuated as long as the parent strain persists. Both temperate phages and bacteriocins exist as episomes but there are many others such as the F factors and the drug-resistant factors (RTF agents). (See Vol. 1, p. 22).

Bacteriophage typing

Because phages are highly specific for the host cell in which they multiply their lytic effects may be used, like serological typing, for the precise identification of strains of bacteria within a genus or species. This method of 'phage typing' is of considerable value in epidemiological investigations of outbreaks of infection in human and some animal populations.

A number of phages, preferably those from lysogenic strains, are selected on the basis of the specificity of their host range. They are then grown on susceptible strains of bacteria which are numbered according to the phages, with the prefix PS for propagating strain. In order to reduce the chance of contamination and variation, the virus and its propagating strain should be preserved by freeze-drying.

Several methods are available for propagating bacteriophages but the freezing and thawing technique on solid medium is preferred when higher titres of virus are required. This consists of seeding the surface of a digest agar plate with a few drops of an overnight broth culture of the appropriate propagating strain. When the culture has been absorbed into the agar, the reconstituted phage is spread evenly over the whole of the dry surface of the agar medium, apart from a small triangular area which serves as a control. After overnight incubation, the bacterial growth in the control zone should show no evidence of lysogenicity, otherwise the plate is discarded. If confluent, the triangular area of surface growth is cut out with a sterile scalpel blade and the remaining agar frozen for one hour at $-60°C$. Thereafter, the agar is allowed to thaw at room temperature and the extruded fluid, containing the phage, is collected and centrifuged to remove bacterial cells and debris. The virus is then titrated by carefully pipetting small drops (0·02 ml) of decimal dilutions in peptone water on to the dry surface of a digest agar plate previously seeded with its propagating strain. After overnight incubation, a plaque count gives the number of virus particles in the preparation. The highest dilution of phage producing almost confluent lysis is taken as the Routine Test Dilution (RTD). If the titre is satisfactory, the phage suspension is filtered through a sintered glass or membrane filter and stored undiluted at 4°C or lyophilized for further propagation (Plates 39.1b and c, facing p. 444b).

In the typing technique, a small amount (0·01 ml) of each virus suspension is placed on separate squares on the surface of an agar plate previously seeded with a broth culture of the bacterial isolate to be tested. Drops of the typing phages are applied in a constant order but without touching the surface of the plate, lest some of the cultures being tested are lysogenic. After overnight incubation at 30°C, or for 6 hours at 37°C, the plates are examined and the complete pattern of lysis for each strain is recorded.

The virus-host cell reaction is not always strain-specific and many phages are active against a number of different strains within a species. However, the 'patterns' of lytic activity are reproducible within narrow limits and are usually sufficiently characteristic to determine the 'phage type' of the test organism.

Further reading

ADAMS M.H. (1952) Classification of bacterial viruses. Characteristics of the T5 species and of the T2, C16 species. *Journal of Bacteriology*, **64**, 387.

ADAMS M.H. (1959) *Bacteriophages*. Interscience: New York.

ARMSTRONG J.A., METZ D.H. AND YOUNG M.R. (1973) The mode of entry of vaccinia virus into L cells. *Journal of General Virology*, **21**, 533.

BALTIMORE D. (1969) The replication of picornaviruses. In, *The Biochemistry of Viruses*, ed. H.B. Levy, p. 101. London: Dekker.

BERTANI G. (1958) Lysogeny. *Advances in Virus Research*, **5**, 151.

BRADLEY D.E. (1971) A comparative study of the structure and biological properties of bacteriophages. In, *Comparative Virology*, eds, K. Maramorosch and E. Kurstak, p. 207. London: Academic Press.

CHAMPE S.P. (1963) Bacteriophage reproduction. *Annual Review of Microbiology*, **17**, 87.

COHEN S.S. (1955) Comparative biochemistry and virology. *Advances in Virus Research*, **3**, 1.

COHEN S.S. (1963) The biochemistry of viruses. *Annual Review of Biochemistry*, **32**, 83.

COLTER J.S. AND PARANCHYCH W. (1967) *The Molecular Biology of Viruses*. New York: Academic Press.

CRICK F.H.C. (1962) The genetic code. *Scientific American*, **207**, 67.

DALES S. (1965) Penetration of animal viruses into cells. *Progress in Medical Virology*, **7**, 1.

DATTA N. (1965) Infectious drug resistance. *British Medical Bulletin*, **21**, 254.

ERIKSON R.L. (1968) Replication of RNA viruses. *Annual Review of Microbiology*, **22**, 305.

FENNER F.J. AND WHITE D.O. (1971). *Medical Virology*. London: Academic Press.

FRAENKEL-CONRAT H. (1969) *The Chemistry and Biology of Viruses.* New York: Academic Press.

HAYES W. (1963) The bacteriophage model. In, *Mechanisms of Virus Infections*, Ed. W. Smith, Chapter 2. London: Academic Press.

HENRY C. AND YOUNGER J.S. (1963) Studies on the structure and replication of the nucleic acids of poliovirus. *Virology*, **21**, 162.

JOKLIK W.K. (1962) The multiplication of poxvirus DNA. *Cold Spring Harbor Symposia on Quantitative Biology*, **27**, 199.

JOKLIK W.K. (1968) The poxviruses. *Annual Review of Microbiology*, **22**, 371.

LURIA S.E. AND DARNELL J.E., JR. (1968) *General Virology*, 2nd Edition. New York: John Wiley.

LWOFF A. (1953) Lysogeny. *Bacteriological Reviews*, **17**, 269.

STANLEY N.F. (1967) Reoviruses. *British Medical Bulletin*, **23**, 150.

TOLMACH L.N. (1955) Attachment and penetration of cells by viruses. *Advances in Virus Research*, **3**, 63.

WATSON J.D. AND CRICK F.H.C. (1953) A structure for desoxyribose nucleic acids. *Nature*, **171**, 737.

WILLIAMS R.E.O. AND RIPPON J.E. (1952) Bacteriophage typing of *Staphylococcus aureus*. *Journal of Hygiene*, **50**, 320.

ZIMMERMANN E.F., HEETER M. AND DARNELL J.E. (1963) RNA synthesis in poliovirus infected cells. *Virology*, **19**, 400.

ZINDER N.D. (1955) RNA phages. *Annual Review of Microbiology*, **19**, 455.

CHAPTER 40

ADDITIONAL PROPERTIES OF ANIMAL VIRUSES AT THE CELLULAR LEVEL

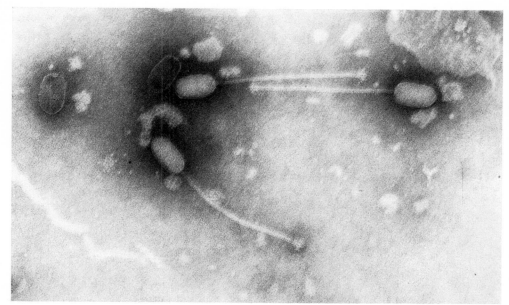

39.1a

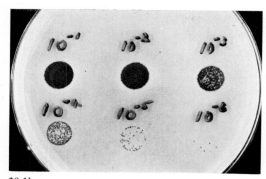

39.1b

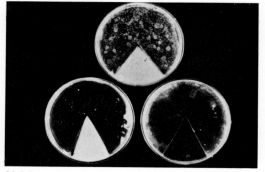

39.1c

39.1a Electron micrograph of staphylococcal phage (strain 3C/1), negatively stained with phosphotungstic acid, showing 'empty' and 'full' heads, long slender tails and terminal fibres, × 120 000.

39.1b Titration of bacteriophage on a nutrient agar plate seeded with a culture of the propagating strain (3C/1) of staphylococcus. Notice the individual plaques produced by the highest dilutions of the virus (10^{-5} and 10^{-6}).

39.1c Steps in the propagation of a bacteriophage. *Bottom left*: The bacterial cells of the propagating strain of staphylococcus have been lysed by the phage, except in the triangular control zone of bacterial growth which was not infected with the virus. *Bottom right*: After removal of the triangular control zone, the plate is 'snap-frozen' and virus-containing fluid expressed from the agar is harvested and sterilized by filtration. *Top centre*: This culture showing numerous foci of lysogenic staphylococcal colonies is unsuitable for propagation of phage and is discarded.

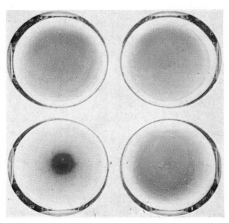

40.1a

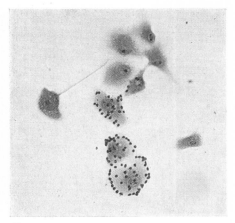

40.1b

40.1a Haemagglutination of fowl red blood cells by allantoic fluids harvested from 3 embryonated hens' eggs infected with Newcastle disease virus. Allantoic fluid from a fourth egg did not contain virus and a small raised button is formed at the foot of the well (lower left) by the normal sedimentation of the healthy erythrocytes.

40.1b A continuous line of sheep kidney cells persistently infected with Newcastle disease virus. The proportion of infected cells can be readily determined by counting the number of cells in the monolayer culture that are capable of attaching (haemadsorbing) normal guinea-pig erythrocytes. Haematoxylin eosin stain, × 106.

Additional properties of animal viruses at the cellular level

Virus mutation

Although viruses such as those of mumps in man and Newcastle disease in poultry are remarkably stable over many years, others like influenza A are strikingly labile and show a marked tendency to variation in some of their properties. Characteristically, all viruses replicate very quickly and, consequently, the less stable forms have high frequencies of variation. In actively growing cultures there is a continuous process of selective proliferation and survival which ultimately determines the dominant virus; and it is for this reason that influenza virus frequently assumes a new form and causes new epidemics. In contrast, mutants that remain antigenically stable but lose their pathogenicity are referred to as being 'attenuated'. An example is vaccinia virus which has retained antigens of variola virus but has lost the ability to produce smallpox.

Of the many different mutations that may occur, loss of virulence is probably the one which is most practically useful; others that have been recognized include increased rate of reproduction, extension of the natural host range, altered haemagglutination activity and changes of antigenic structure, plaque size, morphology or resistance to heat, drugs or other inhibitors. The selection of an attenuated mutant is usually obtained quite empirically, by deliberate rapid serial transfer of large doses of the chosen virus in unusual hosts such as laboratory animals, eggs or cell cultures; but especially in those of diminished susceptibility so that any fast growing mutant will have optimal conditions for survival. After many transfers in the secondary host, the mutant may be separated from the parent strain on monolayer cell cultures using the virus plaque techniques. In most instances the mutation is stable and since it was probably derived from not one but many mutational changes, there is little tendency for it to revert to full virulence in the abnormal host. This was well demonstrated many years ago by Pasteur's classical experiment in which the virulence of the "street" strain of rabies virus was altered to the avirulent fixed form (virus fixé) by serial passage in rabbits. Since then the fixed virus has been passed regularly at monthly intervals in rabbits without alteration in its characters. Thus, by retaining the antigens of rabies but without the power to cause disease, it is ideally suited as a safe and efficient agent for the production of anti-rabies vaccines. Although in general terms, the risk of back mutation is small, mutants can arise spontaneously since even a single passage involves enormous numbers of viral replicative cycles. Thus the possibility remains that attenuated strains of the more labile types of viruses, such as foot-and-mouth disease virus or some members of the myxovirus groups including Newcastle disease virus, may revert in the laboratory or under field conditions to full virulence.

Myxoviruses, and influenza viruses in particular, are extremely variable and it is of interest that the great pandemic of human influenza that swept throughout the world in 1918–19 with a total death role probably exceeding 25 million persons, was probably due to some accident of mutation.

Also about this time a new influenza-like disease suddenly appeared in swine in America which, because of its striking clinical and pathological similarity to human influenza virus, was called swine influenza. Although, at the time, the disease received little attention from virologists, subsequent investigations have tended to confirm the then popular opinion that it had arisen as a result of infection from man during the 1918 human influenza epidemic.

It is also interesting to recall that Newcastle disease, often considered to be a relatively new disease entity of poultry, apparently arose in Java sometime prior to 1926 and again appeared in the Spring of 1926 on a farm near Newcastle-on-Tyne, England. Although it has been suggested that the virus could have been passed to poultry from some unknown animal host with a latent or subclinical infection, it is also possible that the Newcastle disease virus was 'born' as a result of a series of accidental mutations of a related myxovirus or some other unknown virus.

Defective virus

When an intact infectious virus particle makes contact with a susceptible host cell there develop a number of reactions at the surface which lead to the release of the genetic material of the virus (viral genome) within the cell. This is immediately followed by a series of biosynthetic processes which may lead, if the conditions are favourable, to the formation of new viral proteins and nucleic acid and, ultimately, to the assembly, maturation and release of complete infectious virions. However, along with intact progeny virus, many immature forms as well as incomplete viral components may be developed and released into the external environment. On the other hand, in some systems the mature virions are inefficiently released by cultured cells even after a successful productive cycle, and in others a break may occur in the replication cycle prior to the stage of assembly and no mature virus is produced.

Upsets in the regulatory mechanisms associated with viral replication are particularly well illustrated by the temperate bacteriophage which may persist for long periods as prophage in lysogenic bacterial cells in which the viral genome becomes wholly integrated into the bacterial gene, without new virus being produced. Later, virus particles may appear spontaneously in the bacterial cell and the progeny viruses that are released are usually virulent and capable of infecting and lysing other susceptible cells. This sequence of events would suggest that part of the phage genome becomes integrated into and remains in the genetic apparatus of the host and is replicated at cell division. It is possible also that viral DNA may be integrated with the DNA of an animal cell since polyoma virus will transform cells in culture which readily form tumours when injected into another species of animal but do not produce new virus particles. It has also been shown recently that cells transformed by SV40 virus can be fused to other susceptible cells and the resulting heterokaryons give rise to a re-awakening of the viral genes and the release of new virus particles. An important feature of this phenomenon is that the DNA of the transforming virus is very similar to that of the cell whereas the DNA of viruses which do not cause transformation is different.

Similar defects in the replication cycle have been described with certain animal viruses that have lost the ability to perform any one of the essential steps required for successful replication and these viruses or strains have been termed defective viruses. There are a number of examples of defective animal viruses that persist in suseptible cells but, unlike

provirus which is difficult to detect in its host cell, the presence of persistent defective infections can readily be detected by several methods including resistance to superinfection with closely related strains, resistance to the curative effect of specific antisera, the production of interferon, immuno-fluorescent staining techniques and, in the case of myxoviruses in particular, by haemagglutination and haemadsorption methods. In certain circumstances, some defective viruses require the assistance of other so-called "helper" viruses before growth takes place. For example, a very small RNA virus called tobacco necrosis satellite virus grows only in plants already affected with tobacco necrosis virus. It is thought that the satellite virus has only sufficient RNA to code for its protein coat and that it is dependent on the larger virus to code for the enzymes required for RNA synthesis. In animal virology there are a number of similar examples of minute satellite viruses. In the DNA series the adeno-satellite virus (ASV) will only grow in the presence of the intact virion of adenovirus while the RNA-containing Rous sarcoma virus depends on help from a number of Rous-associated viruses (RAV). More recently, satellite viruses have been observed in negatively stained preparations of avian infectious bursal agent (gumboro disease) but their aetiological significance has not yet been determined. Successful replication of defective viruses occurs because the helper virus growing in the same cell provides the missing gene or part of the gene causing the functional abnormality. It has also been postulated that two viruses with defects in different genes can complement each other with the release of complete progeny of both viruses.

Incomplete virus

If embryonated eggs are inoculated with influenza virus at a high multiplicity, i.e. with an inoculum containing a high ratio of infective units to cells, the virus is produced with an abnormally low infectivity : haemagglutinin ratio (the von Magnus phenomenon). The virus produced in those circumstances is called incomplete virus, and although it is very similar in morphology to the standard virus, it is deficient in RNA and the fall in infectivity is even greater than the fall in RNA.

Incomplete virus can readily be produced in cell cultures by deliberate serial passage of undiluted influenza virus and there are now numerous examples of chronic infections of cell cultures, with myxoviruses in particular, where there is a disproportionately small yield of infectious virus relative to the quantity of virus-specific material manufactured by the cell, as demonstrated by haemadsorption and fluorescent antibody staining. In certain circumstances the production of incomplete virus is not only retarded but fails completely, and the terms 'abortive virus' and 'abortive infection' are sometimes used since the fault occurs after the replicative cycle has begun.

Lysogeny and latency
When infective phage nucleic acid enters a susceptible bacterial cell it may, on occasion, fail to initiate the synthesis of progeny virus and instead becomes attached to a specific site on the chromosome of the bacterium. In this state of lysogeny, as it is termed, the bacteriophage is reproduced together with the bacterial chromosome and is regularly transmitted at each cell division to the daughter cells along with the genetic material of the host bacterial cell itself. In this prophage state, the virus is indistinguishable from a specific genetic region of the bacterial chromosome.

In animal virus-infected cells the viral nucleic acid, especially of oncogenic viruses, may become integrated with the host cell chromosomes in a manner similar, but not identical, to lysogeny; and is known as latency.

Infection of the cell with two viruses
Whilst the mechanisms of infection and replication of an animal virus within a susceptible host cell have been described earlier (Chapter 39) it is emphasised that concurrent infection, even of a single cell, with two different viruses may occur. In these circumstances the following outcomes are possible.

Dual infection
That particles of two different viruses can enter the same host cell, replicate independently and produce their own characteristic type of infection is now well-known and has been clearly demonstrated in dog kidney cell cultures infected with canine distemper virus and infectious hepatitis (Rubarth's) virus. In this particular system, infected monolayers stained with anti-distemper serum conjugated with fluorescein isothiocyanate and Rubarth's disease antiserum conjugated with lissamine rhodamine B (RB200), clearly show the presence of particles of green staining antigen of distemper virus in the cytoplasm and areas of orange staining viral antigen of canine hepatitis virus in the nucleus of the same infected cell. In the human field, herpes and vaccinia viruses have also been observed to multiply independently in the same cell.

Recombination and complementation
Another form of interaction which may occur when two viruses are successfully cultivated in the same host cell system is known as recombination. Here the first virus influences the reproductive cycle of the second virus, and *vice versa*, so that if the infecting viruses are fairly closely related, progeny particles may be produced either with the identical characters of each parent or with inheritable properties (phenotype) of both parents. If in the latter case the progeny virus breeds true to itself, showing that it possesses its own genotype, recombination is considered to have taken place. The frequency with which recombination takes place largely depends on how close the genes are linked to one another on the linear viral chromosome. Genes closely linked have a low frequency of recombination whereas those situated further apart tend to have a proportionately higher frequency.

Geneticists have described numerous examples of recombination with bacterial viruses but there are relatively few clear examples of recombination taking place between animal viruses. Nevertheless some may do so, whether RNA or DNA viruses, and conclusive evidence has been obtained with influenza, poliovirus type 1 and several poxviruses. Much of the classical work with recombination between animal viruses has been accomplished with influenza and it has been repeatedly demonstrated, for example, that neuropathogenicity can be transferred from the neurotropic strain of influenza A (MEL) to the non-neurotropic influenza A (NWS). More recently, the fowl plague virus, which is closely related to influenza A, has been shown to recombine but Newcastle disease virus, which is more distantly related, does not combine despite extensive efforts to prove otherwise.

If a virus should lose, by mutation, the ability to perform some of the functions needed for replication it is termed a defective virus. Such a mutation need not be lethal and a virus may be able to survive indefinitely as provirus in the persistently infected host cell system. Should a second but non-defective virus enter the same cell it may supply the defective component for the first virus which can then replicate and mature normally. Moreover, should both viral strains in the same host cell carry defective mutations they may compensate for each other's lack, provided their respective mutations are dissimilar. This reaction of complementation differs from recombination since genetic characters are not exchanged and the newly acquired property of the progeny virus particle is not therefore heritable.

There are now a number of examples of defective viruses utilising the assistance of unrelated viruses to complete their reproductive cycles: and among animal viruses the Rous sarcoma virus is defective in that it depends for help on any one of a number of Rous-associated viruses (RAV).

Reactivation and multiplicity reactivation
If a mixture of heat-inactivated myxoma virus and

active fibroma virus is injected into a rabbit, myxomatosis results and the phenomenon is termed reactivation. This well recognised property of poxviruses can be demonstrated also in the developing chicken embryo or in cell cultures, but it does not occur when the actively multiplying virus is from another group. The reaction takes place whatever method is used to inactivate the virus provided the viral nucleic acid remains intact. Thus, it is possible that the function of the reactivating virus is to supply some essential non-genetic material which is lacking in the inactivated virus.

On the other hand, when a host cell, such as a susceptible bacterium, is simultaneously infected with either an irradiated and an untreated virus (bacteriophage) or with two or more irradiated viruses, 'multiplicity reactivation' may take place. Such reactivation occurs only with virus particles that are capable of recombination. Whilst the nucleic acids of inactivated viruses cannot readily multiply because of damage to specific nucleic acid sites by radiation, the phenomenon is explained by assuming that the damaged parents may exchange certain components (viral genomes) among themselves until a complete molecule is formed which can then replicate to produce intact new virions.

Exaltation

In some mixed infections one virus may enhance the growth of a second virus and the reaction may be demonstrated not only with certain pairs of unrelated viruses but also, on occasion, with different mutants of the same virus. Unfortunately, it is not yet clear whether exaltation is due to interaction of the two viruses at the gene level or whether early penetration of the one virus is facilitated by an enzyme activated by the other virus. In veterinary medicine, exaltation of bovine papular stomatitis virus has been reported with rinderpest virus, while in the so-called 'END-test' there is enhancement between the viruses of Newcastle disease and swine fever in primary cultures of pig kidney cells. In the laboratory there is evidence of the enhancement of rabies virus by the virus of lymphocytic choriomeningitis (LCM), although the latter inhibits the formation of plaques produced in chicken embryo fibroblasts by Newcastle disease virus and some other animal viruses.

Interference

In contrast to 'dual infection', laboratory investigations have shown that in certain circumstances entry of one virus into a cell may so modify the cell that multiplication of a second virus is inhibited. The phenomenon which is termed interference or cell blockage, can readily be demonstrated between many different viruses in several animal species and by various routes of inoculation. The interference phenomenon is not, however, an inevitable result of inoculation of two viruses into a single host, for only certain viruses will interfere with one another.

One of the earliest experiments on interference was carried out in 1935 by Hoskins who discovered that an attenuated neurotropic variant of yellow fever virus protected monkeys against a fatal infection with virulent viscerotropic yellow fever virus. Two years later Findlay and MacCallum confirmed these findings and showed that the phenomenon is in no way related to classical humoral or non-specific forms of immunity. They demonstrated this by protecting monkeys with an injection of the antigenically unrelated Rift Valley fever virus, which caused only mild illness, against a lethal dose of yellow fever virus. In a series of similar experiments it has been shown that monkeys infected with a benign strain of lymphocytic choriomeningitis virus (LCM) do not develop symptoms of paralysis when challenged with virulent poliomyelitis virus. In this case, the protection afforded by the LCM virus lasted for about a fortnight but the animals' susceptibility to the poliomyelitis virus was restored after about a month. Although the viruses used in these two examples are unrelated and immunologically distinct, there are numerous instances of interference occurring between pairs of immunologically related viruses and even between two strains of a single virus. Thus, infection with influenza A virus may protect susceptible host cells against subsequent invasion by a secondary strain of influenza A or by the more distantly related mumps or Newcastle disease viruses. There is evidence also, that under field conditions the use of live attenuated rinderpest vaccine protects cattle by interference against the virulent field strain of virus before active immunity has had time to develop.

The normal procedure for demonstrating interference is to inoculate the first or interfering virus into the susceptible host system, be it animal, embryonated egg or cell culture, allow a few days for viral multiplication to take place in the animal (or hours in the chick embryo or cell culture), and then follow with the inoculation of the second or indicator virus. If the dosage and timing are correct, the full growth of the second virus is prevented and occasionally it can be shown that if the two viruses are given simultaneously, multiplication of both viruses is inhibited; but usually extensive multiplication of the interfering virus is necessary before growth of the challenge virus is totally prevented.

Mechanism of viral interference

Although the mechanism of interference action is not yet clearly understood, it has been shown that animal viruses may interfere with each other at different stages of infection and perhaps in a number of different ways. For example, (1) Newcastle disease virus prevents attachment or adsorption of a second virus by destroying the surface receptor sites of the host cell while, (2) certain leukaemia viruses are thought to inhibit an essential biosynthetic step in viral eclipse. Both of these events take place at a very early stage in the growth cycle of the challenge virus. On the other hand, (3) interference between different antigenic types of poliovirus occurs at a later stage and is probably due to competition of the RNA of the two viruses for certain essential substrates, key enzymes or for limiting replication sites.

Knowledge of the mechanisms involved in viral interference was greatly extended by the discovery that one variety, at least, of interference is due to the formation and release of a soluble protein from virus-infected cells. This virus-inhibiting substance was named interferon.

Interferon

Interferon was discovered by Isaacs and Lindenmann in 1957 during their studies on the effect of ultra-violet irradiated influenza virus on fragments of chick chorioallantoic membrane maintained in an artificial medium. After several hours of incubation the supernatant fluids from the cultures, although devoid of viral particles, contained a soluble substance which inhibited the multiplication of active influenza virus in fresh cultures. It was subsequently shown that interferons were produced by living cells of many different types in cell cultures, embryonated eggs or in laboratory animals infected by almost any animal virus, either DNA or RNA.

Characteristics of the interferon molecule

Studies of purified interferon from various sources show that it is a small protein containing all, or nearly all, amino acids but without nucleic acid and with a low molecular weight of about 25–45 000. It is thermostable at 4°C and resists heating at 50°C for 1 hour. Interferon from chick tissues is somewhat more stable than mouse or rabbit interferon and will retain about half its activity even after one hour at 70°C. Interferon is active through a wide range of pH values, is unusually stable at low pH and, unlike viruses, it can resist a long exposure to pH2. It is relatively non-toxic, is weakly antigenic and cannot be neutralized by the specific antiserum against the virus used to make it. Interferon is not self replicative nor is its activity affected by high speed centrifugation sufficient to sediment most viruses. The interferon molecule possesses the properties of proteins in that it is not dialyzable, but is inactivated by proteolytic enzymes such as trypsin and can be concentrated by precipitation with ammonium sulphate. It is not affected by treatment with receptor destroying enzyme, RNase, DNase or periodate.

Production of interferon

There are many factors which affect the synthesis and mode of action of interferon but the most important are the nature of the inducer virus, the type and species of the infected host cell and the temperature of incubation.

The Virus. In general, viruses that multiply readily and produce marked cytopathic effects (CPE) tend to be poor inducers, whereas viruses that multiply more slowly and do little damage to the cells usually produce fairly large quantities of interferon. Notable exceptions are togaviruses which multiply rapidly, produce a marked CPE and are, together with myxoviruses, amongst the best inducers of interferon. Picornaviruses, including enteroviruses, and many DNA viruses such as herpesviruses are poor inducers; poxviruses occupy an intermediate position but adenoviruses are non-inductive and almost totally insensitive to the effects of interferon. Similarly, inactivated viruses are usually better inducers than live viruses and in certain cases infectious virions will only induce interferon production in cells previously treated with the inactivated virus.

The Cell. Synthesis of interferon begins soon after viral maturation is initiated and, if there is no great damage to the cells, will continue to be manufactured and released extracellularly for 20–50 hours. When the cells survive beyond this time, they cannot produce interferon again, even if re-infected, until they have divided at least twice. Of practical importance in viral titrations is the fact that the dilutions containing large amounts of virus may be less effective than smaller inocula since the former may contain enough interferon to block viral infection and subsequent cycles of multiplication.

Interferon can be produced in many different types of cells varying from embryonic cells from chickens and mammals to primary, secondary and continuous cell cultures of human and animal tissues. The amount of interferon produced by continuous cell lines is low and special assay methods are generally required to detect it. As already mentioned, interferons can be produced by many different types of virus and are not virus specific. On the other hand they show a marked cell species specificity in both their production and in their effects. For example, purified interferon prepared from chick cells infected with influenza virus (a RNA virus) is similar to that produced by *Herpes simplex* (a DNA virus). Also, interferon generally inhibits viral replication most effectively in cells derived from the animal species in which the interferon has been produced. That is to say, interferon produced in chicks will protect chick cells but not mouse cells against a wide variety of viruses; and, conversely, mouse interferon does not protect chick cells.

In a given cell culture, different amounts of interferon are required to provide comparable levels of protection against different viruses. In chick fibroblasts roughly 30 times more interferon is needed to cause the same degree of interference with Newcastle disease virus as with some togaviruses.

The age of the cell may also play a part in determining the amount of interferon produced. Cells from 6-day-old chick embryos have a lower capacity to synthesise interferon than cells from 11-day-old embryos. Similarly, unweaned mice produce much less interferon than adult mice and young animals may, therefore, be more susceptible to virus infections than adults.

Temperature. The temperature at which the preparations are held greatly influences the yield of interferon but in most experiments 35–37°C is preferred. Viruses with a low optimal temperature for growth (35°C) usually produce large amounts of interferon whereas those that replicate best at higher temperatures (40°C) tend to induce little or none. This would suggest that viruses which multiply optimally at 35°C are likely to be seriously affected *in vivo* by pyrexia. It is also of interest that experiments with mice infected with Coxsackie B virus show that large amounts of interferon are produced and there is no mortality when adult mice are held at room temperature; whereas at 4°C interferon is not produced, many of the animals die and high titres of virus appear in the heart and some other organs.

Other factors. The antiviral effects of interferon may also be inhibited by low pH, increased oxygenation or by the addition of certain steroids including cortisone and various chemical carcinogens such as methylcolanthrene.

Assay of interferon

The earlier methods of testing for interferon activity by protecting laboratory animals, embryonated eggs or cell cultures from the destructive effect of a challenge virus have now been largely replaced by the more convenient and much more accurate method of virus plaque reduction. In this technique, monolayers of cells prepared in small disposable Petri dishes are pre-treated with interferon and then inoculated with a known number of plaque forming units (p.f.u.) of a test virus such as vesicular stomatitis. This virus is especially suitable since it not only forms good plaques on many species of cell but is also very sensitive to the effects of interferon.

Many preparations of interferon are of low potency and require to be concentrated in order to increase their activity. This can be done as follows:

(1) dialysis against polyethylene glycol (Carbowax 20M) at 4°C for 3–4 days to obtain a ten-fold concentration of interferon;

(2) simple evaporation of dialysed preparations by an electric fan for 5–6 hours, the residues being dissolved in medium using one tenth of the original volume, and

(3) freeze-drying in the presence of gelatin.

The mode of action of interferon

Little is known either about the mode of action of interferon or even of the specific portion of the virus particle necessary for the stimulation of interferon production, but it is generally agreed that adsorption, penetration and uncoating of the virus proceeds normally in interferon-treated cells. However, since synthesis of progeny virus and even of infectious RNA is prevented, this would suggest that the action of interferon takes place at a relatively early stage in the growth cycle. Whatever the precise mechanisms of interferon action might be it is undoubtedly true that both RNA and DNA viruses can be inhibited. Since in many RNA viruses the viral RNA itself functions as mRNA while in those viruses whose genome is DNA the mRNA is transcribed from the viral DNA, it is possible that interferon acts by preventing the early translation of viral mRNA into virus-specific proteins and other information transcribed from the viral genome. More recent evidence also suggests that interferon may act by inducing a cellular gene to synthesise a cellular mRNA that is not normally produced following viral infection and which, in turn, directs the synthesis of a new cellular protein. This cell-coded protein, known as the 'translation-inhibitory protein' (TIP) is believed to interfere with the combination of viral mRNA with cellular ribosomes to form functional polysomes on which the viral proteins are normally synthesised. Because TIP inhibits the translation of viral mRNA, the proteins required for the replication of the viral RNA are not made and the viral nucleic acid is not replicated. In the case of cells infected with one particular picornavirus, interferon has been shown to prevent even the early inhibition of host RNA synthesis.

The biological significance of interferon

The production of interferon is, in effect, a particular response of a cell to infection with a virus, and frequently occurs *in vivo* as well as *in vitro*. In fact, the formation of interferon is not a rare event to be found only in association with the phenomenon of viral interference but rather it is a very common reaction whereby cells, groups of cells or even whole animals protect themselves against virus multiplication.

The outcome of a virus disease may depend on the balance between the production of infectious virus on the one hand and the synthesis of interferon on the other. If the balance is in favour of the virus the animal may die, but where interferon production predominates the amount of virus is greatly reduced and the animal survives. The relationship between cells, viruses and interferons is complex but there is now little doubt that it plays an important role in non-immune defences and, like the immune mechanism, is an essential factor in the body's defences. The protection afforded by interferon appears to be specially useful because it develops more promptly than antibody formation. However, viral interference is clearly independent of any specific response of the host cell to the antigens of the inducer virus and is, therefore, quite distinct from immunity. Unlike antibody which is produced by specialized cells of the body and which is the other anti-viral protein produced by animals infected by virus, interferon can be produced by virtually any type of cell following suitable stimulation. Antibody combines directly with the virus and its anti-viral activity is specifically directed against the antigenic type of virus which stimulated the antibody formation, whereas interferon shows no viral specificity and will inhibit the growth of virtually all animal viruses. Moreover, the anti-viral action of interferon, unlike that of antibody, is specific for the animal species and interferon produced in cells of one species will generally protect cells from only the same or closely related species. Antibody, unlike interferon, cannot penetrate living cells and cannot, therefore, prevent intracellular viral multiplication or the intracellular transfer of viruses such as *Herpes simplex* that can spread directly from cell to cell. In some instances recovery from viral infections may take place in the absence of antibody and, conversely, there is recent evidence that the formation of detectable amounts of neutralizing antibody may not result in clinical recovery. Moreover, the ability of patients with hypogammaglobulinaemia to recover from viral infection, although they are particularly susceptible to bacterial infection, suggests that other factors apart from the small amount of antibody they produce may be responsible for their recovery.

Interferon is manufactured early in the course of virus infection and appears in the blood stream of experimentally infected animals only a few hours after intravenous inoculation with large amounts of inducer virus. However, due to its rapid uptake by cells lining the vasculature, the high titres of interferon obtained following intravenous inoculation of virus falls approximately thirty-fold every hour. The cells most responsible for the production of interferon include tissue macrophages, blood mononuclear cells and polymorphs. The fact that macrophages from immune animals may produce three times as much interferon as macrophages from susceptible animals when challenged with the homologous virus, suggests also that there may be an important relationship between the mechanisms of interferon production and immunity. Although the production of interferon may be slower in animals inoculated by other routes, it usually continues for about one to three days when the cell becomes refractory to further synthesis for a period of a few days.

In many virus infections, clinical recovery may occur before the development of detectable levels of antibody and in short-lived infections such as influenza this recovery may be due to the very early production of interferon since there is good evidence that the fall in virus titre begins just before the interferon titre reaches its peak. For the same reason, the administration of attenuated rinderpest virus vaccines in the field gives rise to appreciable levels of interferon in the blood within six hours and cattle are protected against virulent strains of rinderpest virus twenty-four hours post-inoculation, long before the development of neutralizing antibodies.

Possible therapeutic uses
There is little doubt that interferons play an important protective role in certain virus infections. Theoretically at least, interferon could be the ideal therapeutic agent in certain virus infections because of its broad anti-viral spectrum, its lack of toxicity for host cells, its poor antigenicity and its very high activity. Its main disadvantages, at present, are that it is difficult to produce in large amounts, is effective over relatively short periods and cannot be used to block viral synthesis once it has been initiated within the cell. Interferons are most likely to be used for prophylaxis rather than cure especially since they are most effective when administered several hours before the virus.

In man, interferon produced on monkey kidney cells infected with influenza type A virus inhibits the development of the lesions of primary smallpox vaccination, and a similar interferon has been used successfully in the treatment of vaccinial keratitis. Also, smallpox vaccination may not 'take' in children recently inoculated with live measles virus vaccine at the peak of the circulating interferon titre. In animal experiments, interferon has been used to protect mice against challenge by ectromelia and mouse hepatitis viruses. Rabbits can be protected against intradermal vaccinia virus infection by interferon produced in rabbit kidney cells, and guinea-pigs can be protected against rabies by the subcutaneous and intramuscular inoculation of interferon. In chickens, interferon appears to inhibit the subsequent progress of Rous sarcoma virus-induced tumour formation and similar inoculations of hamsters inhibit the development of tumours due to polyoma virus. Since they are species-specific, the interferons used must be produced in homologous cells and, in every case, both the interferon and the challenge virus must be given by the same route.

In order to protect animals against systemic viral infections, interferons must reach the vulnerable cells in time to inhibit subsequent viral multiplication. Other difficulties to be overcome are the effects of dilution of the interferon by body fluids and its inactivation by proteolytic enzymes. It seems unlikely, therefore, that interferons will be of much practical value in anti-viral therapy in the immediate future except, perhaps, for the control of localised viral diseases in which greater concentrations of interferon can be maintained.

Non-viral induced interferons (See also p. 465).
Other substances have been discovered that can induce cells to produce interferon. These include certain non-viral nucleic acids, rickettsiae, bacterial endotoxins and bacteria (e.g. *Brucella* and *Haemophilus*). It is emphasised, however, that the interferons produced in a particular host cell are very similar whatever the nature of the inducer.

Stimulon and blocker
Substances having properties entirely opposite to those of interferons have been described in cultures of rat-embryo cells infected with adenovirus type 12. These non-viral substances which also enhance the growth of the rat K virus appear to act by inhibiting the production of interferon, and are called 'enhancers' or 'stimulons'.

An additional inhibitor of interferon production called 'blocker' has been detected in crude preparations of interferon. It differs from stimulon or enhancer since it is not destroyed by pepsin or trypsin.

Haemagglutination
The exciting and all important discovery that many animal viruses are capable of agglutinating red blood cells was described independently by Hirst (1941), and McClelland and Hare (1941) while working with embryonated hens' eggs infected with influenza virus. They observed that the red blood cells in allantoic fluids, harvested without an attempt to prevent bleeding, would clump and quickly settle out of the fluid. No agglutination occurred with similar egg fluids containing no virus and the phenomenon, which is now called viral haemagglutination, was readily reproducible *in vitro* simply by mixing influenza virus with a suspension of freshly drawn chicken red cells in saline. The appearance of the clumps of agglutinated erythrocytes which settled to form a thin, lace-like veil or mesh of cells covering the bottom of the tube provided an easily visible and direct means of recognising the presence

of an influenza virus and, significantly, of measuring its amount. The effect is in marked contrast to the small raised button that is formed at the foot of the tube by the normal sedimentation of healthy erythrocytes in the absence of virus (Plate 40.1a, facing p. 445). It was soon discovered that haemagglutination was not an exclusive property of influenza viruses but occurred with other viruses as well; that erythrocytes other than avian cells were also susceptible and that the phenomenon could be blocked specifically by antisera.

All types of influenza virus and most members of the paramyxovirus group possess the capacity to haemagglutinate. Other haemagglutinating viruses include some poxviruses, e.g. variola, vaccinia and ectromelia, all of the reoviruses, the majority of togaviruses, a few enteroviruses and some unclassified viruses.

The nature of the haemagglutinin varies greatly among the different viral groups and even from virus to virus within a group. In most haemagglutinating viruses, whether they belong to the myxovirus, togavirus, reovirus or adenovirus groups, the haemagglutinin is an integral part of the virus or of the envelope surrounding the virion. In this respect it differs from the haemagglutinin of poxviruses which is separable from the intact infectious particle and consists of a phospholipid–protein complex which is smaller than the virion and is not so readily sedimented by centrifugation.

Mechanism of haemagglutination
The actual mechanism of haemagglutination is not yet fully understood but it is generally agreed that while the haemagglutinating viruses are capable of adhering to the surface of susceptible erythrocytes, they do not penetrate and infect them as occurs with susceptible tissue cells. Electron micrographs clearly show that most haemagglutinating viruses possess a surface fringe of short spike-like processes which function as enzymes and which attach themselves to highly specialized areas on the surface of the red blood cell. These receptive areas on the erythrocyte consist largely of complex carbohydrate groupings called mucopolysaccharides which are sticky substances closely related chemically to the mucins of the air passages. During haemagglutination large numbers of virions become attached to the surfaces of the susceptible red blood cells, and if two erythrocytes each carrying a few virus particles collide, they will stick together. Although it is not clear whether physical adsorption of the virus particle on to the surface of the erythrocyte, or specific attachment due to the interaction of the viral enzyme and the substrate groups, plays the more important role in the mechanism of haemagglutination, a network of protoplasmic bridges is formed between the cells.

These bridges fasten the erythrocytes together until large clumps (aggregates) of red blood cells are formed and gently settle to the bottom of the tube.

Various species of erythrocytes may be used to demonstrate haemagglutination but, in practice, human group 'O', chicken and guinea-pig cells are mostly used. With togaviruses, red blood cells from newly hatched chicks or adult geese are preferred. In general, the composition of the suspending medium and the conditions of pH and temperature are not very critical, and haemagglutination may occur over a wide pH range (5·0–9·0 for most viruses) but a slightly alkaline pH is best. In some cases, however, (e.g. togaviruses) the conditions are critical and even the species of red cell is important. With certain viruses (e.g. influenza and Newcastle disease viruses) the haemagglutinin is formed early in the replication cycle and can be demonstrated in immature or incomplete virus which is not yet infective. Defective and 'incomplete virus' or intact virus particles which have been rendered non-infectious by treatment with heat, formalin or ether retain the ability to haemagglutinate susceptible red blood cells.

Elution

If large quantities of virus are used for haemagglutination and allowed to act on red blood cells for a long period of time, the agglutinated erythrocytes shed the virus particles which then float freely in the suspending fluid and neither attach to the cells nor agglutinate them. This disaggregation of the clumped erythrocytes, which is accompanied by a sudden, sharp rise in the titre of virus in the suspending fluid, is due to the carbohydrate groupings of the receptors on the cell surface having become exhausted or destroyed by enzyme activity. This process of dissociation or elution as it is called, usually occurs most rapidly following incubation at 37°C. (Plate 42.16a–d, between pp. 504 and 505). At 0°C the enzyme

responsible for altering the surface cell receptors is less active and little release of virus occurs.

After elution has been completed the affected erythrocyte is permanently altered and, while the released virus is still capable of haemagglutinating a fresh batch of red blood cells, the 'exhausted' erythrocytes can no longer combine with the virus or even with a new batch of similar virus, because the affected cells have lost their receptors and cannot regenerate them. Thus, red blood cells stabilized for a given influenza virus or other myxovirus are inagglutinable by the same virus although they may be subsequently agglutinated by another virus of these two families. Because of this, it has been possible to arrange the members of the influenza group and some paramyxoviruses in a definite series, called the 'receptor gradient'; thus, any particular virus named in the gradient will destroy the red cell receptors for itself and for those viruses listed below it in the series, but not those above it. It has been shown that red blood cells treated with influenza C virus can be agglutinated by other species (e.g. mumps and Newcastle disease) but not by influenza C again. In the same way, cells treated with Newcastle disease virus can be agglutinated by influenza A or B strains but not by either Newcastle disease, mumps or other myxoviruses lower down the receptor gradient. The order of viruses on the receptor gradient, starting with those having the weakest action on cell receptors, is shown in Table 40.1.

It has been suggested that the order of viruses in the receptor gradient series is due to the presence of individual enzymes for each viral species enabling them to act on different parts of the cellular receptor sites. There is evidence that the enzymes responsible are serologically distinct, and that they differ both quantitatively and in their mode of attachment to the cell receptors. Members of the parainfluenza group, except perhaps Sendai virus (parainfluenza 1) whose activity may lie between Newcastle disease

TABLE 40.1 The receptor gradient.

Strain of haemagglutinating virus	Virus strain applied to treated red blood cells.						
	Influenza C	Mumps	Newcastle disease	Influenza A (MEL)	Influenza B (Lee)	Swine Influenza	Influenza B (Mil.)
Control cells (untreated)	+	+	+	+	+	+	+
Influenza C	—	+	+	+	+	+	+
Mumps	—	—	+	+	+	+	+
Newcastle disease	—	—	—	+	+	+	+
Influenza A (MEL)	—	—	—	—	+	+	+
Influenza B (Lee)	—	—	—	—	—	+	+
Swine influenza	—	—	—	—	—	—	+
Influenza B (Mil.)	—	—	—	—	—	—	—

+ = haemagglutination.

and influenza A, do not appear to fall into the gradient.

The enzyme of the virus particle that is responsible for elution of the virus from agglutinated cells is called 'neuraminidase'. However, not all haemagglutinating viruses possess this enzyme and it is of interest that most togaviruses, 'incomplete myxoviruses' and certain other haemaglutinating viruses do not possess neuraminidase and therefore do not elute from agglutinated red cells.

Studies on viral neuraminidase have shown that enzymes having similar properties can be produced by several types of bacteria. The one most closely resembling the viral enzyme is formed by the bacterium causing Asiatic cholera (*Vibrio cholerae*) and is called 'receptor-destroying enzyme' or, simply, RDE. This enzyme, which can be purified and concentrated by normal chemical methods, renders susceptible red blood cells totally inagglutinable by any of the myxoviruses and also by some others, including polyoma virus, which seem to neutralize the same receptors. Thus, the receptor destroying reaction is enzymic in nature and the cell surface receptor which is a neuraminic acid-containing mucopolysaccharide, is attacked specifically by the virus enzyme, neuraminidase. Haemagglutination and elution are affected differently by higher temperatures of incubation and, with most myxoviruses, heating to 56°C for 30 minutes will destroy the eluting but not the haemagglutinating ability of the virus. Such heated virus is known as 'indicator virus'.

Role of receptor destroying enzyme in infection

Most types of host cells possess receptors for myxoviruses similar to those found on red blood cells, and these receptors probably assist in the attachment of viruses to susceptible host tissue cells. For this reason, haemagglutination can probably be regarded as a model of the first stage of the natural infection of cells.

If it is accepted that certain viruses must first become attached to the surface receptors before they can enter a susceptible tissue cell and initiate infection, then it is theoretically possible to protect an animal against virus attack by temporarily destroying the receptors. Indeed, it has been shown in experiments with mice and chicken embryos that susceptible host cells treated with RDE were rendered insusceptible to virus action and no signs of disease followed the inoculation of a challenge virus. Unfortunately, the beneficial effects were short-lived since the surface of a tissue cell is constantly being remade and the receptor areas destroyed by RDE are usually regenerated in 48 hours' time when the animal again becomes susceptible to infection. Thus, the method seems to have little or no practical advantage. The function of viral neuraminidase is not yet known but its ability to destroy the attachment of intact virions to cells suggests that it plays an important role in the release of progeny virus at the completion of a successful replication cycle. However, in natural infections and with myxoviruses in particular, the viral enzyme may actually assist in overcoming the defence mechanisms of the host by destroying the mucoproteins or inhibitor substances in the film of mucus that lines the respiratory passages, thereby preventing the virus being destroyed and allowing it to adsorb and enter the cell. The importance of the enzyme in the infectious process is supported by recent evidence showing that mature and morphologically complete Newcastle disease virus cannot initiate a replication cycle if it lacks or cannot code for neuraminidase.

Practical applications of haemagglutination

The haemagglutination reaction has a number of important applications in virology. In the diagnostic laboratory it can be used as a rapid method for detecting the presence of a haemagglutinating virus in embryonated egg and cell culture fluids and, indeed, the existence of a number of previously unknown viruses has been discovered simply by adding a few drops of egg or culture fluid to a weak suspension (0·5–1·0 per cent) of red blood cells which are then observed for the development of haemagglutination. Similarly, the amount of virus in a suspension can be estimated (titrated) by a simple dilution technique using healthy erythrocytes as indicator. In most cases approximately 10^6 virus particles are required to give a positive test although the virus particles need not always be in the infectious form. Thus, the method is much less sensitive than titration by infectivity and the haemagglutination titre is not necessarily related to the infective titre.

Viral haemagglutination is readily prevented or blocked by an antiserum specific to the infecting strain, and inhibition of haemagglutination provides a rapid and reliable method of identifying an unknown virus isolate (Plate 42.16, between pp. 504 and 505). The test is highly specific and permits the accurate identification not only of members of different groups of haemagglutinating viruses but also of members of the same group. Among the influenza viruses, the haemagglutination-inhibition test can be used to distinguish, for example, human influenza A from swine influenza or even from other strains of human influenza A. On the other hand, strains of Newcastle disease virus which differ widely in their biological properties cannot be differentiated by haemagglutination-inhibition although their ability to agglutinate chicken but not, say, horse erythrocytes may be helpful in conjunction with some other tests in differentiating lentogenic from velogenic strains (Chapter 43). Since haemagglutination-inhibition is sensitive enough in some instances for distinguishing between variants within the same species, it is especially useful for studies of those virus groups consisting of many serotypes; and cross haemagglutination-inhibition tests are invaluable in delineating subgroups of myxoviruses, togaviruses and adenoviruses. An additional and extremely important practical advantage of viral haemagglutination is its use in testing sera for antibodies which block agglutination. Therefore, the haemagglutination-inhibition test which, as we have seen, is useful for the identification of viruses, also provides a reliable serological test for (1) detecting exposure to infection, (2) assessing the efficacy of viral vaccines, and (3) for epidemiological investigations of diseases caused by haemagglutinating viruses.

Although group specific reactions are obtained with the haemagglutinating strains of chlamydiae and poxviruses, type specific responses are the rule with myxoviruses, adenoviruses and also, to a limited extent with some togaviruses (*vide supra*). In general, haemagglutination-inhibiting antibodies are intermediate in specificity between complement-fixing antibodies on the one hand and serum neutralizing antibodies on the other. Also, the haemagglutination-inhibition test is somewhat more sensitive than the complement-fixation test and about the same degree of sensitivity as the serum neutralization test. In togavirus and some other infections, haemagglutination-inhibiting antibodies usually persist longer than complement-fixing antibodies and the choice of test must be made accordingly.

Since many viruses readily elute from agglutinated erythrocytes under conditions which are not optimal for adsorption, viral haemagglutination can be used as a method of virus purification and concentration. This is done by adding freshly drawn erythrocytes to a crude infected fluid at the optimum temperature for adsorption (e.g. 4°C). As soon as agglutination takes place the deposited red cells are washed, resedimented and the supernatant fluid discarded. A smaller volume, say one-tenth, of fresh diluent is then added to the deposit of red cells and the virus is eluted either by increasing the temperature of incubation to 37°C or, more rapidly, by adding RDE. Thus, the virus has been purified and concentrated approximately ten-fold. The method is simple to perform, and is especially useful for separating virus particles from the particulate matter which abounds in egg fluids and does not adhere to red cells. It can also be used to separate a haemagglutinating virus from a mixed population containing both haemagglutinating and non-haemagglutinating viruses. Moreover, since treated red cells cannot be agglutinated again by the same virus, the eluted erythrocytes can be used to adsorb and remove a second haemagglutinating virus from a mixed population containing the first haemagglutinating virus.

Further discussion of viral haemagglutination and details of the procedure for carrying out haemagglutination-inhibition tests are included in Chapter 42.

Haemadsorption

In 1957, Vogel and Shelokov showed that the addition of red blood cells to monolayer cell cultures infected with an haemagglutinating virus causes the erythrocytes to be adsorbed on to the surface of individually infected cells, but not of healthy cells, in the monolayer. The phenomenon is termed haemadsorption (Plate 40.1b, facing p. 445).

Most haemagglutinating viruses induce haemadsorption of erythrocytes but some such as adenoviruses and reoviruses do not. Conversely, most haemadsorbing viruses haemagglutinate. However, African swine fever virus (which does not appear to haemagglutinate red blood cells) haemadsorbs swine and hamster erythrocytes at 37°C, and the ability of infected swine leucocyte cultures to adsorb healthy pig red blood cells is the basis of an important diagnostic test for African swine fever (Chapter 57). It is interesting also that among the haemadsorbing viruses that haemagglutinate, all but an unassigned virus isolated from the intestinal tract of cattle (the Haden virus) are ether sensitive.

There is, as yet, no clear understanding of the mechanisms of viral haemadsorption, but it is generally agreed that since much of the surface of the infected tissue cell consists of viral protein, the entire cell behaves as if it were a single large virus particle and the indicator red cells are adsorbed directly on to its altered surface. Immunofluorescence studies suggest that haemadsorption is dependent on the amount of viral antigen being extruded from the cell and that when the cytoplasmic stores diminish, haemadsorption is absent. Electron micrographs also show that haemadsorption occurs when red cells adhere to mature virus particles as they are extruded from the surface of the infected cell.

Haemadsorption is of value in detecting the presence in cell cultures of certain viruses, notably strains of the parainfluenza types that do not produce visible cytopathic lesions in infected cultures or which show haemadsorption before the cytopathic effects become apparent. Indeed, the existence of several previously unknown viruses was first discovered by this method.

Compared with haemagglutination, the haemadsorption technique is an even simpler and more direct indicator of infection in tissue cultures, and is performed as follows.

After 2 or 3 days of incubation the infected tissue culture fluids are removed and 0·2 ml of a sterile 0·4 per cent suspension of washed erythrocytes (chick, guinea-pig, sheep or human cells may be used) is added to each tube whether or not a cytopathic effect has occurred. The tubes are inclined for 10–15 minutes at 4°C, 22°C or in an incubator at 37°C, rinsed briefly with sterile buffered saline to resuspend the settled red blood cells, and then examined under low magnification. Positive haemadsorption is detected by firm adhesion of the erythrocytes which must not float across the monolayer when the tubes are gently agitated. Individual infected cells can be demonstrated and the ratio of infected to healthy cells determined in stained coverslip cultures.

Haemadsorption-inhibition tests have been developed on similar lines to those of haemagglutination-inhibition tests. Both reactions are highly specific and the extent to which a serum is able to inhibit haemadsorption or haemagglutination is a measure of its antibody content.

A mixed haemadsorption test (Chapter 42) has also been devised to detect and identify viral antigens in cell cultures infected with certain viruses such as *Herpes simplex*, which do not possess haemadsorbing or haemagglutinating properties.

Further reading

ALMEIDA, J. D. AND MORRIS, R. (1973) Antigenically related viruses associated with Infections Bursal Disease. *Journal of General Virology*, **20**, 369.

ANDERSON K. (1942) Dual virus infection of single cells. *American Journal of Pathology*, **18**, 577.

BARON S. (1967) Host defences during virus infections. In, *Modern Trends in Medical Virology* I, eds. R.B. Heath and A.P. Waterson. London: Butterworth.

BURNET F.M. AND LIND P.E. (1952) Studies on recombination with influenza viruses in the chick embryo. III. Reciprocal genetic interaction between two influenza virus strains. *Australian Journal of Experimental Biology and Medicine*, **30**, 469.

BURNET F.M. AND STONE J.D. (1947) The receptor-destroying enzyme of *V. cholerae*. *Australian Journal of Experimental Biology and Medicine*, **25**, 227.

BURKE D.C. AND SKEHEL J.J. (1967) Interferons and other cell products influencing viral multiplication. *British Medical Bulletin*, **23**, 109.

BUZZELL A. AND HANIG M. (1958) The mechanism of haemagglutination by influenza virus. *Advances in Virus Research*, **5**, 289.

FENNER F. AND COMBEN B.M. (1958) Genetic studies with mammalian poxviruses. I. Demonstration of recombination between two strains of vaccinia virus. *Virology*, **5**, 530.

FENNER F. AND SAMBROOK J.F. (1964) The genetics of animal viruses. *Annual Review of Microbiology*, **18**, 47.

FENNER F. AND WOODROOFE G. (1960) The reactivation of poxviruses. II. The range of reactivating viruses. *Virology*, **11**, 185.

FINDLAY G.M. AND MACCALLUM F.O. (1937) An interference phenomenon in relation to yellow fever and other viruses. *Journal of Pathology and Bacteriology*, **44**, 405.

FRANKLIN R.M. AND BREITENFELD P.M. (1959) The abortive infection of Earle's L-cells by fowl plague virus. *Virology*, **8**, 293.

FRASER K.B. (1967) Defective and delayed myxovirus infections. *British Medical Bulletin*, **23**, 178.

GINSBERG H.S. (1958) The significance of the viral carrier state in tissue culture systems. *Progress in Medical Virology*, **1**, 36.

HIRST G.K. (1941) The agglutination of red blood cells by allantoic fluid of chick embryos infected with influenza virus. *Science*, **94**, 22.

HO M. (1962) Interferons. *New England Journal of Medicine*, **266**, 1313.

HOSKINS J.M. (1959) Host-controlled variation in animal viruses. In, *Virus Growth and Variation*, Eds. A. Isaacs and B.W. Lacey, p. 122, London: Cambridge University Press.

HOTCHIN J. (1971) A concept of persistent virus infection. In, *Viruses affecting Man and Animals*, eds. M. Saunders and M. Schaeffer, p. 213, St. Louis: Warren H. Green.

HUANG A.S. AND BALTIMORE D. (1970) Defective viral particles and viral disease processes. *Nature*, **226**, 325.

ISAACS A. (1963) Interferon. *Advances in Virus Research*, **10**, 1.

ISAACS A. AND EDNEY M. (1950) Interference between inactive and active influenza viruses in the chick embryo. IV. The early stages of virus multiplication and interference. *Australian Journal of Experimental Biology and Medicine*, **28**, 635.

ISAACS A. AND LINDEMANN J. (1957) Virus interference. I. The interferon. II. Some properties of interferon. *Proceedings of the Royal Society, London*, **147B**, 258 and 268.

KLEINSCHMIDT W.J. AND MURPHY E.B. (1965) Investigations on interferon induced by statolon. *Virology*, **27**, 484.

KUMAGAI T., SHIMIZU T., IKEDA S. AND MATUMOTO M. (1961) A new *in vitro* method (END) for detection and measurement of hog cholera virus and its antibody by means of effect of HC virus on Newcastle disease virus in swine tissue culture. I. Establishment of standard procedure. *Journal of Immunology*, **87**, 245.

LOCKART R.Z. (1967) Recent progress on interferons. *Progress in Medical Virology*, **9**, 451.

VON MAGNUS P. (1951) Propagation of the PR8 strain of influenza virus in chick embryos. II. The formation of 'incomplete' virus following inoculation of large doses of seed virus. *Acta pathologica et microbiologica Scandinavica*, **28**, 278.

McCLELLAND L. AND HARE R. (1941) The adsorption of influenza virus by red cells and a new *in vitro* method of measuring antibodies for influenza virus. *Canadian Public Health Journal*, **32**, 530.

RAPP F. (1969) Defective DNA animal viruses. *Annual Review of Microbiology*, **23**, 293.

ROSEN L. (1964) Haemagglutination. In, *Techniques in Experimental Virology*, ed. R.J.C. Harris, p. 257, London: Academic Press.

RUSTIGIAN R. (1966) Persistent infection of cells in culture by measles virus. I. Development and characteristics of HeLa sublines persistently infected with complete virus. *Journal of Bacteriology*, **92**, 1792.

VOGEL J. AND SHELOKOV A. (1957). Adsorption — haemagglutination test for influenza virus in monkey kidney tissue culture. *Science*, **126**, 358.

WALKER D.L. (1964) The viral carrier state in animal cell cultures. *Progress in Medical Virology*, **6**, 111.

WALKER D.L. AND HINZE H.C. (1962) A carrier state of mumps virus in human conjunctival cells. I. General characteristics. *Journal of Experimental Medicine*, **116**, 739.

CHAPTER 41

INACTIVATING AGENTS, CHEMOTHERAPY AND VACCINES

Inactivating agents, chemotherapy and vaccines

The effects of physical and chemical agents on viruses
Some antiviral agents show a more pronounced action on one viral component than on another and, for this reason, they are generally classified as nucleotropic, proteotropic, lipotropic and universal (unselective) agents. Nucleotropic agents include ultraviolet light of 2600 Å wavelength, formalin, nitrous acid and hydroxylamine. Proteolytic substances are ultraviolet light of 2350 Å wavelength, heat, acid pH and proteolytic enzymes such as trypsin. Many viruses possess lipid-containing envelopes and, accordingly, are sensitive to a variety of 'fat-solvents' including alcoholic ether, chloroform, bile salt (sodium deoxycholate) and lipase or other lipolytic enzymes. The unselective group of agents includes x-rays, alkylating agents (e.g. ethylene oxide) and photodynamic action.

The properties of some of these agents are as follows.

Temperature
Many viruses are extremely labile and may survive outside the body for only a few hours. In the laboratory great care must be taken to ensure that virus suspensions and specimens of diseased tissues are stored with a minimum of delay at —40°C or preferably at —70°C. Other viruses including poxviruses and enteroviruses are more stable at room temperature and may survive under ordinary atmospheric conditions for prolonged periods.

Some viruses are partially inactivated by the process of freezing and thawing, and should not be handled oftener than is necessary. Viruses are resistant to extremes of cold and are best preserved by drying from the frozen state, using the method of freeze drying. The majority can be stored for many months or years in sealed glass ampoules in liquid nitrogen (—196°C) or in a refrigeration cabinet at —70° or —90°C. Specimens in containers with loosely-fitting caps must not be preserved in 'dry-ice' because released carbon-dioxide readily destroys most viruses. Pseudorabies is unusual in that it can be stored at +4°C. or —70°C but does not survive for long at —20°C.

Most animal viruses are inactivated by moderate heat at 56°C for 30 minutes, or at 100°C for a few seconds, due to denaturation of the protein component of the viral capsid. Differences in thermo-resistance have been used extensively in virus taxonomy. The addition of either salts containing divalent cations or small amounts of protein increases the thermostability of many viruses.

pH variation
Acid-stability is employed extensively for the differentiation of viruses. In general, most viruses remain viable within the ranges of pH 5–9 but are quickly inactivated by extreme acidity or alkalinity; though there are some notable exceptions. For instance, rhinoviruses are readily destroyed at pH 5.3 whereas enteroviruses retain their infectivity at pH 2.2. On the other hand, certain properties like haemagglutination by togaviruses are greatly influenced by slight variations of pH.

Ultraviolet irradiation
It is well known that direct sunlight exerts a lethal effect on microorganisms due to the ultraviolet rays it contains.

Ultraviolet radiation belongs to the same general category as light, x-rays and radiowaves. They are all forms of electromagnetic radiation and have the same speed of travel, namely 300 000 km (186 000 miles) per second. The difference between these forms of radiation lies in the wave-length concerned. The shortest are x-rays (c. 1Å) and the longest are special radio waves used for radio communication with wavelengths of several thousands of metres. Only a very small range of wavelengths are visible to the unaided human eye. These are ordinary light waves (4000–7000 Å); the range of colours in the spectrum being due to different wavelengths within this band. The 4000 Å waves are the shortest and produce the sensation of violet. Ultraviolet is immediately beyond the violet and extends down to a wavelength of about 40 Å. Just as light displays different effects according to the wavelength so, too does ultraviolet.

For practical purposes the different effects of ultraviolet rays according to the wavelength in question have been classified into three groups:

(1) The u.v.-A group (3150–4000 Å) corresponds to the u.v. rays in sunlight. They pass through most kinds of glass but have no erythemic action.

(2) The rays of the u.v.-B group (2800–3150 Å) have a pigmenting and erythemic action. They also form vitamin D and are mainly used for therapeutic purposes (sunlamps).

(3) The rays of the u.v.-C group (below 2800 Å), sometimes referred to as short-wave ultraviolet, have a strong germicidal action, and may also cause erythema and conjunctivitis. Most kinds of glass absorb rays of the u.v.-C group.

Short-wave ultraviolet light of 2600 and 2350 Å acts on viral nucleic acids and viral proteins, respectively. However, the method is somewhat inconvenient to use because the rays are readily absorbed by substances in biological media and the risk of virus particles escaping inactivation is high.

For air disinfection of a laboratory a relatively low intensity of germicidal radiation is spread evenly throughout the room, the object being to disinfect the air and not to provide high intensity radiation of the surfaces of walls and ceilings. For maximum efficiency of air disinfection each individual ray should travel the maximum distance possible before being absorbed by some obstructing surface. Good mixing of upper and lower air is essential for efficient sterilization but, unfortunately, this does not obtain in many situations and the method may be inadequate and even hazardous. In some laboratories, mercury vapour lamps emitting u.v. light with a wavelength of 2537 Å are inserted in input air ducts to sterilize air. For surface disinfection high intensity radiation is provided by a number of u.v. lamps placed in close proximity to the object or surfaces to be disinfected.

Personnel must be protected from the harmful effects of ultraviolet light and should not be permitted to enter laboratories where more than 90 per cent disinfection of air is desired, since the intensity of the irradiation becomes too high particularly in rooms with low ceilings and highly reflective wall surfaces.

Formaldehyde

A water solution of formaldehyde (formalin) is widely used for the production of inactivated virus-vaccines. It reacts mainly with amino groups in nucleic acids and proteins. However, since those of double-stranded nucleic acids are usually not accessible to formalin, its nucleotropic effects are mainly directed against single-stranded nucleic acids which are present in most RNA viruses. Thus, in the case of double-stranded DNA viruses formalin inactivation depends upon reaction with the amino groups of the protein. In the preparation of inactivated vaccines care must be taken to use the minimum concentration of formalin lest the antigenicity of the virus is impaired. Because of this, correct interpretation of the survival curve is vital.

Lipid solvents

Most viruses with lipid-containing envelopes are readily inactivated with ether, chloroform, sodium deoxycholate, phospholipase or other lipid solvents; and the reaction is widely used in the classification of viruses.

Glycerol

Although most vegetative bacteria are readily destroyed by a 50 per cent solution of glycerol, many viruses survive satisfactorily in glycerol-saline for several months or years. Indeed, the vaccinia virus in calf lymph used for vaccination against smallpox is preserved and kept free of bacteria by this means. It is of interest, however, that *Chlamydia* (PLGV agents) and a few viruses, including rinderpest virus, survive for less time in glycerol-saline than many bacteria.

Disinfectants

The most efficient of the more commonly used disinfectant substances are oxidizing agents such as hydrogen peroxide, potassium permanganate and hypochlorites (e.g. Chloros). Formalin is effective but slower in its action. Phenol and certain cresol disinfectants (e.g. lysol) are active against only a few viruses and are not recommended for material contaminated by foot-and-mouth disease virus. Caustic soda and washing soda are highly effective but have a number of practical disadvantages. The gaseous disinfectant, ethylene oxide, is highly lethal to most microorganisms and spores, and is of particular value for sterilizing plastic and rubber materials liable to be damaged by heat. A mixture of 10 per cent ethylene oxide in CO_2 is useful for the sterilization of viruses. Infected materials are placed in a cabinet from which the air has been withdrawn by vacuum and the mixture containing ethylene oxide is introduced to a pressure of 5–30 lb/in^2 above atmospheric pressure. The cabinet is then maintained at 45–55°C for several hours or overnight.

Antibiotics

Antibiotic and chemotherapeutic substances such as sulphonamides, penicillin, streptomycin and the tetracyclines do not effect viruses and are incorporated routinely in cell culture media to prevent bacterial contamination.

In recent years, a number of substances have been found to inhibit viral replication and field trials with N-methylisatin β-thiosemicarbazone suggest that it has a prophylactic effect in contacts of cases of smallpox. The prophylactic and therapeutic effects of a number of other anti-viral agents have been described but their practical value is uncertain (*vide infra*).

Chemotherapy of viral diseases

The rapid development of antibiotic therapy stems from the discovery by Chain and Florey in 1940 that penicillin could be made into an effective chemotherapeutic substance for the treatment and control of many bacterial infections. Since then, an ever increasing number of antibiotics, e.g. streptomycin, chloramphenicol and the tetracyclines have been discovered that inhibit the growth of a wide range of pathogenic and non-pathogenic bacteria in human and animal hosts. Also susceptible to antibiotics are those obligatory intracellular microorganisms such as rickettsiae and chlamydiae which resemble bacteria in that they have cell-walls, multiply by binary fission and are not wholly dependent on the biosynthetic activities of the host cell for their reproduction. The most effective drugs against this class of organisms are the tetracyclines which largely act by interfering with the synthesis of cell-wall mucopeptides in susceptible strains.

Viruses, on the other hand, do not resemble bacteria either in structure or mode of replication and antibiotics which act by inhibiting cell-wall synthesis (e.g. penicillin) or cell-wall formation (e.g. polymyxin) are wholly ineffective against viral infections. Nevertheless, recent laboratory investigations have shown that the growth cycle of several RNA and DNA viruses may be interrupted in cell cultures and, occasionally, in experimentally infected animals by a wide range of chemical compounds and by a few antibiotics also.

Despite these encouraging observations it is unfortunate that most of the drugs with anti-viral activity have proved to be highly cytotoxic and cannot safely be used in trials against virus diseases of man and animals. Another major obstacle in the search for effective anti-viral drugs is the intimate relationship which exists between virus and cell and, for this reason, it is possible that virus-specific inhibition may function in a number of different ways. Theoretically, the drug may act directly on the virus thereby preventing its adsorption and penetration of the cell, or by interfering with one or more of the complex biosynthetic steps in the replicative cycle, or by blocking the processes of assembly and maturation of the progeny virus.

It is well known that virus particles are frequently present outside the cell or attached to the cell membrane during the period of adsorption, but there is little merit in attempting to attack extracellular virus with antiviral drugs since, in most virus diseases, viral multiplication resulting in cellular damage or death is probably nearing completion by the time the first clinical symptoms appear. For the same reason, specific antibody, which is extremely effective for removing extracellular virus, cannot normally penetrate intact living cells and cannot, therefore, inhibit the virus growth cycle once it has started. Nor can it prevent the successful transfer of infectious virus particles, (e.g. *Herpes simplex*), that pass directly from cell to cell. There is evidence also that the therapeutic potency of an antiserum is not necessarily related to its content of neutralizing antibody and that antibody is not the major factor in the recovery of an animal from a viral infection. Often, in the early stages of recovery, antibody is undetectable in amount, and administration of significant quantities of specific antibody frequently fails to affect the course of the disease. On the other hand, the prophylactic role of antibody is indisputable.

The search for antiviral agents

Since, by definition, the growth of a virus depends on the metabolism of the host cell, it is reasonable to suppose that antiviral drugs offering most chance of success under field conditions will be those that act against one of the many complex biosynthetic steps in the replicative cycle of the virus without causing damage to neighbouring infected cells. This may be achieved merely by blocking or inhibiting one of the virus-specific enzymes that appear in infected cells during the growth cycle of the invading virus.

In recent years, the literature on the subject of antiviral chemotherapy shows that there is an ever-increasing number and variety of chemical compounds that can inhibit viral multiplication, and these substances are being tested for their efficacies in the treatment and control of disease under natural conditions.

The efficacy of chemical or biological antiviral agents is usually tested, in the first instance, in laboratory animals, chicken embryos or cell cultures. In animals, different routes of inoculation may be used but the intraperitoneal method is usually preferred since the test substance is most completely and rapidly absorbed by this means. Mice are generally regarded as the most suitable animals for the study of antiviral drugs since they are susceptible to a wide range of viruses. Rabbits are also useful, especially for quantitative and qualitative studies of drugs applied topically in cases of corneal and conjunctival infections caused by *Herpes simplex* and vaccinia viruses. The use of embryonated eggs has the advantage that antiviral substances injected by different routes persist at a high concentration because they are neither excreted nor degraded to any great extent. In many cases the efficacy of the test drug can be accurately evaluated by significant reductions in the number of pocks formed on the chorioallantoic membrane. As in many other branches of virology, cell cultures are being used increasingly to evaluate the effects of antiviral substances. Quantitative studies can conveniently be carried out by a modified plaque assay method in which filter-paper discs impregnated with the test drug at various concentrations are placed on the surface of an agar overlay. The principle of the test is similar to that of the antibiotic disc-diffusion technique in bacteriology where the effect of the drug is assessed by the degree of inhibition of cytopathogenicity as indicated by the width of the plaque produced on the stained monolayer by the infecting virus.

It must be emphasized that whatever methods are used in the laboratory to evaluate the efficacy of an antiviral agent, the results obtained in field trials may be very different from those *in vitro*. For example, drugs that are active in cell culture systems may be destroyed or rapidly excreted when administered to animals, or may produce toxic effects, allergic reactions and even occasionally anaphylactic shock. Because of these difficulties and the considerable gaps in knowledge of the chemical processes involved in viral replication, the search for reliable therapeutic agents is still almost entirely empirical.

Nevertheless, a number of compounds have been discovered, albeit in many cases by chance, which possess the ability to inhibit viral activity both *in vitro* and *in vivo*, and which offer promise for the future. Not all of these compounds are of practical value, but they are included in this chapter to illustrate principles.

Inhibitors of viral penetration

Amantadine. Very few antiviral substances act directly against extracellular virus but there are a number of chemical agents capable of altering the receptor areas of cell membranes, thereby preventing adsorption of the virus to the surface of the susceptible host cell. It is unlikely, however, that these substances will be of practical value since they would have to be administered before multiplication of the virus has taken place and could not, therefore, alter the course of a clinical illness.

On the other hand, amantadine, a tricyclic amine, while not affecting the process of adsorption is believed to act by blocking or interfering with the penetration of viruses into susceptible cells. Reports on the antiviral range of amantadine show that it inhibits the multiplication of a number of myxoviruses in cultures of chick embryo fibroblasts. Most strains of influenza A and C, Sendai and rubella viruses are sensitive, whereas influenza B, strains of parainfluenza types 1, 2 and 3, measles, mumps and Newcastle disease viruses are resistant. In general, all DNA viruses are also resistant.

Although experiments with laboratory animals show that amantadine does not protect animals completely, it does produce a significant reduction in the mortality rate especially if the drug is given orally or parenterally immediately before viral challenge. Trials with human volunteers during an epidemic of influenza also show that amantadine greatly reduces the clinical illness and the infection rate, but has no effect on the course of the disease. These limited observations suggest that the prophylactic use of amantadine and similar compounds is likely to be more successful than its therapeutic use; as is the case with most other antiviral agents.

Cyclooctylamine hydrochloride. This substance has properties very similar to those of amantadine hydrochloride and is also active against a wide range of RNA viruses.

Isoquinolines. These compounds have an inhibitory *in vitro* effect on the neuraminidases present on the surface of ortho- and paramyxoviruses. However, the effect does not appear to be directly on the viral enzyme but may involve interaction with the virus envelope, thereby blocking the uncoating of the virion and the release of the viral RNA.

Purine and pyrimidine antagonists

Iododeoxyuridine (IUDR). The halogenated pyramidines are a group of substances which have long been known to inhibit nucleic acid synthesis of tissue cells and some of them have been regarded as possible anti-tumour agents. The use of these compounds in human malignant disease led to the discovery that they could block not only cellular DNA synthesis but the replication of viral DNA also. Recent work has confirmed these earlier observations and it is now known that three of the halogenated deoxyuridines, namely 5-iodo-2'-deoxyuridine (IUDR) and its bromine (BUDR) and fluorine (FUDR) equivalents show marked antiviral activity when tested in cell cultures or laboratory animals infected with a wide range of DNA-containing viruses, e.g. vaccinia and *Herpes simplex*. The mechanisms by which halogenated deoxyuridines exert their antiviral activities are not clearly understood, but it is generally believed that IUDR interferes with the replication of DNA viruses either by preventing the incorporation of one of the four bases, thymidine, into the viral DNA strand, or by being itself substituted for equivalent amounts of thymidine into the viral DNA to form 'fraudulent' nonfunctional nucleic acid. Since IUDR normally acts in the final stages of viral replication it is also possible that it inhibits the action of the DNA-dependent RNA polymerases and blocks the formation of messenger RNA (mRNA), resulting in the formation of defective virus enzymes and incomplete capsid proteins. In electron micrographs of cells infected with herpesvirus and treated with IUDR, an unusually large number of the virions are seen to possess hollow central cores indicating a possible fault in the assembly of the viral components.

While there is no doubt of the therapeutic value of IUDR it is, unfortunately, too toxic to be given systemically in man, and evidence of its efficacy for systemic viral infections in animals has not been established. Nevertheless, it can be administered locally without danger and encouraging results have been obtained in the treatment of human cases of herpetic ulceration of the cornea. In animals, experimental infections of the cornea with *Herpesvirus hominis* or vaccinia heal more rapidly if treated with IUDR. Whilst this confirms the practicability of IUDR as a therapeutic substance there is already evidence of the emergence of IUDR resistant strains of herpes and vaccinia viruses.

Unlike IUDR and BUDR, the third member of the complex, FUDR, has no selective action on the virus and shows marked effects on both virus synthesis and cell growth in culture. The difference is due to the fact that IUDR and BUDR do not prevent DNA synthesis but are incorporated into the DNA strand in place of thymidine, thereby producing defective DNA particles, whereas FUDR inhibits DNA synthesis by blocking the synthesis of thymidilic acid.

Thiosemicarbazones

Methisazone Another class of antimicrobial compounds, the thiosemicarbazones, were originally introduced into chemotherapy for use in the treatment of tuberculosis. A later observation that one member of the group, p-aminobenzaldehyde thiosemicarbazone, could partially protect mice or chick embryos against infection with vaccinia virus was the first description of a true antiviral compound. Three years later, in 1953, it was found that isatin β-thiosemicarbazone (IBT) was considerably more active than p-aminobenzaldehyde thiosemicarbazone and, in 1960, the synthetic N-methyl and N-ethyl derivatives were shown to be more active than IBT itself.

In cell cultures, IBT inhibits the multiplication of members of the orthopoxvirus group, but not of other viruses. The drug does not reduce synthesis of viral DNA nor interfere with normal production of the two enzymes thymidine kinase and DNA polymerase which are intimately concerned in DNA synthesis. Instead, it probably acts late in the viral replication cycle at the level of translation and interfers with the normal synthesis of viral messenger RNA (mRNA) which is rendered unstable and prevented from combining with the cellular ribosomes to form polyribosomes and, ultimately, late viral proteins.

Equally encouraging results have been obtained with some of the newer thiosemicarbazone derivatives one of which, N-methylisatin β-thiosemicarbazone (methisazone), has an antiviral activity greater than that of the parent compound. Methisazone, later known as Marboran, has been shown in a successful prophylactic trial to greatly reduce the incidence and severity of smallpox when administered to contacts of human smallpox cases within one to two days after exposure. Although Marboran is of considerable practical use for the control of smallpox in man, it failed as a therapeutic agent in patients already suffering from the disease. This was not unexpected since typical lesions appear and develop into pustules only after viral multiplication has reached a maximum, by which time antiviral chemotherapy is mostly ineffective.

Inhibitors of polyribonucleotide synthetic activity

The appearance of new polyribonucleotide synthetic activity induced by RNA viruses in animal hosts is now well established. Because this enzyme activity appears to be characteristic of RNA virus-infected cells, and is not demonstrable in uninfected cells, it seems possible that some viral inhibitors may function by the inhibition of such enzyme systems.

The discovery of this new class of antiviral compounds has been described recently following studies of the metabolites produced by certain fungi. One of these, aranotin, obtained from the mould *Arachniotus aureus*, inhibits poliovirus replication in cell cultures with relatively low toxicity for mammalian cells, and a similar metabolite (designated LL-S88α) formed by strains of *Aspergillus terreus* inhibits the multiplication in cell cultures of Coxsackie virus A21, parainfluenza virus types 1, 2 and 3 and certain strains of rhinovirus. It also shows some *in vivo* activity and protects mice against lethal infections produced by certain coxsackie and influenza viruses. The mode of action of aranotin, and related mould metabolites, is thought to be due to their ability to inhibit the replication of viral RNA by virus induced RNA-dependent RNA polymerase without inhibiting normal cellular DNA-dependent RNA polymerase.

Other antiviral substances

Hydroxybenzylbenzimidazole (HBB) and guanidine. Other compounds that are active against RNA viruses include 2 (α-hydroxybenzl)-benzimidazole (HBB) and guanidine. These two compounds, which have different chemical structures but similar antiviral activities, inhibit the replication of the single stranded RNA of many enteroviruses including polio, coxsackie and ECHO viruses. Although their spectra of activities are similar and both are completely non-toxic for host cells, neither is of value for the treatment or prophylaxis of viral infections in animals due, it is believed, to the rapidity with which drug-resistant mutants can emerge.

Arabinosyl nucleosides During recent investigations of many other classes of chemical compounds having antiviral or antitumour properties, increasing interest is being paid to the arabinosides, e.g. the 5-halogenated uracil arabinosides, thymine arabinoside and especially 1-β-D-arabinofuranosyl cytosine (ara-C) and 9-β-D-arabinofuranosyl adenine (ara-A).

The most promising of the arabinosides at the present time is adenine arabinoside (ara-A). It is markedly active in cell cultures against human strains of *Herpesvirus hominis*, varicella-zoster, cytomegalovirus and vaccinia. In experimentally infected animals it is effective both topically for *Herpesvirus hominis* conjunctivitis and systemically for encephalitis due to vaccinia or *Herpesvirus hominis* type 1 or 2. It has no apparent effect on RNA viruses. Arabinose cytosine (ara-C) which is inhibitory towards numerous DNA viruses, as well as the RNA rhabdovirus of rabies, has been used effectively against *Herpes simplex* virus and vaccinia virus in the rabbit eye. Although it is cytotoxic for several mammalian cell lines, encouraging results have been obtained against *Herpes simplex* virus keratitis in humans. There is also evidence that it inhibits various neoplasms in mice, rats and humans.

Among other compounds that exert inhibitory activity towards several tumours in mice is one of the xylosides, 9-β-D-xylofuranosyladenine (Xyl-A). This compound also shows marked inhibition of viral multiplication and prevents the cytopathic effect of *Herpes simplex* virus in HeLa cells.

A new anti-tumour agent, designated 173t, has been obtained from the extracellular slime produced by cultures of *Pseudomonas aeruginosa*. There is no detectable *in vitro* effect with this agent, but a single high dose of the drug is active against newly-transplanted sarcoma tumours in mice. The fact that 173t is particularly effective against well established murine tumours suggests that it may also prove useful in the chemotherapy of certain cancers in man. The drug is not cytotoxic to mammalian cells and appears to act by interfering with nucleic acid metabolism.

Rifampicin. Rifampicin is a hydrazone derivative of an antibiotic called rifamycin B which is produced by *Streptomyces mediterranei*. It inhibits the multiplication of bacteria, chlamydiae and bacteriophages by binding to the DNA-dependent RNA polymerase and preventing the stabilization of the DNA-enzyme complex. Recent reports indicate that rifampicin also inhibits the replication of poxviruses in mammalian cells, but drug-resistant mutants have already been obtained.

Inhibition of vaccinia replication requires relatively large concentrations (100 μg/ml) of the agent but this does not have any significant effect on the growth of mouse embryo cells in culture. The activity of the compound appears to interfere with the synthesis of virus-specific proteins, rather than viral RNA, late in infection; but the method by which this is achieved is not yet clear. It has also been suggested that rifampicin may interfere with the synthesis of some viral messenger RNA by a viral RNA polymerase which functions late in the developmental cycle.

Rifampicin has no effect on the multiplication of most RNA viruses nor on the multiplication of herpes- or papovaviruses, but adenoviruses may be sensitive.

It has been reported recently that lymphocytes of human patients with leukaemia contain an enzyme capable of making DNA from an RNA template. This enzyme appears to be an RNA-directed DNA polymerase similar to the 'reverse transcriptase' found in leukoviruses and which is capable of synthesising copies of the virus genome. These virus-induced genes can, in turn, be integrated within the host cell chromosomes. As a result of this discovery it may be possible to purify the viral enzyme and use it as a screen for agents that will inhibit the RNA-directed DNA polymerase but leave the normal cellular DNA-dependent DNA polymerase unharmed. In this connection, it is interesting to note that encouraging results have already been obtained using rifamycin and its analogues, and it is hoped that such substances may form the basis for possible therapy in leukaemia and other virus-induced cancers.

Interferon inducers. Interferons are small soluble proteins produced by many types of cells *in vitro* and *in vivo* within a few hours after infection with living or inactivated virus. They suppress the growth of a wide range of related and unrelated viruses, whether DNA or RNA, in other cells by blocking the synthesis of new viral nucleic acid.

When interferon was first described, it seemed to provide the almost perfect method of curing virus diseases, simply by isolating and administering an inhibiting substance that the body itself produced. Unfortunately, the results of clinical trials with interferon have generally proved disappointing and one of the major difficulties that has arisen is the fact that interferons are species specific so that those produced in chicken cells will cure only poultry while those for use in human ailments must be produced in human or primate cells, and so on. Despite considerable progress in our understanding of the mechanisms of interferon action it seems unlikely that methods will be devised, in the near future, whereby sufficient quantities of long-acting interferon will be produced for use in therapeutic and prophylactic trials against systemic viral infections of man and animals; although pre-formed interferon tested against certain localized infections in man and animals has been used, and with encouraging results.

Apart from using pre-formed interferon, the use of 'harmless' viruses to induce interferon formation is of limited value since the formation of viral antibodies means that each 'inducer virus' can be used only once.

A more recent and probably more rewarding approach to the problem is based on the finding that the administration of 'inducer substances', other than viruses, stimulates cells to produce interferons which are not species specific. Of particular interest, in this connection, was the discovery in 1961 of statolon, a polyionic polysaccharide isolated from cultures of the fungus *Penicillium stoloniferum* and a similar product called helenine which is produced by *Penicillium funiculosum*. Both of these antibiotics have wide antiviral spectra and act by stimulating the formation of interferon in animals and tissue cultures. The precise mechanisms of formation of endogenous interferon by these non-viral inducers remained obscure until it was discovered, in 1969, that the active principle of statolon and helenine was a contaminating fungal virus (mycophage) which has its genetic information encoded in double-stranded RNA. Since that time it has become apparent that naturally occurring double-stranded RNA's, including the double-stranded replicative form of RNA-containing animal viruses, possess greater interferon-inducing capacity than single-stranded RNA's; perhaps because of their greater resistance to ribonuclease. Also, since double-stranded DNA is not an interferon inducer, it has been postulated that a DNA-RNA hybrid may be the inducer of interferon in cells infected with DNA-containing viruses. Thus, in the search for other inducer substances the emphasis has been on compounds which mimic double-stranded RNA. Several such substances have been discovered and investigated but, in most cases, the presence of undesirable side-effects severely limits their clinical value. A notable exception is tilorone hydrochloride, a fluorenone compound derived from coal tar which was shown in 1970 to be an extremely active but non-toxic interferon producer when administered orally to mice, and also an effective prophylactic agent against a number of DNA and RNA viruses. If these preliminary observations are confirmed it is likely that other substances will be found that are also capable of boosting the body's first line of defence against many, if not all, viruses by stimulating the production of substances similar to interferon which will protect the cell against viral challenge.

In addition to its ability to stimulate the formation of interferon, statolon may also possess antiviral activity against a number of oncogenic virus systems. Recent evidence shows that it inhibits the growth of Friend leukaemia virus infection in mice and of mouse sarcoma virus in mouse embryo tissue culture. Optimal protection with statolon against mouse leukaemia viruses is obtained when the drug is administered 24 hours before inoculation, while a single injection of the drug affords significant protection in mice for at least a month. In cell cultures, the antiviral effects of statolon can be demonstrated by adding the drug 24 hours before virus inoculation or by adding the drug at the same time as the virus, or 24 hours later.

At the present time, the most widely used of the various species of double-stranded RNAs known to act as interferon inducers is the synthetic polynucleotide pair polyriboinosinic acid polyribocytidylic acid (poly I·poly C). When given to animals by topical or parental administration, poly I·poly C is associated with a rapid rise in interferon levels and protection against local or systemic viral infections. Not only is the antiviral activity of poly I·poly C intimately associated with its interferon-inducing properties, but recent evidence indicates that it protects mice against a number of bacterial and protozoal infections, suppresses the growth of malignant tumours in mice and may even act as an adjuvant in antibody formation induced by influenza virus-vaccines.

Despite the considerable amount of research being carried out on possible antiviral substances, the reward has been very modest so far, and there are only three classes of chemical substances which may be considered to be of clinical value. These are N-methylisatin-β-thiosemicarbazone for prophylaxis of smallpox, the adamantamines for the prevention of certain upper respiratory tract infections, and metabolic inhibitors e.g. iododeoxyuridine and cytosine arabinose for treatment of corneal infections caused by *Herpes simplex* virus. Recent reports concerning the inhibitory action of rifampicin on members of the pox and, possibly, adenovirus groups are also encouraging.

Viral vaccines

The most important aspect of prophylactic immunization is the production or increase of resistance to specific disease, and this almost invariably implies the artificial introduction of substances that will stimulate the animal's immunological mechanisms to active immunity, so causing the formation of specific protective antibodies.

Immunity, which is the state of resistance of the host to a pathogen may be innate or acquired, and an acquired immunity can be conferred passively or actively by either natural or artificial means. An actively acquired immunity develops as a consequence of either spontaneous or experimental infection, or is stimulated by the use of a live or killed vaccine. Active immunity generally takes several days to develop but tends to persist for years after recovery from infection, and the level of antibodies produced largely depends on the efficacy of the antigen and the degree of its invasiveness of the host. During the course of natural viral infections, or following the use of live attenuated vaccines, a second type of antiviral substance known as interferon may be produced. Synthesis of interferon, however, is only induced by certain viruses and, characteristically, it becomes demonstrable much earlier after viral infection than specific antibody. The protective effect of interferon is of short duration, seldom lasting more than a few days and, unlike antibody, it has no effect on extracellular virus particles but acts by inhibiting viral replication.

The main mechanisms involved in resistance associated with acquired active immunity against viral infections can be defined as follows.

(1) **Humoral immunity** which enhances the removal of virus from blood and extracellular spaces by three immunological processes;

(a) neutralization of receptor sites of the virion, thereby preventing cell attachment and infection,

(b) the formation by precipitins of virus-antibody complexes which may be phagocytosed more readily as particulate matter, and

(c) treatment of the virus with immune-opsonins which renders it more susceptible to phagocytosis.

(2) **Cellular immunity** which is probably involved in patients recovering from infection (e.g. influenza), since there is often a lack of correlation between the development of specific humoral antibodies and immunity. There is also evidence that delayed hypersensitivity reactions may play an important role in viral immunity.

It is emphasised, however, that antibody is only effective against extracellular virus and is unable to prevent direct cell-to-cell spread as occurs in many herpesvirus infections. Also, un-neutralized extracellular virus may persist in affected animals even when specific antibodies are present in large amounts. Thus, the formation of antibodies may not in itself result in clinical improvement and, conversely, recovery may take place in the absence of antibody.

The development of viral vaccines

Although considerable progress has been made in the control of bacterial infections by vaccination and chemotherapy, viral infections are thus far almost wholly resistant to chemoprophylactic and chemotherapeutic control. Preventive immunization is the only effective means of controlling viral diseases in large populations of domestic animals. Fortunately, live attenuated viral vaccines and inactivated vaccines, especially when the latter are combined with an appropriate adjuvant, are usually highly effective and induce lasting immunity.

The history of the development of vaccines is almost 200 years old, beginning with Jenner's first successful vaccinations against smallpox in 1798. Almost a century was to pass before the next vaccine, for the control of rabies, was produced by Pasteur and his colleagues in 1884–85, and it is interesting to note that both of these vaccines were prepared before a virus could be seen and before virology had developed as a science. Although the developing hens' egg was used by Ogston in 1881 for cultivating bacteria and by Copeman in 1899 for the propagation of variola virus, the potentialities of the method for the growth of viruses were not generally recognised for another 30 years or more. Until then, viruses were almost invariably cultivated in susceptible animals, and infected organs or tissue provided the only material for both medical and veterinary vaccines. Despite the costs involved in preparing and testing these early vaccines, the development of technical methods led to the introduction of a large number of reliable live and inactivated viral vaccines. In the veterinary field the most notable were the live goat-adapted rinderpest virus vaccine introduced in 1928 for the control of that disease in zebu and other breeds of cattle having a relatively high degree of innate resistance, and the formalin inactivated tongue-epithelium vaccine for foot-and-mouth disease developed in 1938. While the use of goats, rabbits, ferrets and other laboratory animals was invaluable for the large scale production of rinderpest, distemper and some other virus vaccines of veterinary importance, further general progress in this field had to await the introduction and application of the developing chicken egg and cell culture techniques.

The first chick embryo virus vaccine became available in 1933 for the control of avian infectious laryngotracheitis (ILT), followed in 1938 by formalin-inactivated egg vaccines against Eastern and Western equine encephalomyelitis. Fowl- and pigeon-pox vaccines were introduced in 1939 and, from 1946 onwards, a number of avianized virus vaccines were available for general use against Newcastle disease, avian infectious bronchitis, epidemic tremor and some other diseases of poultry. In mammals, two of the most successful and widely used avianized virus vaccines were prepared on the basis of the original observations by Haig and his colleagues on bluetongue virus of sheep in 1947, and on canine distemper virus in 1948.

There can be no doubt that viruses are responsible for some of the most costly diseases afflicting domestic animals, and Newcastle disease, Marek's disease, rinderpest and foot-and-mouth disease are some obvious examples. Fortunately, progress made in prophylaxis against virus diseases has taken enormous steps forward during the last two decades, particularly since 1949 when Enders and his colleagues first showed that poliomyelitis virus would multiply and produce a marked cytopathic effect in non-neural primate tissue cultures. The discovery that infected cell cultures yielded large quantities of virus led to the production of poliovaccines on a commercial scale. Since that time, the growth of animal viruses in mammalian and avian cells derived from a wide range of host species has been extensively investigated and many cell culture vaccines have been successfully developed. For example, live or inactivated virus vaccines have been produced in primary monolayer cultures of calf kidney cells against rinderpest, foot-and-mouth disease, infectious bovine rhinotracheitis, adenovirus infections, Wesselsbron disease and Newcastle disease. Pig kidney cultures have been employed for the production of vaccines against a variety of diseases including rabies, foot-and-mouth disease, Teschen disease, infectious canine hepatitis (ICH) and Newcastle disease. Dog kidneys have been used for distemper, measles and infectious canine hepatitis vaccines, and a feline panleucopenia virus vaccine has recently been produced in cat kidney cell cultures. Many poultry virus vaccines have been developed in chick embryo or chick tissue cultures including Newcastle disease, fowl pox, infectious laryngotracheitis and Marek's disease.

It will be noted from the above examples that, unlike vaccines prepared for the control of human virus infections, animal virus vaccines are produced in homologous or heterologous tissue systems, in primary and secondary cultures or in continuous cell lines e.g. baby hamster kidney (BHK21). Additional advantages are that the final products can be tested for potency and safety in the species of animal to be vaccinated, that experimental animals can be challenged with virulent virus to test the efficacy of vaccines, and that reliance does not have to be placed solely on the levels of antibodies produced or on the effects obtained in other species of laboratory animals. Despite the usefulness of cell cultures for large scale production of human and animal virus vaccines, there is an increasing awareness that many primary and established cell lines are persistently contaminated with latent or passenger viruses (e.g. foamy agent in monkey kidneys; leukosis virus in chicken tissues). Although the oncogenic potentialities of some chronically infected cell cultures have not yet been generally accepted, no new vaccines for use in humans are produced in monkey kidney cells because of this potential risk. There is also some reluctance to use cultures of cell lines, e.g. BHK21 for the production of human viral vaccines because of their tendency to spontaneous cellular transformation. Nor is it likely that cell-bound virus vaccines of the type used to control Marek's disease in chickens would be permitted in human medicine. Indeed, the fact that most 'normal' chick embryos and chick tissue cultures are latently infected with avian tumour viruses is in itself a danger. In veterinary medicine, the life expectancy of farm animals is limited and the use of such cell culture vaccines may, therefore, be justified: but the logical development would seem to be the use of tissues from animals or birds that have been bred and reared in clean, isolated communities.

Use of viral vaccines
Living viral vaccines are mostly prepared from attenuated strains previously modified by regular serial passages in experimental animals, chick embryos or cell cultures. When vaccines containing living virulent viruses are used they must be adequately tested for safety before use, and the animal protected against untoward reactions by the addition or subsequent administration of specific antisera (serum-virus method) or by previous dosage with appropriate inactivated viral vaccines. Inactivated viral vaccines consist of tissue suspensions obtained from artificially infected animals, embryonated eggs or tissue cultures, which have been inactivated by physical (e.g. ultraviolet irradiation) or chemical agents (e.g. β-propiolactone, formalin, acetylethyleneimine, phenol, etc.) so that the viruses are rendered innocuous while retaining their antigenic properties. Sometimes mixed vaccines are used and these are composed of two or more vaccines, (e.g. live distemper plus live or inactivated infectious canine hepatitis). Different types of monovalent viral vaccines may be added together to give divalent,

trivalent or polyvalent vaccines (e.g. foot-and-mouth disease).

In diseases where both living and inactivated vaccines are available, the former are usually employed because they stimulate a stronger immunity over a longer period of time. Usually only one dose is required and protection may be conferred more rapidly due to the production of a prompt 'interference-like' effect (e.g. rinderpest).

Disadvantages of live viral vaccines include possible adverse reactions resulting from the use of too virulent strains in highly susceptible breeds, transmission of infection to other non-vaccinated animals thereby causing disease, and the presence of latent or passenger viruses which are relatively unstable compared with inactivated viruses.

The immunizing properties of inactivated vaccines may be improved by the addition of adjuvants, particularly mineral gels and oily emulsions or suspensions. The most widely employed are aluminium hydroxide, which is a powerful adsorbent, and stabilized emulsions of an aqueous suspension of virus in liquid paraffin.

There are several methods of immunising animals against viral diseases including the following.

(1) Inoculation of live, non-attenuated virus as in the method of aphthization still practised in certain African territories against foot-and-mouth disease of cattle.

(2) Inoculation of live, non-attenuated virus by a route unfavourable to progressive infection (e.g. cloacal scarification of chickens with avian infectious laryngotracheitis virus).

(3) Inoculation of live, non-attenuated or moderately attenuated virus simultaneously with specific antiserum for partial protection (e.g. swine fever 'blood-virus' together with hyperimmune serum).

(4) Inoculation of living attenuated virus which induces infection but no significant disease, and can be employed at different passage levels in appropriate hosts (e.g. LEP Flury rabies vaccine for dogs and HEP for cats). Living attenuated vaccines are usually most effective when their immunogenicities have not been lost by 'over-passage' and when there is no risk of reversion to virulence or of untoward side effects (e.g. keratitis following live infectious canine hepatitis vaccination).

(5) Inoculation of viruses inactivated by physical or chemical means, with and without adjuvants (e.g. Frenkel's fragmented tongue epithelium foot-and-mouth disease vaccine). These are usually the safest types of vaccines to use because there is no possibility of inoculated virus multiplying in the animal body. Compared to live viral vaccines, the immune reaction is shorter and the degree of response depends on the amount of virus in the inoculum. It is important that the antigenicity of the virus must not be destroyed by the inactivating agent and for this reason β-propiolactone is often preferred to formalin.

A wide range of animal virus infections can now be controlled by vaccination (Table 41.1) but the development of reliable vaccines is still required for the control of a number of more complex diseases including jaagsiekte, equine infectious anaemia and other slow virus infections, acute respiratory disorders associated with mixed infections of viruses and bacteria, avian leukosis and animal leukaemias. Further developments will undoubtedly lead to the use of vaccines of greater purity and efficacy, and the introduction of 'sub-unit' vaccines prepared from highly purified viral fractions.

TABLE 41.1. Some currently available animal virus vaccines.

Disease	Virus group	Form of virus	Source of vaccine	Form of vaccine	Administration	Remarks
African horse sickness	Orbivirus	LA	Mouse brain [Polyvalent, 7 strains]	Freeze dried	S/C 5ml.	Annually in Spring: at least 3 months before disease expected to occur. Not used in passively immunized foals under 6 months, or in pregnant mares.
		LA	TC [Polyvalent, 9 strains]	Freeze dried		
Avian infectious bronchitis	Coronavirus	IN	CE-allantoic	IN: propiolactone, formalin. Al. hydrox. gel	I/M 2x0.5ml.	2 doses separated by 4 weeks before point of lay. Boost at 6–12 months thereafter.
		LA	CE-allantoic [Massachussets or Connecticut strain]	Freeze dried	Drinking water, i/nasal, ocular or spray	HEP- broiler chicks, potential layers and breeding stock: 1–14 days of age. LEP- as booster dose at 10–12 weeks.
Bluetongue	Orbivirus	LA	CE [polyvalent]	Freeze dried	S/C 1.0ml.	Annually during Spring: at least 1 month before service or before disease is expected to occur.
		LA	TC- lamb kidney			
Epidemic tremor	Picornavirus	IN	CE- yolk sac IN: propiolactone, formalin [Al. hydrox gel]	Homogenised embryos	I/M 0.5ml.	Laying or breeding stock before point of lay. Revaccinate annually.
Infectious canine hepatitis	Adenovirus	IN	Infected dog tissues	IN: formalin, adjuvant or none	S/C	Single dose. Volume varies with manufacturer. May be incorporated with living distemper vaccine and dead leptospira.
		IN	TC- pig, ferret kidney	— ditto —		
		LA	TC-pig, ferret	Freeze dried	S/C	Single dose. May be incorporated with living distemper vaccine and dead leptospira.
Equine encephalitis	Alphavirus	LA	CE- yolk sac [Bivalent]	Freeze dried	I/D	Bivalent Eastern & Western encephalitis strains given in 2 doses 7–10 days apart. Revaccinate annually.
Equine influenza	Orthomyxovirus	IN	CE-allantoic [Polyvalent]	IN: propiolactone oily adjuvant [Al. hydrox. gel]	I/M 2x2ml.	Strains A/equi 1 Prague 56, A/equi 2 Miami 63, etc. Vaccinate in-foal mares and their foals at 3 months and 6 months of age. Annually thereafter.

Disease	Virus	Type	Substrate	Preparation	Route/Dose	Notes
Equine rhinopneumonitis	Herpesvirus	LA	Mouse brain		I/M or I/nasal	3 doses during first year of life.
Canine distemper	Paramyxovirus	LA	TC [measles virus]	Freeze dried	I/M 0.5–1ml.	1st dose measles at 4–6 wks., 2nd dose distemper plus infectious hepatitis living vaccines at 12 weeks with booster dose at 18 months.
		LA LA LA	CE TC-chick tissues TC-dog tissues	Freeze dried	S/C 1ml.	Pups of immune dams may not respond if under 8 wks. old. Vaccinate at 8–10 wks. and again at 12–14 wks.
Feline infectious enteritis	Parvovirus	LA	TC- cat kidney	Freeze dried	S/C 1ml.	Kitten: 1st dose at 7 wks., 2nd dose at 12 wks. Adult: One dose at 12 wks. or older. Not in pregnant cats.
		IN	Infected cat or mink spleen	IN: 0.25% formalin [may contain mineral oil]	S/C or I/M 1ml.	2 doses at 14-day intervals. Kittens under 9 wks. old 2 doses, second at 9 wks. Adults: 1 dose only. Mink may react severely to feline strain.
Foot-and-mouth disease	Rhinovirus	IN	Tongue or fragmented tongue epithelium TC-calf, pig kidney	IN: formalin, acetylethyleneimine. Al. hydrox., saponin, oily emulsions	S/C c.30ml.	Volume dependent on nature of vaccine and number of valencies contained in it. 1 dose protects for at least 4 months, 2nd dose for about 1 year. May revaccinate annually. Not permitted in U.K.
		IN	TC-cell lines [BHK21]			
		LA	Various animal tissues	May add glycerin as stabilizer	I/M varies.	Usually protects for 4–12 mths. Boost annually. Not to be used in U.K. or in other disease-free areas. Mono-, bi-, tri- and polyvalent. Virus chosen according to type and sub-type.
		LA	TC-primary and cell lines [BHK21]			
Fowl pox	Poxvirus	LA	CE-CAM [Chicken virus]	Fragmented membrane in glycerine [1:4], or freeze dried.	Needle stab [wing web] 1 ml. = 100 doses	For use in birds not over 4 mths. old. Immunity in 14 days, lasts 12–18 mths.
		LA	CE-CAM [Pigeon virus]	Fragmented membrane in glycerine [1:4] or freeze dried		Fowl pox vaccines [chicken or pigeon strains] should only be used where risk of disease exists. Revaccinate annually.
		LA	Cutaneous pigeon breast lesions [Pigeon or chicken strain]	Powdered scabs in 50% glycerin	Scarify inner aspect of thigh 10 ml. = 50 doses	For use in birds of any age. Solid immunity for 4 mths., partial for 12 mths.
Infectious bovine rhinotracheitis	Herpesvirus	LA	TC- ox or pig kidney	Freeze dried	S/C 2–5ml.	Solid durable immunity in 10–14 days. Do not vaccinate pregnant cows.

Disease	Virus		Source	Preparation	Route/Dose	Notes
Infectious laryngotracheitis	Herpesvirus	LA	CE-CAM	Freeze dry fragmented CAM and fluids	Intraocular, 1 drop.	Use in birds 1 month of age or older. Revaccinate young birds before point of lay; and annually.
Louping ill	Flavivirus	IN	TC-sheep kidney	Precipitate fluids with methanol or acetone	S/C 1–2ml.	Vaccinate sheep [1 ml.] every 2 years and boost cattle [2 ml.] annually.
Marek's disease	Herpesvirus	L	Naturally avirulent strain of turkey herpesvirus	Freeze dried	I/M 0.2ml.	For active immunization of potential breeding and laying stock, vaccinate all 1-day-old chicks.
Mink enteritis	Parvovirus	LA IN	TC- mink kidney Infected mink tissue	IN: formalin	I/M 1 ml. S/C 1 ml.	Single dose for all mink over 9 wks. of age. May use feline panleucopenia vaccine in adult stock.
Myxomatosis	Poxvirus	LA	Rabbit skin injected with Shope fibroma	Freeze dry 20% 'tumour' tissue in saline	S/C 0.5ml. I/D 0.2ml.	Protects within 7 days. Fibroma at site of injection disappears in 4 weeks.
Newcastle disease	Paramyxovirus	IN IN	CE-CAM TC- bovine kidney and other non-avian issues	IN: treat CE fluids with propiolactone or formalin [Al. hydrox. gel]	I/M or S/C Fowl 0.5 ml. Turkey 0.5–1.0 ml.	Any age but preferably not less than 14 days old. Booster dose at 16–20 wks. Repeat at 6–12 month intervals.
		LA LA	CE-CAM TC-non avian tissues	Freeze dried	Drinking water, i/nasal, aerosol or needle stab.	Immune response and side-effects depend on age of bird and strain of virus: Lentogenic [Hitchner B1 La Sota, etc.], mesogenic [Mukteswar, Roakin, Komorov]. Vaccines are infectious to man.
Orf	Poxvirus	LA	Cutaneous lamb passaged strain	Powdered lesions in 50% glycerin	Scarify inner aspect of thigh	Segregate vaccinated animals for 3 weeks. Vaccinate ewes at least 6 weeks before lambing. Immunity lasts 6 months or longer. Infectious to man.
Bovine papillomatosis	Papovavirus	IN	Emulsified natural wart tissue	IN: formalin	S/C 5–10ml.	Autogenous vaccine used therapeutically. Repeat at 10–14 day intervals.
Rabies	Rhabdovirus	IN IN	Neural tissue: sheep, goat, horse, rodents. TC-various tissues, e.g. BHK21	IN: UV radiation, phenol, chloroform, etc. IN: phenol, formalin	S/C various	Used prophylactically but not permitted in UK. 5 ml. of 20% phenolized [Semple] goat or sheep brain protects dogs for 1 year. Cattle dose 50 ml., followed by booster dose.
		IN	Duck embryo	IN: propiolactone	S/C 1ml.	Widely used prophylactically and therapeutically in man. Up to 14 daily doses, plus 2 booster doses, as required.

Disease		Source	Preparation	Dose/Route	Remarks
Rabies (continued)	LA	CE [avianized strains, e.g. Flury, Kelev, etc.]	Freeze-dry emulsified living embryos	I/M 1.5–6ml.	Cattle: 3–5ml. HEP [40–60 pass] Flury or 6ml. Kelev strain. Boost at 30 days. Do NOT use LEP. Dogs [over 3 mths]: 3 ml. LEP [180 pass] Flury. Protects over 3 years. Puppies: 3 ml. HEP or Kelev strains; revaccinate at 1 year. Cats: 1.5 ml. HEP only; revaccinate at 1 year.
	LA	TC-various types infected with LEP, HEP, etc.	Freeze dried		
Respiratory infections in cattle	LA	TC-various types etc.	Freeze dried	I/M 2ml.	Live vaccines incorporating various viruses associated with respiratory illnesses. 2 doses given to young calves 6–10 weeks of age.
	IN	Adeno-, reo-, paramyxoviruses etc.			
Rift Valley fever	LA	Unclassified Togavirus	Mouse brain or TC infected with Smithburn or other suitably adapted strain. Freeze dried 10% brain suspension	S/C 2ml. [Cattle] 1ml.[Sheep, goats]	Annually to cattle, sheep and goats in enzootic areas. Not in pregnant animals, or young animals less than 3 mths. old. Solid durable immunity.
Rinderpest	IN	Paramyxovirus	Infected ox tissues	IN: Al. hydrox. with glycerin, chloroform, etc.	S/C 10ml.	Single dose confers serviceable immunity for several months.
	LA		Tissues of goat [KAG] rabbit or chick embryo	Freeze dried. May add stabilizer	S/C 2ml.	Maternally derived antibodies may interfere with active immunity. Vaccinate all yearlings. Caprine more virulent than lapinized, than avianized. TC vaccine may be used in all breeds of cattle to produce durable immunity.
	LA		TC-bovine kidney			
Sheep pox	LA	Poxvirus	'Lymph' from expt. lesions in sheep	Glycerinated	Scarification or I/D.	Scarification [ovination] or I/D in caudal fold; or virulent lymph plus serum [seroclavelization].
	LA		CE- CAM	Freeze dried	S/C or caudal fold 1 ml.	No side effects. Solid immunity for at least 5 months.
	LA		TC-sheep kidney or testis	Al. hydrox. gel		N.B. Al. hydrox. adsorbed virus inactivated with BPL or formalin may also be used, with oily emulsions.
Swine fever	IN	Non-arbo togavirus	Defibrinated blood or spleen of expt. pig	IN: Ethylene glycol or glycerin with 0.25% crystal violet: or eucalyptol	S/C	5ml./30 kilos body weight. 10 ml. if over 30 kilos. Serviceable immunity for several months. Must not be used in U.K.

Disease		Type	Source	Form	Route	Notes
		LA	Tissues from rabbits or pigs infected with lapinized virus	Freeze dried	S/C	Lapinized high pass vaccine used preferably with antiserum.
		LA	TC- pig kidney			Low pass tissue vaccines should be given together with at least 10 ml. anti-serum. Not permitted in U.K.
Teschen disease	Enterovirus	IN LA	Infected swine tissues TC- pig kidney	IN: formalin	S/C	Both types of vaccine give at least 80% protection.
Wesselsbron disease	Flavivirus	LA LA	Mouse brain TC- lamb kidney	Freeze dried	S/C Cattle 2ml. Sheep, goats 1ml.	Vaccinate annually at least 1 month before disease is due to occur. Pregnant animals may abort. Often given simultaneously with Rift Valley fever.

L[LA]: Living [attenuated]
IN: inactivated
CE: chick embryo
CAM: chorio-allantoic membrane
TC: cell or tissue culture
S/C: subcutaneously
I/M: intramuscularly
I/D: intradermally
LEP: low egg pass
HEP: high egg pass
KAG: Kabete [Kenya] anti-goat.

Further reading

ACKERMANN O. (1965) Comparative experimental studies on vaccines against distemper and canine viral hepatitis. *Journal of Small Animal Practice*, **6**, 171.

APPLEYARD G. (1967) Chemotherapy of viral infections. *British Medical Bulletin*, **23**, 114.

BANKOWSKI R.A. (1957) A modified live Newcastle disease virus vaccine. *Proceedings of the Society for Experimental Biology and Medicine*, **96**, 114.

BAUER D.J. (1965) Clinical experience with the antiviral drug Marboran (1 methylisatin β — thiosemicarbazone). *Annals of the New York Academy of Sciences*, **130**, 110.

BAUER D.J. (1967) Antiviral chemotherapy. In, *Modern Trends in Medical Virology*, eds. R.B. Heath and A.P. Waterson, p. 49. London: Butterworth.

BAUER D.J., ST. VINCENT L., KEMPE C.H. AND DOWNIE A.W. (1963) Prophylactic treatment of smallpox contacts with N-Methylisatin β-thiosemicarbazone (Compound 33T57, Marboran). *Lancet*, **2**, 494.

CABASSO V.J., KISER K.H., STEBBINS M.R. AND COOPER H.K. (1962) Canine distemper vaccine of tissue culture origin. *American Journal of Veterinary Research*, **23**, 394.

CHURCHILL A.E. (1965) The development of a live attenuated infectious laryngotracheitis vaccine. *Veterinary Record*, **77**, 1227.

COX H.R. (1953) Avianized rabies vaccine. In. *Proceedings of the 57th Annual Meeting U.S. Livestock Sanitary Association*, p. 305.

FRENKEL H.S. (1951) Research on foot-and-mouth disease. III. The cultivation of the virus in explantations of tongue epithelium of bovine animals. *American Journal of Veterinary Research*, **12**, 187.

GREEN R.G. (1939) Modification of the distemper virus. *Journal of the American Veterinary Medical Association*, **95**, 465.

HAIG D.A. (1948) Preliminary note on the cultivation of Green's distemperiod virus in fertile hen eggs. *Onderstepoort Journal of Veterinary Science and Animal Industry*, **23**, 149.

HAIG D.A., DANSKIN D. AND WINDMILL A.J. (1962) Studies on an adjuvant Newcastle disease vaccine. *Research in Veterinary Science*, **3**, 236.

HITCHNER S.B. AND JOHNSON E.P. (1948) A virus of low virulence for immunizing fowls against Newcastle disease (avian pneumoencephalitis). *Veterinary Medicine*, **43**, 525.

HILLEMAN M.R. (1966) Critical appraisal of emulsified oil adjuvants applied to viral vaccines. *Progress in Medical Virology*, **8**, 131.

KAUFMAN H.E. (1962) Clinical cure of herpes simplex keratitis by 5-iodo-2'-deoxyuridine. *Proceedings of the Society for Experimental Biology and Medicine*, **109**, 251.

KAUFMAN H.E. (1965) Problems of virus chemotherapy. *Progress in Medical Virology*, **7**, 116.

PECK F.B., POWELL H.M. AND CULBERTSON C.G. (1955) A new antirabies vaccine for human use. Clinical and laboratory results using rabies vaccine made from embryonated duck eggs. *Journal of Laboratory and Clinical Medicine*, **45**, 679.

PLOWRIGHT W. AND FERRIS R.D. (1957) Cytopathogenicity of rinderpest virus in tissue culture. *Nature*, **179**, 316.

PLOWRIGHT W. AND FERRIS R.D. (1962) Studies with rinderpest virus in tissue culture. The use of attenuated culture virus as a vaccine for cattle. *Research in Veterinary Science*, **3**, 172.

ROCKBORN G. (1959) Canine distemper virus in tissue culture. *Archiv für die gesamte Virusforschung*, **8**, 485.

SKINNER R.H.H. (1960) Some techniques for producing and studying attenuated strains of the virus of foot-and-mouth disease. *Bulletin. Office international des épizooties*, **53**, 634.

SUBAK-SHARPE J.H., TIMBURY M.C. AND WILLIAMS J.F. (1969) Rifampicin inhibits the growth of some mammalian viruses. *Nature*, **222**, 341.

TAMM I. AND CALIGUIRI L.A. (1971) Mode of action of antiviral substances In, *Viruses Affecting Man and Animals*, eds. M. Saunders and M. Schaeffer, p. 136. St. Louis: Warren H. Green.

TAMM I. AND EGGERS H.J. (1965) Selective inhibition of viral reproduction In, *Viral and Rickettsial Infections of Man*, 4th Edition, eds. F.L. Horsfall Jr. and I. Tamm, p. 305. Philadelphia: Lippincott.

Tilles J.G. (1974) Antiviral agents. *Annual Review of Pharmacology*, **14**, 469.

YORK C.J., BRITTLE J.L., BURCH G.R. AND JONES D.E. (1960). An effective canine distemper tissue culture vaccine. *Veterinary Medicine*, **55**, 30.

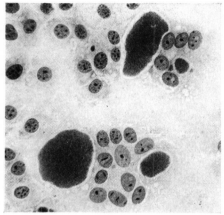

42.1a

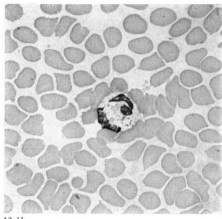

42.1b

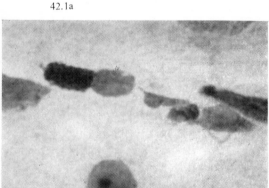

42.1c

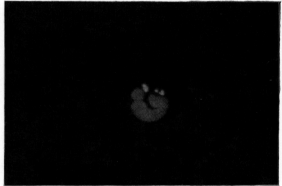

42.1d

42.1a A sheep kidney cell culture infected 4 days previously with the agent of enzootic abortion of ewes, showing large plaques of purple-staining bodies within cytoplasmic vacuoles. The nuclei are not affected. Giemsa stain, × 280.

42.1c Smear prepared from the brain of a goat inoculated with *Cowdria ruminantium* of heartwater fever. The causative organisms form large clusters in the endothelial cells lining the brain capillaries. Giemsa stain, × 1250.

42.1b Blood film prepared from a sheep found suffering from tick-borne fever. The causal organisms (*Cytoecetes phagocytophilia*) are seen as slate-grey particles in an orderly circular pattern within the cytoplasm of a polymorphonuclear leucocyte. The bodies may also occur in clusters as seen in Plate 36.1b. Leishman stain, × 800.

42.1d Blood film prepared from a sheep affected with tick-borne fever, stained with acridine orange and photographed in the ultraviolet light microscope. The causal organisms appear as small clusters of brightly fluorescing orange-red particles within the pale yellow-green polymorphonuclear leucocyte. The erythrocytes are unstained, × 850.

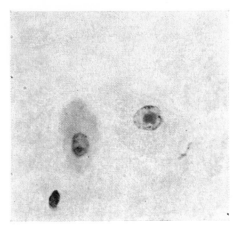

42.2a

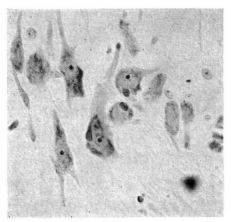

42.2b

42.2c

42.2a   A liver impression smear prepared from a puppy dying from infectious canine hepatitis (Rubarth's disease). Notice the large acidophilic intranuclear inclusion body accompanied by margination of the nuclear chromatin in the infected cell (right). Haematoxylin eosin stain, × 645.

42.2b Section of dog brain affected with rabies. The pale nuclei contain deeply stained nucleoli. The Negri bodies are seen as large round or oval acidophilic inclusions in the cytoplasm of infected nerve cells. Mann stain, × 280.

42.2c   A section through the chorioallantoic membrane of a developing chick embryo infected with cow pox virus. The large regularly shaped acidophilic structures are intracytoplasmic viral inclusion bodies. Phloxine tartrazine stain, × 300.

CHAPTER 42

ISOLATION, CULTIVATION AND IDENTIFICATION PROCEDURES IN DIAGNOSTIC VIROLOGY

Isolation, cultivation and identification procedures in diagnostic virology

The main purpose of the routine diagnostic virus laboratory is to provide the means for achieving a diagnosis as quickly as possible. In other words, specimens from animals suffering from an infectious disease are examined by the most suitable procedures available for evidence of viral infection, followed by a critical assessment as to whether or not the infection is the cause of the patient's disease. Ideally, the methods used should be accurate, rapid, simple and inexpensive.

To the veterinarian the most important feature of an animal virus is its virulence and pathogenicity and, while infections with viruses are similar in many respects to those with bacteria, the means by which viruses injure their hosts is quite different from that of other organisms. The fact that viruses can multiply only within living cells and that the diseases they produce arise from cell damage associated with intracellular multiplication has an important bearing on the methods that are commonly used in the virus laboratory to obtain a specific diagnosis.

General principles

In general, the procedures that are available for the diagnosis of viral diseases fall into two main categories.

(1) Methods for the isolation and identification of the causative virus from clinical specimens, and

(2) Serological tests for the detection and measurement of specific antibodies that develop during the course of the illness.

Although the presence of virus in the tissues of an affected animal is frequently related to the initial febrile stages of the illness, there may be little opportunity in practice of obtaining suitable material for virus isolation or of obtaining a specific diagnosis until after the patient has recovered or succumbed to the disease. For this reason, and on grounds of speed and economy, serological tests for viral antibodies are generally preferred to the isolation and typing of possible causative viruses. Very many

sera can be examined even in laboratories with modest facilities, and the demonstration of a fourfold or greater rising titre of specific antibodies in paired sera (acute and convalescent) generally establishes the nature of the infection.

Diagnostic virology is undoubtedly more expensive, complicated and time-consuming than bacteriology and its usefulness in the clinical field depends almost entirely on close cooperation between the virologist and the clinician, neither of whom, unfortunately, may have received adequate training in the other's discipline.

Before attempting a diagnosis the virologist must, after first consulting his clinical colleagues, decide on the best lines of approach to the problem in hand. For this purpose a good clinical history is highly desirable. This should include the nature of the infection, clinical signs, lesions and other abnormalities, the stage of the illness and details of the geographical location, breed, age and sex of the animals affected, movements on and off the farm, previous vaccinations and so on. When animals have been examined post mortem a provisional but detailed report should be obtained from the pathologist concerning the nature and distribution of abnormalities in tissues and organs.

The above information is necessary to enable the virologist to select the most appropriate procedures and to furnish a meaningful interpretation of the test results.

There is little doubt that many clinicians dealing with infectious disease have an inadequate knowledge of the most suitable material to select, the methods used for collection and how to pack and submit specimens for virological examination. Also, some clinicians may not understand why the virologist requires different material from various cases and how important it is to the success of the laboratory examinations that the specimens must be received in a suitable condition for examination. This is especially important in overseas territories where the clinical laboratory covers a wide geographical area in tropical or semi-tropical conditions.

Microscopic examination

Films and smears

The material should be spread as thinly as possible on clean, grease-free glass slides and allowed to dry. It is important that the smears, although thin, should contain some tissue elements as they will be examined for the presence of pathognomonic cells, such as syncytia in rinderpest, the demonstration of elementary bodies in chlamydial infections (Plate 36.2a, facing p. 388a), rickettsiae or rickettsial-like bodies in Q fever (Plate 36.1a, facing p. 388), heartwater (Plate 36.1c, facing p. 388 and Plate 42.1c, facing p. 474) and tick-borne fever (Plate 36.1b, facing p. 388 and Plates 42.1b & d, facing p. 474), or inclusion bodies such as the Negri bodies of rabies. Smears from infected tissues derived from spleen, liver and brain can be made by impression of a cut surface of the tissue. Slides should be clearly marked, particularly when highly pathogenic microorganisms are likely to be present.

Elementary bodies and rickettsiae are mostly over 200 nm in size and can be demonstrated in stained smears with the light microscope. Almost every type of elementary body can be stained by the Giemsa method (Plate 42.1a, facing p. 474), and the slow or overnight technique using 1 per cent of the stock solution is generally preferred. In veterinary laboratories the modified Macchiavello method (brucella differential or Koster's stain) is particularly useful for identifying the elementary bodies of *Chlamydia* and the rickettsia-like rods of Q fever in tissue smears, because the method stains the infectious particles a contrasting bright red colour against a blue or green background of cells.

Many animal viruses induce the formation of inclusion bodies within the cytoplasm or nucleus of infected cells and some, such as the Negri bodies of rabies, are so characteristic in appearance that their presence is of considerable diagnostic value. Viral inclusions may be basophilic or acidophilic in their staining affinities and their presence in infected tissues and smears can be readily demonstrated by Giemsa, haematoxylin and eosin or other routine histological staining methods (Plate 42.2a, facing p. 474a). Bollinger bodies and other types of poxvirus inclusions stain well with phloxine tartrazine and Mann's method, whereas in rabies diagnosis the recommended staining procedures include those of Sellers, Lepine, Stovall and Black, and Mann.

In certain circumstances films, smears and tissue sections may also be examined for the presence of rickettsial and viral antigens by direct and indirect fluorescent antibody staining techniques. (Plate 42.12a, between pp. 488–9).

Direct electron microscopy

Because of their extremely small size most animal viruses are below the resolving power of the standard light microscope and, until comparatively recently, their presence could only be detected by inoculating specimens into the susceptible host system of animals, fertile eggs or cell cultures. Unfortunately, the effects they may produce on the inoculated host are often not apparent for several days and there may be considerable delay in establishing a prompt and accurate diagnosis. To overcome these difficulties immunofluorescence techniques are being increasingly used to detect viral antigens in specimens taken directly from patients, e.g. swine fever and rabies; and electron microscopy is being adapted for the rapid detection and identification of viruses in clinical specimens, on the basis of their morphology.

There are two major difficulties in using the electron microscope as an additional diagnostic method. The first is that only a very small part of the specimen can be examined at any one time, and the second is that generally the initial concentration of total virus particles must be in the order of 10^9 per ml.

Fortunately, experience has shown that a number of clinical specimens may contain large numbers of morphologically recognisable virus particles, and negative contrast staining with phosphotungstic acid (PTA) has been used successfully to demonstrate paramyxoviruses in nasopharyngeal secretions of human patients suffering from acute laryngitis and of dogs affected with distemper. Other viruses that have been identified by direct electron microscopy include poxviruses from post-vaccination lesions, herpesviruses from whitlows on the finger, adenoviruses from conjunctival washings, mumps from cerebrospinal fluid, reoviruses from ultracentrifuged faecal deposits, and 'orf' from mouth lesions in sheep. (Plate 37.4b, facing p. 431).

The method of preparing specimens, e.g. cerebrospinal fluid, vesicular fluid, throat and eye washings is very simple. One drop of the material is placed on a drop of sterile distilled water resting on a waxed surface. A Formvar-carbon-coated copper grid is held in a fine pair of forceps and touched gently on the surface of the drop containing the virus, and a drop of 2 per cent PTA at pH 6·5–7·0 is added to the grid to act as a negative stain. The grid is then allowed to dry in air before being examined in the electron microscope.

The method can also be adapted for the examination of very small pieces of biopsy or autopsy tissues which are first lysed by alternate freezing and thawing. In the same way, centrifuged deposits of infected cell cultures disrupted by freezing and thawing can be examined for the presence of virus, whether or not a cytopathic effect is present.

Once the morphology of the virus has been ascertained it can readily be assigned to a major virus group and, on the basis of the clinical signs and species of animal affected, will often provide sufficient evidence for a rapid provisional diagnosis which can later be confirmed by serological and other methods.

Histological examination
Biopsy or autopsy material for histological examination must be carefully selected and small pieces of tissue should be placed promptly in a suitable fixative solution such as Bouin's fluid or Zenker's solution containing 10 per cent formalin. The preparation of tissue sections is carried out by standard techniques and the choice of staining methods, which includes those mentioned above, largely depends on the nature of the abnormality that the worker wishes to demonstrate. Fixed tissues taken for histology may also be used to demonstrate specific precipitinogens by means of the agar-gel diffusion technique, (e.g. rinderpest). For a rapid histological examination fresh tissues should be selected and thin sections cut on a cryostat and stained by appropriate methods, including fluorescent antibody staining where necessary. (Plate 42.2b, facing p. 474a).

In general, histological examinations of sections are of limited value in identifying the causative virus although they are frequently of assistance in establishing whether an infectious process of viral origin is present. On the other hand, the value of histopathological methods to the diagnostician has greatly increased with the recent developments in fluorescent-antibody staining techniques where the nature of the causative virus can be established with confidence. On the whole, the conclusions reached after careful histological examination of affected tissues must be confirmed either by isolation and identification of the virus, by demonstrating the presence of a significant increase in specific antibody titres, or by both these procedures.

Collection of specimens for virological examination
The value to the clinician of the service provided by the diagnostic laboratory is almost entirely dependent on the skill and care with which he selects and collects the specimens and transmits them to the laboratory. Specimens most commonly chosen include whole blood, faeces, scrapings from lesions, throat swabs and various tissues taken at biopsy or autopsy; but the choice of material largely depends on the nature of the illness and the possible identity of the causative virus.

The time of collection is also of importance and,

if an attempt is to be made to isolate a virus, the specimens should be collected preferably during the early acute stage of infection because successful isolation is less likely in the later stages of the illness. In some diseases, however, the virus may persist as in the prolonged viraemic stage of African swine fever or in the faeces of animals affected with enterovirus infections. In veterinary medicine, viruses can usually be successfully recovered from lung, liver, spleen and other organs of animals dying during an outbreak, or from the carcases of infected animals that have been sacrificed to facilitate a speedy diagnosis. Since the material is likely to be inoculated into laboratory animals, fertile eggs or tissue cultures, specimens should be collected with sterile precautions. Care should be taken to avoid cross-contamination of tissues collected during the autopsy since it may be important to know not only the identity of the virus but also the tissues or organs from which it was isolated.

In general, specimens should be placed immediately in suitably labelled sterile containers that are airtight, leakproof and resistant to breakage. An appropriate transport medium, with or without antibiotics, may be added and swabs are seldom worth examining unless they are broken off into buffered medium immediately after collection to prevent dessication. Specimens should generally be kept cold unless they can reach the laboratory within one hour of collection because most viruses are unstable above a temperature of 4°C. Freezing and thawing is harmful to many viruses and, although they may be held at 4°C. if they are to be examined within 48 hours after collection, it is preferable for longer periods of time if they are stored in the frozen state at —40°C or below, and should only be thawed when required for testing. In some instances it is essential to send the material by prior arrangement with the laboratory in a vacuum flask, or packed in dry ice and enclosed in an outer container of expanded polystyrene by road, rail or air, whichever is the quickest and most convenient. Transport of materials is greatly facilitated by the use of insulated containers. Plastic picnic bags can be used to hold dry ice but, if so, the virus container must be sealed to exclude the entry of carbon dioxide which is deleterious to many viruses. Glass wide-mouthed universal containers are suitable for holding most specimens but stoppered bottles may be unsatisfactory and cotton-plugged tubes are wholly unacceptable. Current postal regulations regarding the transportation of infectious material must be observed at all times. All containers must be labelled and, since they may be subject to freezing and thawing, white adhesive (zinc oxide) tape marked in pencil or other non-run marker should be used. It is also an advantage if the inner container is carefully wrapped in an excess of absorbent paper or other material to act as a shock absorber and to absorb any fluid that may be spilled should breakage occur in transit. Where dry ice and/or a vacuum flask are neither suitable nor available the material can be transported in a 50 per cent solution of glycerine in saline at neutral pH (7·4) bearing in mind that glycerol may be detrimental to viruses such as rinderpest, or interfere with subsequent immunofluorescence studies.

Since sera from affected and in-contact animals are frequently required to permit a specific diagnosis, the specimens must be collected and prepared with care, and in many cases they must be obtained and handled with aseptic techniques. Dry syringes should be used to avoid haemolysis but anticoagulants or preservatives must not be added to the specimen lest they interfere with the results of subsequent serological tests.

Ideally, serum should be removed from the clotted blood as soon as possible after the sample is taken but it is probably more convenient if the clinician is encouraged to take the sample by means of a sterile vacuum vial and send it without further processing to the laboratory where the serum can be removed without fear of contamination. Since retraction of the blood clot has usually occurred by the time the specimen reaches the laboratory, it is an advantage to use plastic containers with a tapered inner bottom that fit standard centrifuge cups and can be spun down without further handling.

All sera in a diagnostic laboratory are stored either at 4°C or, preferably, in the frozen state since they are frequently required for further examinations weeks or even months afterwards. Moreover, since a diagnosis is often assisted by the appearance of a four-fold or greater rise in antibody titre, at least two and sometimes more specimens of blood are required from a number of animals in the affected herd during the course of the illness; and these must be preserved in a suitable condition. The first sample of paired sera, called the acute phase serum, is obtained as early as possible in the disease. The second, or convalescent phase serum, is usually taken 10–14 days later. Storage of sera in the deep freeze is believed to assist in the preservation of specific antibodies. In a number of instances, the neutralizing capacity of a serum stored in the cold may be restored by the addition of fresh, unheated guinea-pig serum. Whole blood, unlike serum, should never be frozen otherwise haemolysis of the specimen will result.

Strict attention must be given to preventing contamination of serum samples because bacteria or fungi may kill animals, fertile eggs or cell cultures used in neutralization tests, and may also be responsible for the development of anticomplemen-tary effects in sera being examined by complement-fixation tests. Some antiseptics may also render the sera anticomplementary as well as having harmful effects on the virus used in neutralization tests.

Methods of obtaining a confirmatory diagnosis

After due consideration of the clinical history and details of any post-mortem examination, together with the results of microscopical and histological examinations, the diagnostic virologist must select the most suitable procedures for obtaining a confirmatory diagnosis within the limitations of his laboratory. All too often, unfortunately, he must carefully weigh up the cost of the operation in terms of time, effort and expense against the value to the clinician of the results he hopes to obtain.

In attempting a diagnosis two main avenues are open to him, namely, the isolation and identification of the causative virus and the demonstration of a rise in titre of specific antibodies.

Isolation of the causal virus

In recent years the isolation of virus from clinical specimens has been greatly simplified by the increased availability of cell culture systems. Sometimes tissue culture investigations are supplemented with egg and animal inoculations and, indeed, in some instances these alternatives are still the procedures of choice.

Animal inoculation

To confirm the infectious nature of a disease it may be necessary to reproduce the clinical illness in another member of the same species, either by placing healthy susceptible animals in direct contact with those showing symptoms of infection, or by inoculating groups of healthy and immune (vaccinated) animals by a suitable route with material obtained from a sick animal. If the latter procedure is adopted it is necessary to ensure that material capable of transmitting the disease does not contain other microorganisms (e.g. bacteria) which produce a concurrent infection and complicate the clinical picture. To ensure that the inoculum is bacteriologically sterile the material must be filtered or treated with antibiotics.

In medical virology, monkeys are frequently used for inoculation since it is possible to reproduce in these species many human diseases which show similar clinical symptoms and comparable development. In veterinary medicine the same species or at least those closely related to the host animal should be used and in diseases such as swine fever, which show a high degree of host specificity, the use of the same species may be obligatory. On the other hand, many viruses including some members of the togavirus group can be grown successfully and will produce clinical disease in a wide variety of laboratory animals, such as dogs, cats, mice, rats, guinea-pigs, rabbits and hamsters, as well as producing abnormalities of developing chicken embryos and a variety of cell cultures. It is emphasised that whatever procedure is adopted the inoculation of animals for diagnostic purposes may only be performed in the United Kingdom in an approved laboratory by persons holding a Home Office licence and the appropriate certificate or certificates.

Certain procedures such as the intranasal inoculation of mice for the detection of chlamydiae or the intracerebral inoculation of mice for the diagnosis of rabies require that the animals be anaesthetised before use. Suitable long-acting anaesthetics include pentobarbitone sodium (Nembutal); a solution containing 30 mg/kg body weight given intraperitoneally is a suitable dose for a healthy adult rabbit. Short-acting anaesthetics such as ether or a mixture of ether (25 parts) and chloroform (1 part) are suitable for guinea-pigs, rats and mice.

Before using experimental animals the operator should make himself familiar with the general directions for the care and management of laboratory animals and with the conditions laid down under the Cruelty to Animals Act (1876). In their own interests,

preferably, twice daily for the detection of signs of disease or other abnormalities. Wherever possible, rectal temperatures should be taken and recorded daily by means of a blunt-ended clinical thermometer liberally smeared with liquid paraffin. The average rectal temperatures, taken before feeding, of the more commonly used laboratory animals are shown in Table 42.1.

It may be an advantage to withdraw blood samples at regular intervals from experimental animals to detect the possible development of specific antibodies (e.g. Q fever), and to cull and carry out post-mortem examinations of some animals (e.g. rabies diagnosis) during the course of the experiment. Clinical symptoms, the development of visible lesions, abnormal behaviour and all deaths, whatever the cause, should be carefully observed and recorded. At the termination of an experiment involving infectious material, all bedding, utensils, cages, carcases and tissues should be removed, burned, sterilized or thoroughly cleaned by the most appropriate methods. Animals infected experimentally must be held in separate isolation rooms and all persons handling infected animals, cages or other contaminated materials must pay strict attention to personal cleanliness.

TABLE 42.1. Rectal temperatures of some laboratory animals.

Species	°C	°F
Cat	38.5	101.4
Dog	38.6	101.6
Rabbit	38.6	101.6
Rat	37.5	99.5
Mouse	37.4	99.3
Guinea-pig	38.6	101.6
Hamster	37.5	99.5
Fowl	41.5	106.8

laboratory workers in the U.K. should seek the advice of a local Home Office Inspector whose name and address may be obtained from the Under Secretary of State, Home Office, London, S.W.1.

It is imperative that experimental animals must be healthy before they are used and that they be properly cared for during the course of the experiment. Not only are laboratory animals prone to a wide variety of bacterial, viral and parasitic diseases which may complicate the results of a particular experiment, but they are also liable to harbour various 'latent' or subclinical infections which may be activated under the stress of a particular experiment. These difficulties are largely overcome if specific pathogen-free stock or gnotobiotic facilities are available.

Before and during an experiment the operator should personally examine the animals once or,

Special care must be taken when performing inoculations if the material is believed to contain virulent viruses or when specimens obtained from experimentally infected animals are being processed for further passage in animals or inoculated into eggs or cell cultures. This is especially important when tissues such as brain, liver, spleen or kidney are being homogenized in the various types of grinder or blender, or when coarse tissues such as skin are being ground with a pestle in an open mortar.

It may be necessary, as in rabies diagnosis, for the operator to wear rubber gloves although he must realise that these are readily punctured by splintered bone, scalpel blades and syringe needles. A large waterproofed overall should be worn and it may be necessary to protect the face and eyes by means of a surgical face mask and eyeshield, or a light but easily adjusted plastic visor that can be readily fitted to the forehead. It is a good general rule that all carcases should be thoroughly soaked in an antiseptic solution and firmly nailed to a piece of board before starting the post-mortem examination. Soaking of the carcase is particularly important when birds with psittacosis are being examined to prevent airborne spread of chlamydiae from the heavily contaminated feathers.

Various routes may be employed to inoculate experimental animals with virus-infected materials, depending on the virus being studied. The usual methods are intracerebral, intranasal, intradermal, intravenous, intramuscular and subcutaneous. The choice of the route of inoculation is largely determined by the nature of the virus, its possible tissue affinity and the age and species of the experimental animal.

Although animal inoculation has been replaced, in part, by the use of embryonating hens' eggs and cell culture, it is still the most useful method for studying the clinical manifestations, pathogenicity, pathogenesis and epidemiology of animal virus diseases. Animals are also invaluable for the production of antiviral sera as well as for the isolation and identification of viruses which cannot, as yet, be grown by other methods.

Although the natural host species are ideal for the propagation of animal viruses, their value is generally outweighed by practical and economic reasons. Laboratory animals are susceptible to a wide variety of pathogenic viruses but they have a number of disadvantages, not the least of which is the high cost of breeding, raising and maintaining suitable colonies of animals of the same age, weight, sex and breed. The risk of cross-infection to other animals, the presence of intercurrent infections, including latent viruses which may complicate the interpretation of the experimental findings, and the presence of antibodies to the same or related viruses under investigation are additional disadvantages to the use of laboratory animals. Nevertheless, animals are particularly useful for propagating or attenuating viruses required for the production of viral vaccines.

Embryonated hens' eggs
Since the early 1930s, the fertile hens' egg has proved to be a valuable and widely used medium for the cultivation of viruses, rickettsiae and certain other organisms derived from avian or animal sources. Not all viruses grow in the tissues of embryonating eggs but some which do not can be adapted without much difficulty. The method is more economical and convenient than animal inoculation, and with certain viruses it provides the most suitable means for primary isolation and identification, the maintenance of stock cultures and the production of viral vaccines.

The use of fertile hens' eggs in diagnostic virology has a number of advantages over other host systems. For example, eggs are:
(1) readily available, cheap and easily maintained,
(2) sheltered from the natural diseases often observed in laboratory animals, and are relatively free from bacterial and many latent virus infections,
(3) easily manipulated under sterile conditions,
(4) generally free from natural factors of defence, specific or non-specific, that sometimes intervene and prevent passage in adult animals,
(5) sensitive to some viruses that are harmless to the adult birds (e.g. influenza), and
(6) easily identified and labelled with details of the date, nature of the virus and the experimental procedure.

The presence of virus in inoculated fertile eggs can be detected by mortality, deformities and haemorrhages of the embryos, lesions in the form of 'pocks' and oedema of the developing membranes, inclusion bodies in sections prepared from various tissues and the presence of specific antigens in the fluids as shown by haemagglutination-inhibition, complement-fixation, serum neutralization or other serological procedures. Factors which may influence the growth of viruses in fertile eggs include the age of the embryo, the dilution and volume of the virus inoculum, the temperature and humidity of incubation and the route of inoculation.

Preliminary incubation is usually carried out at 38–39°C and inoculated eggs are incubated at 37–37·5°C. In certain cases, however, lower temperatures (35·5°C) may be required. For best results the incubator should be equipped with humidifiers, forced-draught circulation of air, and an automatic egg-turning device.

There are various methods of inoculating embryonating hens' eggs for the growth of viruses and the yolk sac, chorioallantoic membrane and allantoic cavity are the three routes most commonly used. In special cases, the amniotic cavity and intravenous routes are preferred (Fig. 42.1).

Yolk sac. The method of yolk sac inoculation is performed on 6–8-day-old embryos since, at this stage of development, the yolk sac is large, the embryo is small and unlikely to be accidentally damaged, and the eggs can be incubated for a further 10–14 days before hatching. The procedure is as follows. Having first candled the egg and ascertained that the embryo is alive, the shell is disinfected by gentle swabbing with alcohol or a mixture of alcohol and iodine. A small hole is drilled or punched in the shell over the air space. Suspensions of the suspect tissues or dilutions of virus are introduced into the yolk sac by means of a hypodermic syringe fitted with a long (2″) fine-bored needle. The needle is

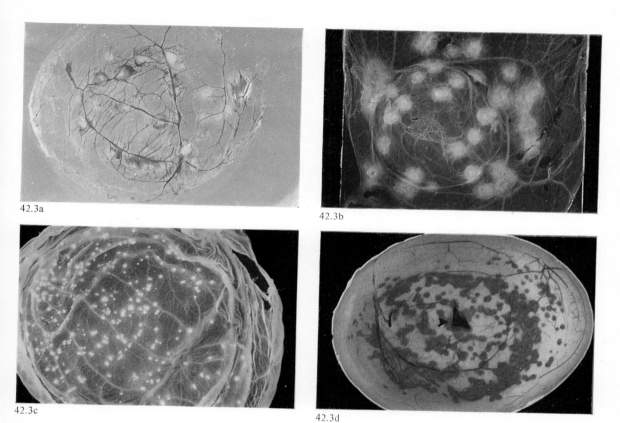

42.3a

42.3b

42.3c

42.3d

Cultivation of viruses on the chorioallantoic membrane of embryonated hens' eggs, after 5 days' incubation at 35·5°C.

42.3a   Unfixed membrane showing the necrotic foci (pocks) produced by fowl pox virus.

42.3b   Formolized membrane containing pocks of avian infectious laryngotracheitis virus.

42.3c   Numerous small pocks produced by Aujeszky's disease (pseudorabies) virus.

42.3d   Haemorrhagic pocks on the chorioallantoic membrane (*in situ*) of an egg inoculated with cow pox virus.

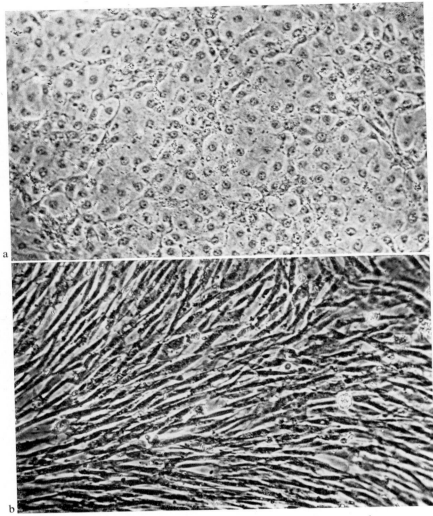

Phase contrast photomicrographs of uninfected cell culture monolayers.

42.4a Continuous culture of pig kidney epithelial cells, ×150.

42.4b Secondary culture of chick embryo fibroblasts, ×230.

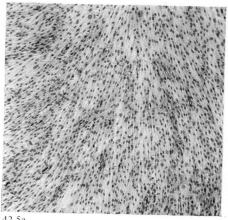

42.5a

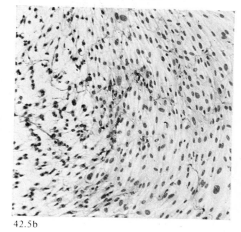

42.5b

42.5c

42.5a   Healthy primary monolayer culture of rabbit
kidney cells showing the cells arranged in a thin, single
layer with parallel orientation. Giemsa stain, ×45.

42.5b A similar uninfected culture of rabbit kidney cells
showing an extensive area (left) of non-specific cellular
degeneration. Giemsa stain, ×70.

42.5c Monolayer culture prepared from a calf kidney
cell line. Three of the cells are undergoing mitosis.
Giemsa stain, ×420.

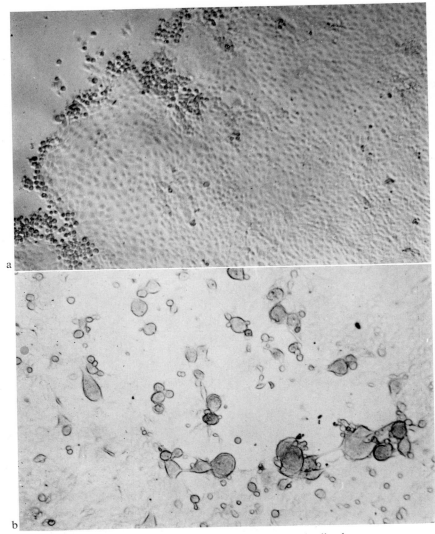

Cytopathic effects on unstained virus-infected cell cultures.

42.6a   Rounding and shrinkage of cells along the periphery of a monolayer culture of pig kidney cells 24 hours after inoculation with a porcine enterovirus, × 75.

42.6b   Development of numerous, large multinucleate syncytia (polykaryons) on a bovine kidney cell culture 72 hours after inoculation with a bovine herpesvirus, × 75.

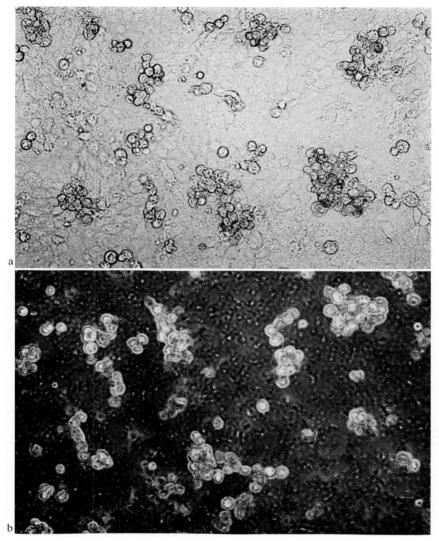

Cytopathic effects on unstained virus-infected cell cultures.

42.7a   Rounding of the cells, increased opacity and aggregation of the cells into irregular grape-like clusters in pig kidney cells inoculated with the Compton 25R strain of porcine adenovirus, × 150.

42.7b   The same as Plate 42.7a, viewed by phase contrast, 24 hours after infection, × 150.

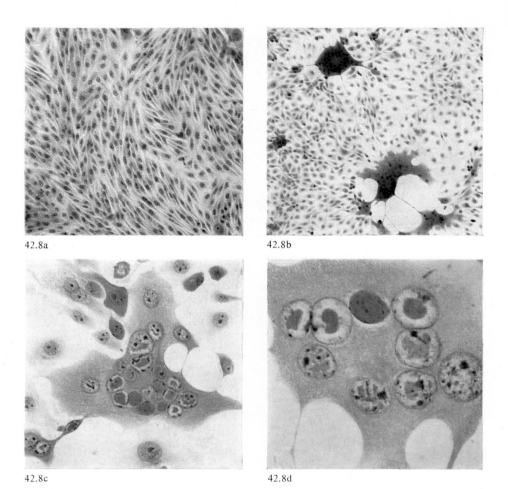

42.8a

42.8b

42.8c

42.8d

Cytopathic effects of bovine mammillitis virus on a secondary monolayer culture of ox kidney cells. Haematoxylin eosin stain.

42.8a Normal culture of growing cells, × 100.

42.8b Three days after inoculation with the virus. Notice the intense staining of the cytoplasm forming the syncytia, and the protoplasmic strands caused by shrinkage of the infected cells, × 70.

42.8c Five days after inoculation. Detail of a syncytium, showing aggregation of nuclei and the presence of a single, large Cowdry type A inclusion in each infected nucleus, × 280.

42.8d A syncytium viewed at higher magnification (× 650), showing the multilobulate appearance of some of the Cowdry type A inclusions. Notice the basophilic staining of the large 'immature' inclusion in one of the nuclei (top centre).

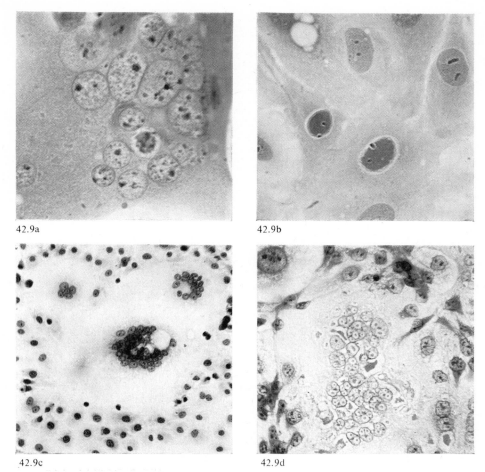

42.9a   42.9b

42.9c   42.9d

Cytopathic effects of viruses: Haematoxylin eosin stain.

42.9a Detail of a syncytium produced on a line of pig kidney cells 5 days after infection with myxoma virus. Notice the large basophilic staining inclusion in one of the nuclei and the crescent-shaped basophilic mass in the perinuclear region of the nucleus immediately above it, × 420.

42.9b A primary kitten kidney cell culture, 3 days after inoculation with feline panleucopenia virus, showing intra-nuclear inclusion bodies which develop through eosino-philia to basophilia, × 420. (Culture by courtesy of Dr R. H. Johnson.)

42.9c Formation of multinucleate syncytia on a growing monolayer of calf kidney cells persistently infected with Newcastle disease virus. Notice the absence of inclusions. Giemsa stain, × 100.

42.9d Monolayer produced by co-cultivating the same persistently infected calf kidney cells as shown in Plate 42.9c with healthy chick kidney cells. After 7 days of incubation the artificially induced syncytia (hetero-karyons) contain large numbers of intracytoplasmic and intranuclear inclusions, × 280.

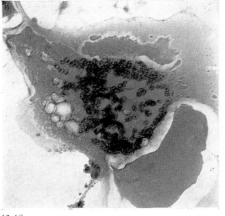

42.10a

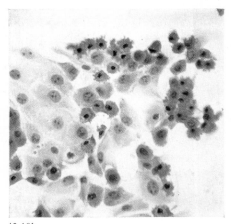

42.10b

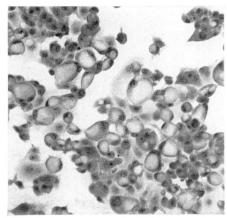

42.10c

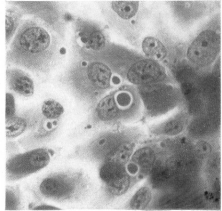

42.10d

42.10a Multinucleate syncytium produced on a primary culture of bovine kidney cells, 11 days after inoculation with rinderpest virus. Notice the very large, homogeneous acidophilic plaques in the cytoplasm. Intranuclear inclusions were not produced in this culture. Haematoxylin eosin stain, ×44.

42.10c Monolayer of sheep kidney cells (MDOK strain) 48 hours after inoculation with an egg-adapted strain of cow pox virus, showing marked vacuolation of infected cells. Haematoxylin eosin stain, ×130.

42.10b Induction of stellate cytoplasmic protrusions in the peripheral cells of a pig kidney cell monolayer infected with a 'V-type' strain of porcine enterovirus. Haematoxylin eosin stain, ×280.

42.10d A growing culture of bovine kidney cells infected 5 days previously with vaccinia virus. Notice the large spherical eosinophilic intracytoplasmic inclusion bodies, each surrounded by a clear halo. Haematoxylin eosin stain, ×420.

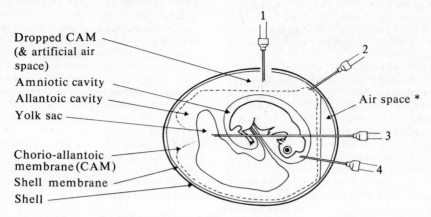

Dropped CAM
(& artificial air
space)
Amniotic cavity
Allantoic cavity
Yolk sac

Chorio-allantoic
membrane (CAM)
Shell membrane
Shell

Air space *

FIG. 42.1. Schematic diagram of developing chick embryo showing routes of inoculation for virus isolation: (1) chorioallantoic membrane inoculation, (2) allantoic cavity inoculation, (3) Yolk sac inoculation, and (4) amniotic cavity inoculation. *Absent in eggs prepared for CAM inoculation.

introduced vertically through the hole in the shell for a distance of about 1¼″ and the virus material inoculated directly into the yolk sac in 0·1–0·2 ml amounts. The needle is withdrawn and the hole over the air space sealed with nail varnish or a mixture of molten wax and petroleum jelly (Vaseline).

The yolk sac route is particularly suitable for the cultivation of agents of the PLGV group (e.g. the agent of enzootic abortion of ewes), rickettsiae (e.g. Q fever) and certain viruses (e.g. louping ill and other togaviruses).

After incubation, infected yolk sacs are harvested, emptied of yolk, gently rinsed in sterile saline and used as an antigen for serological identification. Rickettsiae and chlamydiae can also be detected by preparing multiple impression smears on a clean glass slide, and staining them, after heat fixation, by Koster's method, the modified Macchiavello, or other means. The agent of Q fever and organisms of the *Chlamydia* group stain as small bright red (acidophilic) particles against a pale blue or green background after using Koster's stain, modified Ziehl-Neelsen (Brucella differential) or other modifications of Macchiavello's method.

Allantoic cavity. Many viruses such as influenza, fowl plague and Newcastle disease virus grow readily in the allantoic endoderm of developing chicken eggs. The inoculation method, which is extremely simple to perform, employs embryos of 10–12 days' incubation. Before use the eggs are candled in order to confirm the viability of the embryos and the stage of development of the membranes. The air space is outlined in pencil and a small mark is made on the shell surface above an area free from large blood vessels. The shell is disinfected and a small hole is

drilled or punched over the pencil mark which should be one or two centimetres below the air space. The inoculum which is generally 0·1–0·2 ml is introduced by passing a fine short needle attached to a hypodermic syringe for a very short distance (1–2 mm) through the shell membrane lining the inside of the shell. It is often an advantage to punch a second hole over the air space to allow expansion of the air when the allantoic sac expands during the inoculation of virus, thereby preventing 'blow-back' at the inoculation site. Both holes are then sealed with nail varnish or a mixture of molten paraffin wax and petroleum jelly, and the eggs are reincubated and candled daily. The presence of a haemagglutinating virus can be detected by withdrawing a drop of allantoic fluid, by means of a fine Pasteur pipette, and adding it to susceptible red blood cells. (Plate 40.1a, facing p. 445). Large quantities of virus fluid can be harvested by removing the shell over the air space, carefully reflecting the shell membrane to expose the underlying allantoic cavity and passing a Pasteur pipette into the sac down the inside of the shell. The bulb of the pipette should be expressed before puncturing the allantoic sac membrane to prevent air bubbles and great care should be taken not to rupture blood vessels since the release of red blood cells and absorption of virus onto their surfaces greatly reduces the titre of the virus in the fluid. For this reason, it is an advantage to chill the eggs for an hour or two before attempting to harvest the virus fluids.

Chorioallantoic membrane. This method has been widely used in veterinary virology because many viruses (e.g. some herpesviruses, including infectious laryngotracheitis virus and Aujeszky's disease virus and some poxviruses, e.g. fowl pox, ectromelia and vaccinia) grow readily or can be adapted to grow on the chorioallantoic membrane and produce easily visible foci or 'pocks', inclusion bodies, oedema or other abnormalities.

After 10–12 days of incubation, eggs are examined for viability of the embryos and adequate development of the membranes. The outline of the air space is marked on the shell and also an area well clear of large blood vessels. The shell is disinfected and a small hole punched over the air space. Using a dental drill a triangular or square window is cut in the shell, care being taken not to puncture the underlying adherent shell membrane. The lid of shell is reflected to expose the shell membrane. The intact shell membrane is then split by repeatedly drawing with gentle pressure the point of a blunt hypodermic needle in the direction of the fibres of the membrane. The chorioallantois lying immediately beneath the shell membrane must not be punctured in the process. A small drop of sterile saline or of the desired dilution of the virus fluid is placed on the membrane and introduced into the egg when gentle suction is applied to the hole over the air sac by means of a small rubber teat. As the fluid enters the egg, the chorioallantoic membrane drops away from the shell membrane as seen by a clearly visible 'flash'. If sterile saline has been used to drop the membrane the virus material can be inoculated directly on to the surface of the chorioallantois; and the egg is rotated to disperse the virus inoculum evenly over the membrane. The larger opening is closed and sealed with Scotch tape or by replacing the triangular or square lid of shell and sealing the edges with nail varnish or a mixture of molten paraffin wax and vaseline. After 4–5 days of incubation the shell enclosing the false air space is removed to expose the entire infected chorioallantoic membrane which is picked up by means of sterile forceps and excised intact from the underlying tissue, placed in a Petri dish, washed in sterile saline and examined for the presence of surface 'pocks', oedema, haemorrhages or other abnormalities (Plate 42.3a–d, facing p. 480). The decolourised area of membrane due to the inoculum should not be mistaken for a focus of infected cells.

An alternative method of removing the chorioallantoic membrane intact, is to cut a large hole in the pointed end of the egg and shake out its contents. The chorioallantoic membrane, which usually remains adherent to the shell membrane, can then be removed from the empty egg with sterile forceps, suspended in sterile saline and examined for the presence of characteristic lesions ('pocks'). The formation of a 'pock' begins with the infection of a single cell but the virus quickly spreads to contiguous cells giving rise both to cell proliferation and to cell death. These tissue changes result in the formation of the typical 'pock' which is usually a white opaque area on the transparent membrane. However, the lesions vary in size and shape according to the nature of the infecting virus. Some may be circular, raised and dome-shaped, others may have a central depression whilst with cow pox virus they are often haemorrhagic. Intracytoplasmic or intranuclear inclusion bodies are readily detected in stained sections of 'pocks' (Plate 42.2c, facing p. 474a). and virus can be harvested by grinding the infected membranes in a suitable homogeniser. The chorioallantoic membrane route is also valuable for confirming the identity of the virus or for estimating the antibody titres of unknown sera by means of serum neutralization.

Amniotic sac. The amniotic route is recommended for the primary isolation of mumps virus and influenza virus types A, B and C from throat swabs of human patients but has little application in veterinary virology. Embryos between 10 and 14 days of age are preferred and the methods generally used are as follows.

After dropping the chorioallantoic membrane a pair of sterile forceps is forced through the chorioallantois and a small portion of the amniotic membrane is pulled through the ruptured chorioallantois so that the material can be inoculated directly into the amniotic sac. An alternative and more satisfactory procedure is to cut a large square window over the blunt end of the egg, remove the shell membrane lining the floor of the air space or render it translucent by applying a few drops of sterile liquid paraffin. The needle of the hypodermic syringe containing virus fluid and a top layer of air, is introduced through the allantoic sac towards the beak of the embryo. A small amount of air which is introduced into the egg by slowly depressing the plunger of the syringe indicates whether or not the needle has entered the amniotic sac. If the bubbles come to rest just above the embryo this indicates that the amniotic sac has been penetrated, and the inoculum is then introduced in 0·2 ml amounts. Although a disadvantage of this method is that the volume of fluid in the infected amniotic sac is much smaller than that of the normal egg, the advantage is that virus is introduced directly into the amniotic fluid which bathes the developing lung buds of the embryo whose cells are highly susceptible to infection with myxoviruses. Newly isolated influenza viruses must be passaged via the amniotic sac several times before becoming adapted to growth by other routes. Unfortunately, certain strains of virus can only be propagated by the amniotic route and cannot be adapted to grow in the allantoic sac or on the chorioallantoic membrane (Table 42.2).

TABLE 42.2. Cultivation of viruses on embryonated hens' eggs

Age of embryo	Route of inoculation	Virus or other agent inoculated
6–8 days	Yolk sac	Chlamydiae, [e.g. psittacosis and EAE]. Rickettsiae, [e.g. *Coxiella burnetii* of Q fever]; togaviruses.
10–12 days	Allantoic cavity	Myxoviruses, [e.g. fowl plague and NDV].
10–12 days	Chorioallantoic membrane	Most poxviruses; but not parapoxviruses, [e.g. Orf]. Some herpesviruses, [e.g. ILT; ADV] but not others, [e.g. BMV; MCF].
10–14 days	Amniotic cavity	Myxoviruses, [e.g. Influenza C and mumps].

ADV — Aujeszky's disease virus   ILT — avian infectious laryngotracheitis virus
BMV — bovine mammillitis virus   NDV — Newcastle disease virus
EAE — enzootic abortion of ewes   MCF — malignant catarrhal fever virus

Cell and tissue cultures

The cultivation of viruses in cell or tissue cultures has long been used by a small band of enthusiastic workers but, until comparatively recently, it has remained an extremely delicate and expensive technique because of the difficulties in supplying the cells with a suitable medium and of preventing contamination by airborne bacteria and fungi. However, the introduction of antibiotic and fungistatic substances and their inclusion in nutrient media largely overcame the difficulties of maintaining cell cultures and has led, indirectly, to so many important advances that virology rapidly attained a major position among the biological sciences.

Another important milestone in the development of tissue culture techniques was the re-introduction in 1952 of the method of cell-dispersion, whereby trypsin was used to break down the tissues into small cellular clumps which continued to grow and multiply on glass in a nutritive medium containing antibiotics. These factors, together with recent progress in devising more suitable synthetic media, have ensured that work involving cell and tissue cultures need no longer be considered a luxury and, indeed, it is well within the scope of any laboratory.

There are several methods for growing cells *in vitro*:

(1) Cultures can be prepared from cell suspensions or tissue fragments taken from living or recently killed animals and incubated in a nutrient medium in large well aerated flasks; the so-called Maitland-type cultures.

(2) Cells disaggregated by trypsinization can be incubated in tubes, bottles, flasks or Petri dishes in which the living cells will adhere to the inside of the container and grow to form a sheet or monolayer one cell thick.

(3) Organ cultures can be prepared whereby the growth of tissues or the whole or parts of an organ, can be maintained *in vitro* in a way that allows preservation of its architecture and function.

A culture started from cells, tissues or organs taken directly from an animal is termed a 'primary culture', until it is subcultured for the first time. Secondary or subsequent cultures from primary cell cultures of normal diploid tissues are usually known as 'diploid cell cultures' since at least 75 per cent of the cells usually have the same karyotype as the normal cells. Diploid cells may be grown successfully for many months but generally die out after 50–70 serial cultures unless a mutation occurs producing a polyploid or 'transformed' cell. Cell lines which are derived from transformed diploid cells or neoplastic tissues can be propagated indefinitely in culture and are called 'continuous (or established) cell lines'. Whatever the tissue of origin may have been, most transformed lines are epithelial-like in morphology and their complement of chromosomes is variable (aneuploid). Nevertheless, they are very useful in virology since they can be serially cultured without apparent limit and will support the growth of a number of viruses which may produce cytopathic changes characteristic of particular groups. There are many continuous epithelial or fibroblastic cell lines of various origins in use in laboratories throughout the world. Those from human sources include HeLa cells derived from a carcinoma of the cervix, Chang liver cells established from non-malignant tissue, KB cells from an epidermoid carcinoma of the mouth and HEp-2 cells isolated from tumours that had been produced in irradiated, cortisone treated weanling rats after injection with epidermoid carcinoma tissue from the larynx of a human patient. Continuous cell cultures of animal origin include PK-2a and PK-15 from adult pig kidney, MDBK and MDCK from the kidneys of a healthy steer and dog, respectively, BHK-21 derived from the kidneys of 1-day-old hamsters and VERO cells initiated from the kidney of a normal African green monkey. Cell lines have also been derived from marsupials, rodents, reptiles and fish.

Although primary and secondary cell cultures have

a limited life-span and are, therefore, more costly and less convenient to use, they are usually sensitive to a wider range of viruses than continuous cell lines and are particularly useful for isolation procedures.

Whichever method is adopted, the cells can only be grown and maintained in a satisfactory condition provided a suitable medium is used, the containers are clean and sterile, and the cultures are incubated under optimum conditions for growth (Plates 42.4a, b, between pp. 480–1).

Preparation of glassware. Scrupulous cleanliness of all glassware, (e.g. tubes, bottles, flasks, pipettes and syringes) is of paramount importance in tissue culture techniques, otherwise experiments will be ruined and endless time and labour will be wasted. Not only must the glassware be visibly clean but it is essential that all traces of chemicals or other substances likely to prove toxic to cells are completely eliminated.

There is no generally accepted standard procedure for the cleaning of glassware but the methods used in most laboratories are on the following lines.

Glassware, which may be autoclaved to remove any infectious agent, should then be brought to the boil in stainless steel containers containing a weak solution of sodium carbonate or detergent, (e.g. Pyroneg or Calgon-metasilicate), and allowed to simmer for 20–30 minutes. After thorough brushing with a rinse in cold running tap water, the glassware is immersed in 1·0 per cent hydrochloric acid for 1–2 hours. It is then rinsed thoroughly (6 times) in tap water and 3 times in deionised water and finally dried in a hot air oven. (Deionised water is obtained by passing 'double-glass-distilled' water through a resin cartridge to remove all metallic ions.) After use, it is an advantage if glassware containing serum, cells or other protein is not allowed to dry but is discarded into plastic buckets containing a weak solution of a suitable disinfectant. Pipettes should be discarded into a disinfectant solution if infected, otherwise they may be placed in an automatic pipette washer.

In many instances, there is considerable saving in time and labour if disposable tubes, Petri dishes and bottles are used. Unfortunately, tissue culture grade plastics are still relatively expensive but it is becoming increasingly evident that they have considerable advantages over glassware for a number of special techniques (e.g. virus-plaque assays) and may be more economical in the long term.

It is important to note that red and black rubber may contain substances toxic to cells and for this reason white rubber or, preferably, silicone rubber stoppers and cap liners only should be used: also, silicone tubing should be employed instead of red rubber tubing on all water taps and water-still attachments.

Sterilization. The best method of sterilizing glassware is by dry heat in a hot-air oven at 160°C for 60–75 min. The articles to be sterilized must be dry and should be placed in metal, pyrex or glass containers or wrapped individually in domestic aluminium foil. Rubber stoppers, liners and washers will not withstand the temperature of the hot-air oven and bottles already capped or stoppered should be autoclaved at 15 lbs in^2 for 20 min, although the accumulation of moisture in the containers may be a disadvantage. Cotton-wool must not be used to plug tubes, bottles and flasks since it frequently gives off volatile oils and other substances that condense on the glass and later may interfere with the growth of cells. Slip-on aluminium caps or aluminium foil should be employed instead.

Ultraviolet rays have a strong bactericidal and virucidal action and, apart from their general use in sowing booths, inoculation hoods, etc., they are particularly useful for sterilising plastic WHO haemagglutination trays and certain grades of membrane filters.

Filtration by means of bacteriologically sterile asbestos pads (e.g. Seitz) is useful for sterilizing large volumes of sera or solutions of chemicals but smaller volumes should not be sterilized by this method since the asbestos pads may release substances that are toxic for the cells. Hemming filters may be used for sterilizing small volumes of fluids by centrifugation but their disadvantages are the same as for the Seitz. Kieselguhr and porcelain candle filters of the Berkefeld, Mandler or Chamberland types are often inconvenient to use because their pores are readily blocked by serum or other proteinaceous materials, and they are difficult to clean and may be easily cracked. On the other hand, membrane filters of the Gradocol, Oxoid or Millipore type are clean, non-toxic, absorb only small amounts of material, are of known average pore diameter (APD) and are, therefore, very suitable for sterilization. Before use, most types of membrane filters can be sterilized with steam except for the smaller sizes which are usually sterilized by ultraviolet rays. Sintered glass filters do not alter the pH of the solution being filtered and are suitable for sterilizing salt solutions, although they tend to become blocked when sera or solutions containing many impurities are used. Wet sintered glass filters should not be heated too quickly when being sterilized otherwise small pockets of trapped steam may expand and crack the filter plate.

A number of chemical methods are available for the routine disinfection of virus-contaminated glassware. Of these, a 1–2 per cent solution of sodium hypochlorite is particularly useful, especially in the form of 'indicated Chloros' (ICI LTD), which contains potassium permanganate. This solution indicates the loss of available chlorine as the permanganate oxidises organic materials and, in so doing, loses its red/purple colour. Unfortunately, Chloros is harmful to metal parts and may also produce a skin reaction on the hands of laboratory workers.

Bacterial contamination can be eliminated or greatly reduced by means of antibiotics and, while every precaution must be taken to avoid contamination by means of aseptic techniques, sterile rooms, inoculation hoods, etc., it is customary to incorporate a mixture of penicillin (100 units/ml) and streptomycin (100 μg/ml) or other antibiotic substances in the culture media. Fungal contamination may be overcome by the addition of Nystatin (Mycostatin, Squibb) or amphotericin B (Fungizone, Squibb) at a concentration of 25 μg/ml. A more insidious type of contamination is that caused by mycoplasmas. This is a serious hazard in laboratories handling continuous cell cultures for prolonged periods and it is known that the majority of cell lines are chronically infected with human strains of P.P.L.O. Although kanamycin or tylosin (10 μg/ml) incorporated in the medium may help to overcome the infection, it is extremely difficult to cure the cultures completely and it may be necessary to employ other agents such as standard antisera and sodium aurothiomalate. Tylosin should not be used for more than 3–4 serial passages since prolonged use of this drug may lead to the development of resistant forms of mycoplasmas. Viral contamination is difficult to detect and more difficult to overcome. For this reason strict 'hygiene' is essential in all cell culture laboratories including, perhaps, ultraviolet irradiation of rooms and frequent washing of floors, walls and ceilings with a detergent solution. Wherever possible only one type of virus should be handled or investigated in the laboratory at any one time.

Cell culture media. In the early days of tissue culture the medium or nutrient fluid in which the cells were grown consisted almost entirely of biological fluids. Whilst these provided adequate nutrients for the cells, they could not be defined chemically and it was, therefore, a considerable advance when synthetic media were first introduced.

Today, all synthetic media used for maintaining or promoting the growth of cells in culture employ for their base a mixture of isotonic solutions of a number of refined inorganic salts, known as a balanced salt solution (BSS). Although there are many buffered salt solutions available, and Tyrode's modification of Ringer's phosphate buffer was once the most popular, those most commonly used today include Hanks' and Earle's. (See Appendix 2, Vol. I). Whichever solution is chosen it must be balanced to ensure conditions physiologically acceptable to the cell. In other words, it must contain essential inorganic ions, e.g. sodium, potassium, calcium and magnesium, to maintain the correct pH and osmotic pressure, and it must not contain impurities that are toxic to the cell. The chemicals must be of the highest quality and purity and only salts of analytical reagent quality should be used. Since cells form acid as they grow, buffers are added to stabilise the pH, and sodium bicarbonate is usually included for this purpose with phenol red as indicator. None of the basic salt solutions is significantly better than another but Hanks' and Earle's solutions are less likely than some others to form precipitates of carbonates and phosphates. Hanks' saline, unlike that of Earle, may be sterilized by autoclaving rather than filtration; but it does not have so large a buffering capacity as Earle's and is not suitable, therefore, for cell cultures which grow very rapidly and produce large amounts of acid.

A simple medium that is very useful in a busy diagnostic laboratory usually consists of BSS (e.g. Hanks' or Earle's) with the addition of sodium bicarbonate, phenol red, glucose [as a source of carbon and energy], antibiotics, serum and lactalbumin hydrolysate or, occasionally, yeast extract as a source of amino-acids. In addition to this type of simple medium a number of 'chemically defined' cell culture media have been devised in which a very wide range of amino-acids, vitamins, enzymes, accessory growth factors and inorganic salts are added separately in known concentrations. Although these complex chemically defined media may be used without supplementation to maintain continuous cell cultures for periods of several days when cell multiplication is not required, they are frequently used also with added serum or tissue extracts to promote the active growth of cells. The most widely used of the chemically defined media is probably Morgan, Morton and Parker's Medium 199, or a modification of it. Many attempts have been made to simplify defined media of the '199'-type and the best of these is that devised by Eagle, although this solution is still complex enough to require much time and care in its preparation.

For the growth of cells, 5–20 per cent of heat-inactivated or untreated sterile serum, usually calf serum, is added to the medium, the amount varying with the requirements of the particular cell. Once the monolayer has formed, the cells are sustained on a 'maintenance medium' which is basically the same as 'growth medium' but with only 1–5 per cent of added serum.

Various types of sera may be used but in veterinary laboratories pre- or post-colostral calf, ox or sheep sera are generally preferred. The sera are obtained from the blood of at least six freshly killed animals and, after natural clot contraction has taken place, are pooled to minimise the risks of toxicity for actively growing cells. It is then sterilised by positive filtration through membrane filters with a pore size of 0·22 µm and tested for contaminating micro-organisms by the usual bacteriological procedures. The sterile samples are dispensed in tightly stoppered plasma bottles or individual flats and stored at −20°C until they are required for use.

Plasma, amniotic fluid and tissue extracts are not widely used nowadays but dehydrated tissue extracts such as yeast extract and lactalbumin hydrolysate (LAH) are frequently employed. The latter is a relatively inexpensive form of amino-acids, and a balanced salt solution containing 0·5 per cent lactalbumin hydrolysate plus 2–10 per cent serum is one of the simplest cell culture media to prepare.

Basic requirements for growth of cells

Temperature. The optimal temperature range for most species and types of cell is 37–38°C. Although epithelial cells grow best at temperatures of 35–36°C, many of the cells grow slowly at 20–25°C and will remain dormant but viable for some time at 4°C. Most cell lines will remain in a viable state for prolonged periods when suspended in dimethyl sulphoxide (DMSO) in glass-sealed ampoules, slowly frozen and then stored in a low temperature cabinet at –70°C or in liquid nitrogen at –196°C. On the other hand, animal cells are extremely heat-labile and many will die if the temperature is raised 2 or 3 degrees above 37·5°C.

Hydrogen-ion concentration. Although most cells will tolerate a wide variation in pH (6·6–7·8) this should be avoided wherever possible, and for maximum growth the pH of the medium should be held around 7·2. Because of this, a visible check is kept on the pH of the fluid phase of cell cultures by incorporating 0·1 per cent phenol red as an indicator in the medium. In the acid conditions produced by active growth of healthy cells the medium is bright yellow, whereas in cultures containing few actively growing cells (due to virus action, or loosely fitting stoppers or caps), the medium is alkaline and the indicator turns to a reddish-purple colour. Growth medium is always prepared in a buffered salt solution and in some the pH is maintained by the additional buffering action of sodium bicarbonate.

Gaseous conditions. Oxygen and carbon dioxide are required for satisfactory growth of cells. The required CO_2 tension is produced by the cells' metabolism provided the cell cultures are grown in tightly-sealed or stoppered containers. Alternatively, the containers holding cell cultures (e.g. Petri dishes) are either flushed with air containing 5 per cent CO_2 and firmly sealed with Scotch tape or are placed in an incubator equipped with a constant supply of 5 per cent CO_2 and a humid atmosphere.

Constituents of the medium. The precise role of the inorganic salts incorporated in most cell culture media is not fully understood. Sodium salts are concerned with maintaining the osmotic pressure suitable for cells, and both potassium and magnesium are activators of enzymes involved in the cell's metabolism. Calcium, which is also an activator of enzymes, is intimately concerned with the processes of adhering and spreading of healthy growing cells to glass surfaces.

In addition to inorganic ions the cells require amino-acids, vitamins and serum proteins. The amino-acids which are used solely for incorporation into cell protein, are added to the medium either as individual amino-acids or as crude preparations of biological extracts such as yeast extract and lactalbumin hydrolysate. It is important to use the L forms of the amino-acids since the D forms, although non-toxic, are inactive. Essential vitamins are all of the B vitamin group (e.g. folic acid, choline and thiamine) and are an essential part of the structure of the co-enzymes involved in cell metabolism.

The energy requirements of the cell are provided by carbohydrates of which glucose is most commonly used in tissue culture media. Most media are 'completed' by the addition of animal serum which is a useful source of protein, and is also concerned in adhesion of the cells to the surface of the glass.

Preparation of cell cultures

A number of factors must be taken into account when preparing cell cultures for use in virology. These include not only the size of the culture to be prepared (the number of cells per ml will depend largely on the cell type chosen) but also the number and type of containers that will be most convenient for the work in hand. Suitable containers are neutral glass test-tubes or flat-sided Leighton tubes, plastic or neutral glass Petri dishes, medicinal flasks and Roux flasks. The tubes and Petri dishes may contain round or rectangular 'flying coverslips' which can be removed, stained and examined at any time during the experiment.

The choice of the most suitable tissue to be grown *in vitro* is largely determined by the availability of tissues, the nature of the virus being investigated and even, perhaps, the species of animal from which the virus was isolated.

Tissue cultures can be made either with explants, which are tissue fragments taken from living or recently killed animals, or with cell suspensions obtained by trypsinization.

Tissue explants. The preparation of tissue explant cultures adhering to the surfaces of coverslips or the inner sides of tubes, bottles and flasks is very simple and reliable. Several techniques have been devised for the preparation of these cultures, including explants in sealed 'hanging-drops' in hollow-ground slides; in a 'sitting-drop' within a ring of steel, glass or plastic placed on a slide and sealed with a coverslip; in hollow watchglasses; on plastic film or in plasma coagulum. The last method, which is sometimes called the plasma-clot technique, enables a good growth of explant cells to be maintained for long periods of time and is carried out as follows. A drop of fresh chicken plasma is spread thinly on the surface of a coverslip or is added to the container which is rapidly rotated so that the drop is evenly distributed along the inside wall. Small fragments of tissue are added and over each is placed a drop of chicken-embryo extract. The plasma-chicken-embryo extract mixture coagulates and the fragments remain firmly fixed to the glass. Growth medium sufficient to cover the explants is added and the cultures are incubated at 37°C. A major disadvantage of the plasma-clot method is that the growth of explant cultures may cause lysis of the coagulum with detachment of the tissue fragments from the glass. However, this may be prevented by adding not more than 0·18 mg of Soy bean per ml of medium. Tissue explants or cells in suspension are of value for growing viruses especially if large quantities of cells, not required to be examined microscopically, are needed for viral vaccine production.

The above methods are of limited practical value, however, and in diagnostic virology most of the tissue culture techniques are based on the preparation of cells in suspension which are then cultured in bottles or tubes as single layers of cells (monolayers) so that the effect of the virus on these cells can be examined and measured in a number of different ways. A simple and reliable method of preparing monolayer cultures is as follows.

Cell culture monolayers (Plate 42.14, facing p. 489). A kidney is removed from a young, newly-killed animal using aseptic techniques. Care is taken to avoid damage to the capsule and the kidney is immediately transported to the laboratory, preferably in warm Hank's or Earle's saline containing antibiotics. The capsule is carefully removed and the kidney is cut in half longitudinally with sterile instruments to expose the medulla and cortex. Small fragments of the cortical tissue, which is largely composed of epithelial cells, are collected, rinsed twice in Hanks' solution and transferred to a conical flask containing 50–100

ml of warm (37°C) 0·25 per cent trypsin solution at pH 7·4, for every gram of tissue. The trypsinization flask which contains a small, sterile PVC-coated magnet is placed on the heated plate of a magnetic stirrer. The stirrer is adjusted to give a uniform rate of mixing and the temperature of the medium is maintained at 37°C. The surface vortex should not exceed ¼″ in depth and frothing of the cell suspension must be avoided otherwise a high proportion of the cells may be permanently damaged. After every 10–20 min the stirrer is switched off, the suspension allowed to settle and the supernatant is collected by filtering it through sterile gauze, butter-muslin or a stainless steel gauze, into a flask immersed in ice water. Fresh trypsin is added to the trypsinization flask and the procedure is repeated six to eight times or until sufficient cells have been collected.

The harvested cells are twice washed in Hanks' solution, preferably with 5 per cent sterile serum added to inactivate the action of the trypsin and the further digestion of the cell suspension, and then centrifuged at 1000 rev/min for 5–10 min. The final cell deposit is resuspended in growth medium and the cell concentration is determined by preparing a 1/100 dilution of the cell suspension and counting the cells in a haemocytometer. In determining the cell count it is an advantage to add a weak (1·5 per cent) solution of Trypan blue in distilled water to the cell suspension to facilitate the inclusion of only living cells which, unlike dead cells, do not take up the vital stain. The viable cells are then diluted in growth medium to give a concentration of approximately 500 000 cells/ml and dispensed in 1·0 ml amounts in pyrex cell culture tubes, in 10 ml amounts in 4 oz medicinal flats or in 80 ml amounts in Roux bottles. During the first 2–3 days, or until the monolayers have developed sufficiently, the containers are placed horizontally and incubated at 37°C in the stationary position. Tube cultures are usually incubated in racks inclined at 5–7° to the horizontal. Subsequently, the culture fluids are replenished and the tubes rotated in roller drums, if required.

There are various modifications of the trypsinization procedure. Some workers prefer to discard completely the first two or three cell harvests since they may contain a high proportion of dead cells; while others disaggregate the cells slowly by stirring the finely-chopped tissue fragments in trypsin overnight in the refrigerator or cold room at 4°C. In some laboratories where a large output of cells is required, the cells are harvested automatically by continuous trypsinization, the rate of trypsin flow being regulated according to the type and quantity of the tissue being treated.

Trypsin is a proteolytic enzyme which disaggregates the cells by depolymerization of the intercellular ground substance of the tissue at pH 7·4. The pH of the trypsin solution which acts best at 37°C is checked at all stages of the operation by the incorporation of phenol red in the solution and should never fall below pH 7·2.

For satisfactory growth of cell cultures the tubes and other containers must be tightly stoppered or alternatively, as in the case of Petri dishes, the cultures are incubated in a CO_2 incubator or in plastic boxes flushed with 5 per cent CO_2 and tightly sealed with Scotch tape.

Additional tube cultures can be obtained by dispersing the cells in the medicinal flats or Roux flasks by means of versene or a trypsin-versene mixture in magnesium- and calcium-free saline (STV). Versene, the disodium salt of diaminoethane-tetra-acetic acid, is a chelating agent which acts by binding together the divalent ions of calcium and magnesium which are responsible for the adhesion of living cells to glass. Thus, in preparing versene, it is essential to use a calcium- and magnesium-free salt solution as the diluent to prevent neutralization of the versene, otherwise it will be unable to inactivate the calcium link between the cells and glass. Versene is less toxic and consequently less harmful to the cells than trypsin or other proteolytic enzymes and can safely be left to act on cells for several hours. By itself, versene does not readily disperse cells from tissue whereas trypsin and other proteolytic enzymes will kill the majority of cells in an hour unless precautions are taken to inactivate the enzyme by holding the cells in suspension at 4°C. or by adding serum to the medium.

Use of cell cultures in virology

Since 1949 when Enders, Weller and Robbins first showed that the virus of poliomyelitis would grow and produce a marked cytopathic effect in cell cultures of human embryonic material, tissue cell culture has come to be recognised as the best available method for the isolation and identification of pathogenic animal viruses. Cell cultures have several advantages over animal inoculation and fertile egg techniques, and it is easier and more economical to prepare, maintain and manipulate larger numbers of cell culture tubes than either of the other systems. In general, cells are grown in an environment free of contaminating fungi, bacteria and viruses, and they seldom have antibodies or other inhibitors to interfere with the growth of the virus. The effects of the virus on cell cultures can often be detected in a very short time (hours to days, rather than weeks) and in some cases the cell cultures are more susceptible to the effects of the virus than are animals or chicken embryos. Not every cell type can be used for growing any one virus and there is evidence that certain viruses have a high species

specificity. Thus, human adenoviruses are more likely to grow well in cell cultures of human origin than in cultures derived from tissues of laboratory animals.

The first task of the virologist is the selection of the most suitable cell system for the experiment in hand. Unless the virus and its principal biological characteristics are known the choice is largely an empirical one and more than one species of cell, e.g. bovine or sheep, and more than one cell type, e.g. epithelial or fibroblastic, (Plates 42.4a, b between pp. 480–1). may be required in the hope that the cells will be susceptible to infection by the unknown causative virus, if it is present in sufficient amount and in the infectious state at the time of sampling.

In general, primary or secondary cell cultures originating from the tissue of a host that is susceptible to a particular virus will themselves, be susceptible to that same virus. Thus, human adenoviruses may multiply only on certain tissues derived from human sources and pig enteroviruses will grow only on pig kidney cells. However, the relationship between the response of cells *in vitro* and *in vivo* is not always the rule and viruses that are specific for one species *in vivo* can replicate quite readily in cells of another species. Other viruses that have a wide spectrum of species susceptibility, (e.g. Aujeszky's disease virus), grow well in a wide range of human, animal and chicken cell types. On the other hand, certain strains of poliomyelitis virus that are pathogenic for rodents do not grow in cultures of mouse tissues. In some instances, the same virus may produce different effects in different types of cell derived from the same species of animal. For example, Sindbis virus produces a marked cytopathic effect on human uterine cells but not on HeLa cells, and human respiratory syncytial virus grows well on the 'Bristol' HeLa cell line but not on 'ordinary' HeLa cell cultures.

Infection of cultures

After deciding on the most suitable type of cell to be used the required number of cultures are prepared in tubes, dishes or bottles (with or without cover-slips), with the appropriate concentration of cells to form a uniform but not too heavy sheet of cells. The amount of medium to be used is related to the type of cell and the main aim is to maintain the cells in the best possible condition during the entire period of the experiment. For this purpose it is generally best to use a synthetic medium containing only small amounts of added serum or other biological supplements which is well buffered and will not, therefore, require to be changed too often during the experiment.

Tube cultures are usually incubated horizontally in a fixed rack at 37°C and are examined daily.

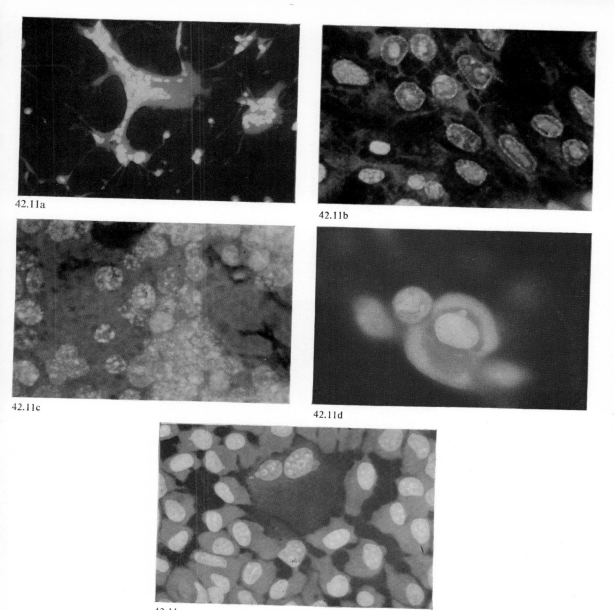

42.11a

42.11b

42.11c

42.11d

42.11e

Infected cell cultures stained with acridine orange and viewed under the ultraviolet light microscope.

42.11a Calf kidney cells, 4 days after inoculation with a bovine herpesvirus. Bright yellow-green fluorescence indicates the accumulation of DNA in the aggregated nuclei. The cytoplasm forming the syncytia is unaffected and fluoresces orange-red (RNA), ×44.

42.11b A line of pig kidney cells (PK15) 2 days after inoculation with a porcine herpesvirus, showing green, DNA-containing intranuclear inclusions, ×500.

42.11c Pig kidney cell culture 10 hours after infection with Aujeszky's disease virus, showing breakdown of nuclear structure and abundance of DNA fluorescence against the red (RNA) background of cytoplasm, ×420.

42.11d Secondary puppy kidney cells, 3 days after inoculation with the adenovirus of infectious canine hepatitis. Notice the apple-green fluorescence (DNA) of the large intranuclear inclusion body and the pink fluorescence (RNA) of the cytoplasm and nucleolus, ×850.

42.11e The same healthy monolayer cell culture as in Plate 42.4a. The orange colour of the nucleoli is clearly visible against the yellow-green of the nuclei. Notice the presence of a small syncytium (polykaryon) in this uninfected monolayer, ×320.

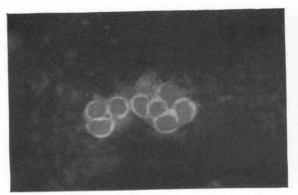

42.12a

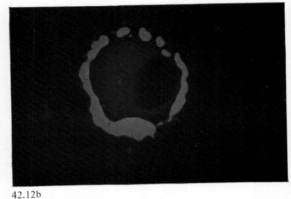

42.12b

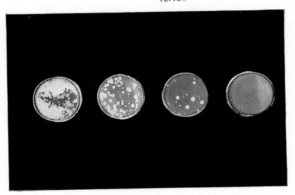

42.12c

42.12a An impression smear from the tonsil of a dog affected with distemper, stained by the indirect method with rinderpest immune serum and an anti-gammaglobulin serum labelled with fluorescein isothiocyanate. Notice specific staining of cytoplasm in peri-nuclear region outlining non-fluorescent nuclei, × 250.

42.12b A single ox kidney cell infected with Newcastle disease virus and stained by the direct method with fluorescein-conjugated rabbit anti-NDV serum. Large intracytoplasmic plaques of specifically stained material surround the nucleus, × 860.

42.12c Plaques produced by inoculating serial dilutions (highest concentration, left) of a porcine enterovirus into Petri-dish monolayer cultures of pig kidney cells. The agar overlay has been removed and the monolayers stained with neutral red, leaving the plaques as discrete foci of dead cells which have not taken up the stain.

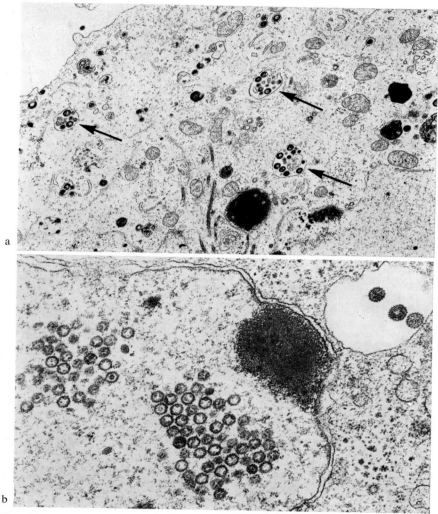

Ultra-thin sections of canine cerebellar astrocytes infected with a strain of canine herpesvirus.

42.13a   Aggregates of virus particles are seen within cytoplasmic vacuoles.

42.13b   Herpesvirus particles are dispersed through the nucleus at random. (Courtesy of Dr H. J. C. Cornwell.)

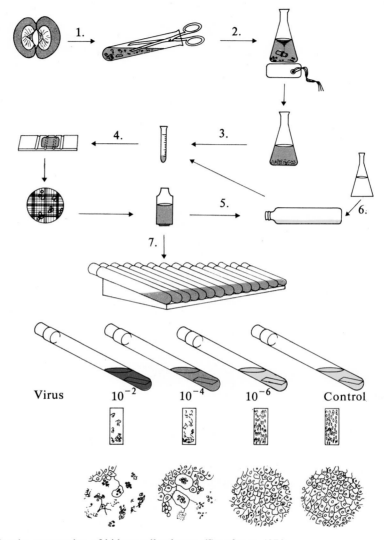

42.14 Procedure for the preparation of kidney cell cultures. (See also p. 487.)

1. Fragmentation of renal cortex.
2. Trypsinization of cortical tissue fragments on magnetic stirrer.
3. Sedimentation of harvested cells by centrifugation.
4. Counting of viable cells in haemocytometer.
5. Distribution of cells in growth medium into Roux flasks.
6. Dispersion of primary cell cultures with trypsin-versene mixture.
   Repetition of sedimentation and cell counting procedures (steps 3 and 4).
7. Distribution of cells in growth medium into tubes; and incubation of cell cultures in the stationary position prior to inoculation with virus.

Note: Healthy growing cells produce acids which lower the pH of the medium and change the colour of the phenol red indicator from red, through orange to yellow. However, in cultures containing few actively growing cells, e.g. due to a cytopathic virus, the medium becomes alkaline and turns to a reddish-purple colour.

When the cell sheets have developed sufficiently the exhausted tissue culture fluid is aseptically removed from each tube and replaced with fresh pre-warmed growth or maintenance medium. The virus to be inoculated may be from another culture or from pathological material. If the virus has originated from another culture showing a marked CPE, the destruction of the infected cells gives rise to the release of infectious virus particles into the tissue culture medium. Virus can be harvested directly from the supernatant culture fluids or, if the CPE is not advanced, the cells may first be disrupted by sonication or by a process of alternate freezing and thawing. In this latter case, the harvest of exhausted culture fluid plus cellular debris is carefully collected, lightly centrifuged for 10 min at 1000 rev/min, and the resultant supernatant is pipetted off and retained as the virus inoculum. The virus infected fluids can be transferred immediately to uninfected cultures or snap-frozen in a mixture of dried ice and alcohol and held at —30 to —70°C.

If the virus is to be isolated from pathological specimens the organ, tissues or excretions to be tested (e.g. brain, lung, skin, muscle, faeces, etc.) are generally made into a homogeneous suspension by means of a pestle and mortar, Teflon grinder or other form of blender. The growth of contaminant bacteria and fungi is prevented by adding penicillin, streptomycin and mycostatin to the 'slurry' of material which is clarified by low speed centrifugation and then inoculated into tubes containing fully formed monolayers of cells.

The inoculum, whether it consists of infected culture fluids or supernatants of homogenised pathological specimens can be inoculated, undiluted or diluted in medium, in several ways. The commonest method is to add 0·2 ml of inoculum to each tube which has been previously re-fed with 0·8 ml of maintenance medium. An alternative method is to remove the exhausted cell culture fluid from the tubes, place 0·2 ml of the inoculum over each monolayer in turn, incubate the tubes at 37°C for 1–1½ hours, leave or remove as much inoculum as possible and re-feed each tube with 0·8–1·0 ml of medium. A third method, which does not require previously prepared monolayers, is to add the inoculum to a suspension of the tissue cells, incubate for an hour at 37°C and dispense the cells in 1·0 ml amounts into clean tubes. The 'infected' cells are incubated in the stationary position at 37°C to allow monolayers to develop. This method is of value for the isolation of certain viruses, e.g. panleucopenia virus of cats, which grow best in young actively-dividing cells.

Whichever technique is used the monolayers are incubated at 37°C. or at the optimum temperature for growth, either stationary in a fixed rack or in a revolving drum which allows the monolayers to be bathed in medium at each revolution. In stationary cultures care must be taken in placing the tubes to ensure that the cell sheet is on the underside of the tube and completely covered by the medium. Roller-drum cultures are preferred by many workers since no care is required in placing the tubes so that the medium covers the cells. It has also been suggested that cell cultures remain in better condition in revolving drums because the regular bathing of the monolayer removes dead cells and other debris which may have toxic effects on the surviving cells.

All tube cultures should be observed daily for evidence of colour change of the medium, cytopathic effects or other abnormalities. Should these occur, a second passage into fresh cell cultures is usually made and, if the abnormalities are repeated, the fluids are harvested and the virus identified by serological methods.

It is important to realise that although massive inocula of virus may produce a high ratio of infected cells the phenomenon of auto-interference may result in an unexpectedly low yield of virus. In this latter case fresh cultures should be inoculated with the material diluted 10^{-1} to 10^{-3}.

Non-specific degeneration of the cells may occur if the inoculated material contains toxic substances as in the case of faecal suspensions (Plate 42.5b, between pp. 480–1). Should this occur the inocula may first be diluted or the culture medium replaced with fresh medium 1½-2 hours after the original inoculation.

Tissue changes due to virus activity are manifest in a number of different ways and, in many cases, are characteristic for each type of virus. In wet or stained cultures they may be seen as:

(1) complete destruction of the cell sheet, e.g. enterovirus infections;

(2) the formation of multinucleate cells, so-called 'giant-cells', and the dissolution of cell membranes with fusion of cell cytoplasm to form syncytia (polykaryons), e.g. myxoviruses and herpesviruses;

(3) the presence of intra-cytoplasmic or intranuclear inclusions, e.g. poxviruses and adenoviruses, respectively;

(4) transformation of the cells as shown by their altered morphology and piled up masses of cells due to loss of contact inhibition, e.g. papovaviruses; and

(5) other changes in the appearance of the cytoplasm, including increased granularity and distortion or fragmentation of the nucleus, e.g. myxoma and some other poxvirus infections.

The multiplication of a virus in the cells can be detected, in the presence or absence of cytopathic changes, in several other ways, viz. by complement-fixation, haemagglutination and haemagglutination-inhibition, haemadsorption and haemadsorption-inhibition, serum neutralization, the production of interferons, agar-gel diffusion, electron microscopy and the detection of specific viral antigen within the cytoplasm or nucleus of infected cells by means of fluorescent antibody staining.

However, if no effects are seen in the cell system after a suitable period of time, the cells should be disrupted by rapid freezing and thawing or by treatment in a sonic oscillator and passed into fresh cultures. A number of such 'blind' passages should be made before the investigation is abandoned. This serves to remove or dilute out any antibodies introduced with the original inoculum, thereby allowing a latent virus to escape and proliferate in the susceptible cell culture.

It is, of course, essential that animal sera incorporated in tissue culture media should first be checked for toxicity and, if possible, for specific antibodies or non-specific inhibitors. Because of these hazards it is preferable, wherever practicable, to use a serum derived from an animal that is not susceptible to the virus being investigated and is of a different species from the cell type of the monolayer.

Identification of viruses

Cytopathic effects

Many animal viruses that replicate in susceptible cells in tissue culture are capable of producing morphological changes, i.e. cytopathic effects (CPE) that are visible, stained or unstained, with the ordinary light microscope. In many cases the rapidity of development and the morphology of the tissue changes are characteristic of a particular group of viruses and are an invaluable aid to diagnosis. The spectrum of cytopathic activity of a virus on cells of one type but not on others may also facilitate subsequent identification. The earliest evidence of cellular damage in infected cultures may be a slower metabolic rate of the cells as shown by the lack of change in the colour of the medium, increased granularity of the cytoplasm, contraction and necrosis or rounding up of the cells. The most drastic type of CPE occurs when replication of the virus results in death and lysis of the host cell. The rapid destruction of cells may occur around the edges of the monolayer or within the monolayer in 8–12 hours after infection (e.g. Teschen and many other enteroviruses). The infection may be rapidly progressive until the entire cell sheet is destroyed within 18–24 hours post-inoculation.

Adenoviruses, herpesviruses and myxoviruses often cause marked cytopathic effects but, depending on the nature of the cell system used, the changes may not be so progressive, and focal areas of necrosis are seen scattered throughout the monolayer. On certain susceptible cell systems, however, the viruses may replicate successfully without producing visible abnormalities.

The type of cellular changes produced by herpesviruses is often an aid to diagnosis. Aujeszky's disease virus gives rise to rounding and ballooning of the affected cells and in many cell cultures large spherical syncytial masses appear throughout the monolayer. Bovine mammillitis virus, a type of herpesvirus, also forms numerous syncytia which are often irregular in shape with numerous cytoplasmic strands bridging the gaps in the monolayer between the healthy and affected cells. Adenoviruses also produce a characteristic cytopathic effect, the infected cells becoming enlarged, rounded and highly refractile with a tendency to clump in grape-like clusters (Plate 42.7a, b between pp. 480–1).

Multinucleated cells which are sometimes called syncytia, giant-cells or polykaryocytes, are produced by many viruses and are probably formed as a result of alterations to the surface membranes of the infected cells. As a result of these changes, infected and non-infected cells may fuse and, following lysis of the fused cytoplasmic membranes, the contents of the cytoplasm of the cells flow together to form the syncytium (polykaryon). The nuclei of the fused cells lie freely and occupy either a central or a peripheral position ('giant-cell' formation) within the cytoplasm of the syncytium. It is of interest that certain viruses such as measles and rinderpest that form syncytia in cell cultures may also produce multinucleated cells *in vivo*, and the presence of these changes in some tissues, e.g. the tonsils, can prove helpful in reaching a diagnosis. Other abnormalities in infected cells include vacuolation of the cytoplasm which is particularly marked in primary or secondary kidney cell cultures of rhesus monkeys carrying a latent SV40 or simian papovavirus infection.

Although the above changes can be observed in living cells in culture, it is often an advantage to fix and stain cells grown on coverslips and to examine them for evidence of virus-induced changes that may assist in identifying the virus (Plates 42.8, 42.9, 42.10, between pp. 480–1).

Tinctorial properties

Monolayers grown on coverslips in tubes or Petri dishes are removed at appropriate intervals following infection, washed thoroughly in warm phosphate-buffered saline (PBS), fixed in alcohol or other suitable fixatives, (e.g. Bouin or Carnoy), stained by haematoxylin and eosin, Giemsa or May-Grunewald-Giemsa, dehydrated by several rapid changes through acetone, acetone/xylol, and xylol, and finally mounted in DePeX on a clean glass slide.

Examination of stained preparations may show not only morphological alterations of the cells, ranging from the earliest changes of the constituent elements of the cell to complete cellular destruction, but also the formation of syncytia and the appearance of viral inclusions.

Not all viruses produce inclusions but many do so, and their distribution and appearance are frequently of diagnostic importance. Inclusion bodies may be formed in the cytoplasm or in the nucleus and may be single or multiple. Vaccinia virus and fowl-pox virus form large round acidophilic intracytoplasmic inclusions, while in rabies the intracytoplasmic inclusions (Negri bodies) are acidophilic with a basophilic inner body.

In herpesviruses, the nucleus contains a single large inclusion which first appears as homogeneous material that stains faintly basophilic. As the inclusion develops it fills the centre of the nucleus and pushes the basic chromatin towards the margin of the nucleus giving rise to the classical basophilic 'signet-ring' appearance of the nuclear membrane. Later, the inclusion appears to shrink to an acidophilic mass surrounded by a clear halo which separates it from the deeply basophilic marginated chromatin (Cowdry type A). A second type of intranuclear inclusion (Cowdry type B) comprises one or more small, circumscribed, acidophilic bodies of various sizes, each surrounded by a wide, clear halo. But, unlike type A, the nucleus shows little disorganization and there is no margination of the chromatin. An example of Cowdry type B inclusions are the Joest-Degen bodies found in neurones in Borna disease of horses. In some virus infections e.g. parainfluenza-3, the cells may contain multiple intranuclear bodies and large irregularly shaped acidophilic masses of inclusion material within the cytoplasm.

Other abnormalities seen in stained preparations include changes in the shape and size of the nucleus and, occasionally, chromosomal abnormalities. For example, in herpesvirus infections the normal mitosis is arrested usually in metaphase which may lead to failure of cell division. In certain adenovirus infections, on the other hand, there may be a marked increase in the mitotic activity of the cells in the infected monolayer (Plate 42.5c, between pp. 480–1).

Other methods which are being increasingly used in virology to study the replication of viruses and the changes produced in infected cells include acridine-orange and fluorescent antibody staining. The fluorochrome dye, acridine-orange, is used on cell monolayers treated as for conventional staining, except that an acid fixative must be used. The dye has a marked affinity for nucleic acids so that when cells stained with this dye are viewed through the ultraviolet light microscope the cytoplasm, nucleoli and other RNA components rich in single-stranded RNA fluoresce with shades of orange and red (Plate 42.11, facing p. 488). Particles containing single-stranded DNA also give an orange-red colour. The nuclei and other double-stranded DNA structures take on shades of green ranging from deep apple-green to a light yellow-green colour.

Fluorescent antibody staining
One of the most elegant and useful staining methods for locating and detecting specific viral antigens in cell cultures is fluorescent antibody staining. Infected monolayers are washed, fixed in acetone and stained by adding a few drops of fluorescent antibody prepared by coupling (conjugating) a fluorescent dye such as fluorescein either to the antibody against the virus, or to a globulin which will react with the antiviral globulin. The excess dye is removed by thorough washing and the preparation is examined in a microscope equipped with an ultra-violet light source. The antibody-coated viral antigens appear as brightly fluorescent particles against a dark background. Care must be taken to include adequate controls to rule out non-specific reactions (Plate 42.12a, b, between pp. 488–9).

Electron microscopy
In recent years the use of phosphotungstic acid (PTA) in negative staining has enabled the electron microscopist to detect the presence of virus in infected cell cultures and to study the ultrastructure of the virions. The virus preparations are obtained either from the supernatant fluids or after disruption of the cells (by distilled water or sonication) if the viruses are not liberated spontaneously. Unless high-titred virus is obtainable it is often necessary to concentrate the virus particles by ultracentrifugation or dialysis. In a number of disease conditions direct electron microscopy of swabs (e.g. from the upper respiratory tract of dogs with acute distemper) or scrapings from lesions (e.g. 'Orf' in lambs or human contacts) may reveal the presence of virions or viral components of characteristic morphology which enable a tentative diagnosis to be made in a very short time (Plates 37.4b, facing p. 431, and 52.1b, facing, p. 676b).

Virus particles can also be detected in ultra-thin sections of infected cells and tissues stained by lead citrate or uranyl acetate, but detailed study of the ultrastructure of the virion is less satisfactory by this method than negative staining with PTA. (Plate 42.13a, b between pp. 488–9). However, a technique has been introduced for specific identification of virus particles even within infected cells. The cells are stained with ferritin-labelled antibody and when examined in the electron microscope the iron core of the ferritin is readily visible and viruses which have taken up the ferritin antibody are surrounded by numerous tiny electron dense molecules of iron.

Haemagglutination and haemadsorption

Viruses that can agglutinate red blood cells may replicate in cell cultures with or without evidence of a cytopathic effect. The presence of such viruses, for example Newcastle disease virus, can readily be detected by adding a small amount of the extracellular tissue culture fluid to a suspension of washed erythrocytes and observing the mixture for haemagglutination. The identity of the virus can then be confirmed by specific haemagglutination-inhibition tests.

Tissue cells infected with viruses of the myxovirus group and some others that possess haemagglutinins, undergo a change whereby chicken or guinea-pig erythrocytes added to the culture adhere to those areas of the monolayer containing virus-infected cells. The phenomenon is probably closely associated with the process of maturation and assembly of the virus resulting in certain changes at the surface of the cell membrane which enable the red cells to adhere to infected but microscopically normal cells. This haemadsorption technique, as it is called, is useful not only for detecting the presence of myxoviruses in cell cultures but also for identification of these viruses and for neutralizing antibody assays.

Haemadsorption is carried out by discarding the exhausted cell culture fluid, rinsing the monolayer gently with warm (37°C) PBS, and adding a weak suspension (0·4 per cent) of washed guinea-pig or other species of erythrocytes to the culture. The treated monolayer is held at room temperature or in the refrigerator (+4°C) for 15–20 min, rinsed gently with PBS, and examined unstained for erythrocytes which have resisted elution by washing. The method can also be used on monolayers grown on cover-slips which can then be stained by Giemsa or haematoxylin-eosin, and the ratio of infected to uninfected cells can be determined by counting the individual infected and non-infected cells.

The method is useful for detecting haemagglutinating viruses that multiply in cells without showing detectable cellular alterations and, possibly, viruses that fail to produce sufficient amounts of haemagglutinins in the extracellular fluids, (e.g. primary isolates of parainfluenza-3 viruses). It is also useful for detecting and identifying viruses (e.g. African swine fever virus) which show haemadsorption although they do not seem to form haemagglutinins. Haemadsorption is inhibited by specific antiviral serum and an inhibition test can be used to confirm a diagnosis. Plate 43.3a, between pp. 518–9.

Mixed haemadsorption

A modification of the haemadsorption technique which may prove useful in detecting viruses e.g. herpesvirus, which do not haemadsorb in the conventional manner, is called mixed haemadsorption. In this procedure, virus-infected cells are treated with, say, rabbit immune serum. The antibodies combine specifically with the virus so that the host cells when treated with sheep erythrocytes coated with anti-rabbit serum permit the sheep red cells to be adsorbed by virtue of the combination between the rabbit gamma globulin (viral antibody) and the species-specific immune serum coating the sheep erythrocytes.

The plaque method

When cell monolayers are infected with certain viruses (e.g. herpes and adenoviruses), cytopathic changes may be produced which are clearly visible to the unaided eye in unstained preparations as localised foci. The presence of these foci or plaques is due to the fact that these viruses are not freely released from the infected cells but are usually transmitted to neighbouring cells by direct cell to cell transfer. With most other types of cytopathic viruses, mature virions are released into the culture fluids and rapidly infect most of the cells in the monolayer producing a progressive rather than a focal type of CPE. However, if a monolayer of cells infected with a markedly cytopathic virus is overlaid with agar after a suitable period of incubation, the released virions are prevented from spreading throughout the monolayer and consequently infect only adjacent cells, giving rise to localised foci which appear as clear areas or 'plaques' in the remaining sheet of healthy cells. The virus plaque is equivalent to the bacterial colony since both are derived from the progeny of a single infectious particle.

The virus plaque method is usually carried out on monolayer cultures grown in tightly-stoppered bottles (medicinal flats) or in disposable plastic Petri dishes either in a sealed container flushed with 5–10 per cent CO_2 or in a CO_2 incubator. When the monolayers have developed satisfactorily, they are infected with suitable dilutions of virus and incubated for two hours at 37°C with occasional rocking of the plate to distribute the virus evenly. After a suitable period of adsorption, the excess virus inoculum is removed and the monolayers of infected cells are covered with an overlay consisting of equal parts of 1·4 per cent agar and maintenance medium. Approximately 4 ml. of agar overlay is sufficient for each 2 in. diameter Petri dish. When, after a further period of incubation, the plaques are large enough to be distinguished by the unaided eye or by means of a hand lens as individual unstained areas or foci, the agar overlay is then removed and the healthy cells remaining in the monolayer are stained with a vital dye such as neutral red. In certain circumstances it may be preferable to incorporate the dye in the agar overlay. The plaques appear as clear zones against a red background and can be counted individually (Plate 42.12c, between pp. 488–9).

The size and shape of virus-induced plaques vary with different viruses and can be a useful aid in diagnosis. Not all viruses produce plaques and, since the ability to form plaques is often proportional to the intensity of the cytopathic effect, a virus that does not induce cell destruction is unlikely to form clearly visible foci of infection. However, viruses that do not produce visible cytopathic lesions may still be titrated by counting other types of foci. For example, oncogenic viruses may form foci of cell proliferation, whilst those that produce haemagglutinins may give rise to localised and countable areas of cells showing haemadsorption. Yet another method which is sometimes applicable with myxoviruses and herpesviruses, is to count the polykaryocytes (or syncytia) produced in infected cell monolayers stained by Giemsa or haematoxylineosin.

When the plaque method is used for titrating virus, the titre of the viral preparation is calculated directly from the number of plaques and the dilution of the sample, and is expressed in plaque-forming units (p.f.u.).

The plaque assay method has a number of important advantages over the end-point dilution methods. Not only does it combine simplicity, accuracy and high reproducibility but it is also highly economical. It has been calculated that one monkey kidney which may be expected to yield 15–30 Petri dish cultures is statistically equivalent to 1000–2500 tube cultures. Thus, to attain a similar degree of accuracy the plaque method is much less demanding in both cells and labour.

The plaque technique is also useful for purifying viruses since the progeny in a plaque area results from infection of a cell by a single virus particle. Provided care is taken to select the virus only from widely separated plaques, and repeating the process once or twice, a clone of pure virus can be obtained by excising a single plaque from a plate. Virus isolated from a single plaque thus represents a genetically pure line. The advantage of this method of cloning is well illustrated by the fact that five serologically distinct porcine enteroviruses were found to produce no fewer than four different types of plaques on monolayers of pig kidney cells. Although not widely applicable to routine virology, the use of specific antiserum which inhibits plaque formation is the basis of a neutralization test which is useful in research work.

Metabolic effects
Healthy, actively growing cells form acids which are liberated into the medium and lower its hydrogen-ion concentration. Since phenol red is incorporated in the growth medium this change in pH of the fluid is visible macroscopically as an alteration in the colour of the indicator which progresses from red through orange to yellow. In infected cultures, on the other hand, and especially where the virus causes drastic cytopathic effects, the amount of cellular metabolism is markedly decreased and the medium remains red. These changes in the pH of the medium form the basis of the metabolic inhibition test since specific antiserum incorporated in the test will inhibit the growth and development of the virus and allow the cells to grow normally, producing the same acid conditions as in uninfected control cells. The test is not suitable for viruses which do not produce a pronounced cytopathic effect or for certain adenoviruses. The replication of some adenoviruses is unusual in that there is increased cellular glycolysis and the accumulation of lactic acid which causes the pH of the medium to fall below that of the healthy control cell cultures.

Interference
All cultures infected with certain types of virus may produce interferons which, even in very small amounts, may protect the cells against a second viral infection. This phenomenon has proved useful for detecting latent or even hitherto unknown infections in monolayer cultures by their reduced ability to support the growth of a challenge virus that is known to produce a cytopathic effect in healthy cells of the same type. Monolayer cultures inoculated with the test material and incubated for several days are super-infected with a virus which is capable of producing a cytopathic effect in the cell system used. The cultures are reincubated and examined at daily intervals. A reduction in titre of 2 logs in the test cultures is held to be significant and indicates the presence of an interfering agent.

The method was used successfully to demonstrate, for the first time, the growth of rubella virus in cell culture, and is also being used in medical virology for the detection of certain non-cytopathic 'common cold' viruses.

Specific methods of virus identification and the serological diagnosis of virus infections
Because of the rapidly increasing use and availability of cell cultures in virology it is now relatively easy to isolate viruses from clinical materials. Nevertheless, failure to isolate a virus does not exclude the possibility of viral infection, nor does the isolation of a virus necessarily establish that the agent is the cause of the patient's illness. It is becoming increasingly obvious that viruses may be present in the animal body without producing disease while others may persist in the tissues for many months

or even years after the animal has made a complete clinical recovery from the infection.

By the time the virus has been isolated from the clinical material it may be possible to give a provisional diagnosis according to the source of the specimen and the rate and nature of the tissue changes in the infected cell cultures, notably the distribution and types of inclusions, syncytia or the morphology of the virion as shown by electron microscopy.

In the majority of cases, however, positive identification of an unknown virus depends upon serology to show that the virus reacts with an antiserum prepared in experimental animals against a member of the serological group or a type to which it belongs. Whether or not the purpose of the exercise is to characterise the virus or to detect and measure the antibodies in the patient's serum, the procedures used involve combinations of viruses with specific antibodies which are measured by one or more serological methods. Thus, the diagnostic virologist must choose between the isolation and specific identification of the causative virus or the use of serological methods for the detection and measurement of specific antibodies that may develop during the course of the illness. In general, group antigens are identified by means of complement-fixation tests, whereas individual serotypes are characterised by serological tests having a narrower reactivity such as haemagglutination-inhibition tests or neutralization tests.

It is again emphasised that, for serological investigations, at least two samples of sera must be obtained if the antibody levels are to be adequately tested and evaluated. The first or acute phase serum ought to be collected as soon as possible after the onset of clinical illness, and the second or convalescent sample should be obtained 2–3 weeks later or at some other appropriate time since antibodies appear earlier in some viral infections and later in others. For complement-fixation tests, and some neutralization tests, it is usually necessary to heat the serum samples for 30 min at 56°C to remove non-specific inhibitors which may interfere with the reading of the test. While the most useful serological procedures in diagnostic virology are undoubtedly complement-fixation, haemagglutination-inhibition and neutralization tests, other methods including immunofluorescence, flocculation and precipitation reactions may also be used. Although the number of basic serological techniques is limited there are, unfortunately, many variations for each method depending not only on the nature of the viral antigen under examination but also on the preferences of the individual investigator.

It is not within the scope of this book to discuss the methods of preparing various viral and other antigens nor to give a detailed account of the different serological techniques that are commonly used in virology. Instead, only the broad outlines of the more important serological methods will be described as they are applied either to the identification of the antigen or to the detection and measurement of specific antibodies.

Complement-fixation

Complement-fixation is probably the most generally useful serological method in virology since the specificity of the reaction is somewhat broader than that of haemagglutination-inhibition or neutralization. Although the complement-fixation test is mostly used for serological diagnosis, it is also of value in confirming the identity of a virus isolate. Almost any viral or soluble antigen, but only certain kinds of antibodies, can be used. One of the main reasons for the wide variety of techniques that are still employed, and the lack of a single standard test, is the difficulty of preparing antigens of sufficient purity and sensitivity. Viral antigens for use in the complement-fixation test may be prepared from the tissues of infected experimental animals but most are derived from allantoic fluids or other tissues of infected embryonated eggs or from infected tissue culture fluids. Cell culture fluids prepared from suspensions of virus-infected cells which have been disrupted by alternate freezing and thawing or by sonication are preferred, since they are generally more easily prepared and tend to be less anticomplementary than extracts of infected animal tissues. For serological assays the antigen must be of adequate potency and show no non-specific or anticomplementary activity at its optimal dilution.

The principles of the complement-fixation test are the same whether the test is used in virology or bacteriology. Thus, when complement is added to a mixture of antigen and specific antibody it is combined or fixed whereas, if no antigen-antibody reaction occurs, the complement remains free. Fixation of a known amount of complement is demonstrated by testing for residual complement by means of an indicator system comprising red blood cells sensitized by specific haemolysin (antiserum to sheep red blood cells). Lysis of the antibody-sensitized sheep red blood cells occurs in the presence of complement after a period of incubation at 37°C whereas absence of haemolysis indicates fixation of complement (a positive result) in the test system (Plate 42.15 facing p. 504).

Complement-fixation tests may be of limited value in certain viral infections, (e.g. Eastern equine encephalitis and other togaviruses), since the complement-fixing antibodies tend to develop rather late (perhaps several weeks) after the onset of clinical symptoms and decline more rapidly than serum neutralizing or haemagglutination-inhibiting antibodies.

One of the problems associated with complement-fixation tests is that some test sera may show anti-complementary activity even after heat inactivation. This may be due to chemical or bacterial contamination of the sera, to an abnormally high content of gamma globulins or to the presence in the serum of inhibitors to complement. The anti-complementary activity that may develop in serum left at room temperature for a few days may be removed by diluting the serum 1/8 in buffer solution followed by heating at 56°C for 30 min. Other anti-complementary activities are not so easily eliminated but attempts may be made to do so by adding one part of fresh inactivated guinea-pig serum to five parts of the test serum which is held at 37°C for 30 min.

Since the general procedure for carrying out a complement-fixation test depends on a large number of variable factors, viz., antigen, complement, haemolysin and test sera, the utmost accuracy is essential. Not only must the reagents be prepared with great care but preliminary standardisation is also essential. This includes titration of the haemolytic system and complement by the 'chequerboard' method in a perspex plate to determine the optimum concentration of haemolytic serum and the haemolytic titre of each new batch of complement; as well as a similar titration of antigen and standard serum to determine the optimum dilution of each antigen required for the test, and the titre of the positive control serum. The test proper can then be carried out for the titration of antibody where two units of antigen are added to a series of twofold dilutions of antiserum, or for the titration of viral or soluble antigen where a selected dilution of antiserum is added to a series of twofold dilutions of antigen.

The short fixation (1½ hours' incubation at 37°C) or the long fixation (overnight incubation at 4° C) methods may be used and in serological diagnosis the results are reported in terms of the titre of each of the paired sera obtained with each antigen. A fourfold or greater increase in the convalescent serum is considered to be of diagnostic significance.

Technical details of the complement-fixation test as used in virology are given in Appendix 2, Vol. I.

Indirect complement-fixation test

Some mammals and many birds including chickens, ducks, turkeys and older pigeons, infected with psittacosis produce antibodies which do not fix guinea-pig complement in the presence of homologous antigens and cannot, therefore, be detected by the direct complement-fixation test. These antibodies can be demonstrated by the indirect complement-fixation test, using the direct complement-fixation test as an indicator. This is carried out by examining the unknown (test) serum for its ability to inhibit fixation of complement by the antigen and a known homologous (indicator) serum obtained from another species. If, under these conditions, the antibodies in the test serum neutralise or saturate the antigens so that none is available for combination with the complement-fixing indicator serum, then fixation of complement fails to occur and the sensitized red blood cells are haemolysed. If, on the other hand, the unknown (test) serum lacks antibodies, the antigens are free to fix complement with the complement-fixing indicator serum, and no haemolysis occurs. The indirect complement-fixation test can also be used in foot-and-mouth disease for detecting low levels of antibodies in convalescent sera. The indirect complement-fixation test is represented diagrammatically on p. 382.

Haemagglutination-inhibition test

Many viruses such as myxoviruses, togaviruses, reoviruses, some enteroviruses, adenoviruses and poxviruses agglutinate red blood cells of various species of animals, and the reaction can be inhibited by antiserum specific for the infecting strain.

Haemagglutination-inhibition tests are of great importance in diagnostic virology because they are extremely specific and can be employed not only to identify freshly isolated viruses but also to determine the levels of antibodies to various strains, sub-strains and even variants of some haemagglutinating viruses. Thus the haemagglutination-inhibition test differs from the complement-fixation test which, as we have seen, is group specific rather than type specific and will only disclose similarities between strains of certain viruses. Although the haemagglutination-inhibition test is extremely reliable and simple to perform it is, like many other serological procedures, not without its difficulties. One of the problems associated with this test stems from the fact that many human and animal sera possess non-specific inhibitors of haemagglutination. The nature of these inhibitors varies for different viruses and also for different animal species, and their presence may add difficulties to the interpretation of the serological findings since they may either prevent haemagglutination at much higher dilutions than does specific antibody or mask a true diagnostic rise in antibody titre. Thus, it is essential before performing the test proper to check all test sera for the presence of non-specific inhibitor substances and to remove them without in any way affecting the titre of specific antibody. Several methods are available for treating sera to inactivate inhibitors. Heat-labile or Chu inhibitors are destroyed by heating at 56°C for 30 min while heat-stable varieties (Francis' inhibitor, or mucoid inhibitor) are removed, or their effects minimised, by treatment with receptor destroying enzyme (RDE), trypsin or potassium periodate. Non-specific inhibitors of togavirus and some other virus haemagglutinins are inactivated by absorption with kaolin or extraction with acetone.

Although haemagglutination and haemagglutination-inhibition were originally described for influenza virus and other myxoviruses, it is now known that these reactions occur with many groups of animal viruses. Indeed, it has been suggested that if the

end-point is read by the pattern of the sedimented red cells; a regular button indicates a negative reaction whereas a diffuse layer or veil of cells covering the bottom of the well indicates haemagglutination. The highest dilution of virus in 0·25 ml volume causing complete (100 per cent) agglutination of chicken erythrocytes contained in 0·25 ml suspension equals one haemagglutinating unit (HAU).

Having established the haemagglutinin titre, the stock virus is diluted appropriately for use in the

TABLE 42.3. Conditions under which haemagglutination and haemagglutination-inhibition occur with some viruses.

Virus	Species of red blood cell	Temperature	pH
Chlamydia	Mouse	20°C.	—
Orthomyxovirus	Chicken, etc.	20°C. (4°C)	7.2
Newcastle disease virus	Chicken, etc.	4, 20, 37°C	7.2
Para-influenza 1, 2 and 3	Chicken, etc.	4–30°C.	7.2
Para-influenza 4	Rhesus. Guinea-pig	20–37°C.	7.2
Measles	Rhesus	37°C.	7.2
Togavirus	Day-old chicken, Gander	20–37°C.	> 6.0, < 7.0
Reovirus types 1, 2	Human 'O'	20°C.	7.2
Reovirus type 3	Bovine	4°C.	7.2
Adenovirus	Rhesus [rat]	37°C. [20°C.]	7.2
Enterovirus	Human 'O'	4, 20, 37°C.	5.8–7.2
Polyoma	Guinea-pig	4°C.	7.2
Pox [vaccinia]	Fowl	20°C.	7.2

right conditions are obtained it may be possible to show that any virus can be made to agglutinate red blood cells of one species or another. The haemagglutination reaction depends on a number of variable factors including the species of red cells, the temperature of incubation and the pH under which the test is carried out. The conditions under which haemagglutination or haemagglutination-inhibition can occur with some representative types of animal viruses is shown in Table 42.3.

In general terms the procedure for the haemagglutination-inhibition test consists of adding either a standard amount of virus to dilutions of the test serum [β method] or a standard amount of the test serum to dilutions of a virus [α method]. The β method is the more usual procedure and is also the more accurate, whereas the α method, using dilutions of virus, has an important place in veterinary diagnostic virology since it enables large numbers of sera to be screened in the shortest time possible during an outbreak of disease in domestic animals.

Test Procedure. Haemagglutination-inhibition test. (*Beta method*). Doubling dilutions (0·25 ml volumes) of the stock virus are made in phosphate buffered saline (pH 7·2) in a WHO perspex plate. To each virus dilution is added 0·25 ml of 0·5–1·0 per cent of freshly drawn pooled fowl red cells and the plate is held at room temperature for 45–60 minutes. The

haemagglutination-inhibition test so as to contain four complete haemagglutinating units (HAU) per 0·25 ml.

Serial twofold dilutions (0·25 ml volumes) are made of each test serum, previously treated for the removal of non-specific inhibitors, from 1/8–1/2048. Virus suspension containing 4 HAU is added in 0·25 ml volumes to each well and allowed to stand at room temperature for one hour. Indicator fowl red cells (0·5–1·0 per cent) are then added (0·25 ml volumes) to all the wells and the test is read after 45–60 min at room temperature. The appropriate virus, serum and erythrocyte controls must be included to establish the specificity and sensitivity of the test. The titre of the serum is expressed as the reciprocal of the highest dilution of serum which causes complete inhibition (100 per cent end-point) of haemagglutination. The serum dilution preventing agglutination when mixed with a standard suspension of virus and erythrocytes is approximately proportional to the amount of antibody present.

It should be noted that increasing or decreasing the amount of virus will proportionately decrease or increase the titre of the serum. In some laboratories where it is the practice to add the red cell suspension immediately after the virus, the serum titres will tend to be slightly lower than by the above method. It is also emphasised that titres *per se* have no absolute meaning and it is important when reporting results

TABLE 42.4.   The haemagglutination-inhibition test [beta method].

STEP 1.   TITRATION OF VIRAL ANTIGEN FOR USE IN THE HAEMAGGLUTINATION-INHIBITION TEST

Reagents	\	\	\	\	\	TUBE OR CUP	\	\	\	\	\
	1	2	3	4	5	6	7	8	9	10	11
Buffer [ml]	—	0.25	0.25	0.25	0.25	0.25	0.25	0.25	0.25	0.25	0.25
Virus [ml] Dil. 1:10	0.25	0.25	0.25	0.25	0.25	0.25	0.25	0.25	0.25	0.25	— (Discard last 0.25)
Buffer [ml]*	0.25	0.25	0.25	0.25	0.25	0.25	0.25	0.25	0.25	0.25	0.25
0.5% fowl RBC	0.25	0.25	0.25	0.25	0.25	0.25	0.25	0.25	0.25	0.25	0.25
Final virus dilution	1:10	1:20	1:40	1:80	1:160	1:320	1:640	1:1280	1:2560	1:5120	Fowl RBC control

STEP 2.   HAEMAGGLUTINATION-INHIBITION TEST (HIT-β method)

Reagents	\	\	\	\	TUBE OR CUP	\	\	\	\	\
	1	2	3	4	5	6	7	8	9	10
Buffer [ml]	—	0.25	0.25	0.25	0.25	0.25	0.25	0.25	0.25	0.25
Serum [1.8]	0.25	0.25	0.25	0.25	0.25	0.25	0.25	0.25	0.25	0.25 (Discard last 0.25)
Viral antigen [4HAU]	0.25	0.25	0.25	0.25	0.25	0.25	0.25	0.25	0.25	0.25
0.5% fowl RBC	0.25	0.25	0.25	0.25	0.25	0.25	0.25	0.25	0.25	0.25
Final serum dilution	1:8	1:16	1:32	1:64	1:128	1:256	1:512	1:1024	1:2048	1:4096

HIT – CONTROLS

	Serum control	RBC control
Buffer [ml]	0.25	0.25
Serum [1:8]	0.25	—
Virus [4HAU]	—	0.25
0.5% fowl RBC	0.25	0.25

VIRUS CONTROL

	4HAU	2HAU	1HAU	0.5 HAU
Buffer [ml]	—	0.25	—	0.25
Virus [4HAU]	0.25	0.25	0.25 (Discard last 0.25)	0.25
0.5% fowl RBC	0.25	0.25	0.25	0.25

*The extra volume of buffer replaces the volume of serum which will be used for the actual HIT.
In both tests the reagents are mixed and left at room temperature for 30–60 minutes.
The titre of the serum is expressed as the highest dilution of serum which completely inhibits viral haemagglutination.

that details are included of the method used. In warm weather, and especially with certain viruses, e.g. influenza virus type C and some strains of Newcastle disease virus which elute rapidly at room temperature, haemagglutination and haemagglutination-inhibition titrations should be carried out at 4°C. The demonstration of a four-fold or greater increase during convalescence of specific Newcastle disease virus antibody by the haemagglutination-inhibition test may be considered significant. The procedure for the β-method is shown in Table 42.4.

It should also be noted that better sedimentation patterns are obtained if bovine plasma albumin is

control serum (diluted 1/5) inhibits haemagglutination through the 1/10 dilution of virus, reading from right to left, then this dilution contains $\frac{640}{10} = 64$ times the amount of virus in the end-point well (or cup), i.e. 64 HAU. Thus, the inhibiting power or the haemagglutination inhibiting titre of the serum will be $64 \times 5 = 320$. Similarly the haemagglutination-inhibiting titre of the negative control serum will be $\frac{640}{640} \times 5 = 5$; that of the unknown serum A will be $\frac{640}{80} \times 5 = 40$; and, that of the unknown serum B will be $\frac{640}{40} \times 5 = 80$.

TABLE 42.5. The haemagglutination-inhibition test. (alpha method)

	Dilution of virus								
	5	10	20	40	80	160	320	640	1280
Virus haemagglutinin titre	+	+	+	+	+	+	+	+	−
Positive Control Serum [Dil.1:5]	+	−	−	−	−	−	−	−	−
Negative Control Serum [Dil.1:5]	+	+	+	+	+	+	+	−	−
Unknown Serum A [Dil.1:5]	+	+	+	+	−	−	−	−	−
Unknown Serum B [Dil.1:5]	+	+	+	−	−	−	−	−	−

added to the diluent (PBS) to a final concentration of 0·1 per cent. Alternatively, normal rabbit serum can be used providing it is known to be free of haemagglutinins and non-specific inhibitors (Plate 42.16, between pp. 504–5).

Haemagglutination-inhibition test. (Alpha-method.)
(Constant serum—decreasing virus). The α-test, using constant amounts of the test serum against serial dilutions of virus antigen of known titre, is commonly used in diagnostic veterinary laboratories where large numbers of unknown sera are required to be examined (Table 42.5). It has the advantage over the β-test in that a limited number of dilutions of stock virus of known titre can be prepared in quantity for the day's run of tests and, apart from the initial dilution to 1/5 or 1/8, there is no need to perform tedious serial dilutions of each serum being tested.

Before carrying out the haemagglutination-inhibition test by the α-method it is necessary to ascertain the haemagglutinin titre of the laboratory stock strain of virus (p. 496). The haemagglutination-inhibition test is then carried out in the same manner except that the serum to be tested is diluted 1/8 or some other suitable dilution and substituted for the saline solution in the haemagglutination test. The titre of the test serum [i.e. the end-point of the inhibiting activity] is the lowest dilution of the virus in which haemagglutination is completely inhibited.

If, as in the example shown in Table 42.5, the haemagglutinin titre of the virus is 1/640 and the positive

In many Newcastle disease investigations large numbers of test sera (diluted 1/5) can be rapidly screened against only two or three dilutions of virus, e.g. 1/20, 1/40 and 1/80, and the haemagglutination-inhibiting titre of the sera can be calculated from the standard formula:

$$\frac{\text{Virus end-point (reciprocal)}}{\text{Serum end-point (reciprocal)}} \times \text{dilution of serum}$$

= Haemagglutination-inhibiting titre.

For practical purposes an inhibiting power of 80 or greater is considered positive for Newcastle disease virus antibodies, more than 10 is suspicious, and 10 or less is taken as negative.

Neutralization tests
Sera from animals that have recovered from a virus infection usually contain immunoglobulins that are capable of reducing or inhibiting the infectious capacity of the causative virus. These neutralizing antibodies are highly specific and their presence provides one of the most useful methods of measuring or assessing the ability of an individual animal to withstand reinfection.

The neutralizing action of an antiserum can be demonstrated in the laboratory by allowing it to combine with the appropriate virus and then inoculating the serum-virus mixture into a susceptible indicator host-cell system. Suitable host systems for demonstrating virus activity include animals, eggs and cell cultures provided they produce a clearly recognisable effect, e.g. death of mice, pocks on egg membranes or cytopathogenicity on cell cultures, so that the end-point of inhibiting activity can readily be determined.

Neutralization tests are very sensitive and are particularly useful not only for detecting a rise in titre of neutralizing antibodies during an illness but also for identifying and typing viral isolates. Although the neutralization test is, today, probably the most widely used serological test in virology, it should be realised that the same information can often be obtained by other simpler and less costly methods. On the other hand, it may be the only test available where the causative virus does not produce haemagglutinins, or if the serum sample is taken at an early or late stage in the illness when complement-fixing antibodies are absent. Moreover, the neutralization test is the only means of investigating the immune status of a population since, in many infections, e.g. Rift Valley fever, the neutralizing antibodies may persist for years in contrast to complement-fixing antibodies.

A major disadvantage of the neutralization test is that it cannot be used like complement-fixation and haemagglutination-inhibition tests to study soluble viral antigens, incomplete or defective antigens, or inactivated virus in preparations such as 'killed' virus vaccines, because these preparations do not cause the development of visible lesions in animals or tissues. A further disadvantage is that the demonstration of infectivity and, consequently, neutralization of infectivity requires living virus and living cells. Thus, it is necessary for the antigen-antibody reaction to occur before the virus penetrates the susceptible host cell system, since the antiserum cannot inhibit replication once the virus has entered the cell. In practice, it is customary to incubate the virus-serum mixture for an appropriate period, e.g. $1\frac{1}{2}$–2 hours, before inoculation into the test system.

The details of performing neutralization tests vary in different laboratories and, although no single procedure can be applied to every virus, the same basic principle underlies all of them. The variations largely depend on the ratio of virus-serum volumes used, and the time and temperature at which the virus-serum mixtures are incubated prior to inoculation.

Titrations can be carried out in two ways; constant virus—decreasing serum or constant serum-decreasing virus, but the former method is most commonly used. Wherever possible, acute and convalescent phase sera should be included in the same run of tests together with a constant virus titration. In general, all sera should first be inactivated at 56°C for 30 min to destroy heat-labile substances that have antiviral activity, and the virus used must first be titrated in the same medium and in the identical manner in which it is proposed to carry out the test.

Neutralization test for measuring antibody (constant virus — varying serum method). In neutralization tests used to assay sera for the presence of antibodies, serial two-fold dilutions of the unknown serum are mixed two-fold dilutions of the unknown serum are mixed with standard volumes of an infective reference virus, incubated together for an appropriate time and temperature, and then inoculated into a suitable cell system. The range of dilutions for unknown sera is from 1/8 to about 1/512 but, if large numbers of sera are to be examined, it may be convenient first to screen them at a single low dilution only and then re-examine any positive sera over a suitably wide range of dilutions. Paired acute and convalescent sera are always examined together.

Method (Titration of reference virus). Before proceeding to examine sera for the presence of neutralizing antibodies, the pool of known virus must first be titrated in order to determine the highest dilution causing a cytopathic effect in 50 per cent of the inoculated cultures (TCD_{50}). If embryonated eggs or animals are employed the end-points are termed EID_{50} (50 per cent egg infective dose) and LD_{50} (50 per cent lethal dose), respectively. In experiments using cell cultures as the indicator system, serial ten-fold dilutions of the reference virus with medium are prepared and added in 1.0 ml amounts to monolayer tube cultures of susceptible cells. The inoculated cultures are then incubated under appropriate conditions and examined daily until a cytopathic effect is observed, and the dilution of virus at which half of the cultures are visibly affected is the titre (i.e. TCD_{50}) of the virus. There are a number of statistical methods available for calculating the 50 per cent end-point of virus activity, but those of Reed and Muench or Kärber are most commonly used. It should be noted that both methods are applicable primarily to a complete titration series and, for this reason, the whole reaction range from 0 per cent to 100 per cent CPE, mortality, etc., should be represented in the experimental data. However, they may also be used satisfactorily even if those conditions are not fulfilled, provided the reactions occur in a uniform manner over the range of dilutions employed, and are not irregularly scattered over a number of dilutions. In Reed and Muench's method an accumulated value for the tube cultures affected is obtained by adding the number showing CPE at a certain dilution to the number infected by lesser doses of virus. A similar addition, but in the reverse direction, is made for the tube cultures showing no CPE (see Table 42.6). The accumulated values of the two critical dilutions between which the 50 per cent end-point lies are now substituted in the formula and the TCD_{50} is obtained.

TABLE 42.6.   Arrangement of data used in calculation of virus titre (TCD_{50}) by the Reed-Muench formula.

Virus dilution	Infected Cultures	Uninfected Cultures	Accumulated Values		Ratio Infected	Per cent. infected
			Infected	Uninfected		
10^{-1}	4	0	13	0	13/13	100
10^{-2}	4	0	9	0	9/9	100
10^{-3}	3	1	5	1	5/6	83
10^{-4}	2	2	2	3	2/5	40
10^{-5}	0	4	0	7	0/7	0

The arrows indicate the direction of addition for the accumulated values.

The data in Table 42.6 illustrates the procedure used in the Reed-Muench method for calculating the accumulated values of infected and uninfected cell culture tubes. In this example, the dilution which would be expected to yield 50 per cent positive (CPE) tubes is seen to lie between 10^{-3} and 10^{-4} and will, in fact, be located at the proportionate distance from 10^{-3}. The necessary proportionate distance (PD) of the 50 per cent infectivity end point is obtained as follows:

$$PD = \frac{(\text{Percentage infected at dilution next above } 50\%) - (50\%)}{(\text{Percentage infected at dilution next above } 50\%) - (\text{Percentage infected at dilution next below } 50\%)}$$

$$= \frac{83 - 50}{83 - 40}$$

$$= \frac{33}{43}$$

$$= 0.77$$

This is 'corrected' by multiplying by the dilution factor (in this case $\log_{10}$)

$= 0.77 \times (1) = 0.77$

Negative log of TCD_{50} titre

= Negative log of dilution above 50% infected + Proportionate distance ('corrected')

$= 3.0 + 0.77$

$\therefore TCD_{50} = 10^{-3.77}$

Alternatively, as in the following example, the 50 per cent end-point can be calculated by the simpler Kärber formula, i.e. Log $TCD_{50} = L-d[S-0.5]$, where L = log lower dilution, d = difference between log dilution steps, S = sum of proportions of tubes showing cytopathic effects.

Virus dilution	Proportion of infected cultures
10^{-1}	4/4 = 1
10^{-2}	4/4 = 1
10^{-3}	3/4 = 0.75
10^{-4}	2/4 = 0.5
10^{-5}	0/4 = 0

Log $TCD_{50} = L - d[S - 0.5]$

$= -1 - 1 [3.25 - 0.5]$

$= -3.75$

i.e. TCD_{50} titre of virus $= 10^{-3.75}$ per inoculum volume.

Test proper. The dilution of reference virus selected for the neutralization test is usually 100 times stronger than the 50 per cent end-point.

Having calculated the virus titre (TCD_{50}) by either of the above methods and prepared 100 TCD_{50} per

0.1 ml, two-fold dilutions of the unknown serum are prepared over the required range, e.g. 1/10 to 1/5120.

To each tube containing antiserum is added 0.1 ml of virus (100 TCD_{50} dilution) and the virus mixtures are gently agitated and incubated at the appropriate temperature and time (e.g. in a water bath at 37°C for $1\frac{1}{2}$ hours, or at room temperature overnight).

After changing the cell cultures to fresh maintenance medium a constant amount of *each* serum-virus mixture is added to five to ten tubes and incubated either in the stationary sloped position or in roller drums at 37°C. The cultures are examined daily for the presence or absence of a cytopathic effect. The serum-antibody titre is taken as the highest dilution of serum in the initial serum-virus mixture which protects 50 per cent of the cultures against 100 TCD_{50} of virus.

In addition to the usual serum and virus controls a check-titration of virus dilutions should, if possible, be included in the test. The uninoculated cell control cultures should, of course, remain healthy throughout the whole period of incubation and the normal serum control tubes should show no signs of toxic or other degenerative changes.

An example of antibody titration in tissue culture tubes is shown below, the titres being calculated by the simple Kärber formula, Log $TCD_{50} = L-d[S-0.5]$ where, in this case, S = sum of proportions of tissue culture tubes protected by the antiserum.

Serum dilution	Proportion of cultures protected
1/16 [$10^{-1.2}$]	4/4 = 1
1/32 [$10^{-1.5}$]	3/4 = 0.75
1/64 [$10^{-1.8}$]	1/4 = 0.25
1/128 [$10^{-2.1}$]	0/4 = 0

Log 50 per cent. neutralization end-point

$= -1.2 - 0.3 [2-0.5]$

$= -1.65$

$\therefore$ 50 per cent. neutralization end-point titre of the unknown serum.

$= 10^{-1.65}$

$= 1/45$

As in most other serological tests employing serial

two-fold dilutions of serum with a standard amount of known virus, the results may contain a two-fold experimental error. Thus, in comparing the antibody titres of acute and convalescent phase sera a two-fold rise in titre is of little diagnostic significance, and for this reason the minimum rise acceptable as significant is four-fold or greater.

Neutralization test for measuring antibody (constant serum — varying virus method). In this test, a fixed quantity of inactivated serum is added to progressing dilutions (usually in serial ten-fold steps) of a known virus, and the mixtures are held at room temperature for one hour or longer before being inoculated into susceptible cell cultures, animals or embryonated eggs. Acute and convalescent phase sera are included in the same batch of tests and a control virus titration is also set up in the presence of a non-immune serum.

The neutralization index of each serum can then be determined by comparing the 50 per cent end-point of the control virus titration with that of the respective virus-serum mixture, as follows:
Logarithm of neutralization index
  = Negative logarithm of virus control titre
  − Negative logarithm of virus serum titre
Neutralization index
  = Anti-log of the figure thus obtained.

A neutralization index of less than 10 is considered to indicate the absence of antibodies, between 10 and 49 is doubtful and over 50 is usually indicative of an infection. Since neutralizing antibodies for many virus infections tend to persist for a long time, it is generally necessary to demonstrate a significant rise in titre in paired sera in order to establish a causal relationship between the virus and a given illness. For diagnostic purposes, the increase in the neutralization index during convalescence should be at least 100.

Neutralization test for identifying virus isolates. Identification of an unknown virus usually necessitates testing with a large number of reference antisera, although it is sometimes possible to narrow the choice of likely sera on the basis of the history of the case, the species of animal involved, the nature of the viral CPE, the type and species of cell culture affected and the morphology of the virion as seen under the electron microscope.

In this test, the unknown virus is prepared in a suitable medium to contain 100 or 200 TCD_{50} per 0.2 ml. To each 0.1 ml of the challenge dose of virus is added an equal volume of the type-specific reference antiserum which has been previously diluted to contain an appropriate number, say, 4 neutralizing units per 0.2 ml. (An antiserum having a neutralizing titre of 1/512 in a test employing 0.2 ml volumes would possess 4 units per 0.2 ml at a dilution of 1/128). The virus-serum mixture is incubated at the appropriate temperature (e.g. 37°C) and time (e.g. $1\frac{1}{2}$ hours), depending on the virus, and inoculated into a suitable host cell system (e.g. five culture tubes). Duplicate sets of cultures are set up, one with cells and antiserum, and a second with cells and virus. The inoculated cultures are examined daily and the tubes containing antisera are read 24 hours after the virus control tubes show complete degeneration of the cell layer. The survival of the cells in the first two groups but not in the third, which contains only cells and virus, indicates protection by the antiserum and, therefore, the identity of the virus.

Plaque-reduction test
The neutralizing activity of an antiviral serum can also be determined by the plaque-reduction test. In this test about 100 plaque-forming units (100 p.f.u.) are incubated with a serial dilution of the test serum and each mixture is added to a monolayer culture of susceptible cells, which is then overlaid with agar and incubated at 37°C. The end-point is an 80 per cent reduction in the number of plaques. In general, the test is only satisfactory with certain viruses that produce a rapid marked cytopathic effect and is not widely used in diagnostic virology.

Metabolic-inhibition test
The metabolic-inhibition test is a colour test which can also be used as a virus neutralization test. Virus-serum mixtures are placed in the wells of plastic trays and, one hour later, known quantities of cell suspensions are added to each. (This eliminates the need for growing monolayer cultures in advance.) In the wells containing an immune serum-virus mixture and in the controls, the cells continue to grow and the acidic changes of their metabolism in normal tissue respiration lower the pH of the medium, especially when glucose is present, and turn the phenol red indicator to a bright yellow colour (pH less than 7·0). In the absence of specific antibodies in the test serum, the virus produces a cytopathic effect on the cells in suspension which cease to grow and the culture medium remains red (pH 7·4–7·8). With cytopathic viruses, e.g. poliomyelitis, the end-point is sharply defined and the colour changes are visible to the unaided eye. This eliminates the need for tedious microscopical examination of unstained tube-cultures for the presence or absence of cellular degeneration.

Since adenoviruses may cause a stimulation of cellular metabolism and a more rapid lowering of the pH than that of the control culture, the colour changes are the opposite of that produced by poliomyelitis and other enteroviruses.

Immunofluorescence

The fluorescent antibody staining technique is a serological procedure which is being increasingly used in veterinary virology not only to detect the intracellular location and sites of replication of virus antigens in infected cell cultures, but also to identify specific virus (e.g. rabies and swine fever) in suitably prepared smears or thin frozen sections of infected tissues. The method is also proving useful in immunological research, experimental pathology and diagnostic bacteriology.

Like most other serological procedures the fluorescent antibody technique has its advantages and disadvantages. One of its main advantages, particularly in veterinary medicine where fresh postmortem specimens are often readily available and usually contain high concentrations of virus, is the rapidity with which an accurate diagnosis can be made. In diagnostic laboratories where skilled personnel are employed, specimens may be received, examined and reported on the same day. The method has a high degree of specificity and, in many cases, a reliable diagnosis can be obtained without the need for cultural examination and the identification of pure cultures of virus which are generally tedious, time-consuming and expensive. Not only can fluorescent antibody staining identify small numbers of virus particles in clinical specimens but it can also detect non-viable pathogens, pathogens which are difficult to isolate and even soluble viral antigens. The main disadvantages to the routine use of immunofluorescence in the diagnostic laboratory include the high cost of the fluorescence microscope, ancillary equipment and reagents, the need for adequately trained personnel who are familiar both with the equipment and the test systems being used and, thirdly, the present scarcity of reliable diagnostic reagents. It is emphasised that a great deal of care is necessary in preparing the reagents and in applying and interpreting the elaborate control preparations, as well as the test itself, before full benefit can be derived from this procedure. Every effort must be made to rule out autofluorescence and other non-specific reactions.

The principle of immunofluorescence depends upon the fact that an antibody may be chemically coupled or conjugated with certain reagents, e.g. fluorescein isothiocyanate (FITC) or lissamine rhodamine B (RB 200) which fluoresce when irradiated with ultraviolet light. A substance is said to be fluorescent if it absorbs light energy of one wave-length and emits light of another wavelength. Thus, suitably conjugated antibody of high titre will combine with its specific antigen to form a labelled antibody–antigen complex which will fluoresce a brilliant yellow-green colour with fluorescein or a bright reddish-brown colour with rhodamine, when viewed in a microscope equipped with an ultraviolet light source. In this way, the procedure can be used either to detect viruses with standardised antisera or to detect antibody against known viruses.

For fluorescence microscopy, a very intense light is necessary. In most modern microscopes the source of ultraviolet light is supplied by a high pressure mercury vapour lamp (e.g. Osram HBO 200) which is fitted with a collecting lens made of fused quartz in order to withstand the considerable amount of heat generated by the lamp.

The length of the life of a bulb varies considerably but the mercury arc lamp has the advantage that it reaches maximum intensity after only a few minutes and can be restarted immediately after switching off. However, it should not be switched off within 15 min of starting otherwise damage to the electrode may occur from residues of non-vaporized mercury. Frequent starting and short periods of use should be avoided since this reduces the lamp life of approximately 200 hours by some 50 per cent. It is extremely dangerous to open the lamp housing when the bulb is hot and, if a replacement is necessary, it is essential to allow the bulb to cool to room temperature before it is removed.

After passing through the quartz collecting lens the ultraviolet light passes through the primary or excitor filter system and is then directed into the condensor by means of a mirror of polished metal which, unlike glass, does not absorb ultraviolet light. The purpose of the excitor filters is to retain visible illumination and to transmit the wavelength of light which the fluorochrome is capable of absorbing.

The secondary, ocular or barrier filter system is inserted anywhere between the object and the observer to arrest the longer wavelengths emitted from the specimen while, at the same time, permitting most of the fluorescent light to pass. The ultraviolet source and the light path to the microscope should be adequately screened to protect the operator from repeated exposure to ultraviolet light.

To overcome some of the problems of non-specific fluorescence, microscopic objectives, slides and coverslips should be made from non-fluorescent glass, and special non-fluorescent immersion oils and mounting media should be used.

The procedure of immunofluorescence can be carried out in two ways: (1) the direct staining method and (2) the indirect staining reaction (Fig. 42.2).

Direct method. In the direct staining reaction the labelled antibody is specific for the antigen in question and is applied directly to the specimen. After the cell culture monolayer or the tissue

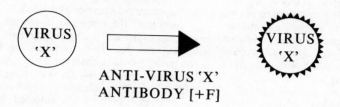

In the direct staining method the labelled [+F] antibodies are specific for the test antigen.

b] Indirect reaction.

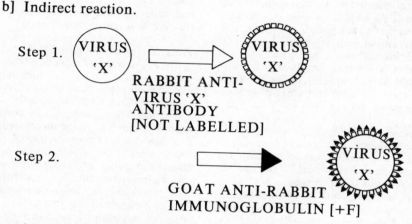

In the indirect staining method, the labelled antibodies are specific for the immunoglobulins which are generally of another species, e.g. goat anti-rabbit immunoglobulin.

Thus, by this method, a *single* labelled immunoglobulin preparation can be used to couple with and stain a wide variety of serologically specific reactions.

FIG. 42.2. Schematic illustration of direct and indirect fluorescent antibody staining reactions.

suspension on a slide has been covered for several minutes with the solution of fluorescein labelled antibody, the slide is thoroughly rinsed to remove all traces of unbound fluorescent protein and then examined with the ultraviolet light microscope. If the antibody is adequately labelled and has combined specifically with the antigen, the location of the labelled antibody and hence the viral antigen can be recognised as small areas of intense fluorescence against a dark background.

The method is more specific than the indirect reaction but it has the great disadvantage from the diagnostic point of view that a specifically labelled antibody is required for each individual antigen. Although more specific than the indirect method it is generally less sensitive unless high titre reference sera are available.

Indirect method. In this method, the specimen of acetone-fixed monolayer, smear or section is first treated with unlabelled specific antibody (which has been produced, say, in a rabbit) to enable the normal antibody-antigen reaction to occur. After removal of excess antibody, the newly formed unlabelled antigen–antibody complex is stained by covering the specimen with fluorescein-labelled antiglobulin which was prepared in another species of animal against the globulin of the animal species providing the original unlabelled antibody (e.g. goat anti-rabbit immunoglobulin). As the labelled antiglobulin is specific for the antiserum under study it will unite with the unlabelled antigen–antibody complex which will then fluoresce brightly in ultraviolet light. Thus, in the indirect method the unlabelled antibody plays a dual role, acting as antibody in the first part of the reaction and as antigen in the second part. In this way, a single labelled serum can be used with a variety of antisera of different specificities provided the antisera are all prepared in the same species of animal, e.g. rabbit. The method is much more versatile than the direct staining reaction since it is not necessary to prepare and standardise a specific labelled antiserum for each antigen being investigated.

Modifications of the indirect staining procedure include the complement staining method. Here, the specific antiserum is allowed to react with the antigen, guinea-pig complement is added, followed by labelled anti-guinea-pig globulin. Specific fluorescence will occur only if the complement has been fixed in the primary reaction.

Specific antisera labelled with different fluorescent markers can also be used to study the possible co-existence of different antigens in the same cell. Thus, distemper antiserum conjugated with FITC and canine hepatitis antiserum conjugated with RB 200 applied to cells infected simultaneously with both viruses will show particles of yellow-green fluorescence in the cytoplasm and areas of orange-red fluorescence in the nucleus.

Procedure for direct staining:

Antibody. The globulins are obtained from a mixture of dye and serum (which must not contain preservatives) by cold precipitation with 50 per cent saturated ammonium sulphate. The deposit of globulin is redissolved in distilled water and conjugation is obtained by passing it through a column of Sephadex G-200 medium. Two main bands will appear, the colour of the faster-moving band, which contains the crude globulin, being the first indication that conjugation has been successful. The material is collected in small volumes and those that are densely and uniformly coloured are pooled. Since the pH is adjusted by the column which also removes excess unwanted fluorochrome, the pooled material is adsorbed with homogenised tissue, e.g. liver of the same species as that to be stained, in order to remove cross-reacting specific antibody and non-specific staining.

The prepared sera are preserved with merthiolate at 1/10 000 final concentration and stored at —20° to —60°C. If non-specific staining develops in a stored conjugate it should either be passed through a Sephadex column again or treated with activated charcoal for 5–10 min.

Antigens. Infected monolayer cultures or smears are fixed by immersion in acetone at room temperature for 10–15 min and dried with a fan at room temperature or in the incubator at 37°C.

Method. The dried preparations, which may sometimes be rinsed in PBS before staining, are covered with a drop of conjugated globulin and held in a moist chamber to prevent evaporation of the conjugate, for a period of 15–30 min at room temperature or, occasionally, at 37°C. When staining is complete, the conjugate is rinsed off with PBS and the preparation thoroughly washed in PBS for several minutes. The coverslips are then removed, the under surfaces dried and they are mounted on thin glass slides in 80 per cent glycerine at pH 6·8 and examined by ultraviolet light in a fluorescence microscope. As controls, infected and uninfected preparations should also be stained with non-immune conjugated sera. Stained films may be kept satisfactory for several months at —70°C.

As an additional check it may be necessary to show that the staining can be inhibited or blocked by pre-treating the coverslip preparation with non-conjugated specific immune serum but not by pre-treating with non-immune serum.

Procedure for indirect staining:

Materials. Infected monolayer cultures (e.g. bovine kidney cells). Immune and non-immune unstained (e.g. chicken) sera. Conjugated anti-chicken globulin absorbed with bovine kidney cells.

Method. The monolayer cultures are prepared by acetone fixation as in the direct staining method.

A few drops of non-conjugated chicken convalescent serum are added to the surface of each preparation and the coverslips incubated in a moist atmosphere for 30 min at room temperature. The coverslips are rinsed thoroughly in PBS (pH 7·2) to remove all the free excess conjugate. Two drops of conjugated anti-chicken globulin are added to each preparation and the coverslips are left for 30 min in a moist chamber. If the staining is accelerated by incubation at 37°C, care must be taken to prevent drying of the conjugate on the surface of the culture which might be interpreted as a false positive reaction. The coverslips are washed thoroughly in fresh PBS for at least 10 min and the undersides are carefully dried with lint-free paper. For examination, the stained coverslips are mounted in glycerine (pH 7·2) or other suitable neutral mounting fluid, care being taken to avoid bubble formation which might interfere with the microscopic examination. A semi-permanent mount can be prepared by ringing the coverslips with clear nail varnish and storing them at —20° to —70°C. Controls of infected cells with negative serum and non-infected cells with positive serum should always be included.

Specific staining should only occur in preparations containing the appropriate antigen and should be confined to the antigen. Moreover, the proof of staining is immunological and does not depend on the brightness of the reaction (Plate 42.18a, b, facing p. 505).

COMPLEMENT–FIXATION TEST

Row 1

Row 2

Row 3

Row 4

Complement titration

(Complement dilutions)

Acute serum

Convalescent serum

(Serum dilutions)

Controls

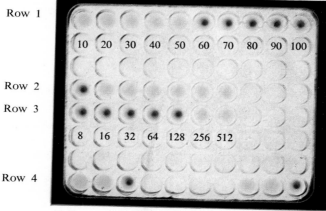

42.15

Row 1: Complement titration (with antigen)
(Titre is 50, therefore 2·5 MHD = 1:20)

Row 2: Acute phase serum (S^A)

Row 3: Convalescent phase serum (S^C)

Row 4: Controls (left to right)

1 = S^A control   8 = complement control
2 = S^C control   9 = antigen control
3 = cell control   10 = haemolytic system control

42.15 COMPLEMENT-FIXATION TEST FOR VIRAL ANTIBODIES
Virus antigen is mixed overnight at 4°C with dilutions
of the patient's sera and complement, before addition of
sensitized sheep erythrocytes. In this example, the titre of
complement-fixing antibody has risen from 8 in the acute
phase to 128 in the convalescent phase serum. A greater
than 4-fold rise in titre indicates recent infection.

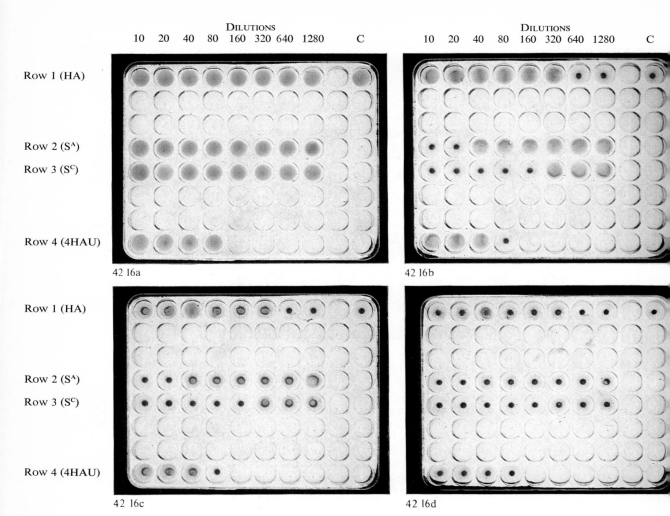

42.16a-d HAEMAGGLUTINATION-INHIBITION TEST FOR VIRAL ANTIBODIES

Row 1:   Titration of viral haemagglutinating activity. The titre is 320 (1 HA unit), thus 4 HAU = 1:80. Notice that well 10 contains red blood cells only (C).

Rows 2 & 3: Wells contain serial dilutions of acute phase serum (S^A) and convalescent phase serum (S^C) plus 4 HAU of virus. The titres are 20 and 160 respectively—a greater than 4-fold rise in antibody titre indicating recent infection.

Row 4:   First 4 wells contain the HAU titration (4, 2, 1 and 0·5 units respectively).

Note: The photographs are of the same test, taken at various intervals after the addition of the red blood cell suspensions:
(a) Zero time: The erythrocytes have not settled in any of the wells.
(b) 40 minutes: Haemagglutination is seen as a diffuse widespread pattern of cells lining the foot of the wells. Erythrocytes not exposed to virus settle in the wells to give a button pattern with a sharp edge.
(c) 1½ hours: Elution of virus from the erythrocytes appears as a ragged edge to the veil of cells lining the foot of the wells.
(d) 3 hours: Elution has proceeded in the majority of wells containing virus, which now resemble the wells containing red blood cells not exposed to the virus.

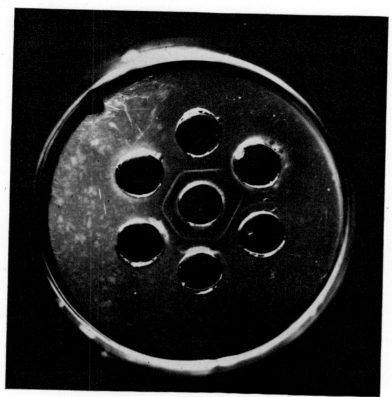

42.17 Agar-gel diffusion test. The lines of precipitation between the positive hyperimmune serum (central well) and the positive control antigens (top and bottom wells) are confluent with the lines between the suspected tissue antigens in three of the lateral wells and the positive serum. There is no line between the positive serum and the fourth lateral well containing the negative control tissue.

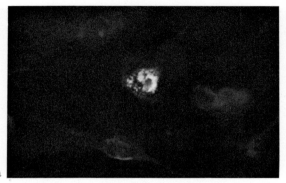

a

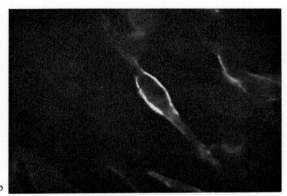

b

42.18a Monolayer of chick fibroblasts infected with influenza-A virus and stained, after acetone fixation, with fluorescent antibody to the viral antigen. Three hours after inoculation, showing the location of viral antigen in the nucleus and the absence of fluorescence in the cytoplasm.

42.18b The same as 42.18a, 5 hours after inoculation. The antigen has left the nucleus and the cytoplasm is fluorescing in the perinuclear region.

Applications of immunofluorescence

Apart from its usefulness in immunological research, experimental pathology and in viral replication studies, the fluorescent antibody staining technique is of value in diagnostic virology where it can assist diagnosis by rapidly detecting specific virus antigens in culture or in material from patients, or by demonstrating specific antibody in the patient's serum against a known virus.

In veterinary medicine the method has given excellent results in the diagnosis of rabies and is superior to conventional staining methods for Negri bodies. Moreover, it is quicker and at least as reliable as biological tests in mice. The reliability of the test depends on the freshness of the brain tissue since advanced autolysis may give rise to false negatives. A similar virus, vesicular stomatitis virus, can be readily detected in infected pig kidney cell cultures and in sections of the tongue of experimentally infected pigs.

A considerable amount of work has been done on the nature and distribution of viral antigens of many species of myxoviruses, especially influenza and Newcastle disease viruses. Although virus can be detected by immunofluorescence in tissue cultures and infected eggs as well as in swabs, sections and tissue imprints of affected birds and animals, there is as yet little justification for its routine use in view of the ability of other simpler tests, e.g. haemagglutination-inhibition, to distinguish between different serological types which are probably below the threshold of sensitivity of the immunofluorescence technique. In fowl plague, swine influenza and other influenza virus infections the antigens may be located in the nucleus or cytoplasm whereas in Newcastle disease, bovine type 3 and other parainfluenza viruses, the antigens are rarely found in the nucleus and are mostly in the cytoplasm or the perinuclear area. Rinderpest virus causes cytoplasmic fluorescence in HeLa cells, bovine kidney and other types of cell cultures while, in distemper, specific antigens can readily be detected in tissue cultures, and even in conjunctival and genital swabs or in lung impression smears from affected dogs.

The viruses of louping-ill, bluetongue and Rift Valley fever of sheep, African horse sickness, equine encephalomyelitis and other arthropod-borne virus diseases of domestic animals lend themselves well to fluorescence staining techniques, especially when high-titred sera are available. Large intracytoplasmic bodies are usually clearly visible in infected cell cultures but direct examination of affected tissues is generally less satisfactory.

Fluorescent antibody staining has also been used successfully in studies of picornaviruses, e.g. foot-and-mouth disease, ECBO and ECSO viruses. In experimentally infected mice, the virus of foot-and-mouth disease is located in the hippocampus, cerebral cortex and choroid plexus, whilst the antigen is distributed in the perinuclear areas of the cytoplasm in infected bovine, calf and rabbit kidney cell cultures. Sera from cattle with lesions of foot-and-mouth disease give positive results to the indirect fluorescent antibody technique although it is not possible to use the method to distinguish between the types of infecting virus.

In calf kidney cells infected with ECBO viruses the antigen appears in the cytoplasm around the nucleus 5 hours post-infection, while direct fluorescent antibody staining of infected tissue impression smears shows that the coronavirus antigen of transmissible gastroenteritis of pigs is present in the cytoplasm of cells of the tonsils, mesenteric lymph nodes and parts of the intestine.

Of the unclassified RNA viruses, that of mucosal disease of cattle, and especially swine fever, have been studied in the greatest detail. In swine fever, fluorescent antibody staining shows that the antigen is most constantly present in the parotid salivary glands and is also to be found in the submaxillary glands, various lymph nodes, spleen, kidney, lungs and brain, and even in the blood and urine of affected pigs. The antigen is initially present in the cytoplasm but there is some evidence of later spread to the nucleus. For diagnostic purposes the best results are generally obtained using fresh tissues, e.g. tonsil, spleen or lymph node from young animals in advanced diseases.

Comparatively little use has been made of immunofluorescence for the diagnosis of poxvirus diseases of domestic animals although rabbit pox, ectromelia and some other pox infections have been studied in laboratory animals. Nevertheless, fluorescent antibody staining has been profitably applied in other DNA virus infections, especially those caused by herpesviruses and adenoviruses. With simian herpes-B virus, impression smears of infected mice show the antigen to be located mainly within and around the nuclei of infected cells whilst, in cell cultures, the antigen can be distinguished from that of *Herpes simplex* by both the direct and indirect staining methods. In animals affected with Aujeszky's disease the antigens appear first in the nucleus and then in the cytoplasm of infected cells in the brain and thoracic spinal cord. They are less obvious in the tonsils and spleen and are rarely present in other tissues. Strains of infectious bovine rhinotracheitis virus have been detected in nasal and vulval smears from cattle affected with enteritis, the antigen being located first in the nuclear membrane, later in the cytoplasm but not, apparently, in the nucleus. On the other hand, the indirect staining method shows that the virus of equine rhinopneumonitis is to be found within the nucleus and in the perinuclear areas of infected kidney cell cultures, whilst in infectious laryngotracheitis of chickens viral antigen can be detected in tracheal swabs and in the cytoplasm or perinuclear areas of giant cells in infected cell monolayers. With the DNA iridovirus of African swine fever, antigen is seen as fine granules within the cytoplasm of infected cell cultures and also in tissue impression smears of spleen, mesenteric lymph nodes and especially the liver of pigs that have died after acute infection. Immunofluorescence can also be used to detect the parvovirus of feline panleucopenia in cell cultures, as well as the antigens of mink enteritis which seem to be confined to the cytoplasm of epithelial cells of the small intestine.

The most frequent use of fluorescent antibody staining in studying adenovirus infections has been in infectious canine hepatitis. Stained sections of infected liver show nuclear staining of hepatic and Kupffer cells, and dogs infected naturally have viral antigen in the tonsils at the time when pyrexia begins. Thus, for reliable diagnosis the tonsil material should be used early in the disease. Immunofluorescence has also proved useful for detecting antibodies to infectious canine hepatitis in unknown sera using positive liver sections.

Immunofluorescence is playing an increasingly important role in studies of RNA and DNA tumour viruses. In infected chicken fibroblasts, the antigens of Rous sarcoma virus are first detected along the borders of an occasional cell, where the virus is concentrated, and later within the cytoplasm. The avian myeloblastosis virus behaves in a similar manner in chicken fibroblasts and antigen appears at the cell surface or in the cytoplasm but never in the nucleus. It is of interest that fluorescent antibody staining is held by some workers to be more sensitive than the COFAL test for diagnosing latent infection by avian leukoses viruses. Immunofluorescence is also being used in studies of animal leukaemias and animal papillomas.

Apart from viruses, the fluorescent antibody technique is of value for the rapid diagnosis of psittacosis and other conditions caused by chlamydial agents, e.g. mouse pneumonitis and enzootic abortion of ewes, as well as some rickettsial diseases such as Q fever.

Agglutination, flocculation and precipitation

Agglutination and flocculation reactions are not widely used in virology since the clumping of virus particles in the presence of specific antibody is often difficult to detect with any degree of accuracy.

Specific tests with rickettsiae, chlamydiae and the larger viruses such as vaccinia, and even some myxoviruses, have been devised but most of them have proved to be impracticable since large amounts of purified antigens are difficult to prepare and relatively large quantities of concentrated virus suspensions are required in macroscopic reactions. With smaller viruses such as the enteroviruses, a number of microflocculation reactions have been developed and slide flocculation tests with poliovirus have given promising results. In the free flocculation method, which is the counterpart of the agglutination test in bacteriology, the highly concentrated virus suspension is added to a serum dilution and incubated at 37°C for a few hours. The presence or absence of fine flocculation can be detected even by direct visual examination or by means of a hand lens.

Compared with agglutination and flocculation tests, modifications of Ouchterlony's original double diffusion gel technique are of considerable value in the qualitative analysis of viral antigens and are now widely used as a simple and rapid method for the diagnosis of many important virus diseases of man and animals.

Although the method is applicable only to antigens that can diffuse through gels and is somewhat less sensitive than other serological procedures, it is simple to carry out and gives satisfactory results with extremely small amounts of reagents. It is especially suited to the analysis of antigenic structure. In veterinary virology, agar-gel diffusion techniques have been used successfully to identify specific precipitinogens in infected tissues, e.g. rinderpest, distemper and infectious canine hepatitis, and an indirect tube method has been devised for the detection of precipitating antibodies for rinderpest.

Procedure for gel diffusion

The principle of the gel diffusion test depends on the ability of antigen and antibody to diffuse freely towards each other in an agar gel resulting in precipitation and the formation of a clearly visible band or bands of precipitate at the junction of the diffusion front, i.e. the zone of equivalence (Plate 42.17, between pp. 504–5). The gel is provided in the form of a thin layer of clear agar on a glass slide or in a Petri dish, in which circular wells are cut to hold the reagents. The optimum diameter of the well and the distance between adjacent wells largely depends on the reactivity of the reagents. For reliable results it is generally necessary to use a high concentration of the antigen together with a high-titre or hyperimmune serum.

The gel consists of 1 per cent high quality agar in phosphate-buffered saline to which 1 per cent merthiolate is added to a final concentration of 1/10 000. If large 4-inch diameter Petri dishes are used, it may be convenient to dispense the agar in 10 ml amounts in universal containers and to store them at room temperature until required. The molten agar is then poured into a Petri dish to give a layer approximately 3 mm deep, and allowed to set. A pattern of circular wells is stamped in the agar gel by means of a cutter made with a set of metal tubes joined together to form the desired pattern. For example, in rinderpest diagnosis each well is about 5 mm in diameter and 5 mm apart. The agar plugs can be removed from the wells by means of a dissecting needle or sucked out by attaching the metal tubes to a vacuum source. The bottom of the wells may be sealed to prevent materials from running under the agar by adding and quickly removing a small amount of molten agar with a fine Pasteur pipette, or left unsealed to individual requirements. Known and control antigens and antibodies are added to

precipitating antigen in the test material, no bands are formed and the test may appear negative. For this reason, only positive reactions are meaningful.

In addition to the above method of double diffusion in two dimensions, precipitin reactions can also be carried out by double diffusion in one dimension. Here a capillary tube containing antiserum in agar is overlaid first by a column of clear agar and then by a column of antigen. The antigen and antibody particles diffuse into the clear neutral or reaction zone and precipitin bands are formed at the point where the antigen and antibody are in equivalent proportions. Single diffusion in one dimension is carried out by placing a solution of antigen over a column of agar gel containing anti-

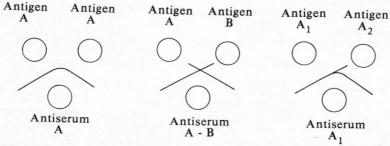

FIG. 42.3. Double diffusion precipitin reactions in agar, illustrating reactions of identity, non-identity, and partial identity

the appropriate wells and the plates are incubated in a humidified chamber either at 37°C or at room temperature. The period varies from one hour to overnight incubation, depending upon the concentration of the reagents used. Readings are facilitated by oblique lighting. In a positive reaction a fine straight line of precipitation appears between adjacent wells and, where more than one antigen is present, several parallel lines are formed. If the same antigen is placed in two adjacent wells and the homologous antibody is present in the common central well, two single precipitin bands are formed which eventually join and fuse at their contiguous ends (reaction of identity, Fig. 42.3). If, on the other hand, more than one type of antibody is present in the central well and different antigens are placed in the lateral wells, the precipitin bands will form independently of each other and cross (reaction of non-identity). On occasion, when cross-reacting antigens (e.g. rinderpest and distemper) are placed in adjacent lateral wells the precipitin bands fuse but, in addition, may produce a spur-like projection that extends towards the cross-reacting antigen (reaction of partial identity).

Precipitation bands form quicker at 37°C than at room temperature, but with weak antigens the reaction may be greatly delayed. If there is insufficient

serum. Provided the concentration of antigen is relatively higher than that of the antibody, the antigen will diffuse downwards through the agar to form a band of precipitation (Fig. 42.4).

Antibodies for myxovirus haemagglutinin and neuraminidase can be assayed routinely in haemagglutination-inhibition and neuraminidase-inhibition tests which involve reaction systems of three components. More recently, antibodies have been detected by gel-immuno-double-diffusion tests using virions disrupted by detergents. In a modification of this latter test, for the quantitation of antibodies, a single-radial diffusion method has been devised whereby only one component, the antibody, diffuses through an agarose medium; the other component, the antigen in the form of intact virus particles, does not diffuse. Dilutions of the test serum are added to circular wells cut in the agarose medium containing suspensions of purified intact virus. After 8 hours' or overnight incubation in a moist chamber at room temperature, the presence of specific antibodies is detected by the appearance of haloes of opalescence surrounding the wells. Although the mechanism of the test has not been fully established it should be noted that the method does not depend on the formation of immune precipitates as in standard agar gel diffusion tests.

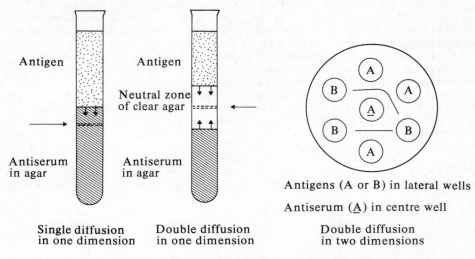

Antigen   Antigen

Neutral zone
of clear agar

Antiserum
in agar

Antiserum
in agar

Antigens (A or B) in lateral wells

Antiserum (A̲) in centre well

Single diffusion
in one dimension

Double diffusion
in one dimension

Double diffusion
in two dimensions

FIG. 42.4. Arrangements for gel-diffusion precipitin reactions.

Further Reading

ANDERSON E.A., ARMSTRONG J.A. AND NIVEN J.S.F. (1959) *Fluorescence Microscopy: observations of virus growth with aminoacridines.* Symposium of the Society of General Microbiology, No. 9, p. 224. London: Cambridge University Press.

BEVERIDGE W.I.B. AND BURNET F.M. (1946) The cultivation of viruses and rickettsiae in the chick embryo. *Medical Research Council Special Report Series,* No. 256. London: Her Majesty's Stationery Office.

BOVARNICK M. AND DE BURGH P.H. (1947) Virus haemagglutination. *Science,* **105,** 550.

BUSBY D.W.G., HOUSE W. AND MACDONALD J.R. (1964) *Virological Technique.* London: Churchill.

CRUICKSHANK R., ed. (1965) *Medical Microbiology,* 11th Edition. Edinburgh: Churchill Livingstone.

DULBECCO R. (1952) Production of plaques in monolayer tissue cultures by single particles of an animal virus. *Proceedings of the National Academy of Sciences of the United States of America,* **38,** 747.

DULBECCO R. AND VOGT M. (1954) Plaque formation and the isolation of pure lines with poliomyelitis viruses. *Journal of Experimental Medicine,* **99,** 167.

ENDERS J.F., WELLER T.H. AND ROBBINS F.C. (1949) Cultivation of the Lansing strain of poliomyelitis virus in cultures of various human embryonic tissues. *Science,* **109,** 85.

FRASER K.B. (1969) Immunological tracing: viruses and rickettsiae. In, *Fluorescent Antibody Tracing,* Ed. R.C. Nairn, 4th Edition, p. 192. Edinburgh: Livingstone.

FRIEND C., PATULEIA M.C. AND NELSON J.B. (1966) Antibiotic effect of Tylosin on a Mycoplasma contaminant in a tissue culture leukemia cell line. *Proceedings of the Society of Experimental Biology and Medicine,* **12,** 1009.

GRIST N.R., ROSS C.A.C., BELL E.J. AND STOTT E.J. (1966) *Diagnostic Methods in Clinical Virology.* Oxford: Blackwell Scientific Publications.

GRUNDBOECK M. (1964) The fluorescence antibody method and its application in veterinary medicine (Trans.) *Medycyna weteryn,* **1,** 36.

HARRIS A.H. (1966) Fluorescent microscopy as aid in diagnosis of infectious diseases. *New York State Journal of Medicine,* **66,** 229.

HARRIS R.J.C., ed. (1964) *Techniques in Experimental Virology.* London: Academic Press.

HIRST G.K. (1941) The agglutination of red blood cells by allantoic fluid of chick embryos infected with influenza virus. *Science,* **94,** 22.

HOORN B. AND TYRRELL D.A.J. (1969) Organ cultures in virology. *Progress in Medical Virology,* **11,** 408.

HOSKINS J. (1967) *Virological Procedures.* New York: Appleton-Century-Crofts.

LENNETTE E.H. AND SCHMIDT N.J., eds (1969) *Diagnostic Procedures for Viral and Rickettsial Infections,* 4th Edition, New York: American Public Health Association, Inc.

LIU C. (1963) Immunofluorescent technique: application in the study and diagnosis of infectious disease. *Clinical Pediatrics (Philadelphia),* **2,** 490.

MERCHANT D.J., KHAN R.H. AND MURPHY W.H. (1964) *Handbook of Cell and Organ Culture,* 2nd Edition, Minneapolis: Burgess.

NEGRONI G. (1964) Tissue culture techniques. In,

Techniques in Experimental Virology, Ed. R.J.C. Harris, p. 327. London: Academic Press.

PARKER R.C. (1960) *Methods of Tissue Culture*, 3rd Edition. New York: Hoeber.

PARSONS D.F. (1964) Electron microscopy of viruses in cells and tissues. In, *Techniques in Experimental Virology*, Ed. R.J.C. Harris, p. 381. London: Academic Press.

PAUL J. (1970) *Cell and Tissue Culture*, 4th Edition. Edinburgh: Livingstone.

PENSO G. AND BALDUCCI D. (1963) In, *Tissue Cultures in Biological Research*. London: Elsevier.

PORTERFIELD J.S. AND ASHWOOD-SMITH M.J. (1962) Preservation of cells in tissue culture by glycerol and dimethyl sulphoxide. *Nature*, **193**, 548.

RAPP F. AND MELNICK J.L. (1964) Application of tissue culture methods in the virus laboratory. *Progress in Medical Virology*, **6**, 268.

REED L.J. AND MUENCH H. (1938) A simple method of estimating fifty per cent endpoints. *American Journal of Hygiene*, **27**, 493.

SCHILD G.C., HENRY-AYMARD M. AND PEREIRA H.G. (1972) A quantitative, single-radial-diffusion test for immunological studies with influenza virus. *Journal of General Virology*, **16**, 231.

STOWARD P.J. (1968) Fluorescence microscopy. *Science Journal*, **4**, 65.

SWAIN R.H.A. AND DODDS T.C. (1967) *Clinical Virology*. Edinburgh: Livingstone.

VOGEL J. AND SHELOKOV A. (1957) Adsorption—Haemagglutination test for influenza virus in monkey kidney tissue culture. *Science*, **126**, 358.

WILLMER E.N., ed. (1965–6) *Cells and Tissues in Culture*, Vols 1, 2 and 3. London: Academic Press.

YOUNGNER J.S. (1954) Studies with monolayer tissue cultures. I. Preparation and standardization of suspensions of trypsin-dispersed monkey kidney cells. *Proceedings of the Society for Experimental Biology and Medicine*, **85**, 202.

CHAPTER 43

MYXOVIRUSES

Myxoviruses

Myxoviruses are medium sized, enveloped, RNA viruses with helical symmetry which generally cause respiratory diseases of man, animals and birds. The name is derived from the affinity of these viruses for mucins in the respiratory tract, and they are characterized by possessing an enzyme, neuraminidase, which cleaves neuraminic acid residues from mucoproteins. Myxoviruses are classified according to their morphology, size and biological characters into two major groups known as orthomyxoviruses and paramyxoviruses.

It will be noted from Table 43.1 that the measles, rinderpest, distemper group of viruses have been separately classified as pseudomyxoviruses in the paramyxovirus group, although rinderpest and distemper viruses do not possess neuraminidase and fail to cause haemagglutination. It has also been suggested recently that two members of the paramyxovirus group, namely respiratory syncytial virus and the pneumonia virus of mice, may occupy an intermediate position between ortho- and paramyxoviruses, and that they should be included in a third myxovirus group named metamyxovirus. This present classification is tentative until further details are known about the chemical and biological characters of these viruses.

ORTHOMYXOVIRUSES

Morphology
Influenza viruses are pleomorphic structures, but in negatively stained preparations they commonly appear spherical measuring 70–120 nm in diameter. The individual virus is often indented on one surface so that it presents an umbilicate appearance. Apart from these spherical particles, a wide range of pleomorphic forms can be found including filamentous virions up to 4000 nm in length. (Plate 43.1 facing page 518).

All myxoviruses possess a limiting membrane or envelope consisting of protein, lipid and carbohydrate; and their most distinctive feature is a fringe of projections on the surface of the outer envelope. This consists of two different types of spikes, one associated with haemagglutinin and the other with

TABLE 43.1. Classification of the myxoviruses.

Orthomyxovirus group	Metamyxovirus group (Proposed)	Paramyxovirus group

INFLUENZA VIRUS A
  Human influenza virus A (AO), A1, A2 (Asian)
  Swine influenza virus
	Pneumonia virus of mice
	Respiratory syncytial viruses
	  of man and animals
		Newcastle disease virus
		Yucaipa virus
		Mumps virus

Equine influenza virus (Equi–1, Equi–2)
  Avian influenza virus
    Fowl plague virus
    Tern virus
    Virus N
  Duck influenza virus
		PARAINFLUENZA VIRUSES
		  Type 1 (Sendai; HVJ: HA–2)
		  Type 2 (CA; SV–5; SV–41)
		  Type 3 (HA–1; SF4; RE55)
		  Type 4 (M25; CH 19503)

INFLUENZA VIRUS B
  Human influenza virus B, B1, B2, B3 (Taiwan)
INFLUENZA VIRUS C
  Human influenza virus C
		PSEUDOMYXOVIRUS
		  Measles
		  Rinderpest
		  Distemper

neuraminidase. The subunits possessing haemagglutinin activity are rod-shaped structures 10–14 nm long by 4 nm wide, and are triangular in cross section. The neuraminidase-containing subunits are cylindrical in shape and measure approximately 9 nm in length and 5 nm in width. They are attached centrally to the distal end of the spike which, itself, is 10 nm in length and bears a small knob about 4 nm in diameter at the proximal end. The haemagglutinin and neuraminidase subunits each have a hydrophilic and a hydrophobic end, and the latter functions in binding the subunit to the viral membrane. It should be noted that both these proteins are of viral origin and are distinct from the proteins of the host cell.

In negatively stained specimens of most influenza viruses the surface of the covering membrane generally contains only a single row of short radiating projections whereas in influenza C virus the envelope frequently possesses three types of morphological unit:

(1) an outer fringe of spikes which is indistinguishable from that of influenza A and B viruses,

(2) an outer reticulum composed of hexagons and occasional pentagons, and

(3) an inner layer which shows no network and appears as an amorphous sheath.

Examination of orthomyxovirus preparations under the electron microscope reveals only intact virions with no obvious central structure. On rare occasions, however, and particularly with high titre preparations, there may be evidence of disruption of some of the virus particles. This allows penetration of the phosphotungstic acid stain which clearly reveals a central core, the nucleocapsid, which has the appearance of a tightly wound spring with a hollow centre running the length of the filament.

Disruption of the outer envelope of the virion is readily achieved by treatment with ether or ether and Tween 80. In this way, the inner nucleoprotein, sometimes called the ribonucleoprotein or S antigen component, can be distinguished from the surface projections containing haemagglutinin and neuraminidase.

The haemagglutinins can be prepared from the aqueous phase of ether-treated virus suspensions by adsorption–elution from red blood cells followed by centrifugation. Electron micrographs of these components show numerous particles measuring 30–40 nm in diameter, which are known as 'rosettes' and consist of star-like aggregates of short, rigid rods indistinguishable from the projections seen on the surface fringe of the intact virion. These 'rosettes', which are derived from the envelope of the virus, carry the strain-specific V antigen and show strain-specific agglutination of red blood cells by the virus particles. They also function in the production of specific neutralizing antibodies. It is

significant, however, that patients recovering from influenza invariably produce antibodies to V antigen components which are not demonstrable in the infecting strain by *in vitro* methods. This observation suggests that some of the components of the V antigen may not be present on the surface of the virion, and recent studies using ether fractionation of influenza virus have confirmed that the haemagglutinin component is present partly on the surface as well as within the intact infectious virion.

The other surface antigen, neuraminidase, is different in appearance from the haemagglutinin (*vide supra*) but its precise function is unknown. Some workers believe that viral neuraminidase is involved in the liberation of virus from infected cells and in elution of virus from agglutinated red blood cells, but others consider that it plays an important role in actual penetration of virus into the cell.

The ribonucleoprotein (RNP) component, sometimes called the 'g' (gebundenes) antigen, which corresponds morphologically to the internal helical nucleocapsid, is antigenically identical to the soluble antigen that is present in infected cells. The 'g' antigen and the soluble antigen are often referred to, collectively, as the S antigen. The soluble S antigen is in the form of elongated structures about 10 nm in diameter and up to 600 nm in length and its ultrastructure probably consists of chains of small subunits arranged in the form of a double helix with five or six subunits to each turn of the helix. Coiled inner components are seen in only a comparatively small number of virions and, in disrupted particles when the phosphotungstic acid stain has penetrated to the interior of the virus, the nucleocapsid appears as an amorphous structure. In some particles (e.g. incomplete and defective viruses) there may be no internal helix whereas in others the nucleoprotein coils are deeply embedded in an haemagglutinin gel and visible only in virions containing less haemagglutinin than normal. When extracted from virions, the tightly wound orthomyxovirus nucleocapsid appears in several distinct short segments, whereas in paramyxoviruses it is a single entity with a larger diameter and a much greater length.

Members of the myxovirus group may be divided into two subgroups on the basis of the diameter of the internal helical component. The first group, possessing a helix of 9 nm diameter, includes the influenza viruses while the second group, with a helix of 18 nm diamter, includes Newcastle disease, mumps and other paramyxoviruses. Members of the recently proposed metamyxovirus group have a helix of between 12–15 nm diameter. The two main subgroups are also distinguished by certain features of their replicative cycles, the orthomyxoviruses showing the phenomena of multiplicity reactivation and genetic recombination which do not occur among the paramyxoviruses.

Physicochemical properties

The orthomyxovirus virion contains virus-coded protein and an inner core of single-stranded RNA of molecular weight 2×10^6 daltons. On the other hand, because the viral envelope is derived by budding from the plasma membrane, the virus particle contains lipids and carbohydrates characteristic of the cell in which the virus was grown.

Orthomyxoviruses are stable at $-70°C$ but are usually inactivated in 30 minutes at $56°C$. They are labile when held at room temperature or at pH 3, maximum stability being between pH 7 and 8. Infected tissues retain activity for months in 50 per cent glycerol-saline at $4°C$, but the virus is inactivated by formalin, phenol, soaps, detergents and oxidizing agents. All orthomyxoviruses are sensitive to ether and other lipid solvents.

Haemagglutination

Orthomyxoviruses are capable of agglutinating the red blood cells of different animal species. Agglutination results from adsorption of virus particles to the mucoprotein receptors on the surface of the erythrocytes and is later followed by spontaneous elution due to the destructive action of the viral enzyme, neuraminidase, on the red cell receptors. Influenza A and B viruses cause haemagglutination at both $4°C$ and $20°C$ of red blood cells derived from man, monkey, guinea-pig, dog, ferret, hedgehog, squirrel rat, mouse, frog, duck and from many other avian species. In contrast, the red blood cells from ox, sheep, goat, pig, rabbit, cat and hamster are agglutinated only at $4°C$. Influenza C virus reacts poorly and only fowl, mouse, rat, frog and ground squirrel red blood cells are agglutinated and then only at $4°C$. Haemagglutination can be inhibited by specific antibody and the haemagglutination-inhibition reaction provides a simple and reliable means of detecting and measuring the antibody content of a serum.

It is noteworthy that red blood cells treated with one strain of influenza virus cannot subsequently be agglutinated by that same strain, although they may remain agglutinable by other myxoviruses. Moreover, there appears to be a graded arrangment of receptors on the erythrocyte surface enabling myxoviruses to be placed in a series in which treatment of cells with any one virus removes all receptors for that virus and for all viruses preceding it in the series, but not for viruses later in the 'receptor gradient' (Table 40.1, p. 453).

Development

Fluorescent antibody techniques have shown that in infected cells the viral S antigen is demonstrable in the nucleus of the cell 3 hours after infection, while the V antigen is not detectable until one hour later in the cytoplasm. After about 5 hours post-infection, both the S and V components appear in the cytoplasm and migrate to the surface of the cell (Plate 42.18, facing p. 505). Here, the haemagglutinating factor becomes associated with the cell membrane and the helical filaments (S antigen) of ribonucleoprotein (RNP) are enclosed within it. Following maturation, viral particles are released by extrusion or 'budding' from the cell membrane. When viral synthesis is incomplete, the virus becomes incorporated in and modifies the cell membrane so that healthy erythrocytes will adhere to the surfaces of the altered cells and show the phenomenon of haemadsorption. (Plate 43.3a, between pp. 518–9).

Antigenic properties

Members of the orthomyxovirus group are antigenically distinct, one from another, on the basis of complement-fixation, haemagglutination-inhibition and neutralization tests; but some overlapping may occur. In general, the group can be divided into three immunological types (A, B and C), on the basis of the S antigens which are specific for each type. In addition, members of the two major types, A and B, can be divided into a number of immunological subtypes on the basis of differences in their haemagglutinin and neuraminidase antigens. Although types and subtypes of orthomyxoviruses are antigenically stable, numerous variants appear from time to time probably as a result of minor changes in the surface envelope antigens by the process known as antigenic or immunological drift.

Cultivation

All viruses included in the orthomyxovirus group can be grown in the amniotic cavity of embryonated hens' eggs. After initial amniotic passage, influenza A and B viruses usually grow readily in the allantoic sac, also; whereas influenza C virus grows only in the amniotic cavity.

Influenza viruses may or may not grow in cell cultures of chicken and mammalian tissues and may produce recognizable cytopathic effects in some. Unlike paramyxoviruses, most species do not readily produce inclusion bodies either in the cytoplasm or the nucleus. In the absence of visible cytopathic changes, the presence of virus can be demonstrated by immunofluorescence staining or by haemadsorption.

Ecology and pathogenicity

Orthomyxoviruses are usually transmitted by droplet infections from the respiratory tracts of infected hosts in close contact with one another, and disease is frequently associated with inflammatory lesions involving principally the respiratory tract. In some instances (e.g. fowl plague) generalised infections develop and most of the viscera become involved.

Human influenza

It is widely believed that the great pandemic of human influenza in 1918–19 was caused by a virus related to swine influenza and that this virus may have been transmitted to pigs at that time. Indeed, the first successful isolation of any influenza-type virus was that reported in 1931 by a group of workers investigating an outbreak of swine influenza. Two years later the first strain of human influenza virus was isolated from throat washings from human patients by the intranasal inoculation of ferrets. The infection was readily transmissible and it seemed that the virus alone was responsible for uncomplicated influenza in man. This strain of human origin has been designated *Myxovirus influenzae -A hominis* and is the type species of the orthomyxoviruses.

In 1940 a second human influenza virus was isolated and was named *Myxovirus influenzae -B* because its antigen was distinct from that of the *M. influenzae -A* strains. More recently, a third antigenically distinct type named *M. influenzae -C* has been described. This is a very mild virus which rarely causes human influenza but often occurs concurrently with influenza A and B infections.

Growth characteristics

The growth characteristics of human influenza A and B viruses are generally very similar and both types are pathogenic for the chicken embryo, ferret and mouse. Embryonated hens' eggs may be infected by a number of routes but primary isolation from human sources and initial adaptation of the virus are best carried out by amniotic inoculation. Influenza viruses recently isolated from human tissues (O phase) grow best amniotically but, after adaptation (D phase), growth of all but type C strains is equally good in the allantoic cavity. Influenza C virus has a long growth cycle in the egg and is difficult to adapt to the allantoic cavity.

Ferrets inoculated intranasally with fluids infected with influenza A or B viruses develop a mild febrile disease with lesions on the nasal epithelium. Mice can be infected intranasally but several passages with chick embryo infected material are needed before lung lesions are regularly formed. Strains of influenza viruses grow on a variety of cell culture systems, including monkey kidney and human embryonic tissues, giving different reactions, and almost all neurotropic variants produce a marked cytopathic effect. Growth of influenza viruses on mammalian or avian cells is characterized by the development of cytopathic effects with intracytoplasmic and, sometimes, intranuclear inclusions. However, cell culture systems are generally less susceptible than fertile hens' eggs and are not recommended for primary virus isolation.

Interference

Interference can be demonstrated on cell cultures or eggs with viruses of types A and B or between different strains of type A. Interference also occurs between influenza viruses, other myxoviruses and unrelated groups including some togaviruses and poxviruses. *Myxovirus influenzae -C* growing in eggs interferes with influenza B and Newcastle disease virus and, in mice, it interferes with western equine encephalitis virus.

Haemagglutination

Influenza viruses haemagglutinate fowl, guinea-pig, ox, human and other species of red blood cells. It is noteworthy that prior treatment of these viruses with heat, formalin or ultraviolet light, which destroys viral infectivity, does not usually interfere with their haemagglutinating capacity.

Antigenic properties

Antigenic differences between strains of influenza viruses can be determined from their surface antigens which are demonstrable by haemagglutination-inhibition, neutralization, flocculation and complement-fixation tests.

The haemagglutinating antigens are specific for each strain of virus and are distinct from the complement-fixing group specific, soluble antigens. All strains of influenza type A share a common complement-fixing antigen which is distinct from the soluble complement-fixing antigen common to all type B strains.

Influenza antibodies formed as a result of childhood infection demonstrate the serological response throughout life. Successive age groups of the population show different antibody spectra and children lack antibodies against the antigens of 'influenza-virus-families' which disappeared before their birth. Thus, those born before 1946 lack the AO antibodies but possess high titres of A1 and A2 (Asian influenza) antibodies. It is likely that those born since 1957 will possess A2 but not A1 antibodies unless new epidemics of A1 viruses occur. Adults now over fifty years of age possess high titres of anti-swine influenza antibodies, whereas these are poorly represented in sera from younger adults. This represents a change from 1935 when anti-swine influenza antibodies were found in most children and adults aged 12 years and over. This finding supports the suggestion that swine influenza virus represents a persistent remnant of the 1918 pandemic virus.

It was reported that sera collected before the Asian pandemic of 1957 from adults over 70 years of age, sometimes possessed antibodies to A2 virus and it was suggested that the latter A2 virus represented a resurgence of the pandemic virus of the 1890 epoch.

Transmission

Natural transmission of influenza virus is by infected droplets which are expelled during speaking, coughing and sneezing and gain entry into the nasopharynx of in-contacts. The incubation period is about 24–48 hours and the patient rarely remains infective after the fifth day.

Control

Much work has been done on the preparation and use of formolised inactivated vaccines prepared from allantoic fluids of virus-infected hens' eggs and injected into or beneath the skin. Similar vaccines combined with mineral oil adjuvants have also been used. A Russian method of immunization has also been investigated whereby living attenuated virus is administered intranasally, but difficulties in achieving standardization and stabilization have still to be overcome.

Swine influenza

Definition

An acute respiratory illness of pigs.

Host and distribution

Swine influenza was first recognised as an epidemic in the U.S.A. during the autumn of 1918. The disease, which was particularly prevalent among swine in the Middle Western States, was thought to be closely associated with the pandemic of human influenza of 1918–19. Although cases of swine influenza have been reported from Europe, including the U.K., the disease occurs mainly in the U.S.A.

Antigenic characters

The antigenic properties of swine influenza virus are related to those of human influenza-A virus and the original American strains form a common antigenic group of viruses. In contrast, the European strains differ antigenically from each other, and from other strains of influenza virus. Slight antigenic variations have taken place over the years, and the strains currently causing epidemics in the United States differ from the classical Iowa strains isolated in 1931 to the extent that minor antigens in the original isolates have now become dominant. The Cambridge strain of virus, which was isolated in the late 1930s from diseased pigs in the U.K., is antigenically distinct from the original Iowa strain and appears to be intermediate between later American isolates and human influenza-A strains. It is interesting to note that antihaemagglutinins and neutralizing antibodies for swine influenza virus are present in many sera from older people who experienced the 1918–19 influenza pandemic, but few of those born after 1923 have antibodies for the virus. It has also been suggested that the Asian strain of influenza virus that appeared in 1957 was capable of infecting pigs, but this hypothesis has not been confirmed.

Pathogenicity

The disease causes influenza and pneumonia particularly when associated with *Haemophilus influenzae-suis*, although the bacterial infection alone causes no detectable illness in experimentally infected pigs. Intranasal instillation of virus produces symptoms of the disease and intramuscular injection renders swine immune to both the mild disease and the severe form caused by the combined effect of virus plus bacterium. When inoculated into the developing chicken egg, the virus-bacterium mixture gives rise to lung infection and a mortality rate several times higher than that produced by either agent separately.

Ecology

At the present time swine influenza occurs annually in many parts of the United States. The disease usually appears during the autumn and early winter months and there is experimental evidence that swine may become symptomless carriers of the virus before developing clinical disease. Transmission occurs from infected respiratory secretions and it is also believed that the virus may be acquired by pigs eating earthworms containing virus-infected larvae of the pig lungworm, *Metastrongylus elongatus*. The sequence of events as suggested by Shope in 1943 is as follows. Infected ova from lungworms carrying the virus in the bronchi of sick or convalescent pigs are coughed up, swallowed and excreted in its faeces. The ova are then ingested by earthworms in which they pass through three larval stages, the third stage being infective for swine. When such earthworms are eaten by pigs the larvae penetrate the intestinal mucosa and migrate via the lymph and blood stream to the lungs. Usually, no ill effects result, but if the animals are given an intramuscular injection of *H. influenzae-suis*, or are exposed to cold conditions, the virus becomes activated and the pigs develop typical swine influenza. This work has been confirmed by some workers but not others who were unable to detect multiplication or persistence of swine influenza virus in pig lungworms.

Diagnosis

Embryonated hens' eggs are used for isolation of the virus from nasal swabs or affected lung tissues in early acute cases of the disease. Rising antibody titres in paired sera can be demonstrated by haemagglutination-inhibition tests.

Control
Immunization with formalized vaccines has been attempted but is of doubtful practical value.

Equine influenza

Definition
An acute respiratory illness of horses.

Synonyms
Epidemic cough: Stable cough: Newmarket cough:

Introduction
Most workers are agreed that equine influenza is caused by a myxovirus closely related to *Myxovirus influenza-A* of man. There are, however, a number of other influenza-like conditions of horses associated with other, unrelated viruses, including the unclassified RNA virus of equine arteritis (pink-eye) and the DNA herpesvirus of equine rhinopneumonitis. In addition, it has been reported that an enterovirus resembling *Coxsackie-A* 21 and also some human rhinoviruses have been isolated from horses in England.

Morphology
The virus of equine influenza has the structure of a typical orthomyxovirus with a mean diameter of 100 nm.

Haemagglutination
Equine influenza-A virus agglutinates horse, calf, pig, rhesus monkey, fowl, guinea-pig and human red blood cells.

Antigenic characters
This virus shares the complement-fixing antigen of the influenza-A group but can be distinguished from the latter by the haemagglutination-inhibition test. The virus was first isolated in Czechoslovakia by Sovinova in 1956 and, subsequently, antibodies to the virus (A/Equi/1/Prague/56) have been identified in horse serum from many other countries.

In 1960, strains of Equi-1 virus were isolated in Canada and America from epizootics in young horses and, in 1963, a virus was isolated in England from cases of 'Newmarket Cough'. All of these strains are serologically closely related to the original A/Equi/1/Prague/56 virus. Also in 1963, a new strain of equine influenza virus (A/Equi/2/Miami/63) was isolated from cases of equine respiratory disease in Florida. Additional outbreaks of disease caused by the Equi-2 strain have occurred in the United Kingdom, South America, France, Germany and other European countries.

It is now accepted that there are only two distinct serotypes of equine influenza virus, designated A/Equi/1 (Prague strain) and A/Equi/2 (Miami strain). These can be distinguished from each other and from some additional members of the influenza-A group by haemagglutination-inhibition, strain-specific complement-fixation and virus neutralization tests. Cross reactions between equine and avian influenza-A viruses are demonstrable by haemagglutination-inhibition and complement-fixation tests, and have shown that A/Equi/1 is related to the classical fowl plague virus; and A/Equi/2 to both Duck/England/62 virus and Wilmot's turkey/Canada/63 virus.

Cultivation
Equine influenza virus grows well in embryonated chicken eggs and in cell cultures of bovine, chick, monkey and human embryo kidney. The cytopathic effect is characterised by an early development of syncytia and the formation of multiple eosinophilic intracytoplasmic inclusions. Infected cell cultures also haemadsorb guinea-pig erythrocytes.

Distribution
The disease is generally widespread and for several years has assumed epidemic proportions in India and many European countries. It spreads quickly and 90 per cent of a group of horses may become infected within a fortnight. During 1955, extensive epidemics of the Prague strain swept through most European countries and, in 1964, another serious epidemic developed in Florida, U.S.A. While it was found that many horses in the United Kingdom had some degree of immunity to the Prague virus they were fully susceptible to the Miami strain. Thus, when the virus of American origin was introduced into the United Kingdom in the following year a severe outbreak occurred due to the lack of immunity amongst British horses to the Miami strain of equine influenza virus.

Pathogenicity
Influenza viruses cause acute respiratory distress in horses but spontaneous recovery usually occurs after 10–14 days provided the animal is given complete rest immediately following the first appearance of the symptoms. In foals the disease is often more severe, the incubation period ranging from 4–11 days. The symptoms of the acute form of the disease include a raised body temperature, loss of appetite, depression, increased respiratory and pulse rates, and nasal discharge which may contain virus. The mucous membrane of the eye may become icteric and hyperaemic.

In experimental mice, the virus has been adapted to cause pneumonia and encephalitis and it is also believed to cause an inapparent infection of ferrets.

Diagnosis

Equine influenza may be suspected from the characteristic clinical symptoms, the high contagiousness of the disease, its sudden onset and rapid spread among all susceptible in-contact horses. The virus can be isolated in the allantoic sac of developing chicken eggs or in various cell culture systems. Specific antibodies can be detected in paired sera by haemagglutination-inhibition and serum neutralization tests.

Control

Horses which have recovered from influenza are generally resistant to reinfection. Inactivated egg-adapted, oil-adjuvant vaccines have been prepared against the Prague, Cambridge and Miami strains of virus, and are believed to confer about 12 months' protection with a solid immunity developing about 3 weeks after vaccination. In-foal mares are vaccinated so that they may pass a temporary protection to their foals via the colostrum, and these foals are vaccinated after the age of 3 months, revaccinated 6 months later, and annually thereafter. Hyperimmune sera can be used to give limited protection of 3 weeks duration to susceptible foals born from unvaccinated mares.

AVIAN INFLUENZA VIRUSES

A number of strains of influenza-A virus have been isolated from several species of birds suffering from severe respiratory infections. All strains are morphologically identical to other influenza viruses and share with them a common S antigen of A-type.

Serological studies based on haemagglutination-inhibition, strain-specific complement-fixation and virus neutralization tests suggest that the avian influenza-A viruses can be divided into five types according to the dominant V antigen present, as follows:

Type 1: the classical fowl plague virus (Dutch strain), including the Turkey/English/62 strain, and Dinter's virus 'N'.

Type 2: strains of duck influenza virus isolated in Czechoslovakia (1956) and in England (1962).

Type 3: a second strain of duck influenza virus isolated in England (1956).

Type 4: the chicken/Scotland/59 virus and the Tern/South Africa/61 virus.

Type 5: the A-virus (Wilmot strain) isolated from turkeys in Canada in 1963.

Fowl plague

Nomenclature

Fowl plague and Newcastle disease are two distinct and unrelated virus infections of birds. While they are recognised as two separate entities in the Diseases of Animals Act of the United Kingdom, both are included in the term 'fowl pest' for administrative and legal purposes, although outbreaks of fowl plague are separately recorded. Newcastle disease is prevalent in England and, consequently, the term 'fowl pest' is frequently used as a synonym for Newcastle disease.

History and distribution

In 1878, fowl plague was first described in Italy by Perroncito as an extremely severe and fatal disease of poultry. Although it did not spread to other countries during the next 10–12 years there are numerous reports that by the turn of the century it was enzootic in southern Europe and widespread throughout Germany. At the present time, the disease is believed to be enzootic in the United Arab Republic, in other parts of North Africa and, occasionally, in some countries of Eastern Europe and the Far East. Fowl plague was reported in the U.S.A. in 1924 and 1929, and in the United Kingdom in 1922, 1929 and 1963. The 1963 outbreak was the first in the United Kingdom since the Fowl Pest (Newcastle disease) Order was introduced in 1936.

Hosts affected

Fowl plague is an acute, highly infectious and generally fatal disease of chickens, turkeys and, occasionally, ducks and geese. A wide range of wild birds may also be affected but reports that pigeons are resistant await confirmation.

Morphology and development of the virus

The causative virus of fowl plague is one of a small group of influenza-A viruses of avian origin which consist of five antigenic types, with various subtypes.

The virus generally consists of spherical particles about 80–100 nm in diameter. When treated with ethyl ether the helical filaments break up into short rods of about 9 nm in diameter; and the envelope disrupts to form numerous small star-shaped rosettes about 35 nm across consisting of haemagglutinin and neuraminidase. The nucleoprotein is formed in the nucleus of the affected cell and the haemagglutinin in the cytoplasm.

Physicochemical characters

The virus contains RNA and is inactivated by heating at 55°C for 1 hour, or 60°C for 10 minutes. It is sensitive to ultraviolet light and to most disinfectants and antiseptics. It resists dessication and has been known to survive in dried dust for 14 days.

Haemagglutination

Haemagglutination takes place with a wide range of animal red cells including chicken, monkey, horse, ox and pig.

Antigenic properties

Fowl plague virus and all other avian influenza-A strains share the complement-fixing antigen of the *Influenzae-A* virus group but are immunologically distinct from other influenza-A viruses by haemagglutination-inhibition, apart from minor crossing with *M. influenzae-A equi*. Although the envelope antigens of avian strains are related to each other, they can be distributed into five antigenic groupings by haemagglutination-inhibition.

Cultivation

The virus grows well in developing chicken eggs and in cell cultures of chicken and various mammalian tissues, including those of rabbit and ox, human embryonic tissues and HeLa cells. A cytopathic effect is generally produced and infected cells haemadsorb red blood cells, but there are often no intracytoplasmic or intranuclear inclusions. Most strains produce plaques on chick fibroblast cultures overlayed with agar. The virus has been transmitted experimentally to mice, ferrets and to some other mammals mainly by intracerebral inoculation.

Pathogenicity

The disease appears with sudden onset and runs a rapid course. Illness is usually so acute that many birds die after showing no more than slight indisposition, inappetance, ruffled feathers and fever. Other birds stop laying and show weakness and staggering gait. The comb and wattles become cyanotic and the eyes are swollen and closed. Sick birds often sit or stand in a semi-comatose state with their heads touching the ground. Oedema of the subcutaneous tissues around the eyes, ear lobes and wattles tends to extend downwards, along the throat and breast. Oedema of the glottis makes breathing difficult and the mouth is held open and breathing is accompanied by a rattling sound. A profuse watery diarrhoea may also be present. Death usually occurs within two days but in less acute cases there is CNS involvement with spasmodic twitching movements of the head and neck, convulsions, ataxia or blindness.

On post-mortem examination, petechial haemorrhages and ecchymoses may be seen throughout the body but especially in the proventriculus and abdominal fat. Petechiae are also to be found in the inner surface of the sternum.

The incubation period is from 3–7 days and the mortality rate varies from 40–100 per cent. The virus invades most tissues and very high titres are obtained.

Blood is so rich in virus that it can cause disease when injected into susceptible hens even when diluted one million times or more. The virus retains its activity in flesh and bone marrow for upwards of 10 months when kept at chilling temperature.

Ecology

The diseased bird is the most dangerous factor in the transmission of this disease and in nearly every fresh outbreak there is a history of new birds having been introduced. Although the virus is present at high titres in most tissues, and is excreted in eye and nasal secretions and in the watery droppings, the precise method of transmission under field conditions has never been precisely explained. The spread of the disease requires close contact with the infection and it appears that both direct and indirect spread of the virus is possible. Thus slaughter and quarantine quickly bring the disease under control. Minute doses of virus administered by any route always results in infection which is usually fatal. Following natural infection of a flock, the disease spreads quickly and is rapidly fatal to the majority of chickens in a flock. The disease often subsides quickly due, in part, to its high mortality which renders the disease somewhat self-limiting.

Diagnosis

Symptoms and lesions are highly suggestive of a peracute form of Newcastle disease. Losses are regular and extensive. Occasionally, sudden deaths may occur where the post-mortem examination reveals egg peritonitis in the absence of characteristic haemorrhagic lesions. Confirmation of the disease can be obtained by applying the haemagglutination-inhibition test to serum samples, and by isolating and subsequently identifying the virus from tissues of dead birds.

Control

Slaughter and quarantine methods can be effective in bringing this disease under control. Sick birds are destroyed, the carcases burned and thorough cleansing and disinfection of premises is essential. In the United Kingdom the disease is notifiable and is subject to compulsory slaughter, with compensation.

The few birds that recover from fowl plague appear to be solidly immune and their sera contain neutralizing and haemagglutination-inhibiting antibodies that will protect susceptible birds for a limited time only. Formaldehyde and phenol inactivated vaccines, alone and with adjuvants of oil, saponins or killed acid-fast bacilli, have given disappointing results. Attenuation of some strains of virus for fowls follows cultivation in chicken, pigeon, or human cells and it has been claimed that attenuated

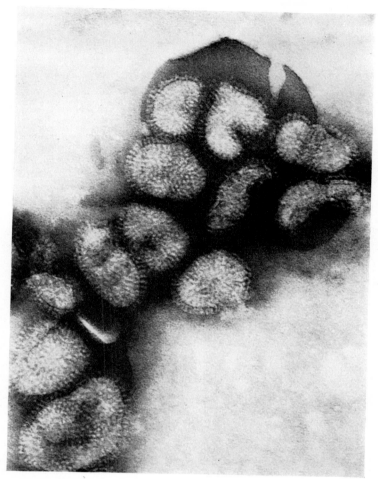

43.1 Electron micrograph of avian influenza-A virus (fowl plague, strain Rostock), showing pleomorphic enveloped virions with a surface fringe of projections 9 nm in length, × 200 000. (Courtesy of Dr C. R. Madeley.)

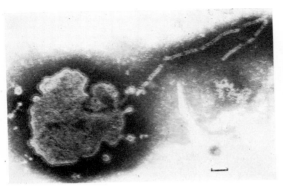

43.2a

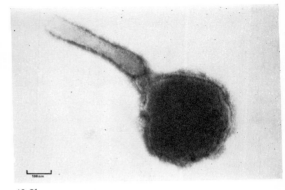

43.2b

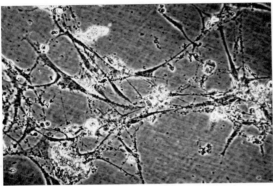

43.2c

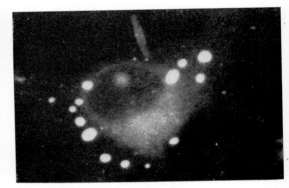

43.2d

43.2a Electron micrograph of a virulent strain of Newcastle disease virus (Herts 33), showing the structure and arrangement of the helical strands forming the internal nucleocapsid and the fringe of evenly spaced, short projections covering the envelope. Bar represents 100 nm.

43.2c Micrograph of chick fibroblasts 24 hours after inoculation with the Herts 33 strain of Newcastle disease virus, as seen in the phase contrast microscope. The infected cells have rounded up and are highly refractile, whereas the dark uninfected cells have retained their fibroblastic appearance.

43.2b Electron micrograph of a defective strain of Newcastle disease virus showing a virion adsorbed to the surface of a chicken red blood cell. Notice the poorly developed fringe of surface projections and the absence of a clearly defined ribonucleoprotein component inside the virus particle. Bar represents 100 nm.

43.2d Distribution of viral antigen in the cytoplasm of a calf kidney cell infected with Newcastle disease virus. Direct staining with FITC-conjugated rabbit anti-NDV serum.

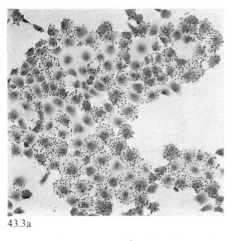

43.3a

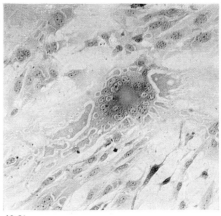

43.3b

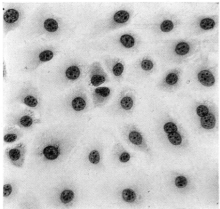

43.3c

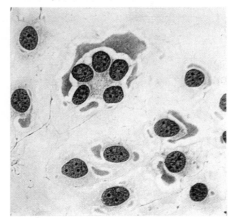

43.3d

43.3a Calf kidney cell line persistently infected with Newcastle disease virus. There is no cytopathic effect, but the presence of infected cells is revealed by their ability to adsorb guinea-pig erythrocytes to their surface, i.e. haemadsorption. Haematoxylin eosin stain, × 44.

43.3c Monolayer culture of healthy bovine kidney cells. Giemsa stain, × 170.

43.3b Bovine strain of parainfluenza-3 virus on secondary calf kidney cells. There are large syncytia containing acidophilic intracytoplasmic inclusions of varied size and shape, and numerous small spherical intranuclear inclusion bodies. Haematoxylin eosin stain, × 90.

43.3d Sub-line of bovine kidney cells chronically infected with Newcastle disease virus. Notice the large plaques of inclusion material in the cytoplasm of infected cells. Giemsa stain, × 350.

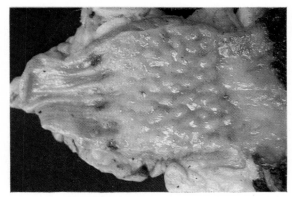

43.4a

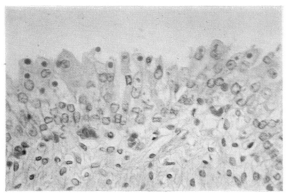

43.4b

43.4a Small haemorrhages in the mucosa of the proventriculus of a chicken dying from Newcastle disease.

43.4b A section through the bladder wall of a dog with distemper. The presence of acidophilic intracytoplasmic inclusion bodies is characteristic of the disease. Haematoxylin eosin stain. × 90.

strains can confer solid immunity against infection with virulent fowl plague virus.

Duck influenza viruses

The Czechoslovakian and British duck influenza viruses are serologically related and classified with members of the avian influenza-type myxoviruses. The Czechoslovakian virus (A/Duck/1/Czech/56) was isolated in 1956 from an outbreak of upper respiratory disease in ducklings when about 30 per cent of affected birds, aged between 10–21 days, died after a short illness. The outstanding feature of the disease was inflammation of the infraorbital sinuses. Laboratory investigations confirmed that the Czechoslovakian isolate possessed the S antigen of influenza-type A virus but differed in haemagglutination-inhibition tests from fowl plague, Newcastle disease or other myxoviruses, and was distinct from the equine influenza-A virus which was widespread in horses in Czechoslovakia at the time of the outbreak of influenza in ducklings.

In 1956, also, a strain of influenza virus was isolated from a mild disease of ducklings on a farm in England and the virus (A/Duck/2/England/56) was readily distinguished from the 1956 Czechoslovakian duck virus by haemagglutination-inhibition, strain-specific complement-fixation and virus neutralization tests. However, in 1962, a second outbreak occurred on the same farm in England and the causative virus (A/Duck/England/62) was isolated from a pool of respiratory tissues from five ducklings affected with sinusitis. This second British strain of duck influenza virus, unlike the Czechoslovakian and British isolates of 1956, did not produce death and extensive lung lesions when passaged intranasally in mice. Serological studies have indicated that it is related to but not identical with the 1956 Czechoslovakian isolates, and it has been assigned to a separate subtype.

Duck influenza viruses grow satisfactorily on tissue cultures and produce cytopathic changes on cultures of chick embryo, duckling, calf, monkey and embryonic human kidney cells.

The chick–tern viruses

In 1959, Wilson isolated a virus from chickens suffering from a disease which resembled fowl plague. Although the virus (A/Chick/Scotland/59) possessed the type-specific influenza-A nucleoprotein antigen, it was serologically distinct from classical fowl plague virus.

Two years later a serious epizootic occurred in the Common Tern in South Africa and the causative virus (A/Tern/S.Africa/61) was serologically indistinguishable from that of A/Chick/Scotland/59. Unlike Wilson's Scotland/59 virus, the South African Tern/61 strain showed the pantropic properties of fowl plague virus and produced high mortality in experimentally infected chickens. There is recent evidence that the tern virus may also occur in Canada.

Other avian influenza viruses

In 1963, Lang and Wells isolated an avian influenza virus (Wilmot virus) from a mild disease of turkeys in Canada. Although strain-specific complement-fixation tests showed the Wilmot virus to be related to Duck/England/62 and A/Equi/Miami/63 viruses, haemagglutination-inhibition tests confirmed that it was distinct from fowl plague and other avian influenza viruses. The Wilmot virus agglutinates chicken and turkey erythrocytes and resembles influenza A2 and A/Equi/2/63 viruses in agglutinating horse and cattle red cells.

Virus N

Virus N was originally isolated in 1949 by Dinter from a dead hen on a farm in Germany where nine chickens had died at fortnightly intervals. The disease was of short duration and the post-mortem picture was similar to that of fowl plague with numerous petechial haemorrhages in the carcase. The causative agent was isolated and serological studies showed that the remaining birds in the flock had antibodies to virus N but not against fowl plague or Newcastle disease viruses. Virus N was unexpectedly avirulent for adult poultry but egg-passaged virus given orally to 1-day-old chickens produced pneumoencephalitis after an incubation period of 8–14 days.

Haemagglutination-inhibition and serum neutralization tests indicate that Dinter's virus N is serologically related to, but distinct from, classical fowl plague virus, whereas the A/Turkey/England/63 strain is related serologically to fowl plague but not to virus N.

METAMYXOVIRUSES

Respiratory syncytial virus (RSV) and the pneumonia virus of mice (PVM) are generally included in the paramyxovirus group. However, this is only a provisional classification because neither of these viruses possess the enzyme neuraminidase nor do they bear any antigenic relationships to other paramyxoviruses. Moreover, it has recently been shown that RSV and PVM may be intermediate between ortho- and paramyxoviruses in that the diameter of their internal helix of ribonucleoprotein is 12–15 nm and, for these reasons, it has been proposed that they be placed in a third myxovirus group called metamyxovirus.

Respiratory syncytial virus
Hosts affected

Respiratory syncytial virus (RSV), formerly called

chimpanzee coryza agent (CCA), was originally isolated from an outbreak of 'colds' in a colony of captive chimpanzees. It is now known that human strains of RSV are frequently associated with minor localized upper respiratory tract infections in adults and that they are important agents of lower respiratory tract infections of young children. Since 1970, a virus antigenically related to human strains of RSV has been isolated from cattle showing mild respiratory disease, in Japan, Switzerland, England and other parts of Europe.

Properties of the virus

Respiratory syncytial virus closely resembles paramyxoviruses morphologically and passes membrane filters of 200 nm APD, but not 100 nm. The virions are mostly 90–120 nm in diameter although larger, pleomorphic forms are found. The central helical nucleocapsid has a diameter of about 12 nm compared with 9 nm for orthomyxoviruses and 18 nm for paramyxoviruses, and is enclosed by an outer lipid membrane with surface projections 10–14 nm in length. Lack of inhibition by halogenated deoxyribosides and inhibition of growth by 5-fluorouracil suggests that the viral nucleic acid is RNA. The virus is sensitive to ether, chloroform, sodium deoxycholate and trypsin, but is labile at pH3 and is readily inactivated at 56°C. Although the virus survives rapid freezing at−70°C, it is more readily isolated from recently obtained clinical specimens and should not, therefore, be held in the refrigerator before examination but should be inoculated into susceptible cell cultures with a minimum delay.

Cultivation

Small laboratory animals are generally refractory to experimental infection with RSV but chimpanzee strains have been propagated by serial passage in ferrets. There is no growth in embryonated hens' eggs. Human strains can be cultivated at 33°–36°C on cell lines of Bristol HeLa, KB and HEp2, as well as in organ cultures derived from human nasal and tracheal epithelium. Cattle strains can be isolated and maintained in primary cultures of bovine kidney, testicle and lung, but not in sheep, human, monkey or hamster cells. In most susceptible cell culture systems, growth of RSV is characterized by numerous foci of ballooned cells and several multinucleate syncytia with small acidophilic intracytoplasmic inclusions. The infectivity titres are generally low. Infected monolayers do not haemadsorb red blood cells and infectious cell culture fluids do not agglutinate erythrocytes of cattle, sheep, guinea-pig and mice. There are no reports of neuraminidase or haemolytic activity.

Pathogenesis

In cattle, RSV is usually associated with an acute febrile (41.5°C) illness involving the upper respiratory tract, with nasal discharge and cough. The course of the disease lasts for 3–5 days in calves and 8–10 days in adults. The infection tends to be more severe in older cattle, but neither deaths nor serious complications have been reported. Neutralizing and complement-fixing antibodies are present in convalescent bovine sera. The virus produces only mild disease in experimentally infected calves and does not appear to be invasive nor destructive. It has been suggested that RSV only causes severe reactions in the presence of an established immune response, such as is found in older cattle. The virus has not been isolated from other species, but a recent survey in Canada has shown that the prevalence of complement-fixing antibodies to RSV is high in sheep sera (81 per cent), relatively low in bovine sera (14 per cent) and in horse sera (6 per cent), but absent in pigs, goats, ferrets and monkeys. There is clear evidence from neutralization and complement-fixation tests of a close antigenic relationship between bovine and human strains of RSV.

Diagnosis

Neutralization and complement-fixation tests are of value for diagnostic purposes; the former is probably the more sensitive method. Bovine strains of virus can be isolated in primary bovine cell cultures and produce a cytopathic effect with syncytial formation in 10–12 days.

It should be noted that other syncytial-forming viruses may be isolated from bovine tissues and should not be confused with strains of bovine respiratory syncytial virus. For example, bovine syncytial virus, (an unclassified virus resembling leukoviruses or, more closely, the simian and feline group of foamy viruses) was first isolated in America from normal and lymphosarcomatous cattle and, more recently, in England from a normal calf.

PARAMYXOVIRUSES

Paramyxoviruses are frequently associated with respiratory illnesses in animals and man, and are the causative agents of a number of important diseases such as mumps in man and Newcastle disease in birds.

Morphology

The virions of most paramyxoviruses are highly pleomorphic in appearance and, compared with orthomyxoviruses, do not seem to have much strength of structure since they are easily disrupted in preparations for electron microscopy. Paramy-

TABLE 43.2.   Differences between orthomyxoviruses and paramyxoviruses.

	Orthomyxovirus	Paramyxovirus
Particle size	75–120 nm	150–450 nm
Diameter of nucleocapsid	9 nm	18 nm
Length of extracted nucloecapsid	50–130 nm	1000 nm
Molecular weight of RNA	$2 \cdot 5 \times 10^6$	$7 \cdot 0 \times 10^6$
Filamentous virions	+	(∓)
Haemolysins	−	+
Site of formation of soluble antigen	Nucleus	Cytoplasm
Cytoplasmic inclusions	(∓)	+
Multiplicity reactivation	+	−
Genetic recombination	+	−
Segmented genome	+	−
Sensitivity to actinomycin D	+	−

xovirus RNA, unlike that of orthomyxoviruses, occurs as a single molecule of molecular weight 7×10^6 daltons. Mature virions have an average diameter of 150–250 nm when examined in the electron microscope by negative staining techniques; but filamentous particles extending to 500 nm or even 1000 nm in length may occasionally be seen. They are, therefore, generally larger than orthomyxoviruses (70–120 nm). Attached to each coil of the internal RNA component are some 15 protein capsomeres [sub-units]. These give the inner nucleoprotein helix a characteristic herring-bone appearance with a diameter of 17–18 nm (Plate 37.2, facing p. 403). This is appreciably wider than the ribonucleoprotein strands of orthomyxoviruses and metamyxoviruses which measure 9–10 nm and 12–15nm, respectively.

The virion is invested by a lipoprotein outer envelope and its infectivity is completely destroyed following exposure to 20 per cent alcoholic ether for 18 hours at 4°C. Most strains agglutinate avian and certain species of mammalian red blood cells and exhibit neuraminidase activity.

Haemagglutination
The projections on the surface of the envelope are composed of glycoproteins, and possess haemagglutinating and neuraminidase activities, as well as the strain-specific antigenicity of the virion. Unlike orthomyxoviruses, most species of paramyxoviruses haemolyse chicken red blood cells and some, including Newcastle disease virus, may lyse the cells after agglutinating them. The haemolytic factor, which is associated with the virus particle and is distinct from the haemagglutinin, has not been described in any of the orthomyxoviruses. Most paramyxoviruses do not fall into the so-called receptor gradient (Table 40.1, p. 453) as cells stabilized with these viruses are agglutinated by all other haemagglutinating myxoviruses. Non-specific inhibitors of haemagglutination present in animal sera may be removed by treatment with receptor destroying enzyme or kaolin.

Physicochemical properties
Paramyxoviruses are relatively unstable at temperatures of 37°C or above, and are inactivated rapidly at pH 3·0. However, they can be stored without loss of infectivity for several years at –70°C particularly if a 'stabilizer' such as 0·5 per cent bovine serum albumin is incorporated in the suspending medium. The virion contains about 70 per cent protein, between 20–40 per cent lipid and approximately 0.9 per cent RNA. There are a number of major and minor polypeptides and an RNA-dependent RNA polymerase has been described in Newcastle disease virus.

Cultivation
Newcastle disease, mumps and Sendai viruses grow well in amniotic and allantoic cells of embryonated hens' eggs but most parainfluenza types and naturally occurring strains of pseudomyxoviruses, such as distemper and rinderpest, multiply poorly or not at all in fertile eggs. Nevertheless, cell culture isolates of many strains of para- and pseudomyxoviruses can be adapted to grow well in the amniotic and allantoic sacs of developing chicken embryos.

Most paramyxoviruses can be propagated in a variety of cell culture systems and all strains, apart from some type 1 and type 4 parainfluenza viruses, produce focal areas of multinucleated syncytia. Unlike orthomyxoviruses, most paramyxoviruses produce numerous, irregularly-shaped, acidophilic aggregates of intracytoplasmic inclusion material and small, multiple, intranuclear inclusions in monolayer cultures. Some, such as Newcastle disease virus may form intracytoplasmic inclusions but rarely intranuclear bodies. Immunofluorescence studies of infected cell monolayers suggest that the synthesis of ribonucleoprotein and surface antigens is confined to the cytoplasm whereas in orthomyxovirus infections the formation of soluble antigen is detected first in the cell nucleus and, later, in the cytoplasm also. This explanation is not acceptable to some workers and recent evidence that nucleic acid synthesis of

Newcastle disease and Sendai viruses occurs in the nucleoli awaits confirmation.

Paramyxoviruses are incapable of genetic recombination, nor do they exhibit multiplicity reactivation, although both of these phenomena are well recognised features of orthomyxoviruses. Another property which helps to distinguish orthomyxoviruses from paramyxoviruses is the suppression of influenza virus replication by the antibiotic actinomycin D which acts by selectively inhibiting the DNA-directed synthesis of RNA.

Antigenic properties

All paramyxoviruses are serologically distinct from orthomyxoviruses. They are probably antigenically stable and, while minor antigens may be shared by at least one, or in some cases two or three members of the family, there is no single antigen which is common to the entire group.

Diagnosis

Diagnosis of paramyxovirus infections can be made by inoculating specimens into susceptible cell cultures and observing them for haemadsorption, haemagglutination and cytopathic effects. Virus isolates are identified, where appropriate, by haemadsorption-inhibition, haemagglutination-inhibition and serum neutralization tests, using standard antisera. The complement-fixation test which is satisfactory for diagnosing distemper and rinderpest is not very useful for identifying 'true' paramyxoviruses since frequent cross-reactions make interpretation difficult.

Newcastle disease

Synonyms

Ranikhet: avian pneumoencephalitis: atypische Geflügelpest (Ger.).

In Great Britain the term 'fowl pest' is often used in a legal sense to include the two diseases of 'fowl plague' and 'Newcastle disease'. It is emphasised, however, that this is a misleading designation since fowl plague and Newcastle disease are distinct clinical illnesses caused by different myxoviruses.

Definition and hosts affected

Newcastle disease is a highly contagious and destructive disease which attacks mostly chickens and guinea fowl but is capable of infecting a large number of species of domestic and wild birds. Turkeys and peafowl are less susceptible, but virulent virus has frequently been isolated from pheasants, pigeons and free-living psittacines. Waterfowl and sea birds are generally refractory but they may act as carriers of the virus. Man is susceptible and there are numerous reports of self-limiting conjunctivitis in laboratory workers and in poultry farmers exposed to diseased birds and living virus vaccines.

History and distribution

In 1926, there was a report of an apparently new disease entity of poultry near Batavia in Indonesia and, in the spring of the same year, there was an outbreak of disease near Newcastle-on-Tyne, England, from which a virus, distinct from any previously known to affect poultry, was identified as the causative agent. The mortality rate was very high, in many cases 100 per cent and, as such, the disease was self-limiting. Newcastle disease was not recognized again in England until 1933, when it was slaughtered out; but in 1947 it reappeared and was only partially contained by a slaughter policy. In the late 1930s, a new disease which was subsequently proved to be Newcastle disease appeared in California and later spread throughout the United States, but the illness was much milder than that in England and Indonesia and was not recognised as Newcastle disease until some 9 years later. No satisfactory explanation has been offered for the apparently spontaneous appearance of Newcastle disease in different parts of the world, and to this extent the origin and source of the virus remain uncertain. Nor has it been ascertained how this new virulent infection first appeared in the United States in a mild atypical form.

At the time of the first outbreak in England, the disease was also spreading in the Far East, and the first recorded outbreak in India occurred in 1927 at Ranikhet. Elsewhere in India the same disease had been called Madras fowl pest. In Australia, Newcastle disease was first reported in 1930 on a number of farms near Melbourne but the last outbreak in that country was in 1933. Today, the disease is almost world-wide in its distribution except in the Scandinavian countries of Denmark, Norway, Sweden and Finland.

Morphology

The causative agent of Newcastle disease is a member of the paramyxoviruses. The mature virus particles are relatively large (100–250 nm) and are less regular in outline than those of fowl plague virus, although generally spherical in shape. Some strains are highly pleomorphic and show elongated, lobulated or annular forms. The coat of the virion has a definite outer membrane and an external surface fringe of spike-like projections each about 8 nm in length (Plate 37.2, facing p. 403). Within the virion is an inner core composed of a coiled hollow filament of ribonucleoprotein about 17 nm in diameter. Newcastle disease virions are much less stable than those of fowl plague and treatment with ether results in total disruption of the virion and the release of rosettes which are both larger (35–65 nm) and more irregular than those of the fowl plague virus (35 nm). The rosettes, which consist of an outer coat fragment of lipoprotein to which the spikes are attached, probably carry the haemagglutinating activity of the virus particle as well as the enzyme neuraminidase. Disruption of the virus particle also reveals a number of released fragments of ribonucleoprotein which have a characteristic 'herring-bone' pattern. These structures consist of protein and ribonucleic acid arranged in the form of helical rods which have a diameter of 18 nm and are about twice as thick as those of fowl plague virus. (Plate 43.2a, between pp. 518–9).

Chemical composition
The coat or envelope of Newcastle disease virus is known to contain lipid as well as protein and is probably a modification either of the surface membrane of the cell or of some internal cellular component such as the endoplasmic reticulum. Chemical analysis indicates that the nucleic acid is a continuous thread of single-stranded RNA, 1 μm long.

Physicochemical characters
Although Newcastle disease virus is inactivated at a temperature of 55°C for 45 minutes, or by direct sunlight for 30 minutes, its infectivity remains unchanged at 4°C for a few days, at –20°C for several weeks, and at –70°C for months or even years. In general, it is a robust virus and well suited to survive in nature. The main factors affecting its ability to survive outside the living bird include the amount of virus present, the strain of virus, the temperature, humidity, rate of drying, exposure to sunlight and other conditions of storage, as well as the presence or otherwise of decomposing organic matter. The viable virus has been recovered from contaminated hen-houses, egg trays, egg shells, feathers and other materials 2–8 weeks after depopulation following an outbreak of Newcastle disease. It also survives in fresh eggs for several months and in frozen poultry carcases for more than 2 years. In unplucked carcases stored at 4°C, virus persists on the skin and in the bone marrow for 4–6 months.

The effects of chemical disinfectants such as sodium carbonate and sodium hydroxide are variable but most detergents rapidly inactivate the virus. Although washing soda has little direct disinfectant action, its detergent properties are excellent and a hot 4 per cent solution is useful for cleaning and general disinfection. Lysol, phenol and cresol at concentrations of 2–3 per cent will inactivate the virus within 5 minutes provided the virus is not protected by tissues, body secretions, faeces or other organic material. The effectiveness of forma-lin is influenced to a very marked extent by variations in temperature and concentration but, at incubator temperature, 0·1 per cent formalin proves effective in 6 hours and a 1/5000 concentration will inactivate purified virus within an hour.

Haemagglutination
All strains of Newcastle disease virus agglutinate a variety of avian and mammalian red cells but chicken, guinea-pig and human group 'O' erythrocytes are most frequently used. Ox and sheep red cells are agglutinated by most strains of virus, whereas horse cells are mostly agglutinated by lentogenic strains but not by velogenic strains (*vide infra*). Haemagglutination tests are best read at 4°C because at higher temperatures elution follows rapidly (Plate 42.16a–d, between pp. 504–5). The pH of the medium is not an important consideration when using paramyxoviruses. Newcastle disease virus can also cause erythrocytes to be adsorbed on to the surface of infected cells in monolayer tissue cultures, a phenomenon that has been termed haemadsorption (Plate 40.1b facing p. 445). High concentrations of Newcastle disease virus will haemolyse fowl red cells — a property which is not possessed by fowl plague virus. Haemagglutination, haemadsorption and haemolysis are all inhibited by specific antibody to the virus.

Antigenic properties
Newcastle disease virus is immunologically distinct from orthomyxoviruses and from other members of the paramyxovirus group. Ether treatment rapidly disrupts the virus into haemagglutinating rosettes (V-antigen) and internal symmetrical helical components resembling the S-antigen of influenza. So far, however, the soluble (S) or nucleoprotein antigen of Newcastle disease virus has been insufficiently characterised and it is not yet possible to differentiate the Newcastle disease group of viruses into subtypes as is done with influenza viruses. A common antigen may be shared with mumps virus because patients with mumps may develop haemagglutination-inhibiting antibodies for Newcastle disease virus.

Unlike many smaller and more simply constructed viruses which contain only virus-specific material, the more complex Newcastle disease virus contains lipoprotein material derived from the surface of the host cell as an integral part of its structure, which possesses normal host cell antigenic activity. This is referred to as the 'normal' component and may amount to about 40 per cent of the total virion mass.

Cultivation
(Plates 43.2c and 43.3d, between pp. 518–9). Newcastle disease virus can be readily cultivated in 10- to 12-day-old embryonated chicken eggs by

inoculation on to the chorioallantoic membrane or into the allantoic sac (Fig. 42.1, facing p. 481). Maximum titres (about $10^{-9.0}$ EID$_{50}$/0·1 ml) are usually obtained after 24–36 hours of incubation and many strains will kill the embryos in 24–72 hours, causing haemorrhagic lesions and encephalitis. Infected allantoic fluids will agglutinate red blood cells. Most strains will multiply, produce haemagglutinins, haemadsorb and cause cytopathic changes in a wide range of secondary and continuous cell cultures including those of rabbit, pig, calf and monkey kidney, chicken tissues and HeLa cells. The most commonly used are chick embryo fibroblast, chick embryo kidney and baby hamster kidney (BHK) monolayer cells. However, the titre of the virus in cell cultures is usually 1 log lower than the corresponding titre in embryonated hens' eggs. In most cases the first evidence of virus infection is the formation of syncytia due to the merging of the cytoplasm of the cells and their nuclei to form large multinucleated masses surrounded by normal cells. (Plate 42.9c, between pp. 480–1). In most cell culture systems the virus produces irregularly shaped acidophilic intracytoplasmic inclusions but only rarely are well defined multiple inclusions seen in the nucleus. Cell cultures may become chronically infected or remain latently infected for prolonged periods with or without the release of complete viruses. These chronically infected cultures frequently show no cytopathic effects and the surviving cells in the monolayer are usually insusceptible to challenge with closely related viruses. In cases where persistent infections are mediated by interferons, super-infection by unrelated viruses is also prevented. Particles of viral antigen can be readily demonstrated in the cytoplasm of persistently infected cells by fluorescent antibody staining techniques, either as small aggregates scattered diffusely throughout the cytoplasm or as large plaques in the perinuclear region. (Plate 43.2d, between pp. 518–9).

Pathogenicity

In the natural disease, the average incubation period is 5–6 days but in severe outbreaks the symptoms may appear within 3 days. In mild outbreaks, several weeks may elapse before the disease becomes apparent. The clinical symptoms vary greatly according to the severity of the outbreak but many other factors also influence the effect of the disease, including the age and immune status of the flock, the strain of virus concerned, the route of infection and the presence of concurrent infections with other species of organisms. In acute cases of the so-called velogenic form there is usually respiratory distress accompanied by rales, gasping and coughing. Depression, prostration and a profuse greenish diarrhoea may also be present and nervous signs may

appear later. The virulent virus usually gives rise to very high mortality and 90–100 per cent. of the flock may die within a period of a few days. In less acute cases, whether they are of the mesogenic or lentogenic types, the mortality rate is generally much lower and the symptoms are less characteristic of the disease. The mesogenic form is sudden in onset, spreads moderately quickly and is associated with drowsiness, mild respiratory symptoms, diarrhoea and a sudden drop in egg production. Eggs may be grossly abnormal and affected birds may show nervous signs and paralysis. The mortality rate is variable but usually does not exceed 25 per cent. In the lentogenic form, the disease is very mild and virtually symptomless but there is generally some decline in egg production. Nervous symptoms are absent and recovery is usually rapid and complete. In certain countries (e.g. Northern Ireland) the disease seldom becomes clinical and can only be detected by serological methods or by recovery of the virus, e.g. McFerran's 'Ulster' strain from carrier birds. Newcastle disease virus affects turkeys of all ages. The symptoms are similar to those in fowls but are generally very mild. In ducks, game birds and other free-living species the disease may be so mild as to pass unnoticed.

In man, infection occurs mostly in poultry processors, veterinarians and laboratory workers as a result of contact with the virus in the laboratory or through careless handling of live virus vaccines. The incubation period is about 48 hours and infection gives rise to an acute self-limiting conjunctivitis involving one and sometimes both eyes and may, occasionally, have serious effects on the cornea. A mild influenza-like illness has sometimes been reported. Most cases run a course of a week to ten days and recover without treatment. There is no lateral spread from one human to another.

Pathology

Lesions associated with natural cases of Newcastle disease in poultry may vary considerably depending on the age and breed of the bird affected and on the virulence of the virus involved. In mild cases, the only abnormalities present may be a cloudiness of the air sacs and congestion of the lungs together with other non-specific lesions of the respiratory tract but, in acute cases, the appearance and distribution of lesions are more characteristic. Petechial haemorrhages may be present in the mucosa of the proventriculus (Plate 43.4a, facing p. 519), on the mesentery, peritoneum, heart and other tissues, while larger haemorrhages often with ulceration of the lymphoid patches may be found in the mucosa of the gizzard and along the length of the intestinal tract. The spleen may be grossly enlarged and the kidneys and other organs cóngested. In the laying hen there is often an accumulation of fresh, watery yolk in the ovules together with congestion of the blood vessels of the ovary.

Pathogenesis

Under natural conditions the virus enters the host by way of the respiratory tract or conjunctiva and less frequently via the digestive tract. Soon after the virus has become attached to the surface epithelial cells, penetration occurs and the virus undergoes a complete cycle of replication within 24 hours. This is followed by release of newly-formed virus, a consequent viraemia and secondary multiplication at the predilection sites in the body. Virus titres reach their peak within about 3 days and multiplication then becomes checked, presumably by the formation of interferon followed by specific antibody. Virulent strains differ from avirulent virus in that they are more destructive to the epithelial cells, are released quicker and pass the blood-brain barrier at an accelerated rate. Most Newcastle disease strains of virus are neurotropic but some are either viscerotropic, pneumotropic or occasionally enterotropic. Tropism can be modified experimentally according to the route of inoculation.

Ecology

The infection may be spread to healthy birds by direct contact or indirectly by inhalation of dust from litter, foodstuffs, drinking troughs and utensils contaminated with respiratory exudates and infected faeces. The alimentary tract is not a common portal of entry of the virus. There is little doubt that the principal methods of spread are associated with traffic in live birds and the movements of dealers or slaughterers on to clean premises from farms where the disease is undetected or in the very early stages of development. The virus can also be spread as a result of inadequate disinfection of diseased premises, unsuitable disposal of swill, offal or contaminated carcases on the farm, or by means of carcases imported from abroad.

There is little reliable evidence that infected eggs play an important role in the spread of infection. Although as many as 30 per cent of eggs laid by a flock during the early stages of the disease may harbour the virus, the embryos invariably die and the only risk of infection arises from breakage of infected eggs and contamination of the incubator.

Mild forms of the disease tend to persist and, consequently, virus is excreted for long periods, greatly facilitating the spread of infection particularly in large flocks confined to poultry houses. Spontaneous infections have been reported among pheasants, gannets and other free-living species and it is probable that wild birds acting as mechanical carriers were the sources of these infections.

Diagnosis

A diagnosis of acute Newcastle disease can generally be made on the basis of the history, clinical symptoms and post-mortem findings. Milder forms are more difficult to diagnose and may be confused, in the absence of nervous symptoms, with other respiratory disorders, especially in flocks where mixed respiratory infections are present.

A confirmatory diagnosis may be obtained in the laboratory by means of the haemagglutination-inhibition test which detects specific antibodies in the sera of recovered birds. (Chapt. 42, pp. 496–498.) Further confirmation can be obtained by isolating the virus from diseased tissues. In the early stages of the acute disease, the virus can be readily isolated from blood, spleen, brain, lungs, trachea or other tissues by the allantoic inoculation of 10–12 days old fertile hens' eggs. The eggs, which are candled daily, are tested for the presence of haemagglutinins by adding one drop of allantoic fluid to a one per cent suspension of fresh fowl red cells. Eggs giving a positive reaction are chilled, the allantoic fluids harvested and the virus identified by the haemagglutination-inhibition test. In less acute cases, or for the purpose of screening a flock, specific antibody to Newcastle disease can be readily detected in convalescent fowl sera by haemagglutination-inhibition. In some instances it may be advisable to run serum neutralization tests while, in vaccinated flocks, it may be necessary to demonstrate a rising antibody titre in paired sera before confirming the diagnosis.

Strain differences in Newcastle disease virus

Virulence is the ability to cause disease or death in the host, and the virulence of a virus may vary from nil to 100 per cent mortality rate. In Newcastle disease the virulence of the virus ranges widely from that of the Herts 33 and Mukteswar strains which cause a velogenic or acute form of the disease, to that of the B1 and F strains which are responsible for the lentogenic or mild form of the disease. In recent years, even 'milder' strains such as the Australian 'Queensland V4' and McFerran's 'Ulster virus' have been isolated from symptomless carrier birds.

Virulence may be assessed according to the ability of the virus and the speed with which it kills chick embryos. The three techniques commonly used to determine whether a virus is a velogenic, mesogenic or lentogenic strain are:

(1) the 'Mean Death Time' of infected 10-day-old embryonated eggs,

(2) intracerebral pathogenicity index in day-old chicks, and

(3) the intravenous pathogenicity index in 6-week-old chicks.

To study strain differences in relation to virulence, particular attention must be given to the morphology and chemistry of the virion, the action of the virus upon different species of erythrocytes, and differences in the speed of growth and sites of multiplication within the cell.

Immunogenicity of strains

The capacity of a strain of virus to bring about immunity to disease, irrespective of the actual serological changes, depends on the amount of virus used, the route of application and the virulence of the strain. Thus Newcastle disease infections induced by virulent strains are more immunogenic among survivors than those caused by less virulent strains; and serum haemagglutination-inhibiting titres are initially higher and last longer. However, immunity is not directly related to the presence of circulating antibodies and birds which no longer possess detectable amounts of haemagglutination-inhibiting or neutralizing antibodies may, nevertheless, be able to withstand exposure to virulent virus. All strains of Newcastle disease virus are closely related on the basis of serological reactions and it is seldom necessary to select a vaccine according to the antigenic type of field virus occurring in any one locality.

Control

The various measures that may be adopted to control Newcastle disease are largely based on policies of slaughter, vaccination or both.

Slaughter

In countries such as Australia, which is geographically isolated and where Newcastle disease is virtually unknown, the slaughter policy has proved completely effective. In other regions, however, where the disease is prevalent in neighbouring countries or in areas where the mild sub-clinical forms exist, the difficulties of complete eradication by slaughter are considerably increased.

In Scotland, where the incidence of Newcastle disease has always been low, a slaughter policy associated with a ban on importation of live birds from England has been markedly successful in controlling the disease, and only isolated outbreaks have been reported from time to time.

England and Wales have been less fortunate and, due to a rapid deterioration of the situation in the late 1950s, it became necessary in 1963 to alter the policy of slaughter with compensation to one of control by the voluntary use of inactivated vaccines. More recently, live attenuated vaccines (La Sota and Hitchner B1) are also being used.

Vaccination

Most countries in which Newcastle disease occurs have adopted a vaccination policy as being the most practical method of control. Different countries have developed various types of living and inactivated vaccines, depending upon local requirements.

An inactivated vaccine has the advantage that the virus is inactivated without destroying its antigenicity, and it is no longer capable of initiating infection or spreading the disease. In addition, the inactivating agents, including ultraviolet irradiation, formalin, chloroform or β-propiolactone, are probably equally capable of inactivating other viruses pathogenic for poultry which may be present in the eggs used to produce the vaccine. Since inactivated vaccines do not usually produce severe reactions they are suitable for use in chickens, young laying stock or birds in poor health. The inactivated virus is administered subcutaneously or intramuscularly and does not multiply in the tissues of vaccinated birds and the immune response is, therefore, less effective than that produced by live virus vaccines. Following vaccination with inactivated virus, the duration of immunity seldom exceeds 6 months. To prolong the immune effect inactivated vaccines usually have an adjuvant base of aluminium hydroxide, or may be used in the form of a mineral or vegetable oil emulsion. A standard programme of vaccination which gives maximum protection and often coincides with the transference of birds to other quarters is as follows: first vaccination 21 days of age, second vaccination 8–10 weeks of age, and third vaccination 16–20 weeks of age (point of lay). Whenever possible, breeding stock should be vaccinated every 5 months.

Although fully virulent strains of virus can safely be used to produce inactivated vaccines, live Newcastle disease vaccines can be prepared only from living attenuated virus. Suitable vaccine viruses include:

(1) *Live lentogenic vaccines.* These include naturally occurring strains of low virulence e.g. Asplin F, Hitchner B1 and La Sota, which are generally harmless although some, including La Sota virus, may cause mild respiratory symptoms and other reactions. In most instances, live lentogenic vaccines are effective for day-old chicks and very young birds. The optimum dose is between $10^{6.5}$ and $10^{7.0}$ EID_{50} per bird.

(2) *Live mesogenic vaccines.* The best known strains are Roakin, Komorov, Hertfordshire (Herts 33) and Mukteswar. The optimum dose is approximately $10^{5.0}$ EID_{50} per bird, administered by the parenteral route. Although mesogenic vaccines provide a long-lasting immunity they are not recommended for the immunization of chickens under 8 weeks of age, nor for adult birds not previously immunized. Roakin strain was isolated in the U.S.A. as a naturally occurring mesogenic strain whereas Komorov vaccine was developed by serial intracerebral passage of virulent virus through

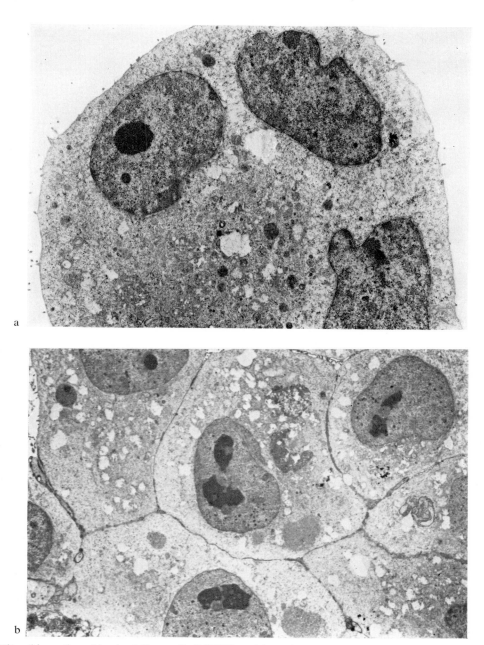

43.5a Ultra-thin section of bovine kidney cells (MDBK strain) persistently infected with Newcastle disease virus. The syncytium (polykaryon) is formed by the fusion of three chronically infected cells, × 9600.

43.5b Five-day-old culture of MDBK cells persistently infected with Newcastle disease virus, showing several intracytoplasmic inclusions composed of a closely woven mesh of fine fibrillar tubules, × 3700. (See also Plates 43.6 & 43.7.)

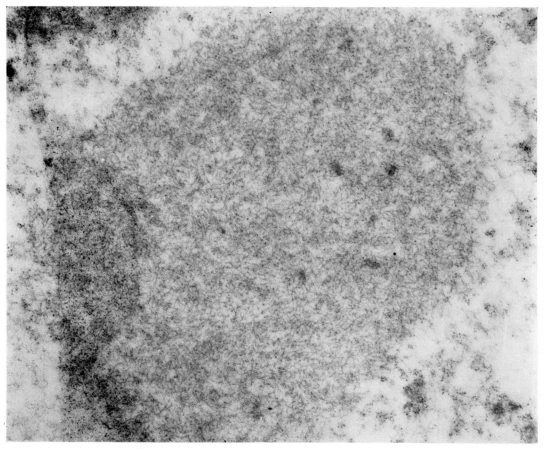

43.6 The same as 43.5b. Detail of an intracytoplasmic inclusion showing the mesh of fine fibrillar tubules, × 37 250.

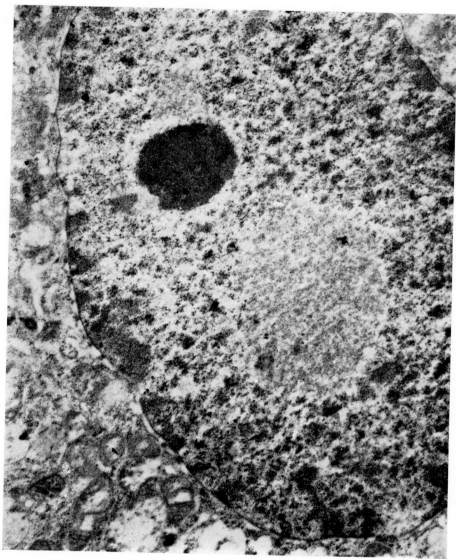

43.7 The same as 43.5b The nucleus, with dark nucleolus, and pale intranuclear inclusion. Notice the amorphous appearance of this inclusion compared with that in the cytoplasm in Plate 43.6, ×21 750.

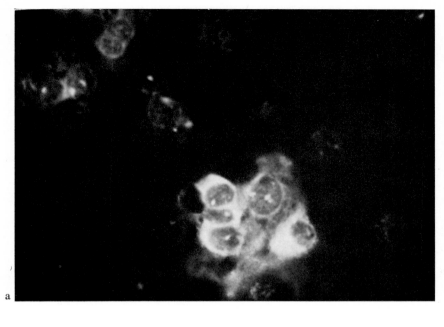

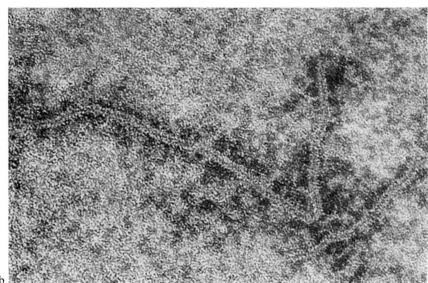

43.8a Impression smear of lung tissue from dog dying with broncho-pneumonic distemper, showing diffuse cytoplasmic fluorescence in a small cluster of infected cells. Direct stain; FITC conjugate.

43.8b Smear of tonsil from puppy with acute distemper, stained with potassium phosphotungstate. The electron micrograph shows a portion of the helical nucleocapsid released from a disrupted distemper virus particle, × 120 000.

ducklings. The Herts 33 strain and the Mukteswar strain (which is the most virulent of the mesogenic vaccine strains) were adapted from virulent viruses by serial passage in chick embryos. All live mesogenic vaccine strains are used for boosting immunity.

The great majority of live virus vaccines are prepared in fertile hens' eggs and are stored by freeze drying. Several methods of administration are in current use. The lentogenic strains (e.g. Hitchner B1) are usually given by instilling a drop of the vaccine into either the nostril (intranasal) or eye (intraocular), or they may be given as an aerosol or by adding vaccine to the drinking water; followed by the more immunogenic La Sota vaccine. It should be noted that the La Sota virus is more potent than most other lentogenic strains and may sometimes cause a severe reaction in young susceptible chickens. For this reason, it should not be given to birds under 28 days of age except in special circumstances. In areas where the virulence of the field virus requires the establishment of a higher and more consistent antibody response, a lentogenic vaccine may be used as the initial dose followed by a mesogenic vaccine for revaccination. The mesogenic strains, on the other hand, are generally given intramuscularly or by the wing-web method of inoculation (intradermal). The use of live virus vaccines produces a mild form of the disease and consequently affords a greater degree of protection than with inactivated vaccines. However, there is the risk that the virus may revert to a more virulent form, that latent infections carried in the eggs used to produce the vaccine may be introduced into a susceptible flock, or that birds may die as a result of severe reaction to the vaccine. The possibility of disseminating virulent virus precludes the use of live Newcastle disease vaccines in non-endemic countries.

The necessity for vaccinating large numbers of birds, and the time and expense involved in repeated vaccinations, has led to the use of combined virus vaccines. Thus, in some countries, Newcastle disease vaccines are combined with either infectious bronchitis virus vaccine or with fowl pox vaccine.

Strains of Newcastle disease virus have been adapted to mammalian tissue culture systems (e.g. monolayer cultures of ox and pig kidney cells), with the production of attenuated vaccines of reduced immunogenicity. They are also non-contagious and must, therefore, be injected into individual birds in selected groups. Lack of satisfactory Newcastle disease cell culture vaccines is particularly disappointing since they would probably be cheaper to produce and overcome the risk of spreading poultry pathogens that might be present in embryonated eggs used for the manufacture of live attenuated virus vaccines.

Immunity to Newcastle disease

In hens carrying a high level of active immunity against Newcastle disease as a result of field exposure or vaccination, the maternal antibodies are passed to the developing ovules and are absorbed from the yolk during the development of the embryo and young chick. Thus, chicks hatched from the eggs of immune hens are passively protected against infection with Newcastle disease virus. Chickens aged 5 weeks or less show a poor response to antigenic stimuli and the resultant immunity is seldom longer than 5 months and may be as short as 2 months. To overcome these difficulties, young chicks which are liable to be exposed to the risk of infection may be vaccinated with a lentogenic strain of vaccine virus at a few days of age. Poor immunity always results when chicks are vaccinated at a day old, and the longer the procedure can be postponed the better will be the immunity produced. To ensure the production of an adequate level of immunity, all chicks are revaccinated a second time with a lentogenic strain of live virus when they are under 4 weeks of age: this will confer protection for 3–5 months. Older birds may be revaccinated either with inactivated virus or with one of the more potent attenuated strains (e.g. La Sota) of vaccine at 8–10 weeks, again at 16–20 weeks, and every 5 months thereafter. In some countries where repeated vaccination is not practical, it may be necessary to use the more virulent mesogenic vaccinal strains only, e.g. Mukteswar or Komorov. The use of living vaccines not only perpetuates the presence of Newcastle disease virus but has also been considered responsible for the greater incidence of chronic respiratory disease and other respiratory disorders, through activating potential pathogens present in a flock at a time of vaccination.

It must be emphasized that if immunized birds are exposed to a field strain of virus they may become temporary carriers without showing clinical symptoms. This is of considerable practical importance since symptomless carrier birds may shed the virus and initiate an outbreak of clinical disease in a susceptible flock.

Myxovirus yucaipa

In 1960 a myxovirus was isolated from the trachea of 3-week-old chickens involved in a serious outbreak of infectious laryngotracheitis on a poultry farm in Yucaipa, California. The presence of both viruses seemed to be responsible for an unusually high rate of mortality and spread of infection.

Laboratory investigations have shown that intra-tracheal inoculation of the virus into young chickens produces a mild respiratory illness with characteristic moist rales. Young mice are not susceptible. Yucaipa virus is serologically distinct not only from influenza types A, B and C, Dinter's virus N and fowl plague virus but also from the paramyxoviruses including Newcastle disease, parainfluenza types 1, 2 and 3, and mumps viruses. Despite these differences, Yucaipa virus is classified as an avian myxovirus since it contains RNA, is readily inactivated by ether and chloroform, and haemagglutinates chicken, guinea-pig and human type 'O' red blood cells. It is cytopathic for pig kidney and HeLa cell cultures and the formation of a viral antigen is restricted to the cytoplasm. Yucaipa virus seems to be closer to the Newcastle disease type of virus in that it forms a haemolysin and is not inactivated by hydroxylamine (as is fowl plague virus), nor by trypsin or a low pH.

Parainfluenza viruses

The parainfluenza viruses form a sub-group of the paramyxoviruses and are important members of the myxovirus family. They are commonly associated with upper respiratory tract infections in man and animals and are especially important as causes of acute respiratory infections in the young.

History

The first recognised parainfluenza virus strain called Sendai, or the haemagglutinating virus of Japan (HVJ), was recovered in 1953 from mice inoculated with lung tissue of newborn children dying from pneumonitis. Since that time it has been shown that mouse colonies are sometimes infected with latent Sendai virus and, consequently, there has been some doubt as to the pathogenic role of Sendai in pneumonias of humans. Soon after this first isolation, other parainfluenza viruses were recovered from cases of human respiratory disease including one which was associated with acute laryngotracheo-bronchitis or 'viral croup', in children. This virus produced syncytia in tissue culture and was originally designated CA or croup-associated virus. Subsequently, three antigenically distinct parainfluenza viruses were isolated in tissue culture from children with respiratory illnesses and these were termed 'haemadsorption viruses' because they produced little or no cytopathic effects but haemadsorbed guinea-pig red blood cells. At the present time, the first of these 'haemadsorption viruses' (HA-1) is known as parainfluenza type 3, the second (HA-2) is included with Sendai virus in parainfluenza type 1 and the CA virus has been designated parainfluenza type 2. Parainfluenza type 4 virus was isolated in 1960 from children with mild respiratory illness.

Morphology

Parainfluenza viruses are roughly spherical in shape and their structure closely resembles that of other paramyxoviruses. The inner helical core is surrounded by a well-defined outer envelope which is rapidly disrupted following exposure to ether, chloroform or a surface-active agent such as Tween 80.

Physicochemical properties

They are relatively unstable viruses losing more than 90 per cent of their infectivity in 2–4 hours when suspended in a protein-free medium at room temperature or at 4°C; and are rapidly inactivated at pH 3 and at temperatures of 37°C and above. Their activity falls off even at temperatures below 0°C.

Haemagglutination

Most strains of parainfluenza virus haemagglutinate avian and certain species of mammalian red cells and exhibit neuraminidase activity. Maximum haemagglutination titres are obtained either with chicken erythrocytes at 4°C (types 1 and 2) or with guinea-pig red blood cells at 25 °C (types 1 and 3).

Unlike orthomyxoviruses, parainfluenza and other paramyxoviruses possess a haemolysin which is inhibited by type-specific antisera. Dialyzable substances in allantoic and cell culture fluids inhibit the haemolytic activity of the virus.

Antigenic properties

Parainfluenza viruses are antigenically distinct but all show minor cross reactions with at least one other member of the group, and with mumps virus. Four distinct serotypes, designated 1, 2, 3 and 4, have been differentiated by haemagglutination-inhibition and serum neutralization tests but only one serotype has been recognised for each of the human type 1, 2 and 3 viruses (Table 43.3).

Pathogenicity

In man, type 1 strains are the most important of the parainfluenza viruses in the croup syndrome but all three types are frequently associated with other acute respiratory illnesses of infancy and childhood. Illness produced by type 4 virus is usually mild and limited to the upper respiratory tract. Parainfluenza viruses associated with infections in lower animals include type 1 (Sendai), which has frequently been isolated from respiratory infections of mice and pigs and can also be present as a latent infection of laboratory mice; simian viruses described as contaminants of 'normal' monkey kidney cell cultures and which are classified as parainfluenza type 2; and strains belonging to parainfluenza type 3 which appear to cause 'transit fever' in cattle (SF4) and an influenza-like illness in horses (RE55).

It is emphasised that reinfections may occur with parainfluenza viruses even in the presence of specific antibodies.

Cultivation

Recently isolated strains of type 1, 3 and 4 parain-

TABLE 43.3. Antigenic types of parainfluenza viruses.

Type	Subtypes	Host
1	Haemadsorption type 2 (HA–2)	Man
	Sendai or HVJ	Mouse, pig and (?) man
2	Croup associated (CA)	Man
	Simian virus 5 (SV5)	Monkey and (?) man
	Simian virus 41 (SV41)	Monkey
		? Man
3	Haemadsorption type 1 (HA–1)	Man
	Shipping fever virus (SF4)	Cattle
	Respiratory illness of horses (RE55)	Horses
4	M–25 strain (Subtype A)	Man
	CH.19503 strain (Subtype B)	

fluenza viruses produce a minimal CPE during primary tissue culture but the presence of viral activity can easily be detected by the ability of infected cells in the monolayer to adsorb healthy guinea-pig erythrocytes. However, naturally occurring strains of type 2 virus and strains of types 1, 3 and 4, serially propagated on cell cultures, produce focal syncytial changes and numerous cytoplasmic inclusions (Plate 43.3b, between pp. 518–9). In most cell culture systems, certain strains of types 1 and 3 parainfluenza viruses may also produce multiple acidophilic intranuclear inclusions. Fluorescent antibody staining shows that parainfluenza viruses replicate chiefly in the cytoplasm but some reports suggest that parainfluenza type 1 strains may replicate in the nucleus, also.

Freshly isolated strains of most parainfluenza viruses grow only with difficulty in embryonated hens' eggs and, in this respect, they differ from paramyxoviruses such as Newcastle disease virus and the orthomyxoviruses. However, they can be adapted to growth in the amniotic cavity of 7- to 9-day-old chick embryos by frequent serial passages, but they generally require 4–6 days of incubation to reach their maximal titre. Thereafter, they can be propagated in the allantoic cavity. There are no reports that type 4 virus can be propagated in eggs.

Intranasal inoculation of parainfluenza viruses into young guinea-pigs and hamsters results in infections which yield high titres of virus in the lungs within 2–3 days; but no pulmonary lesions result.

Diagnosis

Parainfluenza virus infections can be diagnosed in the laboratory by measurement of a rise in serum antibody titres by haemagglutination-inhibition or complement-fixation tests. Identification of the causative virus can be made by isolation of the virus in primary tissue cultures derived from the most appropriate animal species. Because observable cytopathic changes may not be produced or may develop very slowly, the presence of the virus can be recognised rapidly by adsorption of guinea-pig red blood cells to infected cells of the monolayer. The type of parainfluenza virus is finally confirmed by haemadsorption-inhibition or other serological tests using standard antisera.

Parainfluenza-I

It is customary for reasons of antigenic similarity to include the Sendai virus, also known as the haemagglutinating virus of Japan (HVJ) or influenza D, and the haemadsorption virus type 2 (HA-2) in the type 1 parainfluenza virus sub-group.

General properties

Sendai virus haemagglutinates a variety of red blood cells. It also possesses an haemolysin which is active against chicken and guinea-pig red blood cells, especially at 37°C.

Despite the fact that parainfluenza viruses share common antigens, type 1 strains can be differentiated readily from those of types 2, 3 and 4 by complement-fixation, haemagglutination-inhibition, haemadsorption-inhibition or tissue culture neutralization tests, using post-infectional guinea-pig antisera. Even the human (HA-2) and murine (Sendai) strains within type 1 of parainfluenza viruses may be distinguished by the same serological methods using reciprocal and non-reciprocal cross-reactions that may vary in their magnitude. Thus, in complement-fixation tests with Sendai and HA-2 strains, Sendai antiserum will cross-react with human strain antigens whereas HA-2 antiserum may not react with Sendai antigens, or only to a lesser degree.

Sendai virus can be readily isolated and grows well in embryonated hens' eggs, with the production of haemagglutinins. It also grows satisfactorily in primary monkey kidney cell cultures, in human cell lines and in cell cultures of numerous other species, but the cytopathic effects on primary isolation are minimal and the presence of virus can only be detected by haemadsorption. The cytopathic effect that eventually appears consists of a rounding of the affected cells, without syncytia. Although parainfluenza viruses replicate chiefly in the cytoplasm there are reports from fluorescent antibody studies that Sendai and HA-2 viruses may also replicate in the nucleus.

Sendai virus, which may be latent in mice, can be activated to produce fatal pneumonia after mouse-to-mouse passage. Older mice are generally not susceptible to Sendai infections but young and unweaned mice are readily infected by the intranasal instillation of virus or by direct contact with one another. Intracerebral inoculation also causes high mortality but the HA-2 virus is less pathogenic and produces only symptomless infections. Mice dying from Sendai virus inoculated intranasally show partial or, sometimes, complete consolidation of one or more lobes of the lungs; and the macroscopic lesions are similar to those produced by influenza virus. Outbreaks of Sendai virus infection in mouse colonies may persist for several months during which Sendai specific antibodies can be demonstrated and virus can be isolated from both diseased and clinically healthy mice.

The haemadsorption type 2 virus may be one of the main agents producing acute laryngotracheitis in children but it is also frequently associated with pharyngitis, bronchitis, pneumonia and non-specific upper respiratory illness in infants as well as respiratory symptoms in adults like those of the common cold.

In man, formolised egg-adapted virus and an inactivated vaccine produced in primary monkey kidney cell cultures can evoke the formation of specific antibodies and are being used experimentally. It is interesting to note that parainfluenza type 1 has been recently isolated, by cell-fusion techniques, from the brain cells of human patients affected with multiple sclerosis, and that densely packed virus-like tubules have been seen in electron micrographs of tiny early lesions in brain tissues from victims of the disease.

Parainfluenza-2
Parainfluenza virus type 2, formerly known as croup-associated (CA) virus or the acute laryngotracheobronchitis virus of children, is a human pathogen and was first isolated in 1955 in tissue cultures from cases of croup. It is widespread in its distribution but, despite its name, is not as frequent a cause of croup as parainfluenza virus type 1.

General properties
Haemagglutination occurs with red cells from chickens and guinea-pigs but to a lesser degree with human group 'O' cells. The optimum pH for haemagglutination is pH8 and higher titres are obtained with chicken than with guinea-pig red cells at 4°C. Elution of the virus occurs when the cells are warmed to 37°C but the cells re-agglutinate when cooled to 4°C.

The virus is closely related to two simian viruses (SV-5 and SV-41) and to mumps virus, but is unrelated to all other myxoviruses. Serological studies with strains of parainfluenza virus type 2 may exhibit a non-reciprocal relationship; thus, SV-5 antisera may fix complement in the presence of CA virus but not *vice versa*.

Naturally occurring type 2 virus grows well in embryonated hens' eggs. Despite this, the levels of haemagglutinins produced are generally low or even undetectable. They also grow well in cell cultures of various species including man, monkey and dog kidney, and generally produce a recognizable cytopathic effect after 3–4 days of incubation, consisting of intracytoplasmic inclusions and syncytial formation. Infected cells haemadsorb guinea-pig red blood cells but the effect may not occur in monolayers tested during the first 7–10 days of incubation. Plaque assay methods have been developed for type 2 viruses in rhesus monkey kidney cell cultures.

The majority of type 2 strains can infect guinea-pigs and hamsters by the intranasal route of inoculation and inapparent infections can be induced in these, as well as in some other laboratory animals, as shown by the presence of antibodies in their sera. The type 2 simian viruses occur spontaneously in cell cultures prepared from apparently healthy rhesus monkeys, and there are reports of as many as 30 per cent of some culture batches being positive. Neither the simian (SV-5 and SV-41) nor the human CA strains of type 2 virus cause ill effects in adult or unweaned mice.

Promising results have been claimed from preliminary trials of an inactivated CA virus vaccine produced in monkey kidney cell cultures.

Parainfluenza-3

Synonym
Haemadsorption virus 1 (HA-1); bovine SF4 virus; respiratory equine RE55 virus.

Definition and hosts affected
Parainfluenza type 3 viruses are frequently associated with infections of the upper respiratory tract of man, cattle, sheep, horses and occasionally pigs.

History and distribution
The virus was first recovered in cell culture from children with acute respiratory disease in the late 1950s. During initial passage it produced little or

no cytopathic effect but was readily recognised by the phenomenon of haemadsorption when guinea-pig red blood cells were added to infected monolayer cultures. For this reason it was originally designated type 1 haemadsorption virus.

In 1959, the virus was isolated in America from the nasal mucosa of calves showing clinical signs of 'shipping fever' and, a year or two later, a similar parainfluenza virus was isolated in Canada from young horses with acute upper respiratory disease. Since then, strains of parainfluenza virus have been isolated from cattle in many parts of the world including Switzerland, Yugoslavia, the United Kingdom, Sweden and Japan.

Morphology
The virus particle contains RNA and its structure is very similar to that of all other members of the paramyxovirus group. Bovine strains have an average diameter of between 100 and 300 nm and the internal helical component has a diameter of 17 nm.

Physicochemical properties
The parainfluenza viruses are more heat-labile than orthomyxoviruses and other paramyxoviruses, and lose infectivity rapidly after only a few days at room temperature. They are inactivated in 30 minutes at 55°C but survive well at –25°C. Serum proteins added to the suspending medium as stabilizer, slow down the rate of inactivation.

Haemagglutination
Human Group 'O', guinea-pig and some fowl red blood cells are agglutinated by all strains of parainfluenza type 3 virus and maximum titres are obtained with guinea-pig cells when the test is read at 25°C. Haemagglutination occurs more readily with recently isolated strains of bovine origin than with human strains. Equine strains agglutinate human and guinea-pig cells but are less active on fowl red cells. A report that bovine strains of parainfluenza type 3 lack neuraminidase awaits confirmation and there is no clear evidence that bovine sera contain non-specific inhibitors of haemagglutination. Type 3 and type 1 strains of parainfluenza virus produce an haemolysin which lyses chicken or guinea-pig cells, is inhibited by type-specific antisera, and is most active at 37°C. In general, the haemadsorption test is more sensitive than haemagglutination for the early detection of a newly isolated virus in cell cultures, as it is for most other types of parainfluenza viruses. Bovine strains can be divided into two or three subtypes on the basis of haemagglutinating activity for certain species of red cell, and on heat sensitivity.

Antigenic properties
All serotypes of parainfluenza viruses coss-react with one another and with some other paramyxoviruses, but they do not share common antigens with orthomyxoviruses. Despite this antigenic overlap, type 3 strains of human origin can be distinguished from animal strains by haemadsorption-inhibition, haemagglutination-inhibition, complement-fixation and neutralization tests.

Cultivation
Unlike naturally occurring strains of parainfluenza type 3, cell culture adapted strains grow well in the amniotic sac of developing hens' eggs with the formation of haemagglutinins in the egg fluid. They do not grow in the allantoic sac and, in this respect, differ from other types of parainfluenza. Type 3 strains rarely produce obvious cytopathic effects or haemagglutinins in primary cell cultures but virus activity is readily detected in monkey kidney cultures by the haemadsorption technique, and subsequent serial passages give rise to cytopathic change. Multinucleated giant-cells or syncytia are produced on continuous epithelium-like cell lines of human origin. Bovine strains grow well in calf, goat, buffalo, camel, horse and pig kidney cultures as well as on HeLa and HEp2 cells with the formation of large syncytia, acidophilic intracytoplasmic inclusions of varied size and shape, and small regular, spherical-shaped single or multiple intranuclear inclusions (Plate 43.3b, between pp. 518–9). Human strains of parainfluenza 3 do not produce intranuclear inclusions in HEp2 cells. Each intracytoplasmic or intranuclear inclusion is invariably surrounded by a clear zone or halo.

Recently isolated equine strains grow with difficulty in the amniotic fluids of fertile hens' eggs. In monkey kidney cell culture there is no cytopathic effect on the first passage but haemadsorption can be described on the tenth day of incubation. On the subsequent passages the equine strains grow well and produce a marked cytopathic effect with the formation of acidophilic intracytoplasmic inclusions. They also grow in cultures of human amnion, in primary dog, pig and bovine kidney cells, and in continuous cell lines of HeLa and dog kidney cells.

A Swedish report has shown that mixed infections of mucosal disease virus and parainfluenza type 3 virus give rise to severe upper respiratory tract infections of cattle. It has also been shown that parainfluenza type 3 virus infection of tissue cultures enhances the growth of Newcastle disease virus in mixed culture but it is not known whether the synergistic effect of the type 3 virus acts as an enhancing mechanism for other virus infections of domestic animals.

Pathogenicity
Parainfluenza type 3 virus is a common cause of

respiratory tract disease especially in very young children. It is uncommon as a cause of natural respiratory infection in adults although it may give rise to a syndrome resembling the common cold. An outbreak of pneumonia in captive monkeys has been described with a 50 per cent mortality.

Strains of parainfluenza type 3 virus have frequently been recovered from cattle affected with 'shipping fever' or 'transit fever', and serological studies suggest that bovine infections are common in various parts of the world. The incidence of parainfluenza type 3 antibodies in cattle sera in Japan, U.S.A., Yugoslavia and the United Kingdom has been given as 26 per cent, 48 per cent, 77 per cent, and 84 per cent, respectively. It has been shown that in cases of 'shipping fever' the parainfluenza type 3 virus, which may be present in clinically healthy cattle, can assume a pathogenic role in the presence of unrelated viruses or other micro-organisms, in animals that are under stress.

In Umea disease of cattle, named after the township of Umea, U.S.A., parainfluenza-type viruses are thought to be responsible for serious losses in cows during late pregnancy or soon after calving, especially during the winter months of the year. The serological characters of the virus are those of the haemadsorption virus-1 of parainfluenza type 3 and recent work has suggested that it is probably antigenically identical with the parainfluenza strain designated 'bovine SF4'

Parainfluenza 3 virus has been isolated from epidemics of respiratory disease of horses in Canada, and specific antibodies develop in convalescing animals. In some eastern states of the U.S.A., about 20 per cent of horses are said to have antibodies to parainfluenza 3 in their sera.

The isolation of parainfluenza type 3 virus alone or together with *Pasteurella* species has been reported in the U.S.A. and the United Kingdom among lambs and sheep affected with pneumonia. The virus is probably widespread among sheep populations in both these countries.

Parainfluenza 3 virus has also been recovered from bulls' semen and from the genital tracts of cows, and may cause infertility.

Bovine strains of type 3 virus inoculated into experimental calves and cattle may give rise to fever, conjunctivitis, mucopurulent rhinitis and vulvovaginitis, depending on the route of inoculation. On post-mortem examination, there may be large areas of congestion and consolidation of the ventral lobes of the lungs. Microscopical examination shows inflammatory changes in the larger bronchioles and alveoli with fusion of the epithelial cells giving rise to syncytial formation. Both intracytoplasmic and intranuclear inclusions are present.

Parainfluenza type 3 viruses are non-pathogenic to most species of laboratory animal and intranasal inoculation of guinea-pigs and hamsters produces an infection without inducing overt disease.

Diagnosis
The aetiology of respiratory diseases associated with parainfluenza type 3 virus is complex, and virus inoculated into susceptible calves is rarely capable of producing the severe type of clinical syndrome seen in field outbreaks. Significant rising antibody titres to the virus can be detected by appropriate serological techniques, particularly the complement-fixation and haemagglutination-inhibition tests. Most strains from animal sources may be detected by their cytopathogenicity in various cell culture systems, whilst the presence of non-cytocidal strains are readily demonstrable by haemadsorption. Virus isolates can be identified by virus neutralization and haemadsorption-inhibition tests using specific antisera. In human infections the results of serological tests are often difficult to interpret since parainfluenza viruses share antigens with mumps and some other myxoviruses.

Control
Inactivated and living attenuated virus vaccines have been used in calves but opinion is divided on their usefulness. Formolised vaccines combined with an adjuvant can protect calves against infection and give rise to significant antibody titres. Similar vaccines have been used successfully in humans. In Germany, promising results have been obtained by means of several live virus vaccines where the virus has been attenuated by frequent passages in calf kidney cell cultures.

Parainfluenza-4
Parainfluenza virus type 4 has been isolated from young children with minor respiratory illness but its relation to human disease has not yet been established. Although types 1, 2 and 3 are widely distributed in nature, parainfluenza type 4 strains are almost entirely confined to the U.S.A.

Parainfluenza 4 virus agglutinates guinea-pig red blood cells at 4°C, at room temperature, but not at 37°C. Agglutination also occurs markedly with rhesus monkey red cells, poorly with human Group 'O' cells, but not with chicken erythrocytes. The virus is very labile, even at room temperature. There is some evidence of cross reactions between parainfluenza 4 virus and mumps, and recent studies indicate the existence of two separate subtypes (A and B) within the type 4 serotype. The M-25 strain has now been designated as the parainfluenza type 4 prototype.

It is difficult to propagate the virus on embryonated hens' eggs and although little or no growth occurs in HeLa and other cell lines, high virus titres are obtained with a minimal cytopathic effect following passage of the virus in monkey kidney cells. Haemagglutinins are barely detectable in infected cell cultures, but haemadsorption of guinea-pig red blood cells occurs readily.

Parainfluenza 4 virus is non-pathogenic for laboratory animals.

Other parainfluenza viruses

Parainfluenza viruses are frequently present in kidney cell cultures prepared from healthy rhesus and cynomolgus monkeys. Two strains, designated SV-5 and SV-41, which are immunologically dissimilar, have tentatively been classified as simian strains of parainfluenza type 2 because of their close antigenic relationship to the CA virus.

The simian SV-5 virus is very similar, if not identical, to two parainfluenza viruses (DA virus and SA virus) which were believed to be associated with illness in man. The DA virus was obtained from cell cultures of human kidneys inoculated with material from human patients, some of whom had hepatitis. The SA virus was isolated from the brains of hamsters dying from encephalitis following the inoculation of allantoic fluids of eggs previously infected with nasal washings of patients with acute respiratory disease. There is little doubt that the DA and SA strains are identical and that they are closely related to SV-5 virus, but a suggestion that all three be included in a fifth subtype of the parainfluenza group is not acceptable to most workers.

These three parainfluenza strains can be propagated in the amniotic and allantoic cavities of embryonated hens' eggs and will grow well in monkey and bovine kidney cell cultures but not in cultures derived from dog, cat, rat and pig cells. They haemagglutinate chicken erythrocytes at 0 °C, haemadsorb guinea-pig red blood cells and are ether sensitive.

An atypical parainfluenza virus (WB strain) has also been isolated from human sources and is sometimes referred to as parainfluenza type 6; but there seems to be little justification for this classification.

The simian paramyxovirus, SV-41, which was originally isolated from kidney cell cultures of cynomolgus monkeys, cross-reacts with SV-5 and with the CA virus in complement-fixation tests, but not in either haemagglutination-inhibition or haemadsorption-inhibition tests. Although it is sometimes called parainfluenza type 7 virus, most workers believe that presently it should be described as a simian strain of parainfluenza type 2.

PSEUDOMYXOVIRUSES

The Measles — Canine Distemper — Rinderpest Triad

Similarities between the clinical and histopathological features of measles and distemper have been recognised for many years and, in 1954, it was first suggested that a close relationship might exist between the causative viruses of these two diseases. In 1957 it was reported that the presence in human sera of neutralizing antibodies to canine distemper virus was correlated with a history of measles infection, and it was later shown that in measles patients the rise in neutralizing antibodies to measles virus was associated with an increase in titre of neutralizing antibodies for distemper virus. It was also found that measles virus could produce immunity to distemper in ferrets, and that dogs which had recovered from distemper possessed antibodies to measles. Also in 1957, Polding and Simpson in Kenya suggested that an antigenic relationship might exist between the viruses of distemper and rinderpest because dogs fed on rinderpest-infected meat were not affected by canine distemper during a local epidemic of the disease. Since then, there have been a number of reports confirming that rinderpest has some immunizing power against distemper in dogs and that anti-rinderpest sera contain neutralizing antibodies against canine distemper. By implication, a similar antigenic relationship was postulated between measles and rinderpest. This was confirmed by the fact that children with measles developed rinderpest neutralizing antibodies in their sera and, conversely, that cattle infected with rinderpest virus developed measles neutralizing antibodies. Additional evidence of the close but incomplete antigenic relationships between measles, distemper and rinderpest viruses was obtained by means of the gel diffusion precipitation method.

The close relationship between measles, distemper and rinderpest viruses to the myxoviruses is also evident in electron micrographs which show that their general morphology and ultrastructure are very similar to those of Newcastle disease and other paramyxoviruses. All three are RNA viruses showing helical symmetry and measuring between 90–250 nm. The central core of the virion contains helices about 15–18 nm in diameter, with subunits having a 4·5 nm periodicity, and the capsid is surrounded by an outer membrane or envelope which contains numerous radially dispersed projections or spikes. The similarities extend to their kinetic and cytopathogenic properties in cell cultures since they all form multinucleated syncytia containing acidophilic intracytoplasmic and, sometimes, intranuclear inclusions (Plates 43.10a, b, c, facing page 535). They also react in a similar manner to heat, and all three are ether sensitive.

Measles

Definition
Measles or rubeola was first recognised as a clinical entity in the 10th century A.D., and is worldwide in distribution. It is a highly contagious but mainly mild disease of childhood unless complicated by respiratory infections or encephalitis when it becomes severe and even fatal.

Properties of the virus
The morphological, physical and chemical properties of measles virus are very similar to those of the paramyxoviruses. However, in contrast to distemper and rinderpest viruses, it haemagglutinates baboon and rhesus monkey red blood cells but lacks neuraminidase and does not elute spontaneously from agglutinated erythrocytes. Measles virus haemagglutinins consist of five morphological entities each of which can agglutinate susceptible red blood cells, These are the intact fully infectious virus, the partially disrupted non-infectious virus, two smaller portions that are probably empty envelopes without a central core and, finally, small 'rosette' particles of protein that are released when the virion is disrupted with ether and Tween 80. Measles virus usually shows haemadsorption and haemolysis of red blood cells.

Antigenic properties
Strains of measles virus are probably antigenically homogeneous and are closely related, but not identical, to the viruses of distemper and rinderpest. In general, hyperimmune sera to measles, distemper and rinderpest viruses all neutralize heterologous virus to some extent although low titres are usually obtained with distemper antiserum against measles virus. There is recent evidence that the close antigenic relationship between the three viruses is more clearly demonstrated by cross-fluorescent antibody staining than by virus neutralization or complement-fixation tests.

Cultivation
In 1954, measles virus was first regularly cultivated in cell cultures of human and monkey tissues. Human amnion is particularly useful but cell cultures derived from cattle, dogs, ferrets, hamsters, mice or guinea-pigs can also be employed. The cytopathic changes are similar to those produced by distemper and rinderpest viruses, and include the formation of multinucleate syncytial giant cells with intranuclear inclusions and large plaques of acidophilic material in the cytoplasm of infected cells. Recently isolated strains of virus may take about 14 days to produce the typical cytopathic effect but this is shortened to 4–6 days after adaptation. Measles virus has been adapted to growth in developing hens' eggs with the formation of necrotic lesions on the chorioallantoic membrane similar to those produced by egg-adapted strains of dog distemper virus.

Pathogenicity
Measles is usually characterized by two peaks of fever, the second coinciding with the onset of catarrhal symptoms which are quickly followed by a rash on the temples; and affects not only the skin and brain but also the mucous membranes of the respiratory and alimentary tracts. Encephalomyelitis occurs in about 1:1000 cases due to direct invasion of the central nervous system by the measles virus, and in these cases the mortality rate may approach 30 per cent. Encephalitis may also appear many years after recovery from the primary infection and brain sections show inclusion bodies and helical structures resembling those of the measles virion. Immunofluorescence studies in cases of sub-acute sclerosing panencephalitis (SSPE) have confirmed that the inclusions in the neurons and glial cells contain measles antigen and defective strains of measles virus have been released from persistently infected brain cells by cell fusion methods. There is recent evidence also that measles virus-specific immunoglobulins are present in sera and cerebro-spinal fluid (CSF) from cases of multiple sclerosis.

Immunity and control
An attack of measles usually confers a solid, life-long immunity. Second attacks can occur but are very rare. A striking feature of measles epidemics in the United Kingdom is their recurrence every two years, mostly in the late winter or early spring.

A number of vaccines are now employed to control the disease. Inactivated vaccines are prepared from virus grown in dog, monkey or chick embryo cell cultures, with or without a mineral adjuvant, or by the separation of the haemagglutinin fraction by density gradient centrifugation. However, living vaccines are more effective and are prepared in chick embryo or dog kidney cell cultures from the egg-adapted Edmonston strain or one of its derivatives. High levels of antibody are produced which last a lifetime.

Canine Distemper

Synonyms
Maladie de Carré; Hundestaupe; Hard-pad.

Definition
Canine distemper is an acute, highly contagious virus disease which probably causes more deaths in young susceptible dogs than any other infection.

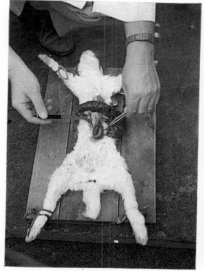

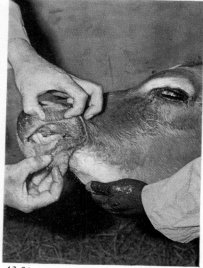

43.9a   43.9 b

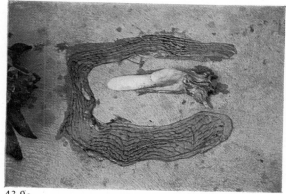

43.9c

43.9a   Response of a rabbit to intravenous inoculation with a lapinised strain of rinderpest virus. Macroscopic lesions are generally seen in the sacculus rotundus, tonsilla caecalis major, appendix and Peyer's patches.

43.9b   Bullock infected experimentally with rinderpest virus. Examination of the mouth on the third day of infection for congestion of the mucous membranes. Oral lesions in the early mucosal phase take the form of small raised greyish pin-head foci with necrotic centres. Lachrymal discharges may also develop.

43.9c   In fatal cases of bovine rinderpest, involvement of the crests of folds of mucous membranes lining the lower colon may result in longitudinal streaks of inflammation and haemorrhage which darken rapidly, following death of the animal.

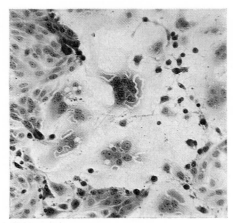

43.10a

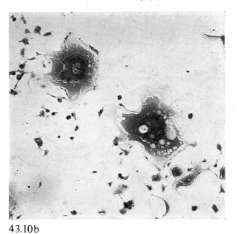

43.10b

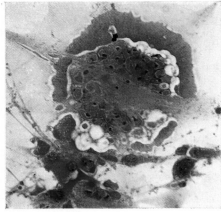

43.10c

43.10a Primary culture of bovine kidney cells 7 days
after inoculation with rinderpest virus. There are small
syncytia with acidophilic intracytoplasmic inclusions.
Haematoxylin eosin stain, × 106.

43.10b The same culture as shown in Plate 43.10a, 11 days
after inoculation. The formation of large multinucleate
syncytia is accompanied by marked cellular degeneration
throughout the monolayer. Haematoxylin eosin stain,
× 80.

43.10c Secondary culture of puppy kidney cells 12
days after inoculation with canine distemper virus. The
multinucleate syncytium shows a large plaque of acidophilic inclusion material surrounding the aggregated
nuclei. Most of the nuclei contain a single acidophilic
inclusion body. Haematoxylin eosin stain, × 280.

Hosts affected

Distemper occurs naturally in all members of the family *Canidae* (e.g. dogs, dingoes, foxes, coyotes and wolves) and the family *Mustelidae* (e.g. mink, ferrets, weasels and skunks) but hyenas (family *Hyenidae*), bears (family *Ursidae*) and members of the family *Felidae* (e.g. cats, lions and tigers) are not susceptible. There are several reports that raccoons (family *Procyonidae*) develop distemper when they assemble in large numbers.

History and distribution

Distemper has been recognised throughout the world for centuries and is still one of the most important infectious diseases of dogs. In Europe the disease appeared in the second half of the eighteenth century and is said to have been introduced from Asia or South America. The filterability of the causative agent of distemper was clearly demonstrated in 1905 by Carré but his findings were not generally accepted until 1926 when Laidlaw and Dunkin unequivocally confirmed the viral aetiology of the disease.

Classification

The causative virus is a member of the measles-distemper-rinderpest group which is closely related to the paramyxoviruses.

Morphology

The virus particle contains RNA and is slightly smaller (90–250 nm) than the typical paramyxovirus virion. Its ultrastructure is very similar to that of other myxoviruses and its central core contains helices that are about 15–17 nm in diameter (Plate 43.8b, facing p. 527). The capsid is enclosed by an envelope which contains an outer fringe of short radiating spikes or projections (peplomers).

Chemical composition

The virus particle consists of a core of single-stranded RNA and is enclosed within an outer lipoprotein envelope which is susceptible to treatment with ether.

Physicochemical characters

Thermal inactivation of the distemper virus is rapid. It survives at 55°C for 30 minutes but not for 1 hour, and is inactivated by heating at 60°C for 30 minutes. Storage at any temperature above 0°C results in the rapid destruction of infectivity but the virus will survive for months at −10°C and indefinitely at −70°C or when lyophilised. It is ether-sensitive and is inactivated in a few hours by 0·1 per cent formalin or 1·0 per cent lysol. The optimum pH for stability is about 7·0.

Haemagglutination

Haemagglutination by distemper virus is uncertain but high concentrations of egg-adapted virus may give an irregular, partial haemagglutination of chicken and guinea-pig red blood cells. There are also unconfirmed reports of agglutination of human and frog erythrocytes.

Antigenic properties

Complement-fixation tests indicated that the Laidlaw and Dunkin dog distemper virus, the Wellcome hard-pad virus, Green's distemperoid virus and some other isolates share a common soluble antigen and are, therefore, antigenically indistinguishable. Although A, B and C-type strains have been described, cross-protection tests convincingly show that there is but a single antigenic type, as is the case with measles and rinderpest viruses.

Specific distemper precipitinogens can be demonstrated within 6–8 hours on agar gel by diffusing infected tissues against anti-distemper, anti-measles or anti-rinderpest hyperimmune serum. Thus, there is a close antigenic relationship between all three viruses. Further examples of this close relationship between measles, distemper and rinderpest viruses are as follows:-

(1) rinderpest virus will give some immunity in dogs against distemper;

(2) sera of rinderpest-immune cattle contain neutralizing antibody against measles;

(3) dogs recovered from distemper show antibodies to measles, and people with a history of measles may have distemper neutralizing antibodies in their sera; and

(4) dogs and ferrets inoculated with measles virus may be immune to distemper.

There is some evidence that the antigenic relationship is less complete with egg-adapted viruses.

Interference

Resistance following parenteral vaccination with attenuated live distemper vaccines may be the result of interference by the attenuated (vaccinal) virus against the field virus. There is no interference with the virus of infectious canine hepatitis, and dual infections with canine distemper may occur. Immunofluorescence studies of infected monolayers have clearly shown the distribution of specific viral antigens of hepatitis and distemper within the nucleus and cytoplasm, respectively, of a single infected cell.

Cultivation

Clinical distemper can be experimentally induced in ferrets, dogs and mink by various routes of inoculation and it is possible to adapt the virus to grow in unweaned mice, baby hamsters and rabbits. In 1939, Green discovered that successive passages of distemper virus in ferrets increased the virulence of the virus for ferrets but reduced it for dogs. This observation led to the development of modified live-virus vaccines for distemper immunization. Green's distemperoid virus was adapted by Haig in 1945 to grow on the chorioallantoic membrane of the developing chicken egg. Haig's Onderstepoort virus and other more recent avianised strains do not produce lesions on initial passage but, after three to ten serial transfers in eggs, the attenuated viruses are capable of producing specific linear lesions and thickening of the chorioallantoic membrane 5–7 days after inoculation. After 80–100 transfers, these egg-adapted strains of virus become attenuated for dogs and ferrets, and are especially useful as vaccines for distemper protection. Distemper virus can be cultivated in primary or continuous cultures of dog or ferret kidney cells as well as in some other types of cell cultures of human or simian origin. The egg-adapted strains grow well in chick embryo cell cultures and in cell cultures prepared from unweaned ferrets. In dog kidney cultures cytopathic changes include granular degeneration and vacuolation of the cells accompanied, usually, by the formation of giant cells and syncytia with cytoplasmic and, occasionally, nuclear inclusion bodies (Plate 43.10c, facing p. 535). Thus, the essential features of the cytopathic effects of measles, distemper and rinderpest viruses are very similar.

Pathogenicity

Characteristically, distemper attacks primarily puppies and seldom older dogs because of natural immunity. The disease has an incubation period of about 3–5 days followed by diphasic fever, the development of discharges from the eyes and nose, vomiting, diarrhoea and catarrhal inflammation of the respiratory tract which often develops into pneumonia. Clinical manifestations of the disease include depression, progressive loss of weight, dehydration, hyperkeratosis of the foot pads and nose, nervous symptoms and muscular spasms or posterior paralysis which may perist for long periods. The mortality rate is variable but, in uncomplicated cases, it is generally low and some observers consider that 75 per cent of cases are subclinical. Complications such as pneumonia and encephalitis occur in about 50 per cent of all cases and these may have a case fatality rate of up to 70–80 per cent. The pattern of distemper is largely dominated by the immune status of the dog population in a given locality at any one time. The situation in an enzootic area is quite different from that of an unvaccinated ferret or mink colony, where an outbreak of distemper in highly susceptible animals is nearly always spectacular and the case fatality rate may rise rapidly to about 90 per cent or more. The age incidence of distemper is usually related to the degree of immunity in the dog population but most of the clinically diagnosed cases occur in puppies between 3–6 months of age. The disease appears to have a seasonal prevalence, with the highest incidence in the winter months, and severe outbreaks tend to occur in 2- or 3-yearly cycles.

Studies on the pathogenesis of canine distemper have shown that during the first 6 days after infection the virus multiplies in the lymphatic system but does not reach the epithelial cells. Immunofluorescence techniques have shown that viral antigen appears within 24 hours initially in the bronchial lymph nodes and tonsils and by the second and third days the virus is present in the mononuclear cells of the blood. About 9 days after exposure, dissemination of the virus occurs throughout the body and destruction of epithelial tissues results in diarrhoea, pneumonia and central nervous system (CNS) involvement by about the 12th–16th day.

In dog distemper the lungs may be unaffected but congestion or interstitial pneumonia is not uncommon. Bronchopneumonia, especially of the exudative type, is due to complicating bacterial infections but cases are becoming less common. Inflammatory changes of the conjunctiva, the upper respiratory passages and the gut occur in association with necrosis of the liver. After 2–3 weeks, post-infection encephalitis is an almost constant feature of the disease but inflammatory or demyelinating lesions of the brain may develop in the absence of clinical signs. Cytoplasmic inclusions are to be found chiefly in the epithelium of the urinary tract and bladder, respiratory system, bile ducts, mucosa of the small and large intestines and in certain cells of the adrenal medulla, lymph nodes, tonsils and spleen (Plate 43.4b, facing p. 519). Intranuclear inclusion bodies are more difficult to observe but usually occur in the bladder. The distribution of distemper inclusions may be related to the presence of viral antigen.

Immunity

In fully susceptible animals infected with distemper virus, neutralizing antibody titres reach a peak in about 30–40 days. As the titres develop the amount of free virus in the blood rapidly declines and usually disappears completely by about the 8th day post-inoculation. Interferons produced by infected cells may also play an important part in the elimination of the virus. In natural infections the virus may persist for much longer periods and there are numerous reports of virus being recovered from the brain tissues of encephalitic cases 6 weeks following the onset of the illness.

Puppies born of susceptible dams do not have antibodies to distemper in their sera and are fully susceptible to infection. Puppies born of immune dams obtain only a limited degree of immunity *in utero* because antibodies do not readily cross the placental barrier of the bitch. Hence, the immune titre in the serum of a newborn puppy seldom exceeds 3 per cent of that of its mother. However, passive immunity is readily transferred to the offspring through the colostrum so that within the first 36 hours after birth the level of antibody in the puppy's serum may rise to between 70 and 80 per cent of the dam's serum antibody titre. The level of passive immunity in the sera of puppies in a litter varies and depends upon the amount of colostrum ingested by each individual puppy. These passively acquired antibodies have a half-life of only 7 or 8 days and, in most cases, the antibody concentration falls below the protective level in about 8 weeks. From this age onwards the susceptibility of puppies to distemper increases markedly and they require further protection by vaccination.

Ecology

Distemper is a highly contagious disease and the infection is readily transmitted between susceptible species. The dog is the principal source and reservoir for the virus.

It seems likely that distemper is spread by direct contact or by droplet infection over very short distances. The portals of entry are the tonsils, other lymphoid tissues, the respiratory epithelium and conjunctiva. In ferrets, specific viral antigen can be detected by fluorescent antibody staining techniques in the cervical lymph nodes 48 hours after intranasal exposure. The viral antigen first appears as tiny fluorescing particles in the cytoplasm of epithelial cells but, at a later stage of infection, the particles aggregate to form large oval structures resembling intracytoplasmic inclusions. On the fourth day following experimental or contact exposure, the virus may be detected in the blood, mediastinal and mesenteric lymph nodes and in the spleen. It usually persists for about 19–21 days in these sites. From about the ninth day onwards mononuclear cells laden with virus appear throughout the body and, in those dogs that fail to develop antibody, the infection develops into steadily progressive and widespread invasion of epithelial cells. The damage sustained by these epithelial cells gives rise to the characteristic clinical symptoms of the disease, e.g. anorexia, diarrhoea, conjunctivitis, convulsions and fits. Attempts to infect animals *per os* and by other routes |give variable results, and when virus is administered directly into the stomach the animals do not show signs of distemper and remain fully susceptible to reinfection.

Mink infected by aerosols excrete virus in their nasal discharges from the 5th–46th day post-exposure. Swabs of conjunctival discharges taken on the 21st and 30th day may also reveal virus. Although most reports suggest that virus is not present in the faeces, distemper inclusions can readily be detected in the intestinal epithelium in Peyer's patches and in the mesenteric lymph nodes. Since these findings are in striking contrast to those of rinderpest in cattle, further work is urgently needed to confirm these observations. During the later stages of catarrhal distemper and early in the course of neurotropic distemper, the urinary bladder often contains many well-defined intracytoplasmic inclusion bodies and there is a report that viruria has been observed in experimentally infected dogs from the 3rd–17th day after the initial rise in temperature. It has also been claimed that virus appears irregularly in the urine up to the 6th and 8th week post-inoculation, although other workers believe that the virus is rapidly inactivated by the acid pH of dogs' urine.

Diagnosis

A provisional diagnosis of distemper is often possible on the basis of the clinical appearance of the disease. Important criteria include respiratory involvement, diarrhoea, catarrhal discharges from the eyes and nose, hyperkeratosis of the foot pads, nervous signs and especially fits in younger animals, and an illness of at least 3 weeks' duration. The demonstration of multinucleated syncytia in stained smears of readily accessible epithelium such as the nares, conjunctiva, tongue, vagina and urethra may be of value in the hands of skilled workers but, as in rinderpest diagnosis, the method is not generally recommended. It is impossible to recognise the disease with any certainty from the gross appearance of the carcase, but microscopical evidence of CNS and other tissue changes may suggest distemper. The presence of intracytoplasmic inclusions in stained smears of the conjunctiva or in smears and sections of urinary bladder and trachea are generally held to be of diagnostic significance. Nevertheless, final confirmation of a provisional diagnosis must depend on laboratory aids. These include the isolation and identification of the causal virus by inoculating nasal and pharyngeal secretions or other suitable specimens into susceptible ferrets or cell cultures prepared from puppy or ferret kidneys: or by the detection of specific distemper antigens using immunofluorescence, complement-fixation or gel diffusion tests with hyperimmune anti-distemper or anti-rinderpest sera (Plate 43.8a, facing p. 527). Alternatively, rising antibody titres in paired sera may be demonstrated by complement-fixation or serum neutralization tests using chick embryos or cell cultures with a suitably adapted strain of virus as the antigen. Attempts can also be made to detect the virus by means of electron microscopy. For this purpose, thin films prepared from nasal or ocular discharges, tonsils, lungs or other suitable material are negatively stained with phosphotungstic acid.

Control

Since animals that recover from distemper develop a solid long-lasting active immunity, the only rational means of controlling distemper under present-day conditions is by vaccination prior to field exposure. To be successful, a vaccine should produce antibodies of the same quality and at about the same level as those induced by natural infection. It must also be appreciated when using vaccines, that dogs differ greatly in their susceptibility to infection and in the readiness with which they develop antibodies.

Irrespective of the type of virus vaccine that is used to protect dogs against distemper, it is well known that puppies cannot be successfully vaccinated until they have lost their maternally derived antibody and become susceptible to distemper. Thus, if only one injection of vaccine is to be given, it should be delayed until the dog is about 12 weeks of age, although it is realised that puppies receiving low levels of colostral antibody at birth will already have been at risk for five or six weeks. Since it is a practical impossibility to test the serum of each puppy for neutralizing antibodies before vaccination, it is often recommended that young animals should be immunized with a suitably adapted strain of virus at 6–8 weeks of age with a further booster dose being given at 12 weeks. To overcome these practical difficulties Baker and his colleagues have devised a nomogram which predicts, on the basis of the pregnant dam's serum neutralizing titre, the age at which the declining passive antibody of her litter ceases to protect them against virulent virus: this being the earliest time at which the puppies can be successfully vaccinated.

Inactivated distemper virus vaccines are rarely used nowadays because the antibody levels they produce decline at a rate similar to that of colostrum-derived antibody, namely, a 50 per cent decrease every 10 days. Moreover, the duration of active immunity produced by inactivated vaccines, with or without adjuvants, is considerably less than that obtained with live virus vaccines.

The first anti-distemper vaccine was produced in 1928 by Laidlaw and Dunkin who immunized puppies with inactivated spleen tissue from affected dogs. These immunized dogs were then used for producing immune sera which was combined with virulent virus to give the so-called 'simultaneous' method of vaccination. In 1939, Green successfully adapted a strain of distemper virus by continued passage through ferrets until it was highly pathogenic for both ferrets and mink but of reduced virulence for dogs and foxes. Not only does Green's distemperoid virus stimulate a high degree of active immunity in dogs, thereby preventing distemper, but it also acts therapeutically by interfering with the field strain of distemper virus. This phenomenon of virus interference or cell blockage also occurs between attenuated vaccine virus and field strains of rinderpest virus. In South Africa in 1948, Haig found that Green's distemperoid virus could be adapted readily to grow on the chorioallantoic membrane of developing chicken embryos, while retaining its immunizing properties. As a result of this discovery, avirulent avianised vaccines have been used on a very wide scale with generally satisfactory results. It was later discovered that cell culture attenuated distemper virus is also a suitable and well-tolerated immunizing agent against dog distemper. Very high antibody titres are obtained and a solid, durable immunity is produced. Moreover, there is very little excretion of the tissue-adapted virus and susceptible in-contact dogs do not acquire the disease from vaccinated dogs.

It is generally agreed that measures to protect puppies against distemper should begin when maternally derived antibody has declined in the puppies to a level which allows them to become susceptible to the virus, and that successful immunization cannot be obtained, even from a good vaccine, until after the temporary colostrum-derived immunity has disappeared. In an attempt to overcome the danger period between the loss of colostral antibodies and the production of active immunity by vaccination, a recent and novel method of heterotypic protection by measles virus has been used and such vaccines are now available commercially. Thus, it may now be possible to protect puppies at an early age against virulent distemper, irrespective of the passive immunity status, by using an avirulent measles virus that is effective within 8 hours and confers protection for at least 8 months. To obtain maximum protection the measles vaccine must contain large amounts of virus (about 10^4 ID_{50}/ml) and should be administered intramuscularly. At approximately 4–6 months of age the passively derived maternal distemper antibody will have declined and young dogs that have previously been inoculated with attenuated measles virus can then be given live distemper vaccine that will produce maximum immunity against distemper. It is emphasised that the formation of distemper antibody is not influenced by the presence of measles immunity and that the secondary response consists of a more rapid development of immunity to distemper compared with the 2–3 weeks that must elapse before the onset of immunity produced by distemper virus is established in susceptible dogs. Although the mechanisms of heterotypic vaccination are not fully understood, it seems that the antibody-producing cells are sensitised by the heterotypic (measles) virus so that following exposure to distemper virus the puppy is able to produce rapidly large amounts of specific distemper neutralizing antibody.

Whatever type of virus vaccine is used to stimulate active immunity to canine distemper, the level of protective antibody reaches a peak about 4 weeks after successful vaccination. The duration of antibody depends on a variety of factors such as the age and immune status of the animal, the strain of virus used, its concentration and even the route of inoculation. While many workers believe that the antibody levels will fall within two years in the absence of restimulation, others have shown that protective levels of antibody may remain for as long as 6 years. However, there is little doubt that exposure to street virus can boost the vaccination titre, and that this is still an important factor in maintaining the immune status of vaccinated dogs in urban areas.

Rinderpest

Synonym
Cattle plague.

Definition
Rinderpest is an acute and sometimes sub-acute or inapparent febrile contagious disease of ruminants, particularly cattle. It is characterised by severe haemorrhagic catarrh of the mucous membranes with necrotic stomatitis and gastroenteritis. The mortality rate is high in animals with a low innate resistance.

Hosts affected
The natural hosts of rinderpest are cattle and other members of the order Artiodactyla, the so-called 'cloven-hoofed' mammals. In addition to cattle, natural infections have been confirmed in water buffaloes, sheep and goats, and the disease has also been reported in pigs in Asia and parts of the Far East. Free-living wild animals, e.g. warthog, African buffalo, eland, wildebeest (gnu), impala and Thomson's gazelle are also susceptible to rinderpest but only a few of these regularly suffer from the disease.

Buffalo, eland, wildebeest and warthog possess a low innate resistance and tend to react severely to the disease, whereas Thomson's gazelle and other wild Artiodactyla have a high innate resistance and seldom appear to develop clinical symptoms. These latter species may become inapparent carriers of the virus and are capable of infecting other more susceptible species of wild game.

History and distribution
Rinderpest was originally recognised in Asia and epizootics of the disease swept over Europe practically every 40 or 50 years, until about the end of the 19th century, thereby considerably reducing the cattle populations in the countries affected. As a result of the serious losses sustained during a series of epizootics in France about the middle of the 18th century, a school for the training of veterinarians was established at Lyons in 1762; the first of its kind in the world. The last disastrous outbreak of rinderpest in Great Britain occurred in 1865, with the introduction of live cattle from Finland to the London market, which resulted in the destruction of no less than 500 000 cattle before being eradicated in 1866 by means of a slaughter policy. Recent outbreaks in Europe occurred in Belgium in 1920, Malta in 1946, Rome in 1949 and Trieste in 1954; and all these outbreaks were associated with the movement of cattle by sea from enzootic areas. The outbreak in Belgium in 1920 was due to Indian zebus being temporarily landed at Antwerp while in transit to Brazil, and the same animals caused the only recorded outbreak on the American continent soon after their arrival at Sao Paulo. A single outbreak occurred in Western Australia in November, 1923, due, it is thought, to sheep being landed at Freemantle as ship's stores and sold for slaughter to local butchers. On the African continent, until the year 1884, rinderpest was known only in Egypt but it was introduced by the movement of cattle during the Italian/Abyssinian War and spread rapidly over the whole of Central and South Africa causing enormous losses in domestic cattle and also among wild game. At the present time the disease is enzootic in certain areas of equatorial and North-east Africa as well as in parts of Asia, including Afghanistan, Pakistan, India, Cambodia and Viet Nam. Despite the widespread use of vaccines, severe epizootics of rinderpest still occur from time to time and, as late as 1949, it was held to be responsible for the deaths of over 2 million cattle each year.

Classification
The causal agent of rinderpest is a member of the measles-distemper-rinderpest triad and, as such, probably belongs to the myxoviruses. On the basis of their physical, chemical and biological characters, the measles-distemper-rinderpest group are closer to the paramyxoviruses, (e.g. Newcastle disease virus and mumps virus), than to the orthomyxoviruses (e.g. influenza virus). Nevertheless, there are a number of important differences and some workers prefer to assign them, for the time being, to a separate subgroup called the pseudomyxoviruses, although this term has no official status.

Morphology
The structure of the rinderpest virus closely resembles that of measles, distemper, Newcastle disease and other paramyxoviruses, and electron micro-

graphs reveal almost identical morphological features. The virus particles are generally spherical in shape and vary in size from 90–250 nm in diameter. Pleomorphic forms are not uncommon and some filamentous particles may measure up to 500–1000 nm in length. The virion consists of an outer envelope of lipoprotein fringed with short radial projections or spikes and an inner coiled helix of ribonucleoprotein. The inner helical component is approximately 18 nm in diameter and consists of single-stranded RNA coated along its length with molecules of protein in the form of capsomeres.

Physicochemical characters

The virus of rinderpest is relatively labile and the infectivity of cell culture preparations has a half-life of 1–3 hours at 37°C but only minutes at 56°C. Nevertheless, small fractions of tissue culture virus may survive heating at 56°C for 60 minutes or 60°C for 30 minutes, Storage of the virus at 4°C results in marked loss of infectivity within a few months and, even at –70°C, some loss of infectivity titre occurs after about a year. Virus preparations are best preserved by lyophilization or by the addition of 2 per cent dimethyl sulphoxide (DMSO) with storage at 4°C or lower. Inactivation by ultra-violet light irradiation or by heat proceeds rapidly in an exponential manner. That is to say, the greater the amount of virus the longer it takes to destroy infectivity. Many strains of rinderpest virus vary significantly in their pH stabilities but most are inactivated below pH 4·0. The optimum stability is probably between pH 7·2 and 8·0. Because of the presence of an essential lipid component in its envelope, the virus of rinderpest is rapidly inactivated at 4°C after treatment with 20 per cent ethyl ether or chloroform. An unique property of the virus is its apparent fragility in glycerine; a fact which was used in the preparation of the first inactivated rinderpest vaccine. In general, the rinderpest virus is not very resistant. It is rapidly inactivated by putrefaction and it soon loses its infectivity when exposed to sunlight or when dried under natural conditions. The virus does not survive in carcases and the risk of spreading the infection abroad by hides and chilled or frozen meat is relatively small even though the virus can survive for several weeks in lymph nodes and spleen held at –25°C. The greatest danger lies in the importation of live animals, especially those with a mild or even sub-clinical infection. Strong alkalis are believed to be the best disinfectants, and glycerol, phenol, formalin or β-propiolactone readily destroy infectivity but not antigenicity.

Haemagglutination

Despite the fact that measles virus agglutinates red blood cells of baboons and various species of monkeys, and that egg-adapted strains of distemper virus partially agglutinate chicken and guinea-pig red cells, the rinderpest virus has not been shown to possess haemagglutinating activity. Nevertheless, the inability to demonstrate rinderpest haemagglutinins may be due to technical difficulties since their presence may be inferred from several confirmed reports that anti-rinderpest sera inhibit measles haemagglutinin and also that the receptor sites for measles haemagglutinin on monkey red blood cells can be blocked by prior treatment with rinderpest virus. Moreover, if measles virus is treated with ether and Tween 80, which disintegrates the viral envelope to form small uniform particles of haemagglutinin, then the agglutination of monkey erythrocytes can be inhibited to high titre by distemper or rinderpest antibodies. In contrast to this, HeLa cells infected with measles or distemper viruses haemadsorb healthy guinea-pig erythrocytes, but rinderpest virus does not.

Antigenic properties

Rinderpest virus is antigenically uniform and vaccines protect against all known strains. Serological studies indicate that the virus contains a number of soluble antigens distinct from the infectious component. These include the complement-fixing antigen which, by Nakamura's method, can be extracted from infected tissues in alcohol, acetone or ether and resists boiling for 20 minutes. There are also a number of precipitating antigens, two of which are heat-stable and the third, the slowest migrating one, is heat-labile. The precipitinogens are readily demonstrable by agar gel diffusion techniques using lymph node and a variety of other tissues from infected animals, as well as in concentrated fluids from infected cell cultures. The precipitinogens, like the complement-fixing antigens, are rapidly destroyed by putrefaction.

Similarities between the clinical and pathological features of measles and dog distemper have been recognised for many years and in 1954 it was reported that distemper neutralizing antibodies occurred in human sera. Three years later it was shown that these antibodies were closely associated with similar increases in measles antibodies in human patients recovering from measles. In 1957, Polding and Simpson reported from Kenya that dogs which had fed on meat from cattle affected with rinderpest resisted infection with field distemper. These and many subsequent reports have amply confirmed that there is a close but not identical antigenic relationship between all three members of the so-called measles-distemper-rinderpest triad of viruses; several experiments have failed to demonstrate cross neutralization between distemper antiserum and measles virus, although neutralization was readily demonstrated with all other combinations. Similarly, cross-protection tests show that dogs infected with measles or rinderpest virus develop an immunity against distemper virus, whereas many workers have failed to protect cattle against rinderpest following inoculation with distemper virus. Measles virus haemagglutinin can be used as a reliable diagnostic method for detecting antibodies against both rinderpest and distemper.

The virus of 'peste des petits ruminants' (PPR), a rinderpest-like disease of sheep and goats in West Africa which does not spread to rinderpest-susceptible cattle, produces a cytopathic effect in sheep kidney cells similar to that caused by rinderpest virus. Moreover, tissue culture adapted PPR virus immunizes cattle against rinderpest while anti-rinderpest ox serum immunizes sheep and goats against the virus of PPR. Thus, PPR virus appears to be a strain of rinderpest virus which has lost its ability to infect cattle by the natural route, but which spreads readily among sheep and goats.

Interference

Interference with Rift Valley fever virus in hamsters is reported. Interference may also occur between attenuated vaccine virus and virulent strains of rinderpest.

Cultivation

The virus of rinderpest has been adapted to grow in sheep, goats, rabbits, golden hamsters, susliks and white mice (Plate 43.9a, facing p. 534), but horses, dogs and guinea-pigs are less susceptible and are not affected by contact with rinderpest-infected cattle. Rinderpest virus has proved adaptable to growth in embryonated hens' eggs by the intravenous, chorioallantoic membrane or yolk-sac routes of inoculation and some strains have become attenuated for cattle after 20 or more passages by the yolk-sac method. Lapinized strains have also been adapted to grow in chicken embryos. Both field and laboratory-maintained cattle strains of rinderpest virus grow well in primary and continuous cell cultures and most produce a marked cytopathic effect, but lapinized and caprinized strains do not. Nor do bovine strains of rinderpest virus replicate or produce cytopathic effects in rabbit cell cultures. Susceptible cells include those from cattle, sheep, goats, chicken embryos, pigs, hamsters, dogs and man. The cytopathic effect consists of large well-defined multinucleated giant cells or syncytia (polykaryons) each containing several large acidophilic cytoplasmic plaques and, sometimes, a number of smaller single or multiple intranuclear inclusions (Plates 43.10a, b, facing p. 535). In addition, infected cultures contain large numbers of stellate or spindle-shaped cells with long, fine anastomosing intracel-lular processes. The formation of multinucleate giant cells seems to be due to fusion of the affected cells rather than abnormal division of the nuclei. Field strains of virus seeded from the buffy coats of the blood of sick animals induce typical cytopathic changes in roller-tube cultures of primary calf kidney cells after 3–12 days of incubation at 37°C. The effects are more easily demonstrable if the cells are infected as trypsin-dispersed suspensions rather than complete monolayer cultures. After about 10–12 days of incubation, 80 per cent of the cell sheet is affected. In most cell systems there appears to be a predominance of cell-associated virus but, unlike cultures infected with distemper or measles, rinderpest-infected HeLa cells do not adsorb guinea-pig erythrocytes. After about 20 passages on cell cultures, there is an appreciable degree of attenuation of the virus for the original donor, and animals immunized with tissue culture virus resist challenge with virulent virus. Tissue culture techniques are particularly suitable for fundamental studies of the size, shape, architecture and resistance of the virus, the economical testing of sera for neutralizing antibodies, as a means of isolating and identifying field strains of virus and for developing live attenuated virus vaccines.

It is generally agreed that rinderpest virus, like the viruses of distemper and measles, multiplies in the cytoplasm of susceptible host cells. Comparative immunofluorescence studies on an established line of African green monkey kidney cells (Vero cells) infected with the three viruses, suggest that all have the same pattern of development of specific viral antigens and, moreover, that their V and S antigens are synthesised exclusively in the cytoplasm. However, further recent studies of the growth cycle of rinderpest virus by means of indirect fluorescent antibody staining indicate that while there is no evidence of intra-nuclear fluorescence in monolayer cultures fixed by the conventional acetone method, fluorescing particles may be seen in the nuclei of infected cells in air-dried preparations. Moreover, the number and size of the fluorescing granules and their distribution corresponds precisely with the inclusions seen in monolayer cultures stained by haematoxylin eosin. If these observations are confirmed, the rinderpest virus can be held to resemble orthomyxoviruses rather than paramyxoviruses by synthesising virus-specific antigens in the nucleus as well as in the cytoplasm.

Assembly and maturation of progeny rinderpest virus takes place at the cell surface and infectious virus particles are released by budding of the cellular surface. The mature viruses are morphologically similar to those of measles and distemper as well as mumps, Newcastle disease and other paramyxoviruses.

Pathogenesis

In natural cases of rinderpest the primary site of entry of the virus is through the nasopharyngeal mucosa but experimental cattle can readily be infected by a variety of different routes.

According to Plowright and his colleagues, the course of the disease can be divided into four phases, namely, incubation, prodromal, mucoid and convalescent. The incubation period or the time between infection and the first rise in temperature usually lasts for two to nine days, according to the strain and dose of virus used. During this period the virus passes through the mucosa of the upper respiratory tract to the associated lymph nodes from which generalisation by the lymph and blood stream occurs in a very short time. The virus multiplies rapidly and produces very high titres, especially in the lymphoid tissues, lungs, bone marrow and intestines. Active proliferation of the virus in many different tissues results in fever.

The second or prodromal phase starts with the first rise of temperature which may reach 105–107°F (41–42°C) and lasts for about 3 days until the appearance of lesions in the mouth. At this stage of infection animals show depression or restlessness and anorexia. The muzzle is usually very dry, the coat staring and most animals are constipated. A leukopenia which begins with the onset of fever becomes rapidly and progressively more marked and usually persists until death supervenes.

The third or mucosal phase begins with the appearance of mouth lesions on the inside of the lower lips and adjacent gums and ends 3–5 days later in death or with the beginning of the period of convalescence. At this stage the visible mucous membranes are often congested and the oral lesions take the form of small, raised, greyish pin-head foci with necrotic centres which enlarge and coalesce and can readily be rubbed away to reveal irregular, sharply-demarcated shallow erosions with raw, red bases due to capillary bleeding. (Plate 43.9b, facing page 534) The presence of the oral lesions invariably produces excessive salivation although smacking of the lips, as in foot-and-mouth disease, is said to be uncommon. In many of the affected animals clear nasal and lachrymal discharges develop which later become purulent.

During the mucosal phase of the illness, the animal is very restless and often shows increased thirst. The temperature remains high until just before the onset of diarrhoea which usually appears about the 4th–7th day, i.e. 1–2 days after the mouth lesions. In fatal cases the diarrhoea becomes progressively worse, the temperature continues to fall and there is rapid dehydration, marked weakness and severe emaciation (Plate 43.9c, facing p. 534). Affected cattle do not die when diarrhoea fails to develop. By the end of the prodromal period only very small quantities of virus remain in the tissues, even at predilection sites, and it is generally believed that all infectious virus disappears from the tissues and secretions by the 9th or 10th days following the onset of clinical symptoms. During the convalescent phase the mouth lesions begin to heal by the 3rd–5th days following their appearance, and there is rapid regeneration of the affected epithelium. In most cases, however, convalescence is prolonged and the return to good bodily condition may take many months. The leukopenia may also persist for several weeks.

Mortality

Virulent field or laboratory strains of virus cause a very high mortality in fully suceptible cattle and, in previously disease-free areas, over 90 per cent of animals can be expected to die. Death usually occurs on the 6th–20th day of the disease following an incubation period of 3–9 days after natural contact infection. Occasional deaths may be delayed until the third week. In resistant breeds of cattle, or with strains of low virulence, the mortality rates may be very small or even negligible.

Pathogenicity

Although there is only one immunological type of rinderpest virus, the virulence of different virus isolates varies widely for different breeds of cattle. Most field strains produce a violent reaction in highly susceptible animals but others have been described which produce only mild or symptomless infections unless there are additional complications from some concurrent debilitating condition e.g. piroplasmosis or trypanosomiasis. Strains of low pathogenicity are often associated with wild game.

A major factor in the epizootiology of rinderpest is the innate susceptibility of different breeds of cattle in enzootic areas. In India, sheep, goats and domesticated pigs are highly susceptible to infection and the 'hills zebu' are more susceptible than the 'plains zebu' because, presumably, the former have been less exposed over the years to rinderpest virus than animals in enzootic areas at lower altitudes. Finer shades of innate resistance amongst moderately-resistant cattle have been revealed during programmes of mass vaccination with different types of attenuated virus vaccines. Thus, Japanese black or Korean native cattle cannot safely be vaccinated with the Nakamura (III) strain of rabbit-adapted virus which induces only mild reactions in most breeds of European origin. In the same way, caprinized virus vaccines which produce marked reactions in Guernseys, the Ankole cattle of Central Africa and other moderately resistant breeds, can safely be used in African cross zebus, The innate resistance of domestic buffaloes also varies considerably. In South-east Asia they are highly susceptible, in India moderately so, while in Egypt and other parts of North-east Africa they possess a high innate resistance. In general, most domestic animals, in enzootic areas have a high innate resistance, the clinical disease is not so severe and the mortality rate is low. On the other hand, the introduction of a virulent strain of virus into disease-free areas invariably results in a disastrous epizootic because of the low innate resistance of the exposed animals.

Wild game play an important role in the epidemiology of rinderpest in Africa and species with a high innate resistance may be responsible for maintaining the virus in enzootic areas, unlike animals with a low innate resistance which generally develop frank clinical disease and die.

Ecology

During the acute illness, rinderpest virus is widely distributed throughout the body, the highest titres occurring in carcase and visceral lymph nodes, the mucosa of the alimentary tract, the spleen and lungs. The virus also occurs in all secretions and excretions during the febrile stage of the disease. Nasal discharges may be the primary route of excretion, particularly during the two days preceding the first rise of temperature (i.e. about one week before the appearance of pathognomonic clinical signs). Conjunctival and oral secretions are also infectious but virus titres are not as high as in the nasal discharges. Urinary excretion of virus seems to be relatively unimportant but the faeces contain concentrations of virus as great as 10^6 ID_{50}/g and the total output may, therefore, be enormous. Despite this, contaminated grass, soil, food and water do not play an important part in the spread of infection because of the labile nature of the virus. Buildings contaminated by the natural discharges of sick animals remain infective for not more than 2–4 days and virus shed in the faeces remains viable in the soil for less than 36 hours.

Successful transmission of rinderpest requires close contact between infected and susceptible animals. Contact infection experiments in cattle suggest that the virus passes through the mucosa of the upper and lower respiratory tracts to establish primary foci in the regional lymph nodes from which a generalized infection develops rapidly via the lymph and blood stream. Transmission is readily effected experimentally by conjunctival instillation of virus, by the intransasal route and by nasal swabbing, as well as by subcutaneous and other parenteral routes. Drenching with infected materials often fails to set up infection and the use of common water troughs seldom results in transmission of the disease. The virus is not airborne over distances greater than a few yards and intermediate vectors such as flies, mosquitoes and ticks do not play an important role in the dissemination of the virus. Thus, transmission of the natural disease is probably due to direct contact between sick and healthy animals and it seems, therefore, that simple quarantine measures are sufficient to limit the spread of infection.

Immunity

There is only one serological type of rinderpest virus and recovery from frank clinical infection produces a lifelong immunity. In animals infected with wild, naturally attenuated strains of virus, the duration of immunity is probably not lifelong and they may suffer a second attack of the disease.

Diagnosis

The conditions under which the disease occurs, the clinical signs and the post-mortem findings generally lead to a strong suspicion of rinderpest, especially in acute cases of disease in highly susceptible animals. In disease-free territories there is usually a history of recent animal movements and rapid spread of infection with a high rate of mortality, but in enzootic areas the symptoms may be less obvious and the mortality rate will depend on the virulence of the the virus and the resistance of the animals at risk. Examination of stained impression smears prepared from the epithelia of the tonsils and other lymphoid tissues may reveal the presence of syncytia and several large pleomorphic plaques of acidophilic inclusion material, similar to those seen in infected cell cultures. The method might be of value in the hands of experienced workers but it cannot be recommended as a routine procedure. In almost every case a provisional diagnosis can only be confirmed by one or more of the following laboratory procedures:

(1) the isolation and identification of the virus

(2) the detection of rinderpest-specific antigen, and

(3) the demonstration of the development of specific rinderpest antibodies.

Wherever possible, samples should be collected in the acute febrile stage of the disease and not from carcases, since the infectivity of the virus and the presence of soluble antigens may be adversely affected by putrefaction.

Isolation and identification of the virus

Rinderpest virus can readily be detected in citrated whole blood, lymph nodes, spleen or other tissues obtained preferably during the prodromal or early mucoid phase of the disease by subcutaneous inoculation of known susceptible and known immune (vaccinated) cattle. If rinderpest virus is present, the susceptible cattle will react in about 2–10 days' time and the survivors from both groups are then challenged 2–3 weeks later with virulent virus. The method, however, is hazardous because live virus is used, and also it is both expensive and time-consuming.

In recent years an equally reliable but simpler and less costly method has been developed whereby the virus is detected in secondary cell cultures of bovine kidney by its characteristic cytopathic effects. The earliest tissue changes appear within 3–12 days and the specificity of the reaction is confirmed by means of neutralization tests with known anti-rinderpest serum. If required, serological identification of the virus can be obtained simultaneously by incorporating rinderpest antiserum in the growth medium of some of the infected culture tubes. Unfortunately, isolation and identification procedures are time-consuming and too slow for the early confirmation of disease which is essential when dealing with fresh outbreaks in clean areas. In such cases, more rapid but less sensitive procedures may be used.

Detection of rinderpest specific antigen
Rinderpest-specific antigen can be demonstrated by complement-fixation and agar gel diffusion tests. The tissues of choice for complement-fixation are fresh carcase or visceral lymph nodes or spleen, taken at the third to sixth day of pyrexia. The method can be carried out by one of several modifications of the standard complement-fixation test and the period of fixation can be one hour at 37°C followed by 30 minutes at 37 °C or, preferably, over-night incubation in the cold (4°C). Both the hyperimmune serum and the susceptible (control) serum are used unheated.

The agar gel diffusion method is simpler to use but is much less sensitive than complement-fixation. Suitable material for the demonstration of diffusible precipitinogens in rinderpest-suspect animals include carcase and mesenteric lymph nodes and many other tissues. The optimal period for collecting lymph nodes for agar gel diffusion tests is during the early acute stages of the disease until the onset of diarrhoea. Results from experimentally infected cattle suggest that diffusible rinderpest precipitinogens are present in many infected tissues and that maximum titres occur on or about the 5th day of pyrexia. For routine diagnosis, carcase and visceral lymph nodes or other suitable tissues are obtained by biopsy, or during autopsy of animals that have been killed or have died recently. Biopsy material from prescapular lymph nodes is readily obtained by means of a syringe fitted with a wide bore needle. Precipitating antigens are difficult to demonstrate in animals that have died 14 days or longer after the onset of fever or in tissues from decomposed carcases.

The agar gel double diffusion test is simple to carry out and requires the minimum amount of materials and reagents. Gels in small Petri dishes are prepared by cutting a pattern of holes (5 mm diameter) so that six lateral depots are placed equidistant (5 mm apart) around a single central depot. Small portions of suspect and known positive tissues are placed in alternate lateral wells and rinderpest hyperimmune serum is added to the central well. After 6–18 hours of incubation at room temperature the plates are examined for the presence of a single, thin but clearly defined line of precipitation between the central well and each of the lateral wells containing rinderpest precipitinogens. The lines should merge without crossing or overlapping. On occasion, two bands of precipitate are formed when crude lymph node extracts are diffused against a hyperimmune rabbit serum. Rinderpest precipitinogens are smaller and distinct from the infectious virus particle and the one which is regularly observed in crude preparations is probably identical with the complement-fixing antigen.

Demonstration of the development of rinderpest antibodies
Specific neutralizing and complement-fixing antibodies develop in the sera of cattle which survive to the fourth day of the disease and later. The concentration is at first very small but increases rapidly to reach maximum levels by about the end of the second week of the illness. Thus, the tests require the simultaneous examination of paired serum samples. The first is taken before exposure or during the early acute stage of the illness and the second 2–4 weeks after the onset of clinical signs. The serum neutralization method is preferred to the complement-fixation test for the detection of rinderpest antibodies (because bovine serum is notoriously anticomplementary) and is carried out in cell cultures, rabbits or cattle. The preferred test is a quantitative one in which dilutions of serum are mixed with a constant amount of tissue culture-adapted rinderpest virus, incubated in the cold overnight and then seeded into dispersed tissue cell cultures. A rise of 0·6 log. units in the antibody titre is held to be significant. If the neutralization test is carried out in rabbits, a lapinised virus must be used as the antigen.

Additional tests
Although fluorescent antibody staining techniques are being used for the early detection of measles and distemper, very little is known about the value of immunofluorescence in the diagnosis of rinderpest. Nevertheless, specific fluorescence has been described in rinderpest infected cultures in which no cytopathic effect is to be seen. Rinderpest serum may also be used to detect antigens of distemper in conjunctival scrapings of suspected cases and in lung impression smears of dogs dying from the disease.

The haemagglutination of monkey red blood cells with measles virus and the inhibition by both measles and rinderpest antibodies has led to the development of a haemagglutination-inhibition test for the detection of rinderpest virus and rinderpest antibodies. More recently, a novel method of diagnosis has been devised whereby the tissue from a suspected case of rinderpest is used to absorb measles haemagglutination-inhibiting antibodies from rinderpest-immune serum, thereby enabling haemagglutination with measles virus to proceed. The reliability of these tests in the diagnosis of rinderpest awaits confirmation.

Differential diagnosis

Several virus diseases resemble rinderpest in their clinical manifestations and a confirmatory diagnosis can only be obtained in the laboratory. Disease conditions which may be confused with rinderpest include viral diarrhoea or mucosal disease, malignant catarrhal fever, foot-and-mouth disease and infectious bovine rhinotracheitis. In sheep, rinderpest may be confused with bluetongue, Nairobi sheep disease and sheep pox.

Control

It is now known that rinderpest virus is nearly always introduced into disease-free territories by living animals, especially those which may have had a mild or even sub-clinical infection. Because of this, rinderpest-free countries remote from enzootic areas ensure their freedom from the disease by imposing a complete embargo on the importation of live animals of susceptible breeds and of unprocessed or frozen animal products from countries where the disease occurs; although the risk from meat products is not as great as it is imagined. Prepared hides are without risk and may be imported. Virgin outbreaks in previously disease-free countries are generally of the acute, fulminating type and are readily controlled by the slaughter of infected and in-contact ruminants and swine, together with the institution of strict quarantine, veterinary and police measures. In enzootic and other areas, stock are safeguarded by vaccination usually with an attenuated rinderpest virus vaccine and the immune status of the herds is maintained by annual vaccination of the previous year's calf crop. Outbreaks of the disease in high risk areas can be controlled and eradicated by slaughtering all infected animals and vaccinating the in-contacts. In Africa, wild-living ruminants, feral swine and some other animal species constitute a permanent reservoir of infection which is quite independent of domestic stock, thereby complicating the problem of eradication. In South East Asia the low innate resistance of the domestic pig constitutes

a serious hazard since it is impracticable to vaccinate all susceptible stock every few months.

Animals that recover from rinderpest may have a lifelong immunity. Calves born of dams that are actively immune through recovery from natural infection or from vaccination acquire passive immunity by the ingestion of antibodies in the colostrum during the first few hours of life. On the other hand, calves that have passed the neonatal period do not absorb rinderpest antibodies from the milk of immune cows and are susceptible to infection. The half-life of maternally derived rinderpest antibody is about 37 days and the duration of the passively conferred protection is related directly to the initial antibody level in the serum of the calf which, in turn, depends on the antibody titre of the dam's colostrum. Calves that ingest colostrum from recently immunized mothers resist infection until they are 8–12 months old, but others, born of dams vaccinated some time previously, in which the antibody level of the colostrum will be lower, are susceptible as early as 4 months of age.

Artificially acquired passive immunity produced by the injection of anti-rinderpest serum may persist for up to 3 months but a single minimal dose of antiserum may protect for only 9 days. The serum-virus simultaneous method of immunizing cattle is no longer popular although it was in vogue for more than 30 years. Inactivated vaccines with or without adjuvants were also used extensively in the past to produce active immunity in cattle. While they were undoubtedly safe to use and helped to eradicate rinderpest from many areas, they were unsuitable for massive vaccination programmes because of their cost and the shortness of the immunity they produced. These earlier methods were, in turn, superseded by vaccines prepared from living rinderpest virus attenuated by passage in goats, rabbits or chick embryos. There is an extensive literature on the results of tests on these various vaccines but it seems that different degrees of attenuation are desirable according to the susceptibility of the different breeds of cattle. For example, the first and most widely used attenuated virus vaccine, the caprinized vaccine, frequently causes severe reactions and deaths in highly susceptible breeds, whereas the more attenuated lapinized vaccines are less reactive but induce only a very short or inadequate immunity in the more resistant breeds. In practice, the use of caprinised vaccine is restricted to animals with a high innate resistance such as the East African zebu. Lapinized vaccines are recommended for use in Ankole, Guernsey and other breeds of moderately high innate resistance, whereas only the milder avianised virus vaccines are tolerated by the highly susceptible Japanese Black and Korean native cattle. The duration of immunity induced by attenuated virus vaccines depends on several factors including the degree of attenuation of the virus. In cattle which react to goat virus the end-point of the duration of immunity is believed to be in excess of 13 years. With lapinized virus vaccine the period varies widely and figures of between 1–7 years have been quoted. Information about the duration of immunity stimulated by avianised virus vaccines is scanty but figures of between 16 and 20 months have been given. In recent years, the high-passaged cell culture adapted virus of Plowright and his colleagues is being used extensively in many parts of Africa and Asia to protect cattle against rinderpest. These high titre cell culture vaccines are particularly suitable for use in mass vaccination programmes since they probably produce a lifelong immunity and do not provoke severe clinical reactions in different breeds of cattle.

Further reading

ABINANTI F., CHANOCK R., COOK M., WONG D. AND WARFIELD M. (1961). Relationship of human and bovine strains of myxovirus para-influenza 3, *Proceedings of the Society for Experimental Biology and Medicine*, **106**, 466.

ALEXANDER D.J., HEWLETT G., REEVE P. AND POSTE G. (1973). Studies on the cytopathic effects of Newcastle disease virus: the cytopathogenicity of strain Herts 33 in five cell types. *Journal of General Virology*, **21**, 323.

ALMEIDA J.D. AND BRAND C.M. (1975). A morphological study of the internal component of influenza virus. *Journal of General Virology*, **27**, 313.

ALMEIDA J.D. AND WATERSON A.P. (1970). In *The Biology of Large RNA Viruses*, eds. R.D. Barry and B.W.J. Mahy, p. 27. London: Academic Press.

ANON. (1966). Vaccination against canine distemper. *Veterinary Research*, **79**, 654.

APPEL M.J.G. (1969). Pathogenesis of canine distemper. *American Journal of Veterinary Research*, **30**, 1167.

APPEL M.J.G. AND GILLESPIE J.H. (1972). Canine distemper virus. *Virology Monographs*, **11**, 1.

ARCHETTI I., JEMOLLO A., STEVE-BOCCIARELLI D., ARANGIO-RUIZ G. AND TANGUCCI F. (1967). On the fine structure of influenza viruses. *Archiv für die gesamte Virusforschung* **20**, 133.

BAKER J.A. (1970). Measles vaccine for protection of dogs against canine distemper. *Journal of the American Veterinary Medical Association*. **156**, 1743.

BAKER J.A., CARMICHAEL L.E., DOUGHTY M.F. AND BENSON T.F. (1958). A serological service for dogs. *Proceedings of the U.S. Livestock Sanitary Association*, **62**, 364.

BARRY R.D., CRUICKSHANK J.G. AND WELLS R.J.H. (1964). The viruses of fowl plague and Newcastle disease. *Veterinary Record*, **76**, 1316.

BARRY R.D. AND MAHY B.W. (1970). *The Biology of Large RNA Viruses*. London: Academic Press.

BETTS A.O., JENNINGS A.R., OMAR A.R., PAGE Z.E., SPENCE J.B. AND WALKER R.G. (1964). Pneumonia in calves caused by parainfluenza virus type 3. *Veterinary Record*, **76**, 382.

BEVERIDGE W.I.B., MAHAFFEY L.W. AND ROSE M.A. (1965). Influenza in horses. *Veterinary Record*, **77**, 57.

BOSGRA O. (1966). Recent developments in the immunization of dogs against canine distemper. *Veterinary Record*, **79**, 739.

BRANDLY C.A. AND HANSON R.P. (1965). Newcastle disease. In *Diseases of Poultry*, eds. H.E. Biester and L.H. Schwarte, 5th Edition, p. 633. Ames: Iowa State University Press.

BREESE S.S. (Jun) AND DEBOER C.J. (1973). Ferritin-tagged antibody cross-reactions among rinderpest, canine distemper and measles viruses. *Journal of General Virology*, **20**, 121.

BREITENFELD P.M. AND SCHAEFER W. (1957). The formation of fowl plague virus antigens in infected cells as studied with fluorescent antibodies. *Virology*, **4**, 328.

Canine distemper supplement (1966). *Journal of the American Veterinary Medical Association*, **149**, No. 5, pt. 2, 599.

Cellular Biology of Myxovirus Infections (1964). CIBA Foundation Symposium, eds. G.E.W. Wolstenholme and J. Knight. Summit N.J.: Ciba.

CHANOCK R.M. AND COATES H.V. (1964). In *Newcastle Disease Virus: an evolving pathogen*, ed. R.P. Hanson. Madison: University of Wisconsin Press.

Committee on Fowl Pest Policy (1962). Report. H.M.S.O. Cmnd. 1664, 108p. London: Her Majesty's Stationery Office.

COMPANS R.W. AND CHOPPIN P.W. (1971). The structure and assembly of influenza and parainfluenza viruses. In *Comparative Virology*, eds. K. Maramorosch and E. Kurstak, p. 407. London: Academic Press.

CORNWELL H.J.C., CAMPBELL R.S.F., VANTSIS J.T. AND PENNY W. (1965). Studies in experimental canine distemper. I. Clinico-pathological findings. *Journal of Comparative Pathology and Therapeutics*, **75**, 3.

CRUICKSHANK J.G., WATERSTON A.P., KANAREK A.D. AND BERRY D.M. (1962). The structure of canine distemper virus. *Research in Veterinary Science*, **3**, 485.

DAWSON P.S. (1964). The isolation and properties of a bovine strain (T1) of parainfluenza 3 virus, *Research in Veterinary Science*, **5**, 81.

DAWSON P.S. (1966). Parainfluenza-3 virus of cattle. In *Veterinary Annual*, ed. W.A. Pool, 7th issue, p. 130. Bristol: Wright.

DITCHFIELD J., ZBITNEW A. AND MACPHERSON L.W. (1963). Association of Myxovirus parainfluenza 3 (RE 55) with upper respiratory infection of horses. *Canadian Veterinary Journal*, **4**, 175.

DOWDLE W.R., YARBOROUGH W.B. AND ROBINSON R.Q. (1964). U.S. Epizootic of equine influenza 1963. *Public Health Reports (Washington)*, **79**, 398.

DOYLE T.M. (1927). A hitherto unrecorded disease of fowls due to a filter-passing virus. *Journal of Comparative Pathology and Therapeutics*, **40**, 144.

DRZENICK R., BOGEL K. AND ROTT R. (1967). On the classification of bovine parainfluenza 3 viruses. *Virology*, **31**, 725.

FISCHMAN H.R. (1967). Epidemiology of parainfluenza 3 infection in sheep. *American Journal of Epidemiology*, **85**, 272.

FRASER G. (1966). The use of rinderpest hyperimmune serum for the detection of canine distemper precipitating antigens. *Veterinary Record*, **79**, 155.

GILLESPIE J.H. (1962). The virus of canine distemper. *Annals of the New York Academy of Sciences*, **101**, 540.

GORHAM J.R. (1960). Canine distemper. *Advances in Veterinary Science*, **6**, 287.

HAIG D.A. (1949). Further observations on the growth of Green's distemperoid virus in developing hen eggs. *Journal of the African Veterinary Medical Association*, **19**, 73.

HANSON R.P., SPALATIN J., ESTUPINAN J. AND SCHLOER G. (1967). Identification of lentogenic strains of Newcastle disease virus. *Avian Diseases*, **11**, 49.

HITCHNER S.B. (1964). Control of Newcastle disease in the United States by vaccination. In *Newcastle Disease Virus: an evolving pathogen*, ed. R.P. Hanson. Madison: University of Wisconsin Press.

HORE D.E., STEVENSON R.G., GILMORE N.J.L., VANTSIS J.T. AND THOMPSON D.A. (1968). Isolation of parainfluenza virus from the lungs and nasal passages of sheep showing respiratory disease. *Journal of Comparative Pathology and Therapeutics*, **78**, 259.

HOYLE L. (1968). The influenza viruses. *Virology Monograph*, **4**, 1.

IMAGAWA D.T. (1968). Relationships among measles, canine distemper and rinderpest viruses. *Progress in Medical Virology*, **10**, 160.

ITO Y., TANAKA Y., INABA Y AND OMORI T. (1973). Structure of bovine respiratory syncytial virus. *Archiv für die gesamte Virusforschung*, **40**, 198.

JENSEN R. (1968). Scope of the problem of bovine respiratory disease in beef cattle. *Journal of the American Veterinary Medical Association*, **152**, 720.

JUNGHERR E.L., TYZZER E.E., BRANDLY C.A. AND MOSES H.E. (1946). The comparative pathology of fowl plague and Newcastle disease. *American Journal of Veterinary Research*, **7**, 250.

KAMMER H. AND HANSON R.P. (1962). Studies on the transmission of swine influenza virus with metastrongylus species in specific pathogen-free swine. *Journal Infectious Diseases*, **110**, 99.

KARZON D.T. (1962). Measles virus. *Annals of the New York Academy of Sciences*, **101**, 527

LIESS B. AND PLOWRIGHT W. (1964). Studies on the pathogenesis of rinderpest in experimental cattle. I. Correlation of clinical signs, viraemia and virus excretion by various routes. *Journal of Hygiene*, **62**, 81.

MATUMOTO M., INABA Y., KUROGI H., SATO K., OMORI T., GOTO Y. AND HIROSE O. (1974). Bovine respiratory virus: host range in laboratory animals and cell cultures. *Archiv für die gesamte Virusforschung*, **44**, 280.

MCCARTHY K. (1959). Measles. *British Medical Bulletin*, **15**, 201.

MCFERRAN J.B., GORDON W.A.M. AND FINLAY J.T.T. (1968). An outbreak of subclinical Newcastle disease in N. Ireland. *Veterinary Record*, **82**, 589.

MCQUEEN J.L., DAVENPORT F.M. AND MINUSE E. (1963). Studies of equine influenza in Michigan. I. Etiology. *American Journal of Epidemiology*, **111**, 271.

MOSES H.E., BRANDLY C.A., JONES E.E. AND JUNGHERR E.L. (1948). The isolation and identification of fowl plague virus. *American Journal of Veterinary Research*, **9**, 314.

PACCAUD M.F. AND JACQUIER Cl. (1970). A respiratory syncytial virus of bovine origin. *Archiv für die gesamte Virusforschung*, **30**, 327.

PEREIRA H.G., TUMOVA B. AND LAW V.G. (1965). Avian influenza A viruses. *W.H.O. Bulletin*, **32**, 855.

PLOWRIGHT W. (1962). Rinderpest virus. *Annals of the New York Academy of Sciences*, **101**, 548.

PLOWRIGHT W. (1964). Studies on the pathogenesis of rinderpest in experimental cattle. II. Proliferation of the virus in different tissues following intranasal infection. *Journal of Hygiene, Cambridge*, **62**, 257.

PLOWRIGHT W. (1968). Rinderpest virus. *Virology Monograph*, **3**, 25.

PLOWRIGHT W., CRUICKSHANK J.G. AND WATERSON A.P. (1962). The morphology of rinderpest virus. *Virology*, **17**, 118.

PLOWRIGHT W. AND TAYLOR W.P. (1967). Long-term studies of the immunity in East African cattle following inoculation with rinderpest culture vaccine. *Research in Veterinary Science*, **8**, 118.

POLDING J.B. AND SIMPSON R.M. (1957). A possible

immunological relationship between canine distemper and rinderpest. *Veterinary Record*, **69**, 582.

REID J. (1961). The control of Newcastle disease in Great Britain. *British Veterinary Journal*, **117**, 275.

REISINGER R.C. (1962). Parainfluenza 3 virus in cattle. *Annals of the New York Academy of Sciences*, **101**, 576.

ROBERTS J.A. (1965). A study of the antigenic relationship between human measles virus and canine distemper virus. *Journal of Immunology*, **94**, 622.

ROBERTSON A. (1964). Methods of control of Newcastle disease and their limitations. In; *Newcastle Disease Virus: an evolving pathogen*, ed. R.P. Hanson. Madison: University of Wisconsin Press.

ROMVARY J., TAKATSY G., BARB K. AND FARKAS E. (1962). Isolation of influenza virus strains from animals. *Nature*, **193**, 907.

SCOTT G.R. (1964). Rinderpest. *Advances in Veterinary Science*, **9**, 113.

SCOTT G.R. (1967). *Diagnosis of Rinderpest*. F.A.O. Agricultural Studies No. 17. Rome: Food and Agricultural Organization.

SCOTT G.R. AND BROWN R.D. (1961). Rinderpest diagnosis with special reference to the agar gel double diffusion test. *Bulletin of Epizootic Disease of Africa*, **9**, 83.

SHAVER D.N., BUSSELL R.H. AND BARRON A.L. (1964). Comparative cytopathology of canine distemper and measles virus in ferret kidney cell cultures. *Archiv für die gesamte Virusforschung*, **14**, 487.

SHOPE R.E. (1941) The swine lungworm as a reservoir and intermediate host for swine influenza virus. I. The presence of swine influenza virus in healthy and susceptible pigs. *Journal of Experimental Medicine*, **74**, 41. II. The transmission of swine influenza virus by the swine lungworm. *Journal of Experimental Medicine*, **74**, 49.

SMITH M.H., FREY M.L. AND DIERKS R.E. (1975). Isolation, characterization and pathogenicity studies of a bovine respiratory syncytial virus. *Archiv für die gesamte Virusforschung*, **47**, 237.

SOVINA O., TUMOVA B., POUSTKA F. AND NEMES J. (1958). Isolation of virus causing respiratory disease of horses. *Acta virologica*, **2**, 52.

SPURRIER E.R. AND ROBINSON R.Q. (1965). Antigenic relationships among human and animal strains of parainfluenza viruses. *Health Laboratory Science*, **2**, 203.

TAJIMA M., MOTOHASHI T., KISHI S. AND NAKAMURA J. (1971). A comparative electron microscopic study on the morphogenesis of canine distemper and rinderpest viruses. *Japanese Journal of Veterinary Science*, **33**, 1.

TAYLOR W.P. AND PLOWRIGHT W. (1965). Studies on the pathogenesis of rinderpest in experimental cattle. III. Proliferation of an attenuated strain in various tissues following subcutaneous inoculation. *Journal of Hygiene, Cambridge*, **63**, 263.

TRAVER M.I., NORTHRUP R.L. AND WALKER D.I. (1960). Site of intracellular antigen production by myxoviruses. *Proceedings of the Society for Experimental Biology and Medicine*, **104**, 268.

WADDELL G.H., TEIGLAND M.B. AND SIGEL M.M. (1963). A new influenza virus associated with equine respiratory disease. *Journal of the American Veterinary Medical Association*, **143**, 587.

WARREN J. (1960). The relationships of the viruses of measles, canine distemper and rinderpest. *Advances in Virus Research*, **7**, 27.

WATERSON A.P., PENNINGTON T.H. AND ALLAN W.H. (1967). Virulence in Newcastle disease virus. A preliminary study. *British Medical Bulletin*, **23**, 138.

WHITE G., SIMPSON R.M. AND SCOTT G.R. (1961). An antigenic relationship between the viruses of bovine rinderpest and canine distemper. *Immunology*, **4**, 203.

WRIGHT N.G., CORNWELL H.J.C., THOMPSON H. AND LAUDER I.M. (1974). Canine distemper: current concepts in laboratory and clinical diagnosis. *Veterinary Record*, **94**, 86.

CHAPTER 44

RHABDOVIRUSES

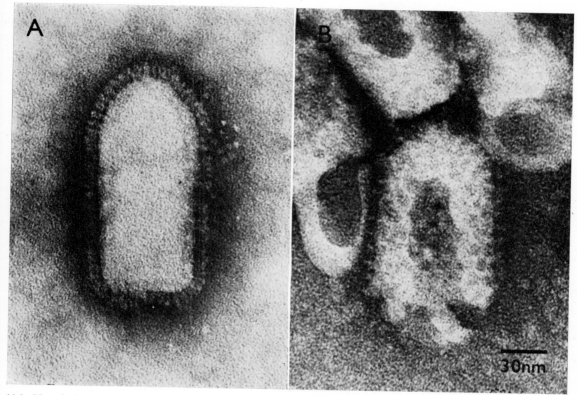

44.1   Negatively stained preparations of (A) vesicular stomatitis virus and (B) rabies virus, showing the bullet-shaped morphology, surface projections and axial channel that are distinctive of rhabdoviruses. The structure of the nucleo-capsid of vesicular stomatitis virus is obscured by the incomplete penetration of the stain, but in (B) the surface of the rabies virus is seen as an arrangement of clearly defined hexomeres. (Courtesy of Dr F. Brown and Mr C. J. Smale.)

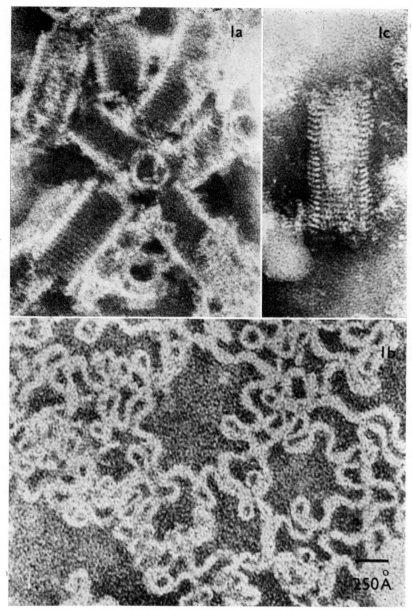

44.2 Electron micrographs of vesicular stomatitis virus showing (1a and 1c) infective skeletons produced by treatment of the virus with the detergent Nonidet P40, and (1b) ribonucleoprotein strands of the virus. (Courtesy of Dr F. Brown and Mr C. J. Smale.)

Rhabdoviruses

The recently proposed Rhabdovirus (Greek, *rhabdos* = rod) group includes members that are uniquely different in morphology from other virus families although they bear a closely similar morphology and structure to each other. They are seen in negative contrast preparations as rod-shaped or cylindrical particles rounded at one end and flat or truncated at the other. These bullet-like structures are about 60×180 nm in size but spherical and irregularly shaped virions may be seen that are not unlike myxoviruses. Members of the genus exhibit a uniform diameter but their length appears to be extremely variable and occasional bacilliform particles may be seen in negatively stained preparations. The shortest is that of the Kern Canyon virus (130 nm) whilst the largest, the Flanders-Hart Park virus, is 210–220 nm long; but a candidate member (Marburg virus) may be up to 2600 nm in length. The central tubular core of the typical virion consists of a tightly wound internal helix not unlike the complex nucleoprotein helices formed by orthomyxoviruses, having a diameter of about 10–20 nm. (Plate 44.2, facing p. 549). The outer layer or envelope which surrounds the axial nucleocapsid is typified as a lipid layer from which protein spikes (about 8 nm in length) protrude. In contrast to the somewhat featureless surface structure of most members of the genus, the surface of the rabies virus is an arrangement of clearly defined hexomeres (Plate 37.1, facing p. 402 and Plate 44.1b, facing p. 548a.)

All members of the group contain single-stranded RNA and are sensitive to ethyl ether and other lipid solvents; and at least three (rabies, vesicular stomatitis and Kern Canyon viruses) possess a lipoprotein haemagglutinin which agglutinates goose erythrocytes. Rhabdoviruses resist freezing and thawing, and some members will persist in the soil for many days at 4–6°C. There is no evidence, at present, that any of the clearly defined members of the group share a common antigen.

The growth of rhabdoviruses in cell cultures is variable. Most replicate and are synthesised in the cytoplasm of a wide variety of cell types with or without visible cytopathic effects. It is a feature of the group that the mature intact virus particles form by budding, either on the outer surface membrane of the cell or from the surface of the membrane lining the intracytoplasmic vacuoles. Recent evidence suggests that the release mechanism differs from member to member depending, to some extent, on the species of host cell—virus system used.

Rhabdoviruses are of special interest because they not only parasitize vertebrates, invertebrates as well as plants, but are also responsible for a number of important diseases of man and animals. Members of the group include:

(1) vesicular stomatitis virus which causes a relatively benign vesicular infection of cattle, horses and pigs,

(2) rabies virus which causes a highly fatal disease of man and all warm blooded animals, including birds,

(3) Sigma virus which is an actual pathogen of insects,

(4) Flanders-Hart Park virus which has been isolated from mosquitoes and birds,

(5) Kern Canyon virus from bats, and

(6) Egtved virus causing viral haemorrhagic septicaemia of trout.

The number of candidates for inclusion in the rhabdovirus group continues to increase and there are reports that the Mount Elgon bat virus and, perhaps, the agent of Marburg or vervet monkey disease may belong to this new and important family of viruses. Other isolates from vertebrate sources having rhabdovirus characters include the Lagos bat virus and the virus of bovine ephemeral fever. By mid 1973 more than five dozen viruses from vertebrates, insects and plants had been tentatively placed in the rhabdovirus group, mainly on the basis of their unique morphology. The properties of some rhabdoviruses are summarised in Table 44.1.

TABLE 44.1.   Some properties of rhabdoviruses from vertebrate sources.

Virus	Site of maturation	Dimensions (nm)	Length of surface projections (nm)	Natural host
Vesicular stomatitis	PM ICM	68 × 175	10·0	Mammals Arthropods
Rabies	PM ICM CM	75 × 180	6–7	Mammals Birds
Egtved	PM	70 × 180		Rainbow trout
Flanders-Hart Park	PM ICM	65 × 220		Birds Arthropods
Kern Canyon	PM	73 × 132	8·0	Myotis bats
Mount Elgon bat	PM	70 × 230	8–10	Insectivorous bats Mosquitoes
Bovine ephemeral fever	PM ICM	80 × 140		Cattle
Marburg	PM	90 × 130–2600		Monkeys

PM = Plasma membrane
ICM = Intracytoplasmic membrane
CM = Cytoplasmic matrix.

Vesicular stomatitis

Synonym
Sore mouth of cattle and horses; pseudo foot-and-mouth disease; stomatite vesiculeuse contagieuse (Fr.); bläschenbildende Mundenzündung (Ger.); pseudo-aftosa (Span.).

Definition
A benign, highly contagious vesicular disease, primarily of horses but also of cattle and pigs in which it closely resembles foot-and-mouth disease.

Hosts affected
The disease occurs naturally among horses, mules, cattle, deer and pigs. Sheep and goats appear to be refractory to natural infection. Accidental infection of man is not uncommon.

History and distribution
It is claimed that vesicular stomatitis was first observed as a disease of horses and mules in South Africa in 1884 but several workers believe that there is no scientific proof of this. It is known that many cases of 'sore mouth' occurred in cavalry lines during the American Civil War and there is circumstantial evidence suggesting that vesicular stomatitis is primarily a disease of Central and North America and may have been carried from there to Africa. There seems little doubt that the virus was introduced to Europe in shipments of American horses but the outbreaks were short-lived and attracted little attention. Originally, vesicular stomatitis was confined to horses and mules but now it is seen more frequently in cattle and pigs. At the present time, the disease occurs sporadically in the United States of America and Canada, and is enzootic in parts of Mexico, Venezuela and Columbia. Its major importance lies in the fact that it closely resembles foot-and-mouth disease in cattle and pigs.

Morphology
The virus particles are cylindrical, bullet-shaped rods with a length about three times the diameter (150–180 × 50–70 nm). The surface of the virion is surrounded by a membranous envelope which is uniformly studded with short spikes, about 10 nm long, not unlike the small projections seen in myxoviruses. The internal component consists of a tightly coiled helical structure which appears as a series of transverse striations surrounding a long hollow axial channel (Plate 44.1a, between pp. 548a and 549). In addition to the characteristic bullet-shaped (B) particles, numerous small truncated (T) particles are present in many preparations of the virus.

Physicochemical properties

Vesicular stomatitis virus contains RNA and a large amount of phospholipid. It has the same degree of resistance to physical and chemical reagents as the foot-and-mouth disease virus. It is inactivated in 30 minutes at 58°C and by visible and ultraviolet light as well as by lipid solvents such as ether and chloroform. The virus is said to survive in soil for many days at 4–6°C. It resists 0·5 per cent phenol for 23 days but is rendered non-infective by 0·05 per cent crystal violet.

Haemagglutination

Vesicular stomatitis virus produces a haemagglutinin in infected cell cultures. The optimum conditions for titration of the haemagglutinin are similar to those developed for rabies, namely, a serum-free growth medium containing 0·4 per cent bovine albumin, a low temperature (0–4°C), pH of 6·2 and the use of goose erythrocytes. There is no spontaneous elution and the apparent lack of receptor-destroying enzyme activity is supported by the fact that the erythrocytes can be used repeatedly.

Antigenic properties

Two serological types of vesicular stomatitis virus have been identified by virus neutralization and complement-fixation tests, and are known as the Indiana and New Jersey strains. Since then, many other isolates have been examined but all have been found to be one or other of these two serotypes. Precipitin reactions are also applicable and two bands of precipitation are formed which are sufficiently specific to distinguish between the two main serotypes.

An agent, called Cocal virus, which was isolated in Trinidad from mites collected from jungle rodents is morphologically indistinguishable from vesicular stomatitis virus and is closely related serologically to the Indiana strain but not to the New Jersey virus. Further studies with several strains of vesicular stomatitis virus, including isolates obtained from equines in Argentina and Brazil suggest that the Indiana serotype can be divided into three subtypes, Indiana 1 for the classical strain, Indiana 2 for the Cocal and Argentina viruses and Indiana 3 for the Brazil isolate.

There is no evidence, so far, that any of the strains of vesicular stomatitis virus share common antigens with other members of the rhabdovirus group.

Cultivation

The virus grows well in embryonated hens' eggs following inoculation by the amniotic, allantoic or yolk sac routes and pocks are produced on infected chorioallantoic membranes. The chick embryos usually die within one or two days. Vesicular stoma-titis virus also grows readily in almost every cell culture system in present use and produces a rapid, destructive cytopathic effect. Variants forming large and small plaques on monolayers of kidney cells have been described. Nearly all mammalian species can be infected with vesicular stomatitis virus under experimental conditions and most develop lesions similar to those in cattle. The virus can also be adapted to grow in mosquitoes.

Development

Studies on the viral growth cycle of vesicular stomatitis virus are limited and there are conflicting reports of the mode of entry of the virus into the host cell. Some workers believe that attachment of the virion to the cell surface (at its truncated end) is followed by fusion of the viral envelope and the cell membrane, with release and penetration of the nucleoprotein into the cytoplasm. Others consider that the cell surface membrane invaginates and closes round the adsorbed virus particles to form an intracytoplasmic vesicle. Once inside the vesicle the virion is degraded by cellular enzyme activity and the viral nucleic acid enters the cytoplasm.

Characteristically, the development of vesicular stomatitis virus is similar to that of other rhabdoviruses and occurs by a process of budding. The site of maturation of vesicular stomatitis virus largely depends on the host cell type and mostly occurs at plasma membranes; but with some strains e.g. the New Jersey serotype, maturation also occurs at intracytoplasmic membranes. Unlike rabies virus, the envelope of vesicular stomatitis virus is not formed intracytoplasmically in association with a viral matrix and there are no readily detectable cytoplasmic inclusions.

An interfering component called the 'T component' has been described in cultures following serial undiluted passage of vesicular stomatitis virus. Electron microscopy shows that the 'T component' consists of small truncated virus particles which are antigenically indistinguishable from the normal bullet-shaped (B) particles. The interfering action of 'T' particles occurs early in the replication cycle of 'B' particles and the effect is very similar to the von Magnus phenomenon which is thought to be due to the presence of 'incomplete' virus particles in the infectious inoculum.

Pathogenicity

In cattle, vesicular stomatitis is characterised by a short incubation period of 3–7 days, mild fever and the sudden appearance of vesicles on the tongue, dental pad, lips and buccal mucosa. The vesicles erupt rapidly and erosion of the surface epithelium follows. The resultant irritation causes profuse salivation and anorexia. In most cases, the lesions persist for only a few days. Outbreaks in milking cows have been described in which the vesicles or erosions extend the full length of the teat with, on occasions, complete sloughing of the teat. Under these conditions, milking is impossible and mastitis may develop. A 'reverse age susceptibility' has been described with vesicular stomatitis since adult cattle appear to be much more susceptible to infection than calves and the disease has seldom been reported in cattle of less than 1 year of age.

In horses, the clinical signs are similar but the lesions are usually confined to the dorsum of the tongue whilst in pigs there are usually vesicles on the snout and lips as well as foot lesions which give rise to lameness. The disease occurs naturally in racoons and deer and these may constitute a reservoir of infection. In man, the virus may be inapparent or it may cause an influenza-like disease which is characterized by fever, sore-throat and general malaise lasting for a few days. In one laboratory fifty-four cases have been reported.

Experimental pathogenicity

Almost all species can be infected experimentally and cattle, sheep, horses, pigs, rabbits and guinea-pigs develop lesions when inoculated into the tongue. Intraperitoneal infection of virus in unweaned mice and intracerebral inoculation of adult mice and guinea-pigs give rise to fatal encephalitis. Guinea-pigs inoculated intradermally into the foot-pads quickly develop vesicles like those of foot-and-mouth disease; and may also show lesions in the liver and kidneys. Cotton-rats, rabbits, ferrets, hamsters and chinchillas are susceptible to the virus and chickens, ducks and geese can be successfully infected in the tongue and foot. Experimental infections of deer show that they are susceptible to the virus and may develop a short term infection somewhat similar to that of swine.

However, exposure of experimental animals to vesicular stomatitis virus frequently produces negative results. Virus swabbed on the intact epithelium of the tongue or gums of cattle, sprayed into the nostrils or ingested by them, fail to produce the disease. Nor are lesions produced by the intradermal, intramuscular or intravenous routes, although cattle exposed to the virus by these methods do produce both neutralizing and complement-fixing antibodies. On the other hand, virus applied to abrasions of the epithelium of the mucosal surface or inoculated intralingually gives rise to vesicles of the typical disease in both young and adult stock.

Pathology

Within a few hours of infection the virus reaches the cytoplasm of the prickle cells in the Malpighian layer causing an accumulation of oedematous fluid. As the fluid accumulates, vacuoles appear which, in turn, coalesce to form vesicles as more and more cells become involved until, finally, large areas of the epithelium may be loosened. About 48 hours after infection the virus enters the blood stream and the temperature of the affected animal rises to 104–105°F (40–40·5°C) by the fourth day. By this time viraemia has disappeared and the vesicles which have reached their maximum size contain very high titres of virus (10^4 to 10^6/ml). There then follows a dramatic fall in the body temperature accompanied by profuse salivation and sloughing of the affected epithelium leaving a raw, bleeding surface. Lesions are also frequently present on the snout and teats, and especially on the coronary band of the hoof which may loosen and slough completely. Repair proceeds with surprising rapidity and within a few days even the most seriously affected animal may be walking about and eating. Recovered animals show high neutralizing and complement-fixing antibody titres and the majority do not succumb to a second infection. Like foot-and-mouth disease, with which it is often confused, vesicular stomatitis causes serious economic losses due to loss of weight and drop in milk yield.

Spread and transmission

In America, the disease occurs sporadically usually in the more northerly states and only in the late summer. It spreads rapidly among pastured animals, slowly or not at all in housed animals and usually disappears with the onset of the autumn frosts and snow. Field observations suggest that it tends to spread along the wooded streams rather than in the open plains and this, together with the seasonal incidence, led to the suggestion that an arthropod vector may be involved in its transmission. The virus has been recovered from naturally infected wild-caught *Phlebotomus* and *Culex* species, and multiplication of the virus has been reported in experimentally infected *Aëdes* and *Culex*. Furthermore, various species of biting diptera have been shown, experimentally, to be capable of mechanically transferring the virus. Although the evidence suggests that vesicular stomatitis virus may be transmitted by an arthropod-vector, its unique morphology and other characters place it outwith the family of togaviruses.

Vesicular stomatitis virus may occasionally be transmitted by indirect means through contact with contaminated objects such as food and water troughs polluted with saliva from cases of the disease; and abrasions of the mucous membrane of the mouth are said to greatly favour the entry of the virus. Although it is generally agreed that direct spread among cattle and other domestic animals does not readily occur there is good evidence to show that contact between animals during an outbreak is at least partly responsible for spreading the disease.

Diagnosis

Although it is a benign disease, vesicular stomatitis is of great interest to veterinarians because of its close similarity to three other vesicular diseases, namely, vesicular exanthema, swine vesicular disease and foot-and-mouth disease. In pigs, the clinical signs of all four of these diseases are so similar that they cannot be differentiated in the field. In the laboratory, the virus can readily be isolated from vesicular fluid or affected tissue fragments by the inoculation of fertile eggs or various tissue culture systems. The recovered virus is identified by virus neutralization, complement-fixation and agar gel

Rabies

Synonyms

Hydrophobia; lyssa; le rage (Fr.); Tollwut (Ger.); rabia (Sp.).

Definition

Rabies is an infectious disease of man and animals caused by a specific virus which is usually transmitted through the bite of rabid animals to other animals resulting in a rapidly fatal encephalomyelitis, after a somewhat lengthy incubation period.

Hosts affected

Man and all warm-blooded animals including birds are susceptible to the virus of rabies but dogs, cats,

TABLE 44.2. The differential diagnosis of vesicular diseases.

		VS	FM	VE	SVD
Intralingual	Horse	+	−	−/+	−
	Cow	+	+	−	−
Intradermal	Pig	+	+	+	−
	Guinea-pig	+	+	−	−

VS = Vesicular stomatitis
FM = Foot-and-mouth disease
VE = Vesicular exanthema
SVD= Swine vesicular disease

diffusion tests. The disease may also be confirmed by the detection of complement-fixing antigens in tissues from suitable lesions or of antibody in the serum. Animal inoculation tests whereby virus material is inoculated intralingually into horses, cattle and pigs are most useful since vesicular stomatitis affects all three species; foot-and-mouth disease virus only the cow and pig, and vesicular exanthema virus usually only the pig. However, cattle inoculated with vesicular stomatitis virus intravenously or intramuscularly fail to develop the disease. Guinea-pigs may also be used since they are highly susceptible to the intradermal foot-pad inoculation of the viruses of vesicular stomatitis and foot-and-mouth disease but not to the viruses of vesicular exanthema and swine vesicular disease (Tables 44.2 and 47.1).

Control

Recovered animals develop high titres of neutralizing and complement-fixing antibodies in their sera and are immune to reinfection by the same type of virus. Despite this, however, artificial immunization is not practised. Although quarantine may be an effective way of controlling vesicular exanthema and foot-and-mouth disease in certain countries, it has not been successful in controlling vesicular stomatitis.

cattle and wild carnivores such as wolves, foxes, coyotes, skunks, jackals and hyaenas are mostly affected. In addition, vampire bats and some insect-eating and fruit-eating bats may also act as natural hosts of the virus.

History

Rabies is one of the oldest diseases known to mankind and there is a report that it existed in India five thousand years ago. Democritus described the disease in dogs and domestic animals in 500 BC and Aristotle (300 BC) was the first to draw attention to the danger of being bitten by a rabid dog.

Various contradictory theories were advanced through the ages to explain the cause and origin of rabies and, less than a century ago, it was generally believed to develop spontaneously. However, in 1804, Zinke first demonstrated the infectious nature of the saliva from a rabid dog by inoculating the material into a healthy dog which later developed the classical symptoms of rabies and this observation, which was subsequently confirmed by other workers, led to the introduction of quarantine regulations and other control measures in Scandinavia in 1826. The next milestone in the history of rabies was the all-important discovery by Pasteur and his colleagues

(1881–89) that the disease was caused by an infective agent and that the central nervous system was the actual seat of infection. Not only did Pasteur and his associates prove conclusively that the agent is invariably present in pure and concentrated form in the central nervous system but they also showed that it could be modified by serial animal passage so as to induce immunity without producing the disease. In 1885 Pasteur performed the first human inoculation with anti-rabies vaccine on a peasant boy who had been severely bitten by a rabid dog. There were no ill effects and the boy did not develop rabies. Later, in 1903, Remlinger demonstrated the filterability of the causative agent and, in the same year, Negri drew attention to the diagnostic importance of the specific intracytoplasmic inclusions, which now bear his name, in the ganglion cells of rabid animals; and which made possible a method for the rapid microscopical diagnosis of the disease.

Distribution
The first recorded epizootic of rabies dates from 1271 when the disease was responsible for widespread losses among wolves and foxes in Southern France and in some other regions of Western Europe. From the late thirteenth century rabies gradually spread throughout Europe and outbreaks are known to have occurred in England in 1613 and among domestic dogs in urban areas in Italy during 1708. By the early part of the nineteenth century the whole continent of Europe, including the United Kingdom, was badly affected. In later years, conditions gradually improved and fewer cases were reported from the more northerly countries including Great Britain, Denmark, Sweden and Norway. The introduction of legislation by the British Government in 1897 resulted in a marked decrease in the incidence of rabies, from an average of 256 human deaths per year in the previous decade to only 8 per annum during the five-year period up to 1902. In the 17-year period prior to 1903 no fewer than 3056 animals, of which 2604 were dogs, are known to have died in the whole of Great Britain. Thereafter, Britain remained free from the disease until the end of the World War I when a dog, which was believed to have been smuggled into the country by a returning serviceman, subsequently developed rabies and caused a new outbreak of urban rabies which lasted until the end of 1922, involving no fewer than 328 confirmed cases in domestic animals, of which 312 were dogs. During the next 45 years, when almost 100 000 animals were imported under licence, Britain remained free from rabies apart from 27 cases that occurred in quarantine. Of these, 25 were dogs and the other two were in a leopard imported from Nepal in 1965 and a cat imported from Kenya in 1969. Nearly all of these cases were of the 'dumb'

variety. The only other case of rabies in animals in Great Britain over the same period occurred in 1966 in a rhesus monkey which had been imported direct to a research laboratory. Eight cases of human rabies were confirmed in Britain during this period but in each case the infection was acquired abroad.

In October 1969 rabies was reported in a dog in Camberley, England; the first to have occurred in imported animals outside quarantine in the United Kingdom for 47 years. This animal showed symptoms of the disease 10 days after its release from a 6 month period of quarantine and died 4 days later. One month later, a second dog in the same kennels developed symptoms of rabies and was destroyed; the disease being confirmed by laboratory examination. Although there is insufficient evidence to show whether the dogs acquired the infection abroad or in the quarantine kennels it is, perhaps, significant that a third dog which died from rabies in the same premises 3 months earlier is known to have been involved in a fight with a stray dog a month before leaving India.

In February 1970, a further case of rabies in a dog following quarantine occurred in another part of England. This animal showed no symptoms of the disease during its stay in the kennels but died from the 'dumb' form of rabies 3 months after its release from quarantine. No further cases have been reported and the infection does not appear to have spread to other animals. These cases, together with three others that died between $6\frac{1}{2}$ and $7\frac{3}{4}$ months in quarantine kennels, suggest that unusually prolonged periods of incubation do occasionally occur in dogs with rabies.

At the present time, rabies occurs in most parts of the world except the continents of Antarctica and Australasia and a few other regions such as Eire, Norway, Sweden, Finland, Portugal, Cyprus and Japan. These territories have remained free from rabies largely because of their stringent regulations concerning the entry of dogs and cats. Several countries including Australia, New Zealand, New Guinea, Iceland and some islands of the Pacific and Caribbean Seas have never had rabies, apart from a few isolated cases in imported animals. On the other hand, severe epizootics are frequently reported in other island communities such as Sri Lanka and the Philippines, and the disease is endemic in many parts of Africa, Asia and both North and South America. Since the end of World War II rabies has again become rife in many regions of Western Europe where red foxes and, to a lesser extent, wolves and badgers are mainly responsible for the spread of infection. In India, the incidence of rabies remains very high and it is estimated that over 200 000 people are vaccinated annually following exposure to infection. In the United States of America there are now few human deaths from rabies but about 20 000 people receive post-exposure treatment every year.

Properties of the virus

Until recently, surprisingly little attention has been paid to the rabies virus despite its importance in both human and veterinary medicine and the recent rapid advances in electron microscopy, cytochemistry and cell culture techniques. Evidence that the viral nucleoprotein contains RNA and that the intact virion possesses helical symmetry similar to a myxovirus led to its being classified as a member of the genus *Rabiesvirus* in the family *Myxoviridae*. Further studies of the virus in infected cell cultures, particularly by electron microscopy, showed that the rabies virus is morphologically very similar both in shape and in size to members of a group of some two dozen RNA viruses which includes vesicular stomatitis virus, Mount Elgon bat virus and, perhaps, vervet monkey or Marburg disease virus (Plate 44.1b, between pp. 548a and 549). As a result of these later observations rabies, vesicular stomatitis and other bullet-shaped viruses have been placed in a single taxonomic group — Rhabdovirus — lying between the myxoviruses and togaviruses.

Morphology

In negatively stained preparations the rabies virus may appear as filamentous, bell-shaped or bullet-shaped structures about 180–250 nm in length by 75 nm in diameter. The bullet-shaped virion is rounded at one end and flat or truncated at the other, the whole being surrounded by a fringe of short, pointed projections (6–7 nm long) similar to that of a myxovirus. Throughout the longitudinal axis of the virus particle runs a central cylindrical core consisting, apparently, of a tightly coiled internal filamentous component arranged in the form of a double helix of ribonucleoprotein. In rabies and vesicular stomatitis viruses, about 30 turns of the strand are evident. The nucleoprotein of rabies virus, as in myxoviruses, is synthesised in the cytoplasm and the virion is assembled on the surface of the infected cell. Its envelope, which is probably composed of two membranes of different densities, is derived from the host cell membrane as the mature particles are released by a process of budding. By negative contrast staining, the surface structure of the rabies virion consists of an arrangement of hexomeres which has been described for some plant viruses but not for other animal rhabdoviruses.

Haemagglutination

Rabies virus produces haemagglutinins when propagated on baby hamster kidney (BHK-21) cells maintained in media containing 0·4 per cent bovine albumin and no serum. The optimum conditions for the test include a serum (inhibitor)–free medium, low temperature (0–4°C), low pH (6·2) and the use of day-old chick or, preferably, goose erythrocytes. It is emphasised that rabies haemagglutinin-inhibitor is present in high titre in sera of many mammals and is difficult to remove even after adsorption by 25 per cent kaolin at pH 9·0. It is also interesting to note that erythrocytes pretreated with rabies virus are still capable of being agglutinated by the same strain of rabies virus and, furthermore, that receptor destroying enzyme has no effect on receptors of the erythrocytes for rabies virus. This latter observation suggests that the rabies virion is deficient or even totally lacking in neuraminidase activity. In both respects, the rabies virus differs from typical myxoviruses.

Chemical composition

The nucleic acid of the rabies virus consists of single-stranded RNA as shown by staining with acridine-orange and by the failure of 5-bromo-deoxyuridine (BUDR) to block replication of the virus in tissue culture. The virus is readily inactivated by lipid solvents and emulsifying agents and probably possesses a lipoprotein haemagglutinin.

Physicochemical characters

The virus is very resistant to autolysis and putrefaction and may remain viable in autolysed brain tissue for 7–10 days. It will also survive lyophilization and will persist for months in infected nervous tissue in 50 per cent glycerol. Infectivity in tissues is also retained at 4°C for several weeks and at lower temperatures for many months but the virus is labile at room temperature after only a few days. Repeated thawing and freezing will inactivate the virus and exposure to ultraviolet irradiation, proteolytic enzymes, acid pH, bile salts, formalin, 20 per cent ether and to ordinary environmental conditions of light, heat and air will rapidly reduce its infectivity. It is usually destroyed by boiling for 2 minutes and is inactivated in about 15–30 minutes at 56°C. Inactivation also occurs following exposure for 15 minutes to 1 per cent formol, 3 per cent cresol or 0·1 per cent mercuric chloride. Infected cell culture fluids are inactivated within 2 hours by a concentration of 1/6000 β-propiolactone which is used in the preparation of some inactivated vaccines. When dried from the frozen state *in vacuo* and stored at 4°C, the virus will maintain its titre for several years. It deteriorates rapidly in dilutions containing less than 0·1 per cent tissue extract unless a stabilising protein is added to the diluent. Phosphate buffered saline at pH 7–9 containing 2 per cent inactivated normal guinea-pig serum or 0·75 per cent bovalbumin fraction V is a satisfactory diluent for studies of the virus.

Antigenic properties

All strains of unmodified virus isolated from naturally occurring cases, so-called 'street virus', resemble each other closely in antigenic structure. Minor antigenic differences may be detected by serum neutralization tests but seldom by cross-protection tests in animals. Like many other virus infections, rabies-infected cells produce a number of soluble antigens of several sizes. Precipitin tests yield a single line when purified virus is allowed to react with anti-rabies serum and two additional lines occasionally appear due, it is believed, to breakdown products of the virion. A soluble complement-fixing antigen has also been described which is about 12 nm in size, is stable between pH 6 and 10 and can be separated into trypsin-resistant and trypsin-sensitive components. These slight variations in antigenic structure are of academic interest only and are of little importance in relation to the efficacy of anti-rabies sera and vaccines. The rabies virus is not related antigenically to other members of the rhabdovirus group although one of the Indiana subtypes of vesicular stomatitis virus and Cocal virus share common antigens.

Strains of the natural disease and attenuated laboratory strains may differ widely as regards their biological characters in laboratory animals, e.g. length of incubation period, invasiveness and histopathology, but individual strains cannot be accurately differentiated by any of the serological tests as yet available. Thus, there is only one immunological type of rabies virus and specific antibodies are readily detected by complement-fixation, serum neutralization and agar gel diffusion tests. The serum neutralization test is the serological test of choice. Complement-fixation is less suitable because of difficulties in obtaining stable antigens and because of the relatively short period during which complement-fixing antibodies are present.

Street virus

Strains of rabies virus occurring in animals under natural conditions ('street virus') form a complete antigenic community but differ from each other in terms of virulence, length of incubation period and type of histological lesion produced. They also vary in their fixation, some become fixed almost immediately, others after 50–60 passages and some not at all. Most strains are highly virulent but a few, such as the African strain known as 'oulou fato' are of reduced invasiveness and are seldom pathogenic for man.

Fixed virus (virus fixé)

Pasteur and his colleagues observed that dogs inoculated intracerebrally with a suspension of brain from a rabid dog developed typical rabies after an incubation period of 1–2 weeks and died within 3 weeks. The same material inoculated into rabbits invariably produced paralysis, followed by death, in about 14–19 days. However, after between 40 and 80 serial intracerebral passages the incubation period was reduced to about 7 days. This procedure produced a number of irreversible changes in the biological properties of the virus which, in its altered form, was designated 'fixed virus' or 'virus fixé'.

Different strains of 'street virus' vary in their virulence and also in their capacity to become fixed; the more virulent they are the easier they become fixed. The phenomenon of fixation is characterised by:

(1) a marked increase in the rate of multiplication as 'fixed virus',

(2) a progressive shortening of the length of the incubation period (4–9 days in rabbits), according to the strain, and which remains constant and irreversible,

(3) increased neurotropic affinities for the rabbit and regularity of symptoms which are exclusively the paralytic form rather than the furious form,

(4) failure to produce typical Negri bodies; the few inclusions present being very small with only small numbers of basophilic granules, and

(5) increased virulence for its host (rabbit) but decreased virulence for other animal species.

'Fixed viruses' can be produced by repeated serial passage through other animals, also. Most anti-rabies vaccines are prepared from, or are derived from, some form of 'fixed virus'.

Growth of rabies virus

Rabies can be transmitted to a wide range of laboratory animals such as hamsters, mice, guinea-pigs, white rats and rabbits in order of decreasing susceptibility. Various routes of inoculation can be used but the intracerebral and intramuscular methods are most widely employed. Although they are not so susceptible as some other species, rabbits are especially suitable for rabies investigations because their constant susceptiblity serves as a standard of comparison for strains and they invariably develop the paralytic form of the disease and are safe to handle. Guinea-pigs are very susceptible and are frequently used for the isolation of virus but they tend to show symptoms of nervous excitement and may be dangerous to handle. Young white mice (e.g. Swiss Albino) and young hamsters are probably used more than any other species because they are cheap, uniformly susceptible, easy to handle and maintain, and have a short (5–7 days) but constant rabies incubation period. Intracerebral inoculation of rabies virus into day-old chicks usually gives rise to a fatal paralysis but older chicks may recover. Strains of rabies virus that grow under natural conditions (street virus) are relatively difficult to cultivate in embryonated eggs and tissue cultures because, presumably, they possess a highly specific neurotropism.

In 1913, Noguchi claimed to have successfully propagated the virus by incubating small pieces of rabid brain tissue together with pieces of rabbit kidney tissue in ascitic fluid but, unfortunately, his results were not confirmed. Attempts to grow the virus in spinal ganglia and other nervous tissues were also unsuccessful. In 1930, five successive transfers of rabies virus were made in chick embryo brain and heart tissues *in vitro*, and it was clearly demonstrated that chick embryo fibroblasts were highly susceptible to rabies virus. Moreover, during the period 1936–37 there were a number of reports that the virus could also be grown in Maitland-type cultures of minced embryonic mouse brain tissue suspended in Tyrode's solution containing added serum or plasma. Since then, rapid progress has been made in the development of cell culture techniques and in 1945 Parker and Hollander were able to maintain rabies virus for 57 passages in suspended mouse-embryo brain cultures. By 1958 the virus had been propagated and serially transferred on cultures of mouse and hamster kidney cells and a cytopathic effect had been observed, albeit irregularly, on monolayer cultures of hamster kidney epithelial cells and mouse fibroblasts. Although many cell-types will support the growth of rabies virus, relatively few cells are infected, the cytopathic effects are poor and the virus titres are low. An important exception to this general rule is provided by continuous lines of the human diploid cell strain WI-26 and baby hamster kidney cells (BHK21 clone 13) in which almost 100 per cent of cells are infected and there is a marked cytopathic effect. In the hamster kidney cultures the highest titres are obtained after 6–7 days of incubation at 33–35°C, rather than at 37°C. Tissue culture methods are ideally suited for the preparation of vaccines although, on occasion, the yields are disappointingly low because much of the virus remains cell-associated. Chick embryo and some other cell cultures infected with rabies virus show interference when exposed to Western Equine Encephalitis, Eastern Equine Encephalitis or poliomyelitis viruses, but it is not yet clear whether the interference is due to small amounts of interferon being elaborated by the rabies infected cells or if some other factor is involved. In general, interferon is detected only in the presence of large amounts of infective rabies virus and the titres of interferon *in vivo* are higher than those *in vitro*. In this respect, rabies and Newcastle disease viruses are very similar.

From 1938, onwards, important advances were also made in the cultivation of rabies virus in the developing chicken embryo. For this purpose 5- or 6-day-old embryonated eggs were preferred and the virus was inoculated on the developing chorio-allantoic membrane. Rabbit-fixed strains grew well on the infected membrane as well as in the central nervous tissue of the embryo until it was about 2 weeks old. From this time on, the virus titres gradually diminished and ultimately disappeared completely.

In January, 1939, Leach isolated rabies virus from the brain, salivary glands and lachrymal glands of a 14-year-old girl who died from rabies after a 4-day illness. Virus was not recovered from whole blood, spinal fluid, kidney, pancreas, liver, spleen or adrenal tissues. An unusual feature of this case is that the patient is believed to have acquired the infection through the mucous membranes after exposure to the licks of a dog that died from rabies 1 week before she became unwell. This, therefore, is a very rare example of transmission of the rabies virus by simple contact of intact mucous membrane. The strain, which is known as the Flury strain, was inoculated in the form of infected human brain tissue, intracerebrally into 1-day-old chicks. In 30 days' time the chicks showed signs of paralysis and the virus was serially passaged in baby chicks until the incubation period fell to approximately 6 days. As the result of this procedure the pathogenicity of the virus was greatly reduced for mammalian hosts. At the 136th chick passage level the Flury strain of Leach and Johnson was adapted by Koprowski and Cox (1958) to the 7-day-old developing chick embryo. During this regime of serial egg passage the virus characters changed and it spread extraneurally, became pantropic and was present in all the embryonic tissues. After 40–50 transfers, a single intramuscular injection of this low egg passage (LEP) virus produced immunity in dogs without harmful effects. Moreover, after about 180 passages the virus, which was termed the high egg passage strain (HEP), produced immunity in cattle and humans, without evidence of disease, when administered by the intramuscular route. A modified avianised strain similar to that of the Flury virus was also developed by Komarov and Hornstein (1953), and was designated the Kelev strain.

Development of the virus

Titres of rabies virus propagated in a wide variety of cell types are often disappointingly low, due to the progeny virus particle being strongly cell-associated. However, higher titres are obtained in certain cell lines (e.g. BHK21) or after adaptation of the virus in other cell systems. Studies of the replication cycle of rabies virus in cell cultures show that many of the infected cells continue to grow and divide although large plaques of specific viral antigen can be demonstrated in the cytoplasm by fluorescent antibody staining methods. In other cell systems the antigenic components appear only as small fluorescent particles scattered throughout the cytoplasm. Intracytoplasmic inclusion bodies may be seen in suitably stained 'flying' cover-slip preparations and there is recent evidence that they consist of viral protein and contain both DNA and RNA. Cell lysis may or may not readily occur and, in some types of culture, chronic infections are obtained where the virus may continue to be produced for prolonged periods, if not indefinitely, without interfering with cellular growth. It is interesting to note that similar kinds of chronic or persistent infections have been observed, or deliberately induced, with many members of the myxovirus group and some other 'membrane-forming' viruses.

Antiserum will specifically inhibit the growth of the rabies virus in cell cultures but may not effect a permanent cure because direct intracellular transmission of virus can occur during mitosis. It is interesting to speculate that direct cell-to-cell transmission of virus in the presence of antibody might also occur *in vivo* and give rise to a state of latency in animals exposed to infection, whether vaccinated or not.

With the animal rhabdoviruses, ribonucleocapsid formation appears to occur exclusively in the cytoplasm and is frequently located near plasma membranes or intracytoplasmic membranes. With rabies, however, the production of ribonucleocapsid is commonly associated with the formation of cytoplasmic inclusions (Negri bodies) and maturation mostly occurs at plasma membranes.

Immunofluorescence studies on the growth cycle of the HEP strain of Flury virus in cultures of chick embryo fibroblasts, show that less than 1 per cent of infected cells contain viral antigen throughout the cytoplasm after 48 hours of incubation. However, the percentage of fluorescing cells gradually increases and reaches 100 per cent by the sixth day. The initial change, as seen under the electron microscope, is the appearance of an homogeneous mass in the cytoplasm on 'day-one' of incubation. These massed accumulations of protein material, or viroplasm, interspersed with numerous dense filamentous ribonucleoprotein structures constitute the ground substance of the intracytoplasmic matrix which appears as an acidophilic inclusion body under the light microscope. Within, or closely contiguous with the matrix, are found large numbers of uniform rod-shaped rabies virions, mostly with 'empty' cores. Immunological fluorescent and ferritin-conjugated antibodies indicate that the filamentous strands in the intracytoplasmic matrices are incorporated into viruses leaving the cellular membrane and constitute the nucleocapsid of the mature virion.

Maturation and release by budding sometimes occur from the inner surface of large intracytoplasmic vacuoles or, more frequently, from the plasma membrane at a late stage in the developmental cycle. Fully mature virions are invested with a double membrane, and the outer layer of this envelope is contiguous with the surface cell membrane or the endoplasmic reticulum of the cytoplasmic vacuole. In contrast to this, assembly of the brain-adapted virus particle is strictly limited to the periphery of the cytoplasmic inclusions and never occurs around the surface of the cell. Thus, the site of rabies virus assembly is neither exclusively within the intracytoplasmic membranous system nor at the surface cell membrane, but varies according to different combinations of virus and host cell.

In spite of numerous similarities found between members of this rapidly expanding genus, it is interesting and, perhaps, significant that the animal rhabdoviruses are bullet-shaped and their ribonucleoprotein site is cytoplasmic whereas the plant strains are bacilliform in morphology and have a nuclear site of ribonucleoprotein synthesis.

Pathology

With the exception of Negri bodies, the gross and histological changes in tissues of affected animals are not pathognomonic for rabies. The most prominent pathological change in cases of natural disease is a non-purulent polioencephalomyelitis associated with perivascular lymphocytic infiltration. The inflammatory lesions occur mostly in the pons, medulla, upper brain stem and thalamus which are also the sites from which the highest titres of virus are obtained. It is also significant that these areas can be reached directly via cranial nerves infected through bites on the head and face or via the peripheral nerves and spinal cord. As with other viral infections of the central nervous system there is usually evidence of varying degrees of neurone degeneration including necrosis (particularly in the hippocampus, cerebral cortex and medulla) together with glial proliferation around damaged nerve cells. These aggregations of glial cells are termed Babes' nodes and have been recognised for many years as a prominent feature of the disease.

The one pathognomonic lesion which distinguishes rabies from all other infections of the central nervous system is the presence of acidophilic inclusions within the cytoplasm of infected neurones. These are the well-known Negri bodies, named in honour of Adelchi Negri who first described them, albeit as protozoa, in 1903 (Plate 44.3c, facing p. 564). These inclusions are specific for rabies and are mostly found in pyramidal cells of the hippocampus and in the cerebellar Purkinje cells of Ammon's horn. On occasion, they may also be demonstrated in the nerve cells of other tissues such as the salivary glands.

For a rapid diagnosis, several impression smears

are made from the cut surface of the hippocampus, cerebral cortex and cerebellum on each side of the brain and stained by Sellers' method but tissue sections generally give a clearer picture and are preferable. With Sellers' method, the Negri bodies are identified as magenta or bright cherry red intracytoplasmic inclusion masses containing a variable number of dark-blue or black granules — the inner bodies or 'Innerkorperchen'. The presence of inner bodies which may appear as small colourless granules against the pink background of the matrix, with some stains, is generally regarded as an essential criterion for the positive identification of rabies and should not be confused with anything else since they do not occur in intracytoplasmic inclusions associated with most other viral diseases, e.g. dog distemper. The natural position of the Negri body is intracytoplasmic but during the process of preparing sections and especially impression smears, this pattern may be distorted and several typical Negri bodies may be found entirely outside the neurone. The Negri body must not be confused with a nucleolus which is intranuclear in position and appears as a small bright red particle against the blue background of the cell. Red blood cells and interstitial tissue stain pink. Negri bodies vary considerably in size and shape but are mostly spherical, oval or elongated structures ranging from 0·24 μm in the smallest to at least 27 μm in the largest forms. As with many other viral inclusions, immunofluorescence staining techniques show that the Negri body may contain specific viral antigens early in the replicative cycle of the virus.

Epidemiological features

Rabies is almost invariably caused by the bite of a rabid animal and the greatest hazard exists when a considerable amount of infected saliva is carried into a deep puncture wound. In exceptional circumstances the virus may pass through intact mucous membranes (vide supra) or be transmitted by aerosol infection as may occur in caves inhabited by large colonies of infected bats.

The amount of virus required to initiate infection varies considerably and depends not only on the virulence of the strain of virus but also, to a large extent, on the susceptibility of the patient. Foxes are believed to be about one hundredfold more susceptible than skunks. Hamsters are particularly susceptible and much more so than guinea-pigs, mice and other rodents. Ruminants are also highly susceptible to rabies but dogs and humans are relatively resistant.

Following exposure, the rabies virus gains access to the subcutaneous tissues where it may persist for 3–4 days before it begins to travel centripetally along the nerve routes to the central nervous system.

However, in the opinion of some workers it enters the nerve cells within 4–5 hours and cannot be detected at the site of infection after 10–12 hours. There is very little evidence that the blood stream is concerned with the dissemination of rabies virus following peripheral infection.

In experimental infections the virus travels along the axons of nerve cells at about 3 mm/hour and reaches the spinal cord in approximately 3–7 days, where it replicates and spreads to the brain. Successful infection of the brain is followed by further replication. The infected brain cells are destroyed and, when a sufficient number have been affected, the classical signs of rabies appear. It is emphasised, however, that clinical symptoms are not always present and there is clear evidence that the virus may persist in the brain of experimentally infected rats, guinea-pigs, bats and foxes for many months after the initial infection.

In naturally occurring cases the virus may spread from the brain along peripheral nerves to reach other tissues and particularly the salivary glands where it multiplies and enters the saliva which is the commonest source of infection in a bite wound.

Susceptible wild-living animals, particularly foxes, wolves, skunks, jackals, racoons and coyotes, constitute the most important residual focus of rabies infection. This sylvatic type, as it is called, is not only the most prevalent form of rabies but also the most difficult to control because mass immunization programmes or significant reductions in the population of proven wildlife vectors are impracticable. Although rabies is more prevalent in wild animals, the domestic dog is still the most important source of human infection, despite the recent decline in the incidence of rabies among urban dogs in many countries throughout the world. The epidemiology of rabies can never be regarded as static and there are numerous examples over the years of changing patterns in the epidemiology of the disease. For example, in Germany during and immediately after the first world war, dogs were held to be responsible for over 70 per cent of the 13 000 confirmed cases in animals and 90 deaths in humans. On the other hand, in the epidemic which followed the end of World War II, foxes, which were not incriminated in the first outbreak, were responsible for more than 60 per cent of all notified cases in animals, although they were still subordinate to dogs as a potential danger to man. (Of 33 human deaths no fewer than 23 were caused by bites of rabid dogs).

Although virus titres in the saliva of confirmed cases of rabies in dogs vary widely, the saliva is believed to be infective in only 50–60 per cent of rabid dogs at the time of the bite, and the presence of virus is generally limited to the few days before death. In a few cases, virus is excreted about 2–4 days before the first onset of symptoms and, on very rare occasions, virulent virus may appear at irregular intervals in the saliva of vaccinated dogs. Recent experimental work has shown that rabies virus may be present in the saliva of skunks for periods of up to 14 days before signs of the disease appear. Only very rarely is virus shed in blood, urine, milk or other secretions and, because the virus is readily destroyed outside the body under normal conditions, it is unlikely that excretions and secretions will remain infective for long periods of time. There is little evidence that animals acquire infection by feeding on the carcases of rabid animals but the possibility cannot be excluded.

The duration of the incubation period varies widely in all species and the ability of the virus to spread to the central nervous system depends on a variety of factors. Different species of animals are more susceptible than others to the virus and younger animals are generally more susceptible than adults. The distance of the bite wound from the central nervous system is important and in man the incubation period following a facial wound (about 30 days) is shorter than when the wound is on the arm (40 days) or the leg (60 days). Other factors which may influence the course of infection include the virulence, invasiveness and concentration of inoculated virus, the amount of nervous tissue near the site of the wound, the degree of trauma and the type of animal inflicting the bite. It is claimed that wolf bites are more serious than urban dog bites because the saliva of wild-living carnivores has a higher hyaluronidase content which has been shown experimentally to increase the permeability of the tissues and to enhance the virulence of certain strains of rabies virus.

Because of the high rate of infection amongst wild animals and domestic cats and dogs, together with the facility of the cell-associated virus to develop chronic infections of cell cultures, there has been a good deal of speculation in recent years concerning the possible existence of symptomless carriers of the virus, and of recovered or abortively infected animals. It is well established that blood-licking bats of the *Chiroptera* family constitute an important reservoir of infection in large areas of Central and South America, that many of them carry the virus without showing clinical symptoms of the disease, and that they frequently infect cattle and man by biting at night. Although bats can infect each other by biting, particularly during fights at mating-time, the mode of transmission of the virus in these densely populated areas of hibernating, latently infected bats has never been fully understood. However, in 1962 our knowledge of the route of transmission and the pathogenesis of bat-rabies was greatly extended by Constantine who showed that all carnivores contracted rabies when held in bat-proof cages placed in densely populated caves. The only possible method of infection was airborne and it has been suggested that latently infected bats in caves acquire the infection from their own kind by the respiratory route. In at least two human cases respiratory infection is thought to have occurred during visits to infected caves. Rabies in insectivorous bats was first reported in California in 1953 and, subsequently, in other species of bats belonging to the sanguivorous and fructivorous groups. Further reports have indicated that the virus may be present in the mouth secretions for as long as 16 months without clinical signs and that bat-rabies is present elsewhere in America and, to a lesser extent, in Europe and other parts of the world. It is emphasised, however, that not all bats are latently infected with the virus and that many show progressive paralysis ending in death.

Throughout its long history, rabies has been one of the most feared infectious diseases of mankind because of its distressing symptoms and the invariably fatal course of the clinical disease. With the exception of two possible recent cases in America, there are no authenticated reports of human patients having recovered from clinical rabies. So far as animals are concerned there has been general agreement, until quite recently, that recovery of dogs and cats from clinical rabies was so rare as to be classified as a biological curiosity. Today, opinion has changed and many workers are of the opinion that some animals may survive and, indeed, that a few may act as symptomless carriers of the virus. In experimentally infected animals the virus has been demonstrated in the brain for many months without producing symptoms, although the clinical disease can be provoked in these animals by trauma. In a report from Ethiopia in 1964, a virus isolation of 'true' rabies virus was obtained from the saliva of a dog which remained clinically healthy for four years after the sample had been taken. Not only do these observations disclose the existence of asymptomatic carriers and shedders of rabies virus but they also provide a clue to the problem of people dying from the disease following the bite of an apparently healthy dog.

Clinical signs

Man

The incubation period of human rabies averages from 30 to 60 days, with a range of 2 weeks to more than 5 months depending on the severity of the bite and its distance from the brain. It is seldom more than 90 days but periods of up to 2 years in length have been recorded. The early symptoms of rabies are headache, anorexia and vomiting. There may also be slight fever and although patients may complain of a dry throat and extreme thirst, they are disinclined to drink. An early symptom of some diagnostic value is a sensation of tingling or pain around the site of infection which gets progressively worse and the patient becomes restless, apprehensive and excitable. This is followed by an obvious fear of swallowing due to painful spasms of the pharyngeal muscles while drinking (hydrophobia), and in rare cases the patient shows maniacal symptoms and violence. Most patients die during a phase of delirium but in some the disease may progress to generalised paralysis and the patient dies in prostration usually 2–6 days after the onset of the clinical disease. Once clinical signs develop death is virtually certain, although a few well-documented accounts of human recovery from the disease have been reported recently.

Dogs

The incubation period in natural outbreaks of dog rabies averages from 3–8 weeks but a high proportion of cases develop the disease within 4 months of infection. On the other hand, it may be as short as 10 days or, in rare instances, as long as a year. In the United Kingdom approximately 50 per cent of the cases occurring in quarantine develop the disease within one month of their arrival, but the incubation periods of these cases are generally unknown. The clinical course of the disease which usually lasts for only 3–7 days, or exceptionally for 10–12 days, can be divided into three phases: the prodromal, the furious and the paralytic or dumb stage.

Towards the end of the incubation period and 2–3 days before the onset of typical clinical signs a number of premonitory or prodromal symptoms set in. The dog has a subtle change in temperament, becomes strange in its behaviour and capricious in its habits. Some become more affectionate than usual but others become more irritable. Additional signs are an alert, troubled look, restlessness, aimless snapping and barking at imaginary objects and licking at the site of the wound. There may also be a slight fever, dilation of the pupils with a wild staring of the eyes, photophobia and decreased corneal reflex. By about the third day after the onset of the illness the dog enters the furious stage which lasts for 3–7 days. It becomes irritable, restless and nervous and tends to shun people and hide in dark corners or under furniture. Sometimes it will snap and bite without provocation or bark repeatedly as if in pain. Often the appetite becomes depraved and the dog refuses its normal food but readily chews unusual objects like stones, sticks, earth and clothing. Most animals are constipated and make frequent strenuous attempts to defecate. Restlessness increases and the dog may stray long distances from home. As it wanders aimlessly it becomes more irritable and vicious and it is at this stage that the animal is most dangerous because it will not hesitate to bite any moving object or anyone who tries to molest it.

During the furious phase there is a characteristic change in its bark or it may howl in an unusual tone due to paralysis of the laryngeal muscles. Salivation and frothing at the mouth become progressively more profuse and the dog has difficulty in swallowing and drinking. Convulsive seizures, delirium and complete muscular incoordination are present shortly before the animal dies. If it does not die at the climax of a convulsive seizure it passes into the paralytic stage during which the disease progresses to paralysis of the entire body, thence to coma and death.

In cases when the second or furious phase is extremely short or absent, the animal rapidly enters into the paralytic or 'dumb' stage when the dog is rarely irritable and seldom bites. The most characteristic symptom of this form of the disease is lower jaw paralysis when the mouth falls open, the tongue protrudes and the dog is unable to eat or drink. Although extreme lethargy develops and the dog is disinclined to bite, it is dangerous to handle the animal or examine its mouth at this stage because the saliva may be infective. Paralysis of the pharyngeal muscles often causes the dog to emit a choking sound which suggests to the owner that there is a bone stuck in the throat. Finally, there is exhaustion and complete incoordination of movement. The animal gradually becomes comatose and dies from the second to the fourth day after the onset of the paralytic stage.

Cats

These animals are very susceptible to rabies and the clinical signs, which are similar to those seen in dogs, last for only 2–4 days before death intervenes. Affected cats tend to hide in secluded corners and mew continually with a hoarse voice. Rabid cats are often more vicious than dogs and readily attack man and other animals by biting or scratching the face of the victim.

Horses

The clinical signs of rabies in the horse are similar to those of tetanus. In the early stages of the illness it often gnaws or rubs the area of the wound, appears easily frightened with staring eyes and dilated pupils and may become aggressive for short periods only. There is progressive paralysis, regurgitation of food and liquid through the nose and stiffening of the hind quarters, ataxia and death.

Cattle

Affected cattle are usually very restless, excited and

aggressive. They paw the ground continuously, bellow loudly, bite or clamber on their stalls as if trying to escape. In many cases there is grinding of the teeth, increased salivation and choking as if a foreign body were lodged in the throat. Veterinary examination of mouth and throat for the presence of 'wooden tongue' or 'choke' can be a hazardous undertaking in endemic areas due to the likelihood of becoming infected through scratches and abrasions on the hands during the examination. Other clinical signs include salivation, abdominal pain, diarrhoea, rectal straining, a drop in milk production, pruritus at the site of the bite and emaciation. Paralysis of the hind quarters occurs followed by death 3–6 days after the first signs of illness.

Sheep and Goats
The clinical signs are similar to those of cattle and the infected animals become unusually restless and aggressive. There is also evidence of dyspnoea, licking of the lips and, as with many other animal species, increased sexual desire with the affected animals continually mounting each other.

Swine
Affected pigs show an early irritative stage, are easily frightened, root up the ground and gnaw or rub at the site of the injury. Later, they may become very aggressive and bite other animals or man. They usually die in 2–4 days with paralysis.

Poultry
Adult hens have a high natural resistance to rabies virus, and affected birds frequently recover. In the fatal form of the disease they show fear, run around wildly with the feathers ruffled, cry hoarsely and will attack other birds, animals and man, with beak and claw. Ataxia develops, they frequently fall and die after 2–3 days with paralysis.

Clinical diagnosis
In human cases there should be little difficulty in obtaining a clinical diagnosis if there is a reliable history of a rabid animal bite several weeks or months prior to the patient showing the characteristic symptoms of the disease. However, the diagnosis may be missed in cases where there is no history of exposure due, perhaps, to forgetfulness on the part of the patient or his relatives or where the clinical signs resemble those of poliomyelitis, other virus diseases affecting the central nervous system and, even, tetanus which is not unknown following bites by animals. In these circumstances, a confirmatory diagnosis can only be obtained by the isolation of virus from the saliva (blood and other tissues are invariably negative) or from the brain and spinal cord at autopsy. Serological tests for the detection of rabies antibody in the serum of a patient during the clinical illness are generally unsatisfactory, but promising results have recently been reported with an indirect fluorescent antibody technique. In the great majority of cases the laboratory is chiefly concerned with obtaining a diagnosis in urban dogs or other animals known or suspected to have bitten a patient. Speed and accuracy are essential since the action to be taken may largely depend on the outcome of the laboratory examinations.

It is emphasised that every effort should be made to trace the source of infection and the animal suspected of being rabid must be captured and placed under strict quarantine. This is necessary so that the clinical signs can be closely observed and the disease permitted to run its full course. To some extent the size and abundance of the Negri bodies, and the clarity of the inner bodies, are related to the length of the clinical illness and for this reason premature killing of suspected cases should be avoided. In special circumstances when it may be necessary to destroy the animal the head, which must not be mutilated by shooting, is removed and rapidly despatched to the laboratory in a suitable, waterproof, metal container which must be sealed tightly and clearly labelled. The head should not be treated with disinfectant or deep-frozen because of damage to the cells and consequent hindering of the histological examination. The sealed container should be placed within a second larger watertight container holding cracked but not 'dry ice'. A detailed clinical history should accompany the specimen and it is an advantage if the clinician or field officer is able to communicate directly with the diagnostician.

In general terms, the laboratory diagnosis of rabies involves histopathology, biological examination and serology but, since there is often a public health hazard, the procedures adopted will largely depend on whether a person has been bitten or not.

The procedure to be adopted *in cases of bite* can be considered under four headings:

If the animal is alive and apparently healthy
The animal must be confined and observed closely for clinical signs of the disease. These usually develop within two days and almost always within the first week. Should symptoms not appear by the fourteenth day the case can be considered negative and no further action is necessary. Treatment of the human patient may be postponed until this stage unless the bites are on the head, face or neck by an animal in a known endemic area.

If the animal dies in quarantine or if the animal was ill at the time of the bite

A provisional diagnosis can generally be made on the basis of the history and clinical examination of the animal. Suitable fresh material is sent to the laboratory and treatment of bitten persons is started immediately, without awaiting confirmation of rabies. If the sick animal is suffering from rabies it will usually die within two or three days. If not, and the symptoms are suggestive of rabies, the animal should be destroyed and the head and neck despatched by the most expeditious means for laboratory diagnosis.

If the animal is found dead

The whole carcase should be sent promptly to the diagnostic laboratory accompanied by as detailed a history as possible. The treatment of persons at risk depends on the clinical history unless the animal has died in an endemic area and the bite wounds are on the head, face or neck. In most cases treatment is withheld for approximately 48 hours until a provisional diagnosis has been obtained by histological or immunofluorescence methods.

If the animal escapes or cannot be identified

During an epizootic of rabies, it may be suspected that the biting animal is one of the recognized wild animal vectors that transmit rabies among themselves and to other animals. Under these circumstances, the patient should receive a course of anti-rabies treatment.

In other cases when there is no history of a bite but where the patient has been in close contact with a rabid dog, careful consideration of the circumstances must be given to decide whether or not treatment should be commenced.

Laboratory Diagnosis

When removing the brain from the cranium of a suspected animal, every precaution must be taken to protect the operator from the possibility of infection. It should be borne in mind that the wearing of rubber gloves does not afford complete protection against splinters of infected bone. If the brain has been removed under field conditions where facilities for animal inoculation are not available, portions of the brain should be sent to the laboratory for confirmatory diagnosis. The brain tissues selected should include portions of the hippocampus, cerebellum and cerebral cortex from each side, and these should be placed in 50 per cent glycerol-saline to preserve the virus. No refrigeration is required. On arrival, the pieces of brain are thoroughly washed in several changes of sterile physiological saline solution. Since glycerinated tissues do not usually produce satisfactory smears on a slide and are generally unsuitable for immunofluorescence staining, a number of freshly prepared unstained brain smears fixed in acetone-free methyl-alcohol and dried at room temperature without blotting should also be despatched to a laboratory where fluorescent antibody tests are available.

Microscopical demonstration of Negri bodies

Freshly prepared smears or histological sections of tissues are stained and examined for the presence of Negri bodies. Tissue sections can be stained suitably by a large variety of methods including Schleifstein's modification of Wilhite, Stovall and Black, phloxine-tartrazine or Mann's method. A good deal of practice may be required to obtain the best results and for this reason many workers still prefer haematoxylin and eosin for routine use (Plate 44.3a, facing p. 564). For impression smears, the differential staining method of Sellers is widely used because of its accuracy and simplicity but other stains such as Giemsa are also suitable. With Sellers' stain, the Negri body may be recognised as a well-defined magenta or reddish purple mass, generally rounded in shape with a variable number of dark-blue to black basophilic inner bodies clustered within its matrix. The inclusions are normally within the cytoplasm but frequently may appear outside the affected cell due to cell damage in preparing the smears. Nevertheless, they are readily identified by their characteristic morphology and staining reaction which contrasts well with the blue stain of all parts of the nerve cell and the background of interstitial tissue which stains rose-pink. Red blood cells can be differentiated from the reddish purple inclusions by their bright red or orange-red colour. In most positive tissue sections Negri bodies are located within the cytoplasm of the affected cell, usually between the nucleus and one corner of the neurone and, because of the variation in size, the larger forms may distort the outline of the cell. It is emphasised that in smear examinations the intracellular position of the Negri body is not required as a diagnostic criterion. A serious drawback to the histological method is the difficulty of differentiating some Negri bodies from other viral or non-specific inclusions in the preparations. For example, acidophilic inclusions of canine distemper also occur in the cytoplasm but do not possess basophilic inner bodies. In fox encephalitis and infectious canine hepatitis, acidophilic inclusion bodies are formed but are situated intranuclearly. Negri bodies must also be distinguished from small acidophilic bodies that occur in the outer loops of the hippocampus and which have been designated 'lyssa bodies'. These do not contain inner bodies and are thought to be indicative only of degenerative changes of the neurones. Other types of non-specific inclusions are not infrequently present in the brains of non-rabid cats and adult white mice.

When typical Negri bodies are identified there can be no doubt about the presence of rabies (Plate 42.2b, facing p. 474a, and plates 44.3a, c, facing p. 564). However, a positive diagnosis is not always easy by this method and in doubtful or even some negative cases a confirmatory diagnosis must be obtained by animal inoculation and other means.

Animal inoculation

For isolation of the virus, the brain or other tissue specimens are prepared as a 10 per cent suspension, by grinding in a suitable physiological solution or in 10 per cent guinea-pig serum saline. It is not usually necessary with brain tissue to add sterile sand as an abrasive but the operator should exercise great care while mincing and macerating tissues such as salivary gland. Bacterial contamination must be avoided and the tissue suspensions are generally treated with 500 units of penicillin and 1 mg. of streptomycin per ml. The material is allowed to stand for 1 hour or is centrifuged at low speed for 10 minutes to sediment the coarser tissue particles which might block the fine needle of the syringe used for inoculation. White laboratory mice or hamsters are generally used for the isolation and identification of rabies virus. Young animals 3–6 weeks old are preferred since the skull is soft and because they are more susceptible to rabies than adult mice. It should be noted, also, that certain strains, such as the high egg passage (HEP) Flury vaccine virus, are pathogenic for infant mice, but not for mature mice, and will produce paralysis and death with an infectivity titre comparable to that obtained with street virus. Groups of 6 mice are inoculated intracerebrally under ether anaesthesia using a half-inch 26 gauge needle with 0·02–0·04 ml of the suspension. Mice which die during the first few days are discarded, death being attributed to trauma or other non-specific cause while healthy survival for 3 weeks is generally interpreted as a negative diagnosis. The mice are examined daily and, if the specimen contains rabies virus, some of the mice will show signs of obvious malaise between the sixth and eighth days post-inoculation. The usual symptoms are muscular tremors, incoordination of gait and paralysis terminating in death. Other clinical signs to look for are ruffled fur, arching of the back, flaccid paralysis of the legs and, sometimes, conjunctivitis. (Rabies virus may be present in the epithelial cells of corneal smears taken from mice several days before death). Infected mice almost always develop clinical symptoms within 17 days of inoculation and in the routine laboratory it is customary to discard the surviving mice at the twenty-eighth day. Occasionally the incubation period may be as long as 21 days and if the circumstances warrant it the mice must be held for 40–60 days or even as long as 90 days. In such cases, it is advisable to re-test the original material in larger groups of mice including infant mice under 5 days of age. This procedure enables one mouse to be sacrificed daily, after the sixth day, and examined for the presence of infection.

To establish a positive diagnosis the mouse brains are removed and examined microscopically for Negri bodies. These are usually quite numerous after intracerebral inoculation especially in mice showing paralysis for 24 hours before death. A confirmatory diagnosis can be obtained by serum-neutralization tests in mice or by immunofluorescence. The complement-fixation test is seldom used in routine rabies diagnosis due to difficulties in obtaining a satisfactory standard antigen. It should be borne in mind that there are a number of specific viruses and other microorganisms that produce encephalitis and paralysis in mice. These include *Listeria monocytogenes*, toxoplasma species and such viruses as lymphocytic choriomeningitis, Aujeszky's disease and some other herpesviruses, ectromelia, vaccinia, poliovirus type II and several togaviruses.

Immunofluorescence

Fluorescent antibody staining is now widely used in rabies diagnosis since it provides a rapid, reliable and highly specific means of detecting the viral antigen. In experienced hands, the results are at least equal to mouse inoculation tests and are infinitely superior to microscopical examinations for the presence of Negri bodies.

Antibody in the form of hyperimmune serum is obtained by inoculating horses with a series of injections of an attenuated strain of rabies virus. The globulin is then precipitated by ammonium chloride and conjugated with fluorescein isothiocyanate (F.I.T.C.). In the diagnostic test, one portion of the conjugated antibody is diluted with a suspension of normal mouse brain, another with a suspension of rabid mouse brain. Duplicate smears of test brain and positive control smears from known rabid brains are fixed in acetone for about 4 hours at –20°C and then flooded with one or other of the conjugated serum-mouse brain suspension mixtures. The smears are then incubated in a moist chamber for 30 minutes at 37°C, washed carefully for 10–20 minutes in buffered saline, air dried and examined under the ultraviolet light microscope. The mixture of fluorescein-antibody conjugate plus the suspension of normal mouse-brain will produce particles or plaques of bright yellow-green fluorescence in those areas in the test and control positive smears containing specific viral antigens, thereby indicating a positive diagnosis of rabies. In contrast, the **control** mixture of fluorescein-antibody conjugate absorbed

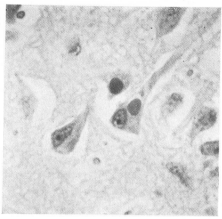

44.3a

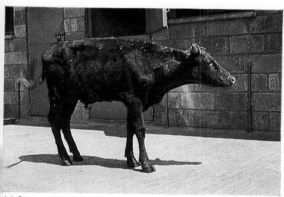

44.3b

44.3c

44.3a Street rabies. Section of dog brain showing large acidophilic inclusions (Negri bodies) in the cytoplasm of affected neurones. Haematoxylin eosin stain, × 420.

44.3b Naturally occurring case of bovine ephemeral fever. The short febrile reaction is associated with inappetance, loss of bodily condition, lameness, joint pains and general stiffness. (Courtesy of Dr W. B. Martin.)

44.3c Detail of section of hippocampus of brain of dog dying from rabies. The pale internal structure of the acidophilic intracytoplasmic inclusion is a characteristic feature of the Negri body of rabies. Mann stain, × 480.

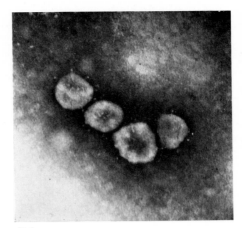

45.1a

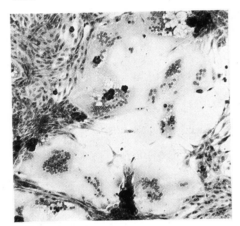

45.1b

45.1a Electron micrograph of coronavirus of avian infectious bronchitis. Notice the loss of many of the club-shaped surface projections after storage at 4°C for 18 hours. Direct examination of infective allantoic fluid, ×80 000. (Courtesy of Dr J. B. McFerran.)

45.1b Formation of numerous large multinucleate syncytia by primary pig kidney cells inoculated four days previously with the haemagglutinating encephalomyelitis virus of swine. Notice the absence of inclusion bodies. Giemsa stain, ×44.

with the suspension of mouse rabid brain will **not** produce fluorescence in either the test or known positive smears. This modification of fluorescent antibody staining has the advantage that it includes two controls in the test system (Fig. 44.1.) As with all fluorescent antibody staining methods the test is highly specific in the hands of experienced workers although interpretation of the results may sometimes prove difficult because of non-specific fluorescence. An additional advantage of the method is that specific viral antigens can be detected in mice as early as the third day following inoculation and before infective virus can be demonstrated by other methods.

Other procedures which are useful for confirmatory diagnosis are serum-virus neutralization tests performed in mice or in susceptible cell-culture systems, and agar gel precipitation. The latter is not highly sensitive and negative results are frequently misleading, but a positive reaction with adequate controls is significant.

cination is usually carried out after exposure with the object of aborting virus before it attacks the central nervous system. Prophylactic vaccination is recommended for veterinarians and other persons in occupations where there is a high risk of exposure to rabies. In man the incubation period is relatively long (30–90 days) and there is usually sufficient time available for the development of active immunity. Nevertheless, vaccination should be started within seven days of the patient having been bitten by a rabid animal or by an animal suspected of having been rabid; or it should be commenced immediately if the wounds are in the region of the head, face or neck. Hyperimmune serum or immune gammaglobulin obtained from horse or sheep serum may be administered to advantage within 48 hours, especially in severe bites of the head, because the incubation period is usually too short for vaccination to be effective. Twenty-four hours later a course of vaccine injections is started. About 20 per cent of human

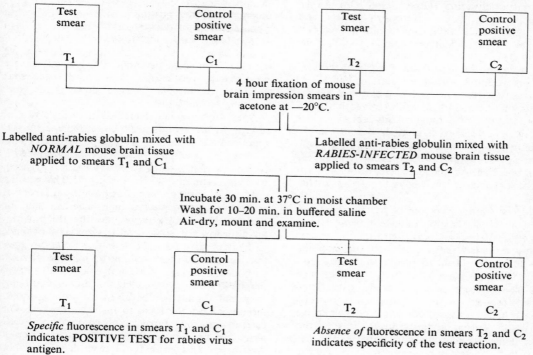

FIG. 44.1. Fluorescent rabies antibody (FRA) test.

Control by vaccination

There is only one antigenic type of rabies virus and antibodies can be induced by vaccination. The immunization procedures applied to animals and man usually differ because in animals they are generally prophylactic, whereas in humans vac-

patients develop serum sickness following treatment with horse or sheep antisera, but this will largely be overcome when purified human immune globulin becomes available. There is little doubt that passive-active immunization by the administration of anti-rabies serum and 14 daily inoculations of vaccine is still the most effective treatment for the exposed human subject. However, if the patient is already showing symptoms of rabies or if clinical signs develop during the course of vaccination, all efforts at treatment will be in vain as the patient will almost certainly die.

Various types of vaccine have been used since the original vaccinal method of Pasteur in 1885 and more are still being developed. They are of two main types, live and inactivated. The strain used by Pasteur to produce his dessicated rabbit spinal cord vaccines had first been passaged over 100 times in rabbits. This attenuated or 'fixed-virus' strain, which is safe to handle, has been maintained solely in the rabbit since November, 1882, and is the basis of many of the present attenuated or inactivated anti-rabies vaccines.

The methods used to inactivate the Institut Pasteur rabbit fixed-virus in the preparation of anti-rabies vaccines include the following: heat (Babes, 1912), phenol (Fermi, 1907; and Semple, 1911), phenol-glycerine (Umeno and Doi, 1921), ether (Alivisatos, 1922), chloroform (Kelser and Schoening, 1930), ultraviolet irradiation (Webster and Casals, 1940; and others) and β-propiolactone (Peck, 1955).

Until recently, the Fermi and Semple phenolized fixed-virus vaccines with their variants, an ultra-violet irradiated fixed-virus vaccine and Peck's beta-propiolactone-treated duck embryo vaccine comprised almost the entire range of anti-rabies vaccines employed in man. Each is given in a course of 14 single daily subcutaneous injections but pain, swelling and acute discomfort may occur around the point of injection. An adequate level of immunity is said to be conferred about 14 days after treatment has started.

Semple or Fermi type phenol inactivated fixed-virus vaccines have the disadvantage of being derived from nervous tissue and may sensitize about 1 in 4000 to 1 in 10 000 patients who will develop side effects during a course of injections varying from transient nervous signs and paralysis to serious allergic reactions, encephalitis and, even, death. These distressing sequelae occur more frequently in people who have had a previous course of rabies vaccine. The risk of neuroparalytic accidents is such that nervous tissue vaccines should not be given unless there is clear evidence of exposure to rabies. Thus, in Great Britain and other rabies-free countries the use of Semple-type vaccine is not recommended save in the most exceptional circumstances.

In view of the fact that latent rabies infection can be activated by adrenocorticotropic hormone and that the development of immunity from rabies vaccines is depressed by corticosteroids, these substances should not be used for the treatment of allergic reactions to rabies vaccines or antisera.

Inactivated nervous-tissue vaccines have proved of value in veterinary medicine and the inoculation of phenolized infected sheep or goat brain affords protection for horses and wild animals up to a year.

Because of the risks of neuroparalytic accidents, repeated attempts are being made to eliminate the encephalitogenic factor from anti-rabies vaccines either by chemical means or by cultivating the vaccine-virus on embryonated eggs or cell cultures derived from hamster, pig or dog kidney cells. Of these, Peck's duck-embryo, freeze-dried virus vaccine is the most widely used in human medicine. Not only is it inactivated with β-propiolactone and rendered safe to use, but it causes fewer local reactions and constitutional upsets than sheep or rabbit brain vaccines. While Peck's vaccine is now in general use and is recommended for pre-exposure immunization of veterinary surgeons and others in 'high-risk' occupations, evidence from field experience during the 1969–70 outbreaks in Great Britain suggests that it has a weaker antigenic potency than nervous-tissue vaccines. The recommended course of duck-embryo vaccine consists of at least 14 daily injections followed by booster doses 10 and 20 days after the last daily dose. Wherever possible, serological tests should be carried out after prophylactic vaccination of humans and, when necessary, additional booster doses given until neutralizing antibodies are detected.

Apart from the inactivated duck-embryo vaccine, several living avianised vaccines have also been produced. Of these, the low egg passage (LEP) and high egg passage (HEP) Flury strains, developed by Koprowski and Cox in 1948, and the Kelev vaccine strain of Komarov and Hornstein (1953) have proved invaluable for the pre-exposure immunization of dogs and other domesticated animals. The fact that dogs inoculated intramuscularly into the thigh with 3 ml of the low egg passage (LEP) virus resist challenge with street virus for as long as three years, suggests that the vaccine is very suitable for mass prophylactic vaccination in dogs. It is emphasised, however, that the LEP strain is intended for use in adult dogs only and should not be given to puppies under 3 months of age, to cats or to any other species. When used in cats, the animal may become ill and vaccine virus can be demonstrated in the central nervous system. The LEP strain is of low virulence for rabbits but is pathogenic for cattle, mice, hamsters and guinea-pigs. The HEP strain of Flury virus is more highly attenuated and is recommended for use in puppies, adult dogs, cats, wild animals and cattle. Indications for the use of the Kelev avianised virus vaccine are similar to those for the HEP (Flury) strain.

It is emphasized that in preparing non-inactivated rabies virus vaccines for use in animals care must be taken to ascertain if the living modified virus is excreted in the saliva since the excretion of such a strain may create a public health hazard for man and some species of animals.

Use of the HEP strain, as a living modified virus vaccine for humans is still in the experimental stage but, in a vaccination trial, serum neutralization studies showed that a single intradermal dose produced a good immune response. The HEP strain has also been adapted to human diploid cell cultures and reasonably high neutralization titres are obtained when tested in monkeys.

More recent developments in the field of anti-rabies vaccines include an inactivated, purified rabies vaccine (PRV) of mouse brain origin from which the encephalitogenic factor has been removed by chemical methods. The PRV vaccine does not cause a local reaction and may prove suitable for use in human patients.

Since 1960, several rabies vaccines have been produced in a variety of cell culture systems including hamster kidney cells, chick embryo fibroblasts and hamster fibroblasts. One of these, the ERA strain of rabies vaccine, was passaged in chick embryos and then adapted to pig kidney cells, and produces immunity for up to five years in dogs and four years in cats. A second strain of vaccine grown in the NIL line of hamster fibroblasts and inactivated with β-propiolactone has good immunogenicity for dogs, cats and cattle, and has been imported into the United Kingdom for use in quarantine kennels. All hamster kidney cell vaccines are highly immunogenic and the Flury LEP virus grown in BHK-21 cells and inactivated with acetylethyleneimine is an excellent immunogen for dogs and cattle.

Cell culture systems suggested for human use include primary hamster kidney, sheep embryo kidney, chick embryo fibroblasts and the human diploid cell strain WI-38. Inactivated vaccines from Flury HEP virus adapted in WI-38 cells are much more antigenic in monkeys than HEP virus grown in chick embryos.

Work is currently in progress to produce purified subunit rabies virus vaccines for human prophylaxis in an attempt to overcome the harmful side-effects which may accompany nervous tissue vaccines. In the United Kingdom an immunogenic subunit vaccine has been recently prepared by disintegrating rabies virions grown in BHK-21 cells, by means of detergents. The vaccine is then inactivated with acetylethyleneimine.

Field control

The success of any control programme for rabies depends on the eradication of the disease from domesticated dogs and cats and the limitation of the spread from wild-living animals, so far as is practicable. The urban type of rabies is best controlled by firm legislation demanding the ruthless destruction of all stray animals, strict confinement, restraint and muzzling of domestic pets while the campaign is under way, mass vaccination within a wide radius of the infected focus, the provision of adequate diagnostic facilities and a continual and energetic publicity campaign. In rabies-free countries there are regulations imposing severe restrictions on the importation of dogs, cats and some other animal species together with compulsory vaccination and/or quarantine for periods of 6 months or longer. The effective control of rabies in wildlife reservoir hosts is extremely difficult to achieve but every effort should be made to reduce the numbers of possible wildlife vectors by poisoned baits, trapping, shooting and gassing of earths, burrows and setts. In rural areas where sylvatic rabies is endemic, stray dogs should be eradicated and prophylactic immunization of domestic dogs and cats carried out to prevent further spread and to protect their owners.

In the United Kingdom, the importation of some mammals, including dogs and cats, is controlled by Orders made under the Diseases of Animals Acts. Insofar as rabies is concerned, the Importation of Dogs and Cats Order of 1928 requires all imported *Canidae, Felidae* and *Hyaenidae* to be detained in approved quarantine premises for a period of 6 months. Other Orders restrict the importation of bats, primates and certain other species to approved zoological gardens and research establishments, and rare animals to certain approved institutions. Additional legislation includes Orders governing the importation of destructive animals such as musk rats, mink and coypus, with a view to preventing them establishing themselves in the wild.

Vervet Monkey Disease

Synonyms

Green monkey disease; Marburg virus disease.

Definition

A severe febrile infectious illness of man, especially laboratory workers, handling infected monkey tissues or cell cultures.

Hosts affected

Man is chiefly affected but the monkeys from which the infection is usually acquired rarely show clinical signs of disease.

History and distribution

A previously unknown infectious disease of monkey handlers and laboratory workers occurred with dramatic suddenness in the autumn of 1967 in the European cities of Marburg, Frankfurt and Belgrade. Seven of 31 patients died of an acute febrile illness which was subsequently traced to direct contact with the tissues or cell cultures of a single batch of African green monkeys (*Cercopithecus aethiops*) imported via London airport from Uganda.

Aetiology

The precise nature of the causative agent has not yet been fully established and all attempts to isolate rickettsiae, bacteria, toxoplasms, fungi and mycoplasms have been unsuccessful. Recent laboratory investigations have resulted in the isolation, in guinea-pigs and in a baby hamster kidney (BHK) cell line, of a virus having properties similar to those of rhabdoviruses.

Pathogenicity

In man, the incubation period probably lies between 4 and 9 days and the clinical symptoms include malaise, headache, high fever, vomiting, diarrhoea and involvement of the central and peripheral nervous systems with impairment of consciousness. The period of convalescence is usually prolonged. In the 1967 outbreak there were 31 human cases of severe illness with 7 deaths, but there were no overt cases of illness in the monkeys. Experimentally infected monkeys all develop a uniformly fatal infection irrespective of the dose or route of inoculation. In the early stages of the illness, even though the animals are febrile, they appear to be quite healthy until after the incubation period of 6–13 days when their condition rapidly deteriorates and death supervenes. In the later stages of the illness most affected monkeys show a petechial rash affecting principally the face, arms and thighs. The infective agent can be isolated from the blood, saliva and urine, often in considerable quantities. Guinea-pigs are highly susceptible and the intra-peritoneal inoculation of blood or other tissues from human patients results in a high temperature. Serial passage produces enhanced virulence of the agent and affected guinea-pigs show necrotic changes in the liver, spleen and lungs. Small, basophilic inclusion bodies of unknown origin occur in many of the liver cells. The infection has also been successfully transmitted to hamsters, but only after at least 9 consecutive hamster passages following initial inoculation of monkey material previously passaged 9 times in guinea-pigs and 3 times in monkeys. The disease in hamsters can be distinguished from that produced in guinea-pigs and monkeys by the development of an encephalitis and the brain contains a high concentration of the infectious agent. Intra-cytoplasmic inclusion bodies are found not only in the liver but also in the kidneys and lungs. The inclusions are pleomorphic, vary in size from 1 to 4 μm in diameter and are either round, elliptical or ring-shaped structures.

Ecology

It is generally accepted that the 1967 outbreak of Vervet Monkey Disease in man was due to direct contact with the tissues or tissue cultures of a batch of African green monkeys that were infected in Uganda, the country of origin, prior to their shipment to Europe. There is also evidence that at least one infected monkey reached each of the three European cities concerned and that they, in turn, infected other monkeys. A number of secondary cases occurred amongst staff in hospital as a result of contact with the blood of patients. It is of interest that animal attendants who cared for the monkeys during life did not acquire the infection. Little is known about the reservoir of infection, the excretion of virus from infected animals or its mode of transmission. In the United States of America, serological studies have shown complement-fixing antibody titres ranging from 1/8 to over 1/256 in about 50 per cent of African green monkeys, chimpanzees, gorillas and orang-utangs.

Properties of the virus

Tissues from infected guinea-pigs and monkeys inoculated into baby hamster kidney cells produced cytopathic effects including nuclear budding, giant-cell formation and, later, intracytoplasmic inclusions. Further studies by means of electron microscopy have shown the presence of numerous sinuous, elongated filaments frequently bent in the shape of a horse-shoe, but of variable length (150 nm to more than 2500 nm). Both ends of the filament are usually rounded but sometimes a blob of membranous material is seen attached to one end. An inner central core is surrounded by a membrane having cross-striations at right angles to its long axis, suggestive of helical symmetry. The agent is sensitive to ether and, since its growth in cell culture is not inhibited by 5-bromodeoxyuridine, its nucleic acid is probably in the form of RNA. Morphologically, it is said to closely resemble vesicular stomatitis virus, rabies virus and other members of the rhabdovirus group, but the frequent presence of several unusual morphological features, together with certain other properties, suggests that the agent may belong to a hitherto unrecognised group of microorganisms. Heat inactivation at 56°C for 30 minutes fails to inactivate the agent completely and higher temperatures or longer periods are required to bring about complete inactivation. Ultraviolet light produces complete inactivation within 2 minutes. There is little, if any, loss of infectivity on storage at room temperature (20°C), 4°C or –70°C over a period of up to 5 weeks.

Diagnosis

The organism is usually present in the blood of human

patients during the febrile phase of illness and can be isolated in primary green monkey kidney cell cultures or by the intraperitoneal inoculation of guinea-pigs. Throat washings and urine may also contain the organism and, on one occasion, it has been isolated from human seminal fluid. The agent can also be grown on a continuous line of baby hamster kidney cells with the production of acidophilic intracytoplasmic inclusions but no other cytopathic changes. In green monkey tissue cultures the cytopathic effect consists of nuclear budding, giant-cell formation and basophilic intracytoplasmic inclusions resembling those of rickettsiae and chlamydiae. Immunofluorescence is a useful aid to the identification of antigen in cells of infected cell cultures as well as in the liver, spleen, lungs, testes and the peritoneal exudates of infected guinea-pigs. Complement-fixation and serum neutralization tests may also prove of value in diagnosing the illness in human patients and in detecting carrier monkeys. Electron microscopy can be used to identify the characteristic sinuous filaments of the organism in infected tissues and in cell cultures.

Control

Adequate safety precautions are essential for the protection of laboratory workers coming into contact with the blood and other tissues of monkeys and in the preparation of cell cultures. Broad-spectrum antibiotics are ineffective in the treatment of the clinical disease.

Ephemeral fever

Synonyms

Bovine ephemeral fever: Three-day sickness: driedaesiekte: bovine epizootic fever: stiff sickness: stywesiekte.

Definition

A benign, non-contagious arthropod-borne viral disease of cattle characterized by sudden fever, stiffness, lameness and spontaneous recovery within a few days.

Hosts affected

The natural disease appears to be specific to cattle. Sheep and other domestic animals are not susceptible.

History and distribution

The disease was first described amongst native cattle in Central Africa in 1867 and may have occurred in Egypt in 1895. It was later recognized as being widespread in Rhodesia, the Transvaal, Natal and other regions of South Africa. By the late 1920s it was reported in the Dutch East Indies, Sumatra, India

and Japan, and in 1936 it was recorded over extensive regions of Australia. At the present time it appears to be enzootic in South Africa, India, Japan and parts of Australia.

Morphology

Electron microscopy reveals that the virus of bovine ephemeral fever possesses some of the characteristics of rhabdoviruses. The bullet-shaped virions have a fringe of fine surface projections and measure about 80×120–140 nm. Virus maturation takes place by budding from the cell surface and cytoplasmic vacuoles, and the progeny virions appear as rod-, bullet- or cone-shaped particles.

South African strains are mostly conical rather than bullet-shaped but serological studies indicate that they are closely related to those from Asia and Australia. The inner electron-dense core of the cone-shaped virion is in the form of a spiral rather than the tightly-wound striated component seen in bullet-shaped particles. The average height of the conical particles is 175 nm and the average basal diameter is 88 nm, giving a ratio of 2:1. From height and pitch measurements it is concluded that the internal component has approximately 10 turns per spiral, and the total length of the spiral is approximately $2 \cdot 2$ μm. The envelope surrounding the virus particle is derived from the host cell membrane.

Physicochemical properties

The virus contains RNA and is ether-sensitive, suggesting the presence of a lipid-containing envelope. Although the nucleic acid of rhabdoviruses is single-stranded RNA, it has recently been shown that bovine ephemeral fever virus contains double-stranded RNA and may not, therefore, be a 'true' member of the rhabdovirus genus.

Citrated whole blood from affected cattle remains infective for 8 days when stored at 2–4°C, but infected mouse brain suspensions in PBS with 10 per cent bovine serum show little loss of titre after 30 days at 4°C. The virus can be stored for several years at −70°C or in the lyophilized state at 4°C. Low pH (2·5) or high pH (12·0) destroys the infectivity of bovine ephemeral fever virus within 10 minutes. The virus is inactivated within 10 minutes at 56°C, 18 hours at 37°C and 120 hours at 25°C.

Cultivation

The virus has been adapted to growth in the brain of unweaned mice or hamsters. Virulent strains become stabilized after only 6 serial intracerebral passages, causing paralysis and death 2–3 days post inoculation. Propagation in new-born hamsters or mice leads to rapid loss of pathogenicity for calves. The virus can also be grown in a baby hamster kidney cell-line (BHK-21) and has recently been adapted to monkey cell-lines. Roller tube cultures prepared from the monkey kidney stable line (MS) show a cytopathic effect after 48 hours of incubation which is characterized by a granular appearance of the cytoplasm and rounding of the cells, followed by their detachment from the glass. In vervet monkey kidney cell cultures (VERO), however, minute pinpoint plaques develop 2–4 days post-inoculation and reach an average size of 1–1·5 mm diameter by the 8th–10th day. The plaques produced in the MS cells are less clear and less sharply circumscribed.

Pathogenicity

The natural disease is characterized by sudden onset of fever, stiffness, lameness, short duration and rapid recovery within a few days, as the name of the disease implies. The sharp febrile reaction is accompanied by listlessness, inappetance and a staring coat, followed by lachrymation, serous, oral and nasal discharges, lameness, joint pains and general stiffness (Plate 44.3b, facing p. 564). The stiffness often passes from one leg to another and the animal may go down and remain prostrate for 3 days or more. The clinical signs are usually accompanied by leucocytosis and marked neutrophilia. In spite of these alarming signs the animal appears perfectly normal a few hours after regaining its feet. The morbidity in enzootic areas seldom exceeds 5 per cent and the mortality rate is often less than 2 per cent. The greatest loss is in the milk yield which remains low for long periods and may be permannetly reduced. Pathological lesions may include serofibrinous polysinovitis, polytendovaginitis, periarthritis, cellulitis and focal necrosis of skeletal muscle.

Ecology

Bovine ephemeral fever is most prevalent during the rainy season when insects are very numerous, and epizootic spread is markedly influenced by wind movement. The virus is closely associated with the leucocyte fraction of the blood and the disease is readily transmissible by intravenous inoculation of as little as 0·002 ml of blood taken from animals at the height of the febrile reaction. Transmission by direct contact does not occur and the virus does not persist much beyond the fourth day after subsidence of the fever. Although definite proof is lacking, it is widely believed that mosquitoes or other biting insects are vectors.

Diagnosis

A diagnosis can readily be made from the sudden appearance of a febrile disease of cattle lasting for 2–5 days with spontaneous recovery. The seasonal occurrence and symptoms of oropharyngeal secretions, stiffness and joint pains are of value. A confirmatory diagnosis can be obtained by demonstrating neutralizing and complement-fixing antibodies in convalescent sera or by inoculating blood from viraemic patients into susceptible cattle. The virus can also be isolated from clinically affected cattle by intracerebral inoculation of unweaned mice.

Control

Recovered cattle are immune for up to 2 years but the disease is regarded as being of little consequence and prophylactic vaccination has not been attempted. Dairy cattle should be carefully nursed and provided with shade, water and food.

Rhabdoviruses of fish

Viral haemorrhagic septicaemia virus (VHSV)

Rainbow trout, brown trout and possibly other salmonid fish are subject to an acute or subacute disease called viral haemorrhagic septicaemia. It occurs during the cold months at the end of winter and beginning of spring and mainly affects young salmonids between 1–2 years of age. The incubation period is 5–20 days. The causal agent has been placed in the rhabdovirus group and is known as Egtved virus, after the name of the village in Denmark where the disease was first recognised in 1950.

Serological studies indicate that Egtved virus is predominantly of one type although a second and less frequently found serotype may exist. High-titred rabbit antisera neutralize most isolates and fluorescent antibody staining shows specific Egtved viral antigen in affected cell cultures.

Electron microscopy has shown that the virus is morphologically very similar to vesicular stomatitis virus and matures at the cell surface by a process of budding. In negatively-stained preparations, the virions show the characteristic cylindrical or bullet-shape of rhabdoviruses with a rounded end and a flat or truncated base which often carries a tail-like appendage following detachment from the surface of the host cell membrane. The viral particle measures approximately 180 × 60–70 nm and is enclosed in a membranous envelope or sheath which is studded with very fine projections.

The virus has been propagated in primary cell cultures of rainbow trout ovary and on a few continuous lines including RTG-2 (rainbow trout gonad) and epithelioid FHM (fathead minnow) cells, grown in Eagle's medium incorporating 15 per cent calf serum. Optimal growth occurs at 12–14°C and in FHM cells progeny virus first appears at 7 hours and the plateau is reached at about 24 hours. According to some workers cell lines infected with Egtved virus contain intracytoplasmic inclusions similar to those produced by rabies virus. Electron microscopy of thin sections shows filamentous helices within the cytoplasmic matrices consisting of viral nucleocapsids which, like rabies virus, probably form the internal tightly-wound striated component of the mature virion. Although the virus persists in infected cell cultures for several weeks at 20°C and for much longer periods at 4°C, affected fish appear to lose all infectivity after storage on ice for 24 hours. In freshly-obtained carcases the virus can be readily recovered from the liver, spleen and kidneys. Egtved virus is markedly ether-sensitive but does not agglutinate red blood cells. It is also sensitive to pH change and produces cytopathic effects in RTG-2 cells at pH 7·4–7·8 but not at pH 7·0–7·2.

Infectious haematopoietic necrosis virus (IHNV)

In 1941, an acute highly-fatal disease was described in young Chinook salmon in a hatchery in California. Since then the disease has been identified in Washington, Oregon and Australia. In 1953 an extensive hatchery epizootic producing mortality as high as 90 per cent in young Sockeye salmon, and involving millions of fish, was reported on the West Coast of the U.S.A.

When comparisons of the causative agents of Chinook and Sockeye salmon disease were made it was found that both possessed similar biophysical properties and produced almost identical histopathological changes which were most severe in the renal and pancreatic tissues. In both diseases the clinical signs of exophthalmia, haemorrhages and abdominal swelling were also similar. In 1967, epidemics again occurred among Rainbow trout and Sockeye salmon in British Columbia and, because of the histopathological changes and the affinity of the causative virus for haematopoietic tissues, the disease was named infectious haematopoietic necrosis (IHN).

Subsequently, it was found that the causative viruses of Chinook salmon disease, Sockeye salmon disease and IHN produced similar cytopathic changes in fish cell cultures although the effects were markedly different from those produced by VHS or Egtved virus. Nevertheless, all three viruses and that of VHS, show the characteristic bullet shape of members of the rhadbovirus group and the mean dimensions are also very similar (90 × 160–180 nm). In 1970 reciprocal neutralization tests clearly showed that the three viruses were closely related and it is now generally agreed that IHNV and the agents of Sockeye and Chinook salmon disease are one and the same. On the other hand, their relationship to the European Egtved (VHS) virus is not yet known. The available evidence suggests that Egtved virus is a distinct entity which differs from IHNV in plaque morphology and by the fact that it produces a fatal infection in both young and sexually mature salmonids whereas IHNV mostly affects fish less than 6 months old.

Spring viraemia of carp (SVC)

In 1971 a fifth fish virus was added to the rhabdovirus group when it was discovered that a bullet-shaped virus named *Rhabdovirus carpio* was the causal agent of Spring viraemia of carp (SVC) hitherto called the acute form of infectious abdominal dropsy or Carp dropsy. More recently it has been shown that *R. carpio* is also responsible for the condition known as infectious swim bladder inflammation (aerocystitis) of carp. Although Egtved and SVC agents are both bullet-shaped rhabdoviruses occurring in fish in Europe, they appear to be two distinct entities. For example, Egtved replicates best at 12–14°C and not above 22°C whereas SVC virus grows best at 20–22°C but will multiply at 31°C, also. Moreover, RTG-2 cells support good growth of Egtved but only low titres of SVC virus.

Further details of rhabdovirus diseases of fish are given in Appendix 1, Vol. 1.

Further reading

ALMEIDA J.D., HOWATSON A.F., PINTERIC L. AND FENJE P. (1962), Electron microscopic observations on rabies virus by negative staining. *Virology*, **18**, 147.

ACHA P.N. (1967). Epidemiology of paralytic bovine rabies and bat rabies. *Bulletin. Office international des épizooties*, **67**, 343.

BACHMANN P.A. AND AHNE W. (1974). Biological properties and identification of the agent causing swim bladder inflammation in carp. *Archiv für die gesamte Virusforschung*, **44**, 261.

BEATON W.G. (1969) Control of rabies. *Tropical Animal Health Production*, **1**, 56.

BEAUREGARD M., BOULANGER P. AND WEBSTER W.A. (1965). The use of fluorescent antibody staining in the diagnosis of rabies. *Canadian Journal of Comparative Medicine and Veterinary Science*, **29**, 141.

CAMPBELL J.B., KAPLAN M.M., KOPROWSKI H., KUWERT E., SOKOL F. AND WIKTOR T.J. (1968). Present trends and the future in rabies research. *Bulletin of the World Health Organization*, **38**, 373.

CHALMERS A.W. AND SCOTT G.R. (1969). Ecology of rabies. *Tropical Animal Health Production*, **1**, 33.

CONSTANTINE D.G. (1962). Rabies transmission by non-bite route. *Public Health Reports*, **77**, 287.

COX H.R. (1949). Review of chick-embryo adapted living rabies virus vaccines, with primary emphasis on use in dogs. *Proceedings of the 53rd Annual Meeting*, U.S. Livestock Sanitary Association, p. 264.

CRICK J. (1973). The vaccination of man and other animals against rabies. *Postgraduate Medical Journal*, **49**, 551.

DEAN D.J., EVANS W.M. AND McCLURE R.C. (1963).

Pathogenesis of rabies. *Bulletin of the World Health Organization*, **29**, 803.

FEDERER K.E., BURROWS R. AND BROOKSBY J.B. (1967). Vesicular stomatitis virus. The relationship between some strains of the Indiana serotype. *Research in Veterinary Science*, **8**, 103.

FERNANDES M.V., WIKTOR T.J. AND KOPROWSKI H. (1963). Mechanism of the cytopathic effect of rabies virus in tissue culture. *Virology*, **21**, 128.

GOLDWASSER R.A. AND KISSLING R.E. (1958). Fluorescent antibody staining of street and fixed rabies virus antigens in mouse brains. *Proceedings of the Society for Experimental Biology and Medicine*, **98**, 219.

GOLDWASSER R.A., KISSLING R.E., CARSKI T.R. AND HOSTY T.S. (1959). Fluorescent antibody staining of rabies virus antigen in the salivary glands of rabid animals. *Bulletin of the World Health Organisation*, **20**, 579.

GORDON SMITH C.E., SIMPSON D.I.H., BOWEN E.T.W. AND ZLOTNIK I. (1967). Fatal human disease from vervet monkeys. *Lancet*, **2**, 1119.

HACKETT A.J., ZEE Y.C., SCHAFFER F.L. AND TALENS L. (1968). Electron microscopic study of the morphogenesis of vesicular stomatitis virus, *Journal of Virology*, **2**, 1154.

HALONEN P.E., MURPHY F.A., FIELDS B.N. AND REESE D.R. (1968). Haemagglutinin of rabies and some other bullet-shaped viruses. *Proceedings of the Society for Experimental Biology and Medicine*, **127**, 179.

HANSON R.P. (1952). The natural history of vesicular stomatitis. *Bacteriological Reviews*, **16**, 179.

HILL B.J., UNDERWOOD B.O., SMALE C.J. AND BROWN F. (1975). Physico-chemical and serological characterization of five rhabdoviruses infecting fish. *Journal of General Virology*, **27**, 369.

HOWATSON A.F. AND WHITMORE G.F. (1962). The development and structure of vesicular stomatitis virus. *Virology*, **16**, 466.

HUMMELER K. (1971). Bullet-shaped viruses. In *Comparative Virology*, eds. K. Maramorosch and E. Kurstak, p. 361. London: Academic Press.

HUMMELER K., KOPROWSKI H. AND WIKTOR T.J. (1967). Structure and development of rabies virus in tissue culture. *Journal of Virology*, **1**, 152.

JENSEN M.H. (1963). Preparation of fish tissue cultures for virus research. *Bulletin. Office international des épizooties*, **59**, 131.

JOHNSON H.N. (1965). Rabies virus. In, *Viral and Rickettsial Infections of Man*, ed. Horsfall and Tamm, 4th Edition, p. 814. Philadelphia: Lippincott.

JONKERS A.H., SHOPE R.E., AITKEN T.H.G. AND SPENCE L. (1964). Cocal virus, a new agent in Trinidad related to vesicular stomatitis virus, type Indiana. *American Journal of Veterinary Research*, **25**, 235.

KNUDSON D.L. (1973) Rhabdoviruses. *Journal of General Virology*, **20**, 105.

LECATSAS G., THEODORIDIS A. AND ERASMUS B.J. (1969). Electron microscopic studies on bovine ephemeral fever virus. *Archiv für die gesamte Virusforschung*, **28**, 390.

MARKSON L.M. (1969). The laboratory diagnosis of rabies. *Tropical Animal Health Production*, **1**, 65

OLBERDING K.P. AND FROST J.W. (1975). Electron microscopical observations on the structure of the virus of viral haemorrhagic septicaemia (VHS) of rainbow trout [*Salmo gairdneri*]. *Journal of General Virology*, **27**, 305.

PLUMMER P.J.G. (1954). Rabies in Canada with special reference to wildlife reservoirs. *Bulletin of the World Health Organization*, **10**, 767.

Report of the Committee of Inquiry on Rabies (1971). Final Report. Cmnd. 4696. London. Her Majesty's Stationery Office.

SCHINDLER R. (1961). Studies on the pathogenesis of rabies. *Bulletin of the World Health Organization*, **25**, 119.

SIEGERT R. (1972). Marburg virus. *Virology Monograph*, **11**, 97.

SIMPSON R.W. AND HAUSER R.E. (1966). Structural components of vesicular stomatitis virus. *Virology*, **29**, 654.

TIERKEL E.S. (1959). Rabies. *Advances in Veterinary Science*, **5**, 183.

VAN DER WESTHUIZEN B. (1967). Studies on bovine ephemeral fever. I. Isolation and preliminary characterization of a virus from naturally and experimentally produced cases of bovine ephemeral fever. *Onderstepoort Journal of Veterinary Research*, **34**, 29.

WOLF K. (1966). The fish viruses. *Advances in Virus Research*, **12**, 35.

World Health Organization (1966). *Laboratory Techniques in Rabies*, 2nd Edition, Geneva: World Health Organization.

World Health Organization (1966). W.H.O. Expert Committee on Rabies. Fifth Report. *W.H.O. Technical Series No. 321*. Geneva: World Health Organization.

ZLOTNIK I., SIMPSON D.I.H. AND HOWARD D.M.R. (1968). Structure of the vervet-monkey-disease agent. *Lancet*, **2**, 26.

ZUCKERMAN A.J. (1970). In *Virus Diseases of the Liver*, p. 140. London: Butterworth.

ZWILLENBERG L.O., JENSEN M.H. AND ZWILLENBERG H.H.L. (1965). Electron microscopy of the virus of viral haemorrhagic septicaemia of rainbow trout (Egtved virus). *Archiv für die gesamte Virusforschung*, **17**, 1.

CHAPTER 45

CORONAVIRUSES

CHAPTER 45

Coronaviruses

In 1965 a new type of virus was isolated from naso-pharyngeal washings from human patients with common colds. Electron microscopy showed that the virus particles were very similar in shape to those of infectious bronchitis of chickens and murine hepatitis. They differed, however, from myxoviruses in that the fringe of radiating projections on the surface of the lipoprotein envelope consisted of petal or club-shaped spikes that were more widely spaced than the short slender rods of myxoviruses. The characteristic appearance of this ring of projections surrounding the virion is reminiscent of a crown, and the name coronaviruses has been suggested for this new group of viruses (Plate 45.1a, facing p. 565).

At the present time, the group includes a number of viruses that cause common colds in man, as well as avian infectious bronchitis virus, murine hepatitis virus and, probably, the virus of transmissible gastroenteritis (TGE) of pigs and the haemagglutinating encephalomyelitis virus (HEV) of pigs. Coronaviruses have also been reported in cases of neonatal calf diarrhoea and turkey bluecomb disease.

General properties

Coronaviruses are medium sized (80–160 nm) roughly spherical and sometimes pleomorphic viruses. The club-shaped projections cover only part of the surface of the virus and are less densely packed than in myxoviruses. The central core of the virion is composed of single-stranded RNA but electron micrographs have failed to reveal the presence of an internal tubular or helical nucleocapsid. Hence, their symmetry is undetermined. The viruses have lipoprotein envelopes and are sensitive to ether, chloroform and other fat solvents.

Several human serotypes have been identified some of which cross-react with murine hepatitis virus but not, so far as is known, with avian infectious bronchitis and other animal coronaviruses.

Human strains of coronaviruses are usually associated with mild upper respiratory tract infections, indistinguishable from the common cold. They can be grown in organ cultures of epithelium from the human trachea, the earliest sign of infection being the cessation of ciliary motion, and some can be isolated in monolayers prepared from an established line of human embryo lung (fibroblast) cells — L132. The cytopathic changes, which include cytoplasmic vesiculation, develop slowly and seldom involve the whole of the monolayer. A common feature seen in ultra-thin sections of infected cells is the accumulation of virions in cytoplasmic vesicles.

Avian infectious bronchitis

Definition
An acute, highly contagious viral infection of the upper respiratory tract of chickens which is characterized by depression, coughing, sneezing, tracheal rales and the accumulation of excess mucus in the bronchi.

Synonyms
Gasping disease. Infektiosen bronchitis der Hühner (Ger.): La bronchite infectieuse des gallinae (Fr.): la bronquitis infecciosa (Sp.).

History and distribution
Avian infectious bronchitis was first described in 1931 and again in 1933 as a highly fatal respiratory disease of young chickens, 3 days to 4 weeks old, occurring in certain parts of the U.S.A. The viral aetiology of the disease was confirmed in 1936 and, in the following year, the virus was successfully propagated in embryonated hens' eggs. At the present time the disease is known to occur in all parts of the world where large numbers of poultry are raised. Chickens of all ages, sexes and breeds are susceptible, but other avian species and mammals are not known to be naturally infected.

Morphology
The virus particles are roughly spherical in shape

573

and measure about 80–120 nm in diameter. They are sometimes pleomorphic, and many pedunculate forms with bulbous ends have been observed in negatively stained specimens of infected allantoic fluids. In many respects they resemble ortho- or paramyxoviruses except that the radiating spikes (20 nm in length) are widely separated and cover only part of the surface of the lipoprotein envelope. They are also more bulbous in appearance than the tightly packed fringe of slender spikes that surround the periphery of a typical myxovirus. The centre of the virion appears as an amorphous mass and there is presently no evidence that it contains a helical, tubular, internal component of nucleoprotein.

Physicochemical properties

The virion contains a central core of single-stranded RNA, which is sensitive to RNAse, and is enclosed within a capsid of undetermined symmetry. It is sensitive to treatment with alcoholic ether, bile-salts and other lipid solvents but disruption of the virion by ether or Tween 80 does not release segments of ribonucleoprotein or rosettes as occurs with ortho- and para-myxoviruses.

The stability of avian infectious bronchitis virus at 56°C varies from one strain to another. Newly isolated strains are inactivated after 15–30 minutes whereas laboratory stock cultures of chicken embryo-adapted virus may survive for up to 3 hours at this temperature. The virus retains its infectivity in water (pH 7·4) for at least 24 hours at room temperature, but will not survive for 36 hours at 37°C. It can be stored for several months at –60°C as infective allantoic or cell culture fluid. Virus in allantoic fluid is stable at pH 3·0 for 14 days and shows maximum stability at pH 7·8. It is inactivated within a few minutes at room temperature in 1 per cent formalin, 1 per cent cresol, 70 per cent alcohol and 1/10 000 $KMnO_4$.

Haemagglutination

Allantoic fluid infected with infectious bronchitis virus does not haemagglutinate erythrocytes unless it is first treated with trypsin or ether. It is believed that trypsin acts by blocking a trypsin-sensitive haemagglutinin inhibitor in normal egg fluid which may be adsorbed on to the virus or the red cell receptor surfaces, thereby preventing attachment of the virus to the erythrocyte. The inability of infectious bronchitis virus to elute spontaneously from agglutinated fowl red blood cells suggests that the virus does not possess neuraminidase. Despite the fact that virus modified by trypsin will agglutinate fowl erythrocytes held at room temperature for 45–60 minutes, haemagglutination-inhibition by specific antiserum has not yet been demonstrated.

Interference

Infectious bronchitis virus interferes with the replication of Newcastle disease virus in chickens, chicken embryos and chicken embryo kidney cell cultures; and avian encephalomyelitis virus interferes with infectious bronchitis virus in chicken embryos. It has been claimed that infectious bronchitis virus produces a synergistic effect when co-cultivated with *Mycoplasma gallisepticum* and *Haemophilus gallinarum* in chickens.

Antigenic properties

Strains of infectious bronchitis virus vary in antigenicity, and neutralization tests using death of inoculated embryos as an end-point suggest that there are at least two main antigenic variants — Connecticut and Massachusetts. Other serotypes probably exist and these may include the strains designated JMK, Cuxhaven and Australian 'T' virus. The egg-adapted Beaudette strain is antigenically related to the Massachusetts serotype and is widely used as the reference virus for neutralization tests. At least three distinct soluble antigens can be detected by immunodiffusion in virus suspensions treated with ether and fractionated by CsCl density gradient centrifugation. One of the antigens may reside in the virion while the other two are probably distributed over the surface of the virus.

Cultivation

Strains of infectious bronchitis virus are readily isolated from infected chickens by intra-allantoic inoculation of 9- to 12-day-old embryonated hens' eggs. The virus will grow on the chorioallantoic membrane without producing pocks, but the yolk sac route is unreliable because of the possibility of maternally derived antibodies in the yolk. Infected embryos are stunted or curled tightly into balls, and the volume of amniotic fluid is markedly decreased. Other abnormalities include necrotic foci in the liver, pneumonitis and nephritis. The mortality rate is generally low for the first few passages but egg-adapted strains usually kill the embryos within 48 hours.

A few strains, (e.g. Beaudette and Massachusetts,) can be grown intracerebrally in unweaned mice, producing ascending paralysis and death 3–4 hours after inoculation. Two-day-old rabbits may also be infected by intracerebral inoculation of the virus.

Different isolates of infectious bronchitis have been grown with varying degrees of success in cultures of chicken embryonic tissues but without inducing marked cytopathic changes. Some strains can be propagated in monkey kidney cell cultures but not in other mammalian cell systems. Isolates of the virus in high chicken embryo passage, such as the egg-adapted Beaudette strain, grow well in chicken kidney cell cultures with the formation of multinucleated syncytia but without the production of inclusion bodies. Plaques may be produced on agar-overlay cultures either as a result of necrosis of the infected cells or of syncytial formation. There is recent evidence that tracheal organ cultures infected with infectious bronchitis virus show rounding and sloughing of ciliated cells and complete cessation of ciliary movements.

Replication
Infectious bronchitis virus replicates within the cytoplasm of the susceptible host cell. The developing virus particle first appears 6–15 hours after infection as a crescent-shaped bulging of the cytoplasm into the vesicular lumen. As the virion matures the vesicular membrane becomes incorporated into the outer coat of the virus. There is no evidence of budding on the surface cell membrane and the replication cycle is entirely cytoplasmic by budding into the cisternae of the endoplasmic reticulum. These vesicles, in turn, open to the surface of the cell in order to release the mature virions.

Pathogenicity
Infectious bronchitis is a highly contagious respiratory infection which may involve a whole flock within a few days. Young chickens of between 1–4 weeks of age are principally affected. Clinical symptoms include marked depression, respiratory distress, tracheal rales, coughing, sneezing and nasal discharge, but the severity of the symptoms may vary considerably. The course of the illness is from 7–21 days and the mortality rate is usually about 25 per cent but may be as high as 75 per cent or more in very young chicks. In older birds, the disease is generally milder and may pass unnoticed, but economic losses result from a marked drop in egg production with many malformed, thin or soft shelled eggs of poor internal quality.

Young chickens dying from the disease show sinusitis, catarrhal tracheitis, bronchitis, congestion and oedema of the lungs and, occasionally, cloudiness and thickening of the air-sacs. In fatal cases, there are often catarrhal exudates in the nasal passages and caseous plugs in the bronchi. Intracellular inclusions are not present in stained sections of infected tissues.

Ecology
The virus is highly infectious and may be shed in the respiratory discharges for as long as 4 weeks after infection and in the faeces for up to 3 weeks. Virus may also be present in fertile eggs laid by fowls in the acute stage of the illness but the chicks that hatch from these eggs are usually not infected. Nevertheless, some workers believe that congenital infection does

occur and that it is an important factor in initial outbreaks of the disease. In most cases the virus is spread by droplet infection but indirect transmission may also occur by contaminated feed racks, water troughs, clothing and equipment.

Immunity
Active immunity results from natural and artificial infection and neutralizing antibodies are generally well developed by the third week after infection. Recovered birds are immune for about a year and do not remain carriers of the virus. Naturally acquired passive immunity is provided by the maternal antibodies in the yolk of eggs laid by hens recovered from natural or artificial infections. The serum antibody titres of chicks hatched from immune eggs remain high for about 14 days after hatching but then decline to negligible levels at about a month when the chick is again susceptible to infectious bronchitis.

Control
A variety of active and inactivated vaccines have been developed for the control of avian infectious bronchitis. Live attenuated vaccines are mostly prepared from selected serotypes which have undergone 25 or more serial passages in eggs. They are usually administered in the drinking-water or as dust or spray in the form of monovalent or bivalent vaccines. Broilers are usually vaccinated during the first week of life and again at a month old, but better results are claimed if the first exposure is delayed until the birds are 6 weeks of age or older by which time they are fully susceptible and immunologically more mature. Attenuated bronchitis vaccine combined with one against Newcastle disease have been used successfully without apparent interference with the immune response to either.

Inactivated vaccines have not been particularly successful, although a β-propiolactone vaccine has been used with some success to prevent the marked drop in egg production which is a feature of infectious bronchitis in laying birds.

Diagnosis
The history of an acute, highly contagious, respiratory infection with high mortality in chicks and a decrease of 50–100 per cent in egg production with a proportion of malformed eggs, is good presumptive evidence of infectious bronchitis. The birds do not show nervous symptoms and haemagglutination-inhibition tests do not reveal the presence of antibodies against Newcastle disease.

A confirmatory diagnosis can readily be obtained by the isolation of the causative virus. Tissue suspensions of lungs, trachea and bronchi inoculated into the allantoic cavity of 9- or 10-day-old eggs produce dwarfing and curling of the embryos. Serum neutralization tests performed in embryonated eggs or chicken kidney cell cultures are useful for detecting antibodies in serum samples collected at least 3 weeks after the onset of the clinical disease. Immuno-diffusion tests are particularly valuable for the rapid diagnosis of infectious bronchitis. The antigens used are prepared from infected allantoic fluids or other tissues. Since precipitating antibodies for infectious bronchitis are transient, the sera should be collected between the 7th–21st day after infection; the optimum time being about the 15th day.

Infectious bronchitis virus (IBV) does not cause direct haemagglutination of chicken erythrocytes and the haemagglutination-inhibition test is not suitable for detecting specific antibodies in sera of recovered birds. However, an indirect test has been described whereby anti-IBV chick serum agglutinates tannic-acid treated horse erythrocytes to which the egg adapted virus has been previously adsorbed.

Direct fluorescent antibody staining methods are of value for detecting infectious bronchitis antigen in tracheal smears of acutely affected chickens. An interference test has also been devised for testing sera for the presence of antibodies to infectious bronchitis virus, based on the inability of infectious bronchitis virus infected cell cultures to be super-infected with Newcastle disease virus. The test is carried out by adding mixtures of two-fold dilutions of the test serum and equal parts of infected allantoic fluid to preformed monolayers. After 30 hours of incubation at 37°C, the cultures are infected with 10^6 EID$_{50}$ of Newcastle disease virus, reincubated and examined for the presence or absence of New-castle disease virus CPE.

Transmissible gastroenteritis of swine

Definition
A highly contagious viral disease of swine, charac-terised by profuse diarrhoea, vomiting, dehydration and a high mortality rate in piglets infected during the first few weeks of life.

Hosts affected
Species other than swine are insusceptible and numerous unsuccessful attempts have been made to infect a wide range of experimental animals including horses, cattle, sheep, rabbits, guinea-pigs, chickens, mice, cats, dogs and occasionally human volunteers.

History and distribution
A disease resembling transmissible gastroenteritis was described in Scotland and England in 1953 and 1958, respectively; and the first detailed account was recorded in the U.S.A. in 1964. The disease has now been described in many European countries, and may also exist in Japan and the U.S.S.R. Reports that it occurs in Australasia and Africa await con-firmation.

Morphology
Filtration, ultracentrifugation and electron micros-copic studies indicate the size of the virus particle to be between 90 and 200 nm in diameter. In nega-tive contrast preparations the intact virions are mostly circular in outline but pleomorphic forms are also present. Each particle is surrounded by a double membrane which is covered with distinctive projections about 18–24 nm long. These projections are mostly petal-shaped in outline and appear to be attached to the surface of the envelope by a very narrow stalk. The distal bulbous end of the spike measures approximately 10 nm in diameter. The projections are easily detached from the virus particle during preparation of the specimen and are often seen in only a limited area of the outer mem-brane. (Plate 45.1a, facing page 565). In some particles, penetration of the phosphotungstic acid stain (PTA) into the interior of the virion reveals an electron opaque central area or nucleoid which is somewhat featureless and quite distinct in its morphology from the tubular or helical ribonu-cleoprotein inner component of the myxovirus. More recently, particles have been described with an internal beaded filament. Thus, from electron microscopic observations of carefully prepared specimens the virus of transmissible gastroenteritis is morphologically similar to avian infectious bronchitis and other coronaviruses.

Physicochemical properties
The failure of 5-fluoro 2′-deoxyuridine (FUDR) and 5-iodo 2′-deoxyuridine (IUDR) to inhibit replication of the virus in cell culture suggests that the nucleic acid core consists largely of RNA. Moreover, the infectivity of the virus is completely destroyed by ribonuclease but is resistant to deoxyribonuclease. All strains of transmissible gastroenteritis virus are inactivated by exposure to detergents, ether and other lipid solvents which suggests that there are essential lipids in the envelope surrounding the capsid.

The virus will survive in frozen tissues for several weeks and at −30°C for over 3 years. It also survives drying for 3 days at room temperature but is heat-labile to the extent that it is completely inactivated by exposure to 56°C for 30 minutes or 65°C for 10 minutes.

The pH stability of the virus has not been ad-equately studied but most workers agree that it is stable at pH 4–9, and of limited stability at pH 3. Most strains are inactivated within 1 hour at pH 2. The virus is rapidly inactivated by ultraviolet light but is not affected by exposure to 0·5 per cent trypsin for 1 hour at 37°C.

Haemagglutination

The virus does not agglutinate erythrocytes from various species of animals, and does not haemadsorb guinea-pig red cells added to infected monolayer cell cultures.

Interference

Certain non-cytopathogenic strains of transmissible gastroenteritis virus may interfere with the replication of Aujeszky's disease virus in cell cultures; and interference between transmissible gastroenteritis virus and the cytopathic effects of mucosal disease virus has been used as an indicator system for the presence of non-cytocidal strains of transmissible gastroenteritis in pig kidney cell cultures.

Antigenic properties

Serological studies, including cross-neutralization between pig-propagated and cell culture-propagated strains suggest that there is only one major serotype of transmissible gastroenteritis virus, and that there is a close antigenic relationship between strains isolated from field cases of the disease in the U.S.A., Great Britain and Japan.

Cultivation

Although earlier successful attempts to grow the virus in primary pig kidney cultures were not accompanied by visible cellular abnormalities, more recent findings suggest that most strains produce various cytopathic changes including swelling and vacuolation of the cytoplasm, rounding off and detachment of infected cells. Inclusion bodies are not produced but some workers have observed well marked condensation of the chromatin around the periphery of the nucleus. Other strains, including the Purdue TGE virus, produce a marked cytopathic effect in primary tissue culture cells of pig kidney, pig thyroid, pig testis and pig salivary gland; and some strains produce macroscopic plaques by the agar-overlay technique. The virus has also been propagated in dog kidney cell cultures.

Virus at low cell culture passage levels may produce typical clinical symptoms and high mortality when inoculated into very young specific-pathogen-free piglets, whereas virus of the 125th passage shows attenuation of pathogenicity as indicated by a prolonged incubation period and diminution of clinical symptoms in susceptible piglets.

The virus cannot readily be grown in embryonated hens' eggs or in a wide range of laboratory animals. A recent report of experimental infection of dogs awaits confirmation by other workers.

Pathogenicity

Transmissible gastroenteritis is most prevalent during the cold months of winter and early spring.

It usually affects every litter in the farrowing house simultaneously and then spreads rapidly to adjacent herds.

The morbidity rate is high in pigs of all ages and, in young unweaned piglets under 5 days of age, the mortality rate may reach 100 per cent. Fortunately, however, there is a steady decline with age and in piglets over 16 days old the mortality may be as low as 0–10 per cent. The virus is highly contagious and tends to spread rapidly both within the affected group and to neighbouring farms. The incubation period is very short, 12–18 hours, and ailing piglets show profuse foetid diarrhoea, weakness and incoordination of gait. In many cases the onset of diarrhoea is preceded by vomiting which is less frequent after the first day of the disease. Affected piglets are dehydrated and may lose up to 20 per cent of their body weight within the first few days of illness. In older pigs the disease runs a more chronic course and, although clinical symptoms are generally absent, failure to gain weight is of economic importance. Sows infected late in pregnancy may show elevated temperatures and act as carriers of the virus, although abortions and stillbirths are rare.

Experimental infection can be induced in young susceptible pigs when the virus is administered *per os*, but not by parenteral inoculation, and the virus can be recovered from the intestinal tract and kidneys.

Post-mortem examination of young piglets dying in the early stages of the disease shows the stomach to be filled with coagulated milk, and the intestines to be distended with yellow foamy fluid and undigested particles of milk curd. In later stages of the illness the carcase is dehydrated, the intestines are less distended but the stomach remains filled.

The most significant pathological changes are found in the intestinal tract. These include acute enteritis accompanied, on occasion, by petechiation and, in the case of some older pigs, by severe ulceration. In the terminal stages of the disease the fundus of the stomach is often very congested and the wall of the intestinal tract is thin and almost transparent. Extensive atrophy of the intestinal villi in the jejunum and ileum, as seen with a dissecting microscope or hand lens, is said to be characteristic of transmissible gastroenteritis as is the absence of chyle from the mesenteric lymphatics. Degenerative lesions and haemorrhages may be found in the spleen, kidney, urinary bladder and heart, and there may be congestion and some evidence of encephalitis in the central nervous system.

Immunity

The immune response to transmissible gastroenteritis infection in pigs has a number of unusual features. Experimental and field observations show that piglets born to sows exposed to infective material 40 or more days before farrowing are immune to natural infection or develop only a mild form of the disease and usually survive. The immunity is probably transmitted through the colostrum since piglets are highly susceptible when removed from the sow before they have sucked. However, antiserum administered parentally does not protect piglets against infection and it is suggested that the protective effect of colostrum is due to the presence of antibody in the lumen of the intestines. Piglets removed from an immune sow are susceptible to rechallenge within 4 hours. This suggests that transmissible gastroenteritis is due to a viral infection of the superficial cells of the intestine and that antibody protection can only occur by neutralization of the virus within the lumen of the gut.

Ecology

It is generally assumed that the small intestine is the primary site for the replication of the virus and that ingestion is the natural route of infection.

Experimental evidence shows that virus titres in the gut lumen fall appreciably within the first 3–5 days post-infection, and that the virus continues to be excreted in the faeces of recovered pigs up to 8 weeks or longer. There is no evidence, however, that the virus is shed in the urine although it has been recovered from the kidneys and urinary bladder of the majority of experimentally infected pigs. Persistence of the virus in farm buildings, in swill and, perhaps, in recovered 'carrier' sows may play a major role in the spread of the disease. Several workers have reported that aerosol dissemination of the virus is also likely.

Diagnosis

A presumptive diagnosis of transmissible gastroenteritis is generally based on the sudden appearance of a rapidly spreading, highly fatal disease of young piglets accompanied by vomiting and diarrhoea. A confirmatory diagnosis can be obtained by the demonstration of rising antibody titres in paired sera from sows with affected litters or from pigs that have recovered from the disease, by means of neutralization tests in primary pig kidney cell cultures. In the case of young piglets dying during the acute stages of the illness, the causative virus may be isolated in cell cultures and identified by neutralization, cross-immunity and fluorescent antibody staining methods. The presence of non-cytopathogenic strains may be detected by interference in cell cultures of the growth of mucosal disease virus. It has also been reported that some non-cytopathogenic strains can be induced to produce visible changes in the cell culture monolayers by cultivation under increased atmospheric pressure in 95 per cent O_2

and 5 per cent CO_2. The presence of specific viral antigens in sections or smears of small intestine and mesenteric lymph nodes can also be confirmed by immunofluorescence techniques.

Control

Control measures are usually ineffective because there is inadequate knowledge of the immunological and epidemiological nature of the disease. Adequate management and strict hygienic measures together with intervals between farrowings help to eliminate the virus from infected premises; and, in some herds, an interval as short as 4 weeks between two successive farrowings may be sufficient to control the disease.

A number of live attenuated tissue culture vaccines have given promising results in laboratory and field trials but few have been approved for general use. These have mostly been given by the intramuscular route to pregnant sows 1–2 months before farrowing. An inactivated vaccine prepared in dog kidney cultures has been shown to be effective when given 4–11 weeks before farrowing.

Since sows affected during pregnancy are capable of conferring a passive immunity on their piglets via colostrum, it has become a popular practice in certain areas to vaccinate pregnant sows by deliberately exposing them to infective material. In some herds a purified virus is given orally in the form of a frozen capsule to all pregnant swine and the method is believed to confer adequate protection. It is emphasised, however, that planned exposure to the virus should only be considered on those farms with a known history of the disease and where there is no danger of spreading the infection to neighbouring farms.

There is some evidence that herds which are badly affected one year and then immunized, rarely show the disease in the following year.

Vomiting and wasting disease of piglets

Synonyms

Haemagglutinating encephalomyelitis virus disease of pigs: Ontario encephalomyelitis: Canadian vomiting and wasting disease of pigs.

Definition and hosts affected

An acute, highly infectious virus disease of young pigs; other species are not susceptible. Affected piglets show symptoms of vomiting, anorexia, constipation and progressive emaciation. In some cases, the disease progresses rapidly to a fatal encephalomyelitis.

History and distribution

In 1958, a hitherto unknown vomiting and wasting

syndrome was described in unweaned piglets in Ontario, Canada. A year later further outbreaks were described in Ontario involving illness in suckling piglets similar to the vomiting and wasting disease except that most affected animals rapidly developed an encephalomyelitis followed by death in 3–5 days. In 1962, an haemagglutinating virus was isolated by Greig and his colleagues from brains and other tissues from several cases of encephalomyelitis in week-old piglets. This agent, which was capable of reproducing clinical and pathological manifestations of encephalitis in unweaned piglets was named the haemagglutinating encephalomyelitis virus (HEV) of swine. Towards the end of 1968 numerous outbreaks of a disease resembling the Canadian vomiting and wasting syndrome were reported in England and Wales and a virus (FS 2063/68) with properties similar, if not identical, to those of HEV was isolated from a 10-day-old piglet. Serological surveys have suggested that a similar virus was present in pigs in England, Wales and Scotland as early as 1966. In 1972, the virus was isolated from the nasal cavity of an apparently healthy pig in Iowa.

The precise relationship between vomiting and wasting disease and encephalomyelitis due to HEV in Canada, the U.S.A. and the United Kingdom has not been fully established, but the available evidence suggests that the two diseases are different clinical manifestations of the same infection.

Properties of the virus

Electron microscopy indicates that the virus of vomiting and wasting disease is a coronavirus of about 150 nm in diameter but smaller particles have been described by Canadian workers. In general, mature virions are composed of a dense featureless core surrounded by an envelope containing a surface fringe of pear-shaped projections 20–20 nm in length. The virus is heat-labile and sensitive to lipid solvents including ether and sodium desoxycholate. It grows well in pig kidney cell cultures and produces numerous large foci of multinucleated syncytia (Plate 45.1b, facing p. 565). There is little evidence of intercytoplasmic or intranuclear inclusions but infected cultures stained by fluorescent antibody techniques show the presence of viral antigen in the cytoplasm.

All known strains of HEV are believed to be antigenically homogeneous and the British isolates (e.g. F.S. 2063/68) are probably identical to those obtained from Canadian outbreaks. It should be noted, however, that the unrelated strain (HEV-18), which also produces multinucleate syncytia in pig renal cell cultures is now considered to be a strain of parainfluenza-3 virus. There is general agreement, that HEV is unrelated to transmissible gastroenteritis virus and all other coronaviruses.

Haemagglutination

HEV haemagglutinates and haemadsorbs several species of erythrocytes, including those of chicken, turkey, rat, mouse and hamster; but does not cross-react with Newcastle disease or fowl plague viruses in haemagglutination-inhibition tests. Neuraminidase activity is absent and there is, therefore, no spontaneous elution of the virus from agglutinated red blood cells.

Pathogenicity

The vomiting and wasting syndrome appears to be confined to young piglets of about 1–3 weeks of age. In the initial stages of the illness there is vomiting, depression, anorexia and constipation. In some herds affected pigs may be seen sneezing, coughing and grinding their teeth, while others may show hyperaesthesia. In Canada, the disease frequently progresses rapidly to a fatal encephalitis with death in a few days, whereas in vomiting and wasting disease a high percentage of animals may recover. In outbreaks in the United Kingdom, clinical encephalomyelitis is often inapparent although brain lesions are frequently found at necropsy. Surviving piglets usually become very emaciated and a number survive for several weeks before dying from starvation or secondary disease, but others remain stunted and are commercially valueless. In some Canadian outbreaks many surviving piglets make a complete clinical recovery without any wasting.

There are no gross lesions at postmortem and, apart from abnormalities in the brains of some animals, no other significant histological changes have been observed.

Piglets experimentally infected with United Kingdom isolates show temperature rises and vomiting by the fifth to sixth days post-inoculation. Thereafter, they become depressed, hairy and emaciated and some may die 2–4 weeks later. All develop neutralizing antibodies in their sera. Studies of the distribution of the virus in piglets infected by the oral and intranasal routes showed that the virus was present in the tonsil, larynx, trachea, lung, oesophagus, stomach and duodenum by the 48th hour, and in the hind brain by the 72nd hour. There was no evidence of virus in faeces or rectal swabs. It is generally believed that the normal habitat of the virus is the upper respiratory tract and that the virus is transmitted by means of infected nasal secretions.

Diagnosis

The clinical signs of vomiting and wasting disease are hardly pathognomonic and permit of a tentative diagnosis only: but the absence of scouring and the variable mortality rate help to distinguish it from transmissible gastroenteritis (TGE). A confirmatory diagnosis can only be obtained by laboratory methods. These include isolation of the virus from the respiratory tract, hind brain and spinal cord and the demonstration of typical cytopathic effects including syncytial formation and haemadsorption of red blood cells, together with the presence of haemagglutinins in the fluid phase of infected primary pig kidney and thyroid cell cultures. Histopathological examination of the brain may also prove helpful. The quickest and most reliable method for obtaining a confirmatory diagnosis is by the serological examination of sera obtained from surviving litter mates or from the dams of affected litters. Antibodies to HEV can be detected in those sera by haemagglutination-inhibition, haemadsorption-inhibition or by serum neutralization tests. In outbreaks in the U.K., neutralizing antibodies develop from about the 7th day post-infection and reach their maximum titres between 2–3 weeks Specific antigen can be detected by fluorescent antibody staining of infected cells, and the virus can be identified under the electron microscope by negative staining of infected culture fluids.

Control
Vaccines are not yet available for the control of wasting and vomiting disease in piglets. Exposure of breeding sows to HEV, 2–3 weeks before farrowing, will ensure the development of active immunity within a few days so that the piglets will be protected by colostral antibodies.

Further reading
ALMEIDA J.D., BERRY D.M., CUNNINGHAM C.H., HAMRE D., HOFSTEAD M.S., MULLUCI L., MCINTOSH K. AND TYRRELL D.A.J. (1968). Coronaviruses. *Nature*, **220**, 650.
MCINTOSH K. (1974) Coronaviruses: a comparative review. *Current Topics in Microbiology and Immunology*, **63**, 85.
TYRRELL D.A.J., ALMEIDA J.D., CUNNINGHAM C.H., DOWDLE W.R., HOFSTAD M.S., MCINTOSH K., TAJIMA M., ZAKSTELSKAYA L. Ya., EASTERDAY B.C. AND BINGHAM R.W. (1975) Coronaviridae. *Intervirology*, **5**, 76.
BISWAL N., NAZARIAN K. AND CUNNINGHAM C.H. (1966). A haemagglutinating fraction of infectious bronchitis virus. *American Journal of Veterinary Research*, **27**, 1157.
CARTWRIGHT S.F. (1969). Vomiting and wasting disease of piglets. In *Veterinary Annual*, 10th Issue, p. 196. Bristol: Wright.
CARTWRIGHT S.F., HARRIS H.M., BLANDFORD T.B., FINCHAM I. AND GITTER M. (1964). Transmissible gastroenteritis of pigs. *Veterinary Record*, **76**, 1332.
CUNNINGHAM C.H. (1970). Avian infectious bronchitis. *Advances in Veterinary Science*, **14**, 105.

GARSIDE J.S. (1967). Avian infectious bronchitis. *Veterinary Record*, **80**, Clinical supplement No. 7.
GEILHAUSEN H.E., LIGON F.B. AND LUKERT P.D. (1973). The pathogenesis of virulent and avirulent avian infectious bronchitis virus. *Archiv für die gesamte Virusforschung*, **40**, 285.
GIRARD A., GREIG A.S. AND MITCHELL D. (1964). Encephalomyelitis of swine caused by a haemagglutinating virus. III. Serological studies. *Research in Veterinary Science*, **5**, 294.
GREIG A.S. AND GIRARD A. (1963). Encephalomyelitis of swine caused by a haemagglutinating virus. II. Virological studies. *Research in Veterinary Science*, **4**, 511.
HOFSTAD M.S. (1965). Infectious bronchitis. In *Diseases of Poultry*, eds. H.E. Biester and L.H. Schwarte, 5th Edition, p. 605. Ames: Iowa State University Press.
MCINTOSH K., KAPIKIAN A.Z., HARDISON K.A., HARTLEY J.W. AND CHANOCK R.M. (1969). Antigenic relationships among the coronaviruses of man and between human and animal coronaviruses. *Journal of Immunology*, **102**, 1109.
MEBUS C.A., STAIR E.L., RHODES M.B., UNDERDAHL N.R. AND TWIEHAUS M.J. (1973). Calf diarrhoea of viral aetiology. *Annales de Recherches vétérinaires*, **4**, (1), 71.
MENGELING W.L., BOOTHE A.D. AND RITCHIE A.E. (1972). Characteristics of a coronavirus [strain 67N] of pigs. *American Journal of Veterinary Research*, **32**, 297.
NAZERIAN K. AND CUNNINGHAM C.H. (1968). Morphogenesis of avian infectious bronchitis virus in chicken embryo fibroblasts. *Journal of General Virology*, **3**, 469.
PENSAERT M.B. AND CALLEBAUT P.E. (1974). Characteristics of a coronavirus causing vomition and wasting in pigs. *Archiv für die gesamte Virusforschung*, **44**, 35.
STONE S.S., STARK S.L. AND PHILLIPS M. (1974). Transmissible gastroenteritis virus in neonatal pigs: intestinal transfer of colostral immunoglobulins containing specific antibodies. *American Journal of Veterinary Research*, **35**, 321.
TAJIMA M. (1970). Morphology of transmissible gastroenteritis virus of pigs. *Archiv für die gesamte Virusforschung*, **29**, 105.
WITTE K.H. AND EASTERDAY B.C. (1967). Isolation and propagation of the virus of transmissible gastroenteritis of pigs in various pig cell cultures. *Archiv für die gesamte Virusforschung*, **20**, 327.
WITTE K.H., TAJIMA M. AND EASTERDAY B.C. (1968). Morphologic characteristics and nucleic acid type of transmissible gastroenteritis virus of pigs. *Archiv für die gesamte Virusforschung*, **23**, 53.
WOODE G.N. (1969). Transmissible gastro-enteritis of swine. *Veterinary Bulletin*, **39**, 239.

CHAPTER 46

LEUKOVIRUSES
(AND OTHER ONCOGENIC VIRUSES)

Leukoviruses (and Other Oncogenic Viruses)

Viruses and tumours

In its restricted sense the word 'tumour' denotes an abnormal growth of new tissue arising from existing body cells and characterized by a tendency to autonomous and unrestricted growth. Two main types are recognised:

(1) a permanently or temporarily uncontrolled growth of cells which may be generalised (metastatic), culminating in the death of the host (malignant tumour), or

(2) a growth of altered cells which may remain localized and eventually regress (benign tumour).

Neoplasms can be classified histologically according to the type of cell predominating in any particular instance. Thus, it is possible for tumours to be composed of epithelial tissue, (e.g. carcinoma), connective tissue, (e.g. sarcoma) and tissues of mixed or uncertain type, (e.g. certain embryological tumours).

The proliferation of cells is a process that normally occurs in health and it is presumed that the reparative process of cell proliferation is initiated by a normal stimulus and is arrested by a similarly normal process. Hence, tumours may arise by a proliferation of cells in the absence of a normal stimulus, or, alternatively, in the presence of an abnormal stimulus, but the precise nature of both processes is unknown. One important difference from the normal reparative process is a tendency for the daughter tumour cells to assume characters of a nature more primitive than those of their predecessors.

A number of factors are believed to favour the initiation of tumour formation. These are carcinogenic chemical agents such as the cyclic hydrocarbons, physical agents including ultraviolet light and X-rays, hormones, inherited predisposing characteristics and infection by microorganisms.

Following the discovery of latency, lysogeny and transduction in bacteriophages, the suggestion that animal viruses may play an important role in the aetiology of cancer has gained considerable support in recent years. The idea that viruses might cause tumours is not new since Ellerman and Bang demonstrated the viral aetiology of the erythromyeloblastic form of fowl leukaemia as long ago as 1908. This important discovery was followed three years later by the first successful transmission of a solid malignant tumour, the Rous chicken sarcoma, by means of cell-free filtrates. Despite these convincing demonstrations of virus-induced tumours in chickens, little attention was paid to the possible oncogenic role of viruses until nearly 20 years later when Shope, in 1932, succeeded in transmitting rabbit fibromas and papillomas with cell-free filtrates. Also of considerable interest was Bittner's discovery in 1936 that the mouse mammary carcinoma agent could be transmitted from mother to offspring through the milk and, subsequently, that adult female mice which are latently infected with the virus develop malignant growths only after the mammary tissue has received an hormonal stimulus either artificially or during pregnancy. In the 1950's a large number of virus-induced leukaemias of mice were reported by Friend, Moloney, Rauscher, Graffi and others and the causative viruses were found to contain RNA. Within the past few years certain RNA viruses have also been shown to cause leukaemia in a wide range of animal hosts including rats, hamsters, guinea-pigs, cats, dogs and, possibly, cattle.

Further interest in the oncogenic role of viruses arose from the discovery that several DNA-containing viruses could cause tumours in experimentally infected lower animals although they seldom did so in the host species. One of these, polyoma virus, was isolated from leukaemic mice while another, the simian vacuolating (SV40) agent was discovered as a latent virus in apparently normal rhesus monkey kidney cells. Other DNA viruses with oncogenic potential include certain human and animal strains of adenoviruses which induce tumour formation when inoculated into baby hamsters, mice or rats, and some herpesviruses one of which is believed to be the causative agent of Marek's disease of poultry. In spite of the abundant evidence that certain RNA and DNA viruses can cause a variety of types of cancer in many different species of lower animals there is, as yet, no conclusive evidence that human cancers are caused by viruses.

The tumour-inducing viruses can be classified into two main groups with differing physical, chemical and biological properties; those that contain RNA as their genetic material and those that contain DNA. Although only one of the 7 or 8 major groups of RNA viruses, the leukoviruses (Table 46.2), has been unequivocally associated with neoplastic disease, certain viruses belonging to 3 or possibly 4 of the 5 major groups of DNA viruses are capable of inducing tumour formation (Table 46.1).

sarcoma viruses cause transformation of cells in tissue culture. Cells rendered neoplastic by RNA tumour viruses, whether transformed or not, usually elaborate infectious extracellular virus indefinitely; but solid tumours in chickens or in certain species of rodents caused by the RNA Rous sarcoma and murine sarcoma viruses, respectively, do not release easily detectable quantities of infectious virus. In some instances where there is little or no infectious virus, the defective viral genomes can be induced or rescued from affected cells by superinfecting them with certain strains of chicken or mouse leukaemia viruses due, it is thought, to the fact that these

TABLE 46.1. Some oncodna or DNA tumour-forming viruses.

Taxonomic group	Virus	Natural host	Artificial host
Poxvirus	Myxoma	Rabbit	Rabbit (domestic & wild)
	Shope fibroma	Cottontail rabbit	Domestic rabbit
	Squirrel fibroma	Squirrel	—
	Yaba virus	Monkey	Human
Papovavirus	Polyoma	Mouse	Baby mouse, rat, hamster and rabbit
	SV40	Rhesus monkey	Baby hamster
	Human wart	Man	—
	Rabbit papilloma	Cottontail rabbit	Domestic rabbit
	Bovine papilloma	Cow	Horse, hamster
	Canine papilloma	Dog	—
Adenovirus	Sub-group A (Highly oncogenic) 12, 18, 31	Man	Hamster, mouse, rat
	Sub-group B (moderately oncogenic) 3, 7, 14, 16, 21	Man	Hamster
	Sub-group C (weakly oncogenic) 1, 2, 5	Man	—
	Numerous simian viruses	Monkey	Hamster
	Bovine, 3	Cow	Hamster
	Chicken (CELO)	Chicken	Hamster
Herpesvirus and herpes-like viruses	Marek's disease virus	Chicken	—
	Burkitt's lymphoma virus & Hodgkin's disease virus	Human	?
	Herpes type 2	Human	Hamster
	Equine herpes type 3	Horse	Hamster
	Herpesvirus saimiri	Squirrel monkey	Owl monkey, Marmoset
	Herpesvirus ateles	Spider monkey	Marmoset
	Lucké frog carcinoma virus	Frog	—

Virus properties

All leukoviruses resemble each other in structure, chemical composition, reaction to chemical and physical agents and in their mode of reproduction; whereas the properties of oncogenic DNA viruses are similar to those of their respective groups.

The leukaemia members of the leukovirus group do not usually cause cytopathic effects whereas the

'helper' viruses provide the functions missing or not expressed in the sarcoma viruses.

Most RNA tumour-forming viruses, e.g. feline leukaemia virus, are pathogenic in their natural hosts, unlike DNA viruses, e.g. polyoma virus, which are highly oncogenic in young experimentally infected laboratory animals but seldom cause tumours in the host of origin. A notable exception is the type-B herpesvirus which is generally regarded as the causative agent of neurolymphomatosis or Marek's disease of poultry.

Infection of a tissue cell by a cytocidal virus results in death of the cell, but infection by a tumour virus usually leads to a synchronous virus-cell relationship resulting in a profound change in some of the properties of the infected cell. In many tissue culture systems, cells infected with sarcoma and certain other tumour-producing viruses are actively transformed due to loss of contact inhibition between contiguous cells in the monolayer. These transformed cells behave like cancer cells when inoculated in young susceptible laboratory animals and may metastasize to distant organs and tissues resulting in death of the affected host. Viral induced cellular transformation can be recognised by:

(1) an increased rate of cellular metabolism and multiplication,

(2) chromosomal abnormalities and marked changes in the morphology of the cells,

(3) loss of contact inhibition with the formation of isolated foci of 'heaped-up' cells in monolayer culture,

(4) ability to divide indefinitely in serial culture,

(5) capacity to grow in suspension or in semi-solid agar,

(6) formation of novel virus-specified antigens (e.g. transplantation and 'T' antigens) and production of tumours when inoculated into young susceptible isologous animal hosts (Plate 46.1a, facing p. 584).

One of the most significant discoveries in recent years was the observation that oncogenic DNA viruses may become permanently integrated with the genes of the host cell and remain in their hosts for long periods of time without releasing infectious virus or producing symptoms of overt disease. There is also evidence from nucleic acid hybridization studies in cell cultures that the continued presence of the DNA viral genome in malignant cells is necessary for the maintenance of the transformed state. Nevertheless, induction of infectious virus from certain DNA transformed cells has been accomplished with chemical agents (mitomycin C) and by co-cultivation techniques with healthy indicator cells. In these latter experiments, fusion of infected and normal indicator cells may occur spontaneously or with a much higher frequency if the mixed cell populations are treated with inactivated Sendai or other myxoviruses (Plates 46.2a, b; 46.3a, b between pp. 584 and 585).

Although the DNA cancer-producing virus is no longer recognizable in the host cell by its normal properties of antigenicity and infectivity, recent studies have shown that its presence can be detected by the formation of new antigens in the nucleus (T-antigen) and on the plasma membrane (transplantation antigen) of the cell. These and other non-viral proteins may arise by translation of some of the virus-specified mRNA formed by continuous transcription of the oncogenic viral DNA which is integrated with the chromosomes of the cancerous cells.

Oncodnaviruses

Oncogenic viruses are widely distributed among the DNA virus groups, ranging from the large poxviruses, through adeno- and herpesviruses, to the small papovaviruses. Unlike oncorna- or leukoviruses, most DNA tumour-forming viruses are highly oncogenic under laboratory conditions but do not usually produce malignant tumours in their natural host, in which they mostly cause only inapparent infections or mild disease.

Poxviruses

Some of the oldest known oncogenic viruses belong to the poxvirus group, but the tumours they produce are usually benign. One member, the Shope fibroma virus is exceptional in that it can give rise to malignant tumours in young experimentally infected rabbits, and the causative virus can be recovered from affected tissues. Myxoma virus of rabbits is not a 'true' oncogenic virus and produces only local swellings in its natural host (Sylvilagus). However, in wild and domestic (Oryctolagus) rabbits it causes a highly fatal infection which is characterized by subcutaneous gelatinous 'tumours' (myxomata) consisting of proliferations of undifferentiated mesenchymal cells (Plate 52.5c). Yaba virus disease was first reported in a colony of monkeys at Yaba, Nigeria, in 1958. It causes subcutaneous tumours particularly of the head and limbs of rhesus and cynomolgus monkeys.

Papovaviruses

Almost all member of the *PA*pilloma-*PO*lyoma *VA*-cuolating group are potentially oncogenic but only the papilloma viruses cause natural tumours in their hosts of origin. Most of these are benign (e.g. warts in man and domestic animals) but others (e.g. rabbit papilloma) are benign in their natural hosts (cottontail rabbits) but may give rise to malignant tumours of the carcinoma type in artificial hosts (domestic rabbits). Papilloma virus particles are present in large numbers in warts, and autogenous vaccines have been used therapeutically in severely affected horses and cattle.

Latent infections with polyoma virus are widespread among colonies of laboratory and wild house mice. Young mice are infected naturally during the first few weeks of life following inhalation of particles contaminated by urine and saliva of adult carrier mice; but without producing demonstrable disease. Naturally occurring tumours are rarely encountered in mice but the virus is highly oncogenic when inoculated into susceptible newborn mice, hamsters, rabbits, guinea-pigs and ferrets. A wide variety of histologically diverse tumours, including spindle-shaped sarcomas or epithelial tumours, may occur in a number of different sites, hence the name 'poly-oma'. Intra-uterine infection is not known to occur. There is recent evidence that polyoma virus can integrate its DNA directly into the host cell chromosome. During infection the appearance in the nucleus of 'tumour antigen' correlates perfectly with the beginning of chromosome duplication, and it is suggested that this virus-specified protein is the molecule responsible for initiating the DNA synthetic machinery and is, in effect, one of the main factors in the induction of cancer.

The vacuolating agent or Simian virus 40 (SV40) is frequently to be found in apparently healthy monolayer cultures of rhesus and cynomolgus monkey kidney cells. Tissue culture fluids inoculated into kidney cell cultures of green African monkeys produce a dramatic cytopathic effect which is characterized by the presence of multiple vacuoles of both large and small dimension giving the cytoplasm a 'foamy' appearance (Plate 54.1b). Since SV40 virus produces malignant tumours when injected into newborn hamsters, the presence of viruses like SV40 as contaminants of viral cultures to be used for the preparation of live attenuated vaccines, e.g. poliovirus vaccine, constitutes a potential danger to human health. It is of interest that a small DNA virus resembling SV40 has been found, together with measles virus, in the brain cells of patients suffering from subacute sclerosing panencephalitis [SSPE] and that large numbers of SV40-like particles have been observed in brain tissues of patients with a slow, progressively fatal brain disease called progressive multifocal leukoencephalopathy [PML]. This is the first evidence that SV40 may be involved in human disease. More recently, in 1974, a second group of workers have produced strong evidence that a human malignant melanoma was caused by SV40. In a detailed study of a patient dying of a melanoma with metastasis to many parts of the body including lung, liver and muscle, they found both 'T' antigen and SV40 in tumour material, but not in tissues which were unaffected by cancer. Antibodies against 'T' antigen and SV40 were also present in sera taken a few days before the patient's death. However, the amounts of virus present in the tumour tissues was small due to the fact that the viral DNA becomes integrated with the cellular DNA and is only occasionally released from transformed tumour cells. The circumstances in which SV40 virus may or may not produce cancer are not known and it is emphasised that monkey handlers are frequently infected with SV40 and produce antibodies against the virus, but do not develop cancer.

Adenoviruses
Following the discovery, in 1962, that human adenovirus type 12 produces sarcomas when inoculated into baby hamsters, it has been found that several other adenoviruses of human and animal origin are also oncogenic. Human types 12, 18 and 31 have the highest oncogenic potential and produce sarcomas in newborn hamsters, rats and mice in about 90 days. Type 7 causes lymphomas and lymphosarcomas in young hamsters in 160 days or more, while types 3, 14 and 21 are weakly oncogenic and induce sarcomas in artificially infected rodents only after a variable but lengthy incubation period. Adenovirus tumours do not contain infectious virus, nor can virus be released from cells transformed *in vitro* either by chemicals or by co-cultivation.

Herpesviruses
Apart from the Lucké virus associated with renal carcinomas of the leopard frog, which was formerly classified with the herpesviruses, there are a number of 'true' herpesviruses with oncogenic potential. These include the Epstein-Barr (EB) virus associated both with Burkitt's lymphoma and Hodgkin's disease of man, herpes type 2 virus from carcinomas of the human cervix and two species occurring in monkeys. There is also evidence to show that the great majority of human patients affected with a type of nasopharyngeal carcinoma have high antibody titres to the EB virus. In birds, a herpesvirus may be the causative agent of Marek's disease.

Leukoviruses (Oncornaviruses)

In contrast to the DNA oncogenic viruses, the RNA tumour-forming viruses comprise an homologous group called leukoviruses or oncornaviruses, but a recent report suggests that they are members of a larger group and should be included as the genus *Oncornavirus* in a family designated *Retraviridae*, together with a number of other reverse transcriptase containing RNA viruses, e.g. visna-maedi viruses (*Lentivirus*) and the foamy viruses (*Spumavirus*).

Oncornaviruses are responsible for the majority of naturally occurring neoplasms of animals known to be of viral origin. All are strikingly similar in structure, chemical composition, reaction to chemical and physical agents and in their mode of reproduction. Cells rendered neoplastic by most strains of leukoviruses usually elaborate detectable amounts of extracellular virus, whereas in neoplasms associated with DNA viruses the virions are generally cell-associated. Most RNA tumour viruses are patho-

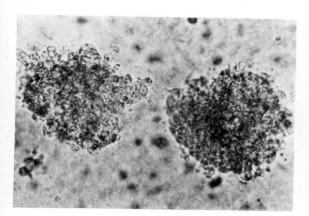

46.1a

46.1a Multilayered colonies on agar of transformed cells from a line of pig kidney cells (Stice 2-a strain) persistently infected with Newcastle disease virus, ×18.

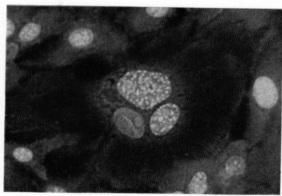

46.1b

46.1b Small heterokaryon produced in co-culture of persistently infected (NDV) bovine kidney cells and healthy chick fibroblasts. The two large bovine nuclei are readily distinguished from the smaller avian nucleus when the culture is stained with acridine orange and viewed in the ultraviolet light microscope, ×380.

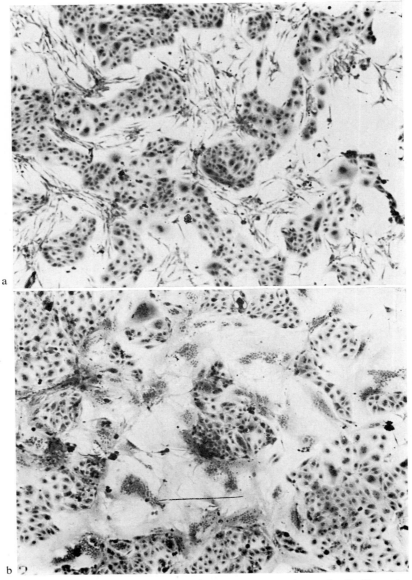

a

b

Co-cultivation with mixed cell populations, showing fusion of infected and normal cells. Haematoxylin eosin stain.

46.2a Mixed suspensions of healthy bovine kidney epithelial cells and chick fibroblasts grow independently and do not fuse. After 3 days' incubation, ×64.

46.2b Mixed cell populations of a line of bovine kidney cells (MDBK) persistently infected with Newcastle disease virus and healthy chick fibroblasts, after 48 hours' incubation. Notice the multinucleate syncytia (heterokaryons) caused by fusion of healthy fibroblasts and chronically infected epithelial cells, ×64.

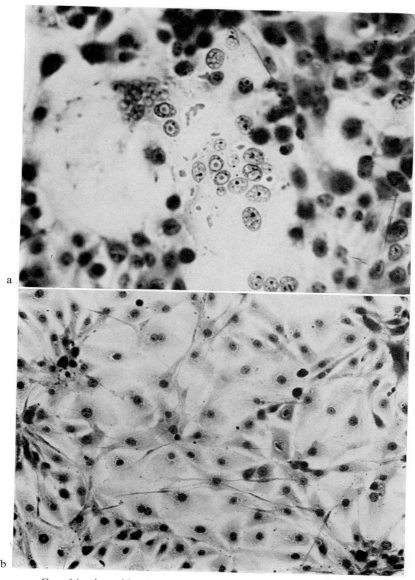

Co-cultivation with mixed cell suspensions. Haematoxylin eosin stain.

46.3a Heterokaryons induced by co-cultivation of healthy chicken kidney cells and the persistently infected MDBK line contain large numbers of acidophilic intracytoplasmic and intranuclear inclusion bodies, × 350.

46.3b Cell fusion and heterokaryon formation does not occur if cells persistently infected with Newcastle disease virus and healthy chick fibroblasts are co-cultivated in medium containing specific anti-viral serum. Cell fusion, similar to that shown in Plate 46.2b, occurs within 24 hours after the antiserum is replaced with normal serum, × 175.

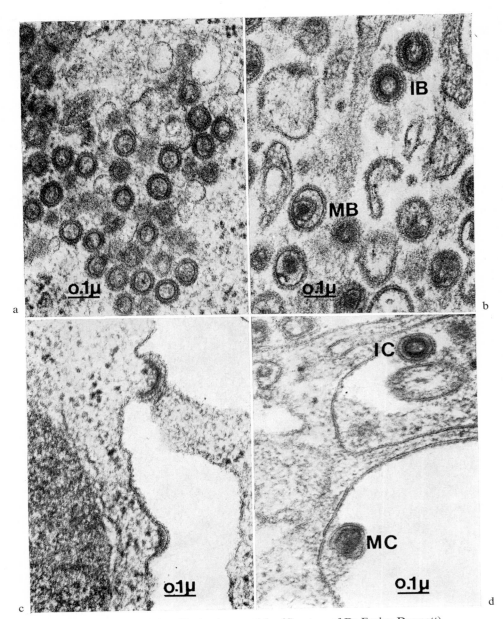

Electron micrographs of leukovirus particles (Courtesy of Dr Evelyn Dermott).

46.4a Type-A particles within the cytoplasm of a mammary tumour cell.

46.4b Immature (IB) and mature (MB) type-B particles in mouse mammary tumour (Bittner virus).

46.4c Early stages of formation of type-C particles at the cell membrane.

46.4d Immature (IC) and mature (MC) type-C particles.

genic in their natural hosts, unlike DNA oncogenic viruses which are highly oncogenic in experimentally infected laboratory animals but seldom cause natural tumours in the host of origin.

Classification

Leukoviruses can be separated into two main groups. The first includes those viruses that are capable of inducing leukaemia in a variety of avian and mammalian species, e.g. avian lymphoid leukosis virus and avian myeloblastosis virus; while the second includes those oncornaviruses which cause solid tumours in susceptible host animals as well as foci of altered cells in tissue cultures of susceptible fibroblasts, e.g. murine, feline and avian (Rous) sarcoma viruses.

The avian leukovirus group contains many strains of RNA viruses which do not cause disease in poultry. Some of these occur in laboratory stock cultures of Rous sarcoma virus and act as helper viruses in 'rescuing' defective Rous sarcoma particles from cell cultures. These have been designated Rous associated viruses (RAV). Other non-pathogenic strains of avian leukoviruses may interfere with the growth of Rous sarcoma virus in eggs or cell cultures and are named 'resistance inducing factor' or Rous inhibiting factor (RIF).

Some members of the leukovirus group are shown in Table 46.2.

Morphology

All leukoviruses are strikingly similar in size and structure. Negatively stained preparations reveal roughly spherical, pleomorphic virus particles surrounded by an outer envelope carrying a fringe of short radially projecting spikes. Mature virions range in size from 70–110 (200) nm. The central core of the virus particle has an amorphous appearance although, in some preparations, penetration of the phosphotungstic acid reveals an internal helical component similar to the nucleocapsid of myxoviruses.

Electron micrographs of ultrathin sections, or centrifuged pellets, of infected cells may show virus particles belonging to three morphological types. These are termed the A, B and C particles. The type A particles are spherical or doughnut-shaped with a double membrane, approximately 75 nm in diameter, surrounding an electron-lucent central core. They are always located intracellularly and may be found either in the cytoplasmic matrix, usually in the region of the Golgi apparatus, or inside the cisternae of the endoplasmic reticulum. Immature B particles resemble A particles except that they are slightly larger, about 100 nm, and are present in the extracellular spaces. They may be formed in two ways, either by envelopment of intracytoplasmic A particles or by budding directly from the surface membrane. Mature B particles are located extracellularly although they are sometimes included in phagocytic vacuoles of infected cells, and are especially prevalent in cases of mouse mammary cancer. They are fairly large, spherical particles (90–200 nm in diameter) containing an eccentrically positioned electron-dense nucleoid (about 35 nm in diameter) surrounded by two membranes of about the same electron density. The nucleoid is separated

TABLE 46.2. Some members of the leukovirus group.

Subgroup		Members of the subgroup
Avian leukovirus	ALV:	Avian lymphomatosis (lymphoid leukosis) virus. Avian myeloblastosis virus. Avian erythroblastosis virus. Rous associated virus (RAV) Rous inhibiting factor (RIF)
	RSV:	Rous sarcoma virus (many strains) e.g. Carr-Zilber, Schmidt-Ruppin, Bryan, Harris, Fuginami. RSV (ALV): Rous sarcoma virus with envelope derived from ALV.
Murine leukovirus	MLV:	Murine leukaemia virus. At least 14 strains including — Gross, Moloney, Friend, Graffi and Rauscher.
	MSV:	Murine sarcoma virus. Several strains including — Harvey, Moloney, Kirsten. MSV (MLV) Murine sarcoma virus with envelope derived from MLV. MSV (FeLV) Murine sarcoma virus with envelope derived from FeLV.
Other leukaemia viruses	FeLV:	Feline leukaemia (lymphosarcoma) virus — including Jarrett, Rickard and Kawakami strains.
	BoLV:	Bovine leukaemia virus.
	CLV:	Cavian leukaemia virus.
Mouse mammary tumour virus	MTV:	Murine mammary tumour virus (Milk factor) of Bittner.

from the two distinct layers of the outer membrane by a wide electron-lucent zone. The C particles vary in size from approximately 85–110 nm in diameter and are similar to B particles except that the electron-dense nucleoid is positioned centrally and has considerably greater electron density than the overlying intermediate layer. The type C particles occur extracellularly or occasionally within phagocytic vacuoles, and it is widely believed that their internal components are formed at the site of budding on the surface membrane rather than by envelopment of intracytoplasmic A particles. (Plates 46.4 a–d, facing p. 585).

Infectivity of type A particles has not been demonstrated but B particles are regularly associated with mammary tumours and are the aetiological agent. Type C particles have been observed in tissues from chickens, mice, rats, hamsters, cats, snakes, cattle, sheep, monkeys and, perhaps, from man; and are the causative agent of avian, murine and feline leukaemias and sarcomas. It should be noted, however, that there is no scientific proof that B and C particles are the only ones capable of inducing viral neoplasia in animals.

Physicochemical properties

Leukovirus particles contain a central core of single-stranded segmented RNA with an exceptionally high molecular weight of about 9–12×10^6 daltons; together with a small double-stranded DNA molecule apparently of cellular origin. They are sensitive to ether and bile salts, and most strains are readily inactivated by heating at 56°C for 30 minutes. They are also inactivated by mild acid treatment (pH 4·5) and by most commonly used disinfectants, e.g. 0·5 per cent phenol and 1/4000 formalin.

Antigenic properties

The RNA tumour viruses are relatively weak antigens but neutralizing and complement-fixing antibodies are generally present in the sera of tumour-bearing animals, and in animals artificially inoculated with live or inactivated virus. All avian and mammalian C-type particles contain 3 major structural polypeptides and 2 glycopeptides derived from the viral envelope. These include a group-specific 'gs-a' virion protein of avian leukoviruses, a 'gs-l' antigen which is the main marker for the species of origin (chicken, mouse, cat, etc.) of the virus, and a 'gs-3' antigen shared by all mammalian C-type oncornaviruses. Avian leukoviruses possess an RNA-directed DNA polymerase with antigenic determinants which also may be shared by various mammalian viruses.

Growth and development

Many strains of leukoviruses grow readily in embryonated hens' eggs or in cell cultures prepared from susceptible species, but without producing noticeable cytopathic effects: others, e.g. Rous sarcoma virus, produce 'pocks' on the chorio-allantoic membrane of fertile eggs and induce visible cellular transformation in certain tissue culture systems. In the absence of cytopathic changes, the presence of leukovirus infections in cell cultures can often be revealed by the production of viral antigens in the supernatant fluids using complement-fixation tests with sera from tumour-bearing animals.

All RNA tumour-bearing viruses grow in the cytoplasm, but not the nucleus, of the susceptible host cell. The virus emerges along the edge of membranes lining the cell and its cytoplasmic vacuoles, and is released continuously by a process of budding without drastic impairment of the cell's viability.

It is well known that the antibiotic actinomycin D inhibits the synthesis of RNA made on a DNA template, but not the synthesis of RNA on the RNA template. Thus, when it was found that actinomycin D added to cells infected with Rous sarcoma virus inhibited the production of all RNA this seemed to indicate that the virus was different from other RNA viruses and might replicate through a DNA intermediate. Further experiments showed that cells treated with 5-fluoro-2'-deoxyuridine [FUDR] and cytosine arabinoside, to inhibit cellular DNA synthesis, were protected from infection with Rous sarcoma virus; and this additional evidence supported the suggestion that Rous sarcoma virus requires the synthesis of new viral DNA produced on an RNA template. Considerable progress has been made during recent years in understanding the molecular events during replication of RNA tumour viruses, and the means by which these unusual activities take place has largely been explained by the discovery that the virions of Rous sarcoma and other RNA oncogenic viruses contain a series of novel enzymes including RNA-dependent DNA polymerase, DNA-dependent DNA polymerase, DNA endonuclease and DNA ligase. The fact that all oncornaviruses contain RNA-dependent DNA polymerase, or more precisely, RNA-directed DNA polymerase (reverse transcriptase), suggests a reversal in the 'normal' flow of information in so far as the viral RNA genome can be copied to produce a DNA strand giving an RNA/DNA hybrid. This, in turn, may be copied by another polymerase to produce small pieces of double-stranded DNA which can be further replicated and inserted into the chromosome of the host cell. In this way, the genome RNA of oncornaviruses may persist in an integrated DNA copy (provirus state), and may continue to be replicated with the host DNA. At a later stage in the replicative cycle, continuous transcription of DNA into RNA is necessary for new viral nucleoprotein and envelope protein as well as the assembly and release of mature infectious virus.

Theories of viral carcinogenesis

In recent years a great deal of attention has been paid to the possible role of C-type particles and viral genomes in the induction of tumours in animals. It is becoming increasingly clear that certain viruses can integrate their genetic material with that of the host cell they invade, and that this material is replicated and passed to the daughter cells when the host cell divides. According to one current theory of viral carcinogenesis, every vertebrate is born with the genetic information for producing C-type viruses dormant in its cells, and inherited from its parents. The virogenes (genes for the production of C-type particles) and the oncogenes (that portion of the virogene responsible for transforming a normal cell into a tumour cell) are maintained in an unexpressed form by repressors in normal cells. Thus, the basic cause of cancer could be failure of the host cell's natural repressor to keep the tumour-inducing gene switched off. Failure of the repressor, which probably blocks the transport of mRNA into the cytoplasm and prevents synthesis of various proteins on the polyribosomes, might be due to a spontaneous mutation of the cell concerned or might result from the action of various agents including radiation and chemical carcinogens or infection by other viruses. It is also possible that the chances of the repressor mechanism failing will tend to increase with age. Evidence in favour of the oncogene hypothesis includes the following:

(1) very few established mouse colonies are entirely free of C-type viruses, and infectious particles can be induced in apparently normal mice by various physical and chemical carcinogens

(2) C-type viruses appear spontaneously in healthy mouse embryo cells cultured intensively for many generations

(3) single cell clones from normal and transformed cells can be induced to release infectious C-type virus.

An alternative hypothesis for viral carcinogenesis is based on the fact that the RNA Rous sarcoma virus replicates through a DNA intermediate (protovirus) which is not sensitive to inhibitors of protein synthesis, and that the virus contains an RNA-directed DNA polymerase (reverse transcriptase) which is responsible for transferring information from viral RNA to the DNA protovirus. Thus, in the protovirus hypothesis, unlike the oncogene hypothesis, the genetic information required for cell transformation does not exist in the germ cell, and is not inherited. Instead a normal process of RNA to DNA to RNA information transfer is deranged to give rise to the formation of genes for neoplastic transformation.

Pathogenicity

Leukaemia viruses are almost ubiquitous in mice and poultry, and many animals appear to harbour virus for a considerable span of their life-time before they are affected by the disease, if at all. The proportion of infected cells that becomes transformed is very small and there is good evidence that actively multiplying virus can be widespread in the animals' tissues without producing symptoms of illness. Thus, tumour formation may only arise when certain specialized target cells are transformed by the virus.

It is not known whether different forms of leukaemia are due to a single virus or whether they are caused by distinct, although possibly related, oncogenic viruses. The generally accepted view that a single strain of avian leukosis virus can give rise to lymphoid leukosis, osteopetrosis, myeloblastosis and, even, sarcoma cannot be confirmed until further experiments have been carried out with clones of purified field strains of virus in animals that are not themselves latently infected.

Most natural infections with leukoviruses remain latent for prolonged periods but they may eventually cause fatal diseases, usually of the lymphoid or haemopoietic systems. A few strains cause the rapid production of solid tumours, notably Rous sarcoma virus in birds and Moloney and Harvey sarcoma viruses in rodents.

Ecology

Transmission of many avian and mammalian leukaemia viruses occurs congenitally through the embryo and in mice they may pass through the milk. In general, RNA oncogenic viruses are poorly transmitted from animal to animal by horizontal contact.

Avian leukosis

The term 'avian leukosis complex' is generally used to describe a number of contagious conditions of poultry which are characterized by neoplasms of the haemopoietic system. These include avian sarcomas, lymphoid leukosis, myeloblastosis, erythroblastosis and, probably, osteopetrosis. The causative viruses are all members of the RNA avian tumour virus or leukovirus subgroup; but it is not clear whether the above conditions are manifestations of a single disease or if they are caused by different but closely related species of leukoviruses.

For many years the avian leukosis complex included fowl paralysis or Marek's disease, but recent work suggests that the lymphoid lesions in the peripheral nerves and other tissues of birds affected with fowl paralysis are due to an infection with a DNA virus of the herpesvirus group and are not in any way associated with avian leukosis, sarcomas or other RNA virus-induced tumours.

Synonyms
Fowl leukosis, erythroblastosis, myeloblastosis, granuloblastosis, myeloid leukosis, fowl leukaemia, aleukaemic myeloid leukosis.

Osteopetrosis, hypertrophic osteitis, marble bone, thick leg disease.

History and distribution
There can be little doubt that diseases of the avian leukosis complex have been present in domestic poultry from the middle of the 19th century. Since then, the incidence of virus-induced tumours has increased rapidly until, at the present time, they constitute one of the most important disease problems in poultry in all parts of the world. In recent years, the avian leukosis complex has been observed more frequently in younger birds of about 4–5 months of age and, in some laboratories, avian leukosis has been diagnosed in about 25–30 per cent of all birds examined. At present, leukosis viruses are so widespread in poultry flocks that supplies of virus-free chickens for research and other purposes can only be obtained by selective breeding under conditions of strict quarantine. It has been estimated that the loss to the British poultry industry due to all forms of the disease is not less than £10m. per annum whilst in the U.S.A. the annual loss from leukosis alone is about 75–100 million dollars.

Species affected
The spontaneous occurrence of avian RNA virus-induced tumours is almost entirely confined to domestic poultry but the presence of the clinical condition in turkeys is becoming more common. Pheasants, ducks, quail, pigeons and guinea-fowl are susceptible to experimental infection.

Morphology and physicochemical characters
The causative viruses of the avian leukosis complex are similar in structure, and fully developed particles bear a close resemblance to ortho- and paramyxoviruses. In negatively stained preparations the virions are roughly spherical in outline and measure about 80–110 nm in diameter. The symmetry of leukovirus is undetermined but a number of reports suggest that the inner component consists of a coiled tubular structure with a helical arrangement of protein subunits similar to the nucleocapsid of myxoviruses. In electron micrographs of ultrathin sections of infected cells the avian leukovirus particles consist of an outer membrane and an inner, electron-dense, featureless core of about 45 nm in diameter. A second membrane may sometimes be seen between the outer envelope and the dense central core giving the virion the typical appearance of the so-called C-particle.

The mature virus particle contains single-stranded RNA with an unusually high molecular weight of about 1.3×10^7 daltons. The outer envelope exhibits a surface fringe of short, radially projecting spikes, but the virions appear to be devoid of haemagglutinating activity. All avian leukoviruses are ether-sensitive and do not survive outside the host cell for more than a few hours. They are thermally unstable and are inactivated by heating to 56°C for 30 minutes. They are also inactivated by formaldehyde and by common disinfectants such as 0.5 per cent phenol. Viability of virus preparations can be maintained for long periods at –70°C or in 50 per cent glycerol-saline. An unusual feature of many avian RNA tumour viruses is their comparatively high resistance to inactivation by ultra-violet light, although they are sensitive to X-rays.

Antigenic properties
The envelope of avian leukoviruses contains virus-specific proteins which are antigenic in the host and are capable of stimulating the production of neutralizing antibodies. Neutralization and cross-neutralization tests are especially useful for detecting different strains of avian tumour viruses and recent evidence suggests that the majority of field strains of avian leukoviruses can be separated into two main antigenic groups (A and B) by cross-neutralization and immunofluorescence tests. According to this method of classification, each of the two groups contains a number of different leukaemia viruses and several different Rous sarcoma strains also. More recently, the presence of a third antigenic group has been postulated.

Studies of the antigenic relationships between avian leukoviruses is further complicated by the rapidly increasing number of new virus strains and by the presence of antigenic heterogeneity in many strains previously thought to be pure.

Strains of avian leukoviruses capable of producing tumours that are histologically different may be closely related antigenically, yet not identical, while others may be antigenically distinct. Nevertheless, all share a group-specific antigen associated with the internal helical component of the virion which can be demonstrated with sera of rodents bearing Rous sarcoma tumours by means of the COFAL (complement-fixing avian leukosis) test, or by either immunofluorescence or immunodiffusion tests.

COFAL test
Sera of hamsters and guinea-pigs carrying tumours induced by Rous sarcoma virus contain specific

complement-fixing antibodies. These antibodies react not only with other strains of Rous sarcoma virus but also with several strains of avian leukosis virus, including myeloblastosis and erythroblastosis viruses. It is stressed that the complement-fixation reaction occurs despite antigenic differences demonstrated in neutralization tests between some Rous sarcoma strains and the avian leukosis viruses.

The group-specific complement-fixation reaction has been used for quantitative assays of avian leukosis viruses in chick fibroblast cell cultures and is particularly suitable for detecting latent avian leukosis viruses which produce little or no cytopathic effect in tissue culture. The test has also been applied to the demonstration of viral antigens in the tissues of naturally infected chickens and chicken embryos. This COmplement-Fixation test for Avian Leukosis virus (COFAL) is said to be as sensitive as the RIF test, which detects interference between the avian leukosis virus and the Rous sarcoma virus, as an assay system for avian leukosis viruses.

Growth and development

Most strains of avian leukoviruses grow well in 11- or 12-day-old embryonated hens' eggs and many, but not all, produce foci of ectodermal proliferation (pock-like tumours) on the chorioallantoic membrane of susceptible eggs. In general, avian leukoviruses, unlike Rous sarcoma virus, can be cultivated successfully in chicken fibroblast cell cultures without inducing malignant transformation or other cytopathic changes of the affected cells. The presence of virus in these non-cytocidal steady-state infections may be detected by failure of the cells to undergo cellular transformation when superinfected with Rous sarcoma virus. The interfering property of strains of leukosis virus for Rous sarcoma virus is due to the so-called *Resistance-Inducing Factor* (RIF). The term 'RIF-positive' has been used to designate chickens carrying a 'resistance inducing factor' which induces such birds to resist inoculation with the Rous sarcoma virus. Since this transmissible resistance-inducing factor is, in fact, a strain of avian leukosis virus there seems little need to designate these chickens as other than natural carriers of a latent leukosis virus.

Despite the lack of cellular transformation, cultures infected with leukoviruses continue to produce large quantities of virus which can induce tumours when inoculated into young susceptible chickens. The route of inoculation is very important for the successful reproduction of erythroblastosis and myeloblastosis in chickens, and the intravenous route is more effective than intramuscular, intraperitoneal or subcutaneous inoculation. Different routes of infection are much less important for the induction of avian leukaemia.

Pathogenicity

It is a well known feature of the avian leukosis complex that a single bird may be affected with more than one type of tumour or that a bird bearing one type of tumour may transmit virus which is capable of inducing a histologically different tumour. It is not yet known whether different types of tumour are caused by one or several strains of virus excreted by the same hen, but recent evidence suggests that each strain of avian tumour virus can, in fact, induce a wide spectrum of diseases. For example, the RPL12 strain of virus originally isolated from a solid lymphoid tumour, can induce erythroblastosis, osteopetrosis and sarcomas as well as lymphomatosis, while a second strain of fowl leukaemia virus has been shown to produce erythroblastosis, osteopetrosis, sarcomas, haemangiomas and adenocarcinomas as well as lymphomatosis. Despite the fact that many strains of avian leukoviruses can induce several distinct neoplastic diseases, in most instances only one particular response prevails. Since it is seldom possible to isolate field strains of lymphoid leukosis virus causing a single disease it seems likely that the different types of tumours are produced by the same strain infecting a number of different types of target cells.

There are, undoubtedly, a number of factors which influence the onset and development of avian leukosis. Genetic characters play an important role in the susceptibility of chickens to the disease and some breeds or lines are extremely resistant to tumour formation while others are highly susceptible. The age at exposure is also an important consideration and young chickens are more susceptible than older fowls. Females are more susceptible than males although castration of cockerels is said to increase the incidence of leukaemia. On the other hand, the use of testosterone and diethylstilboestrol may reduce the incidence.

The majority of chickens in a diseased flock become infected and many birds remain symptomless carriers throughout their lifespan. Birds may die suddenly or the disease may run a protracted course with loss of bodily condition. Most affected birds become pale and listless and some may show diarrhoea in the terminal stages of the illness. At autopsy, the disease is characterised by enlargement of the liver, spleen, kidneys and gonads with diffuse or miliary lesions due to massive infiltrations of the tissues by lymphoid or other types of tumour cells (Plates 46.5, facing p. 592 and 46.6, facing p. 593). A proportion of birds may be affected with osteopetrosis, a nonmalignant tumour produced by excessive activity of osteoclasts leading to gross thickening of the long bones. The avian myeloblastosis virus which usually produces a myeloblastic leukaemia, can also give rise to the development of osteopetrosis and teratomas of the kidneys.

Despite the fact that avian tumour viruses grow readily in almost all tissues of the susceptible host, there is a very strict tissue specificity for the production of virus-induced tumours. This suggests that viral carcinogenesis, but not viral replication, is dependent on the availability of specific target cells in the body. A good example of tissue specificity in avian viral carcinogenesis is the role of the bursa of Fabricius in the pathogenesis of avian lymphoid leukosis. Several workers have shown that surgical removal of the lymphoid bursa prevents the development of visceral lymphomatosis after injection of virulent lymphoid leukosis virus, whereas removal of the thymus has no such effect. Other neoplasms induced by the same virus are not affected by removal of the bursa. These observations suggest that cells of the bursa of Fabricius play a crucial role in the development of virus-induced lymphoid tumours in chickens.

Ecology

The most susceptible host for avian leukosis virus is the domestic chicken and there is good evidence that almost all birds become infected with field strains of the virus sometime during their lives. Nevertheless, not all birds show symptoms of the disease and there can be little doubt that different lines and breeds of chickens show different degrees of susceptibility to infection. Evidence for genetic resistance can be demonstrated in chickens, developing chicken embryos and, even, in cell cultures derived from resistant birds.

The avian leukosis virus is widely distributed in poultry flocks and is excreted in the droppings and saliva of both clinically affected and apparently healthy carrier birds. Contact spread is highly efficient among young susceptible chickens and can even occur by airborne transmission, but adult birds exposed to the virus for the first time generally produce an active immune response and seldom develop the clinical disease.

Adult hens in commercial flocks may be divided into two broad groups. The first includes viraemic birds which have detectable amounts of neutralizing antibody and the second consists of hens which do not carry the virus but have neutralizing antibodies in their blood as a result of previous exposure to the virus. Viraemic hens frequently carry an ovarian infection and pass the virus to their offspring through the egg. Chicks developing from congenitally infected embryos are immunologically tolerant and have large quantities of infectious virus in their blood and tissues. Despite this, they hatch and grow up normally and remain viraemic throughout their lives. Large amounts of virus are shed in their droppings and saliva, and they are a constant source for the horizontal spread of the virus through contact infection. Chicks from immune hens are virus-free upon hatching and are partially protected against contact infection for the first few weeks of their lives by passively transferred maternal antibody. At maturity, the presence of viraemic and non-viraemic birds in the same flock usually results in a high incidence of contact infection in the latter group. Male birds play no part in the transmission of avian leukosis virus and even viraemic cockerels with active foci of infection in the testis do not produce infected chicks when mated with non-viraemic hens. Thus, an infected flock may consist of (a) non-infected immune birds, (b) infected immune birds, (c) tolerant viraemic birds and (d) non-infected non-immune birds.

Diagnosis

In most laboratories the distinctive character and the distribution of gross lesions in affected carcases is usually sufficient for a diagnosis of avian leukosis. Confirmation of the diagnosis is based on histopathological studies and on the identification of the causative virus.

In most cases of lymphoid leukosis, tumours do not occur before 16 weeks of age and the lesions are composed of an homogeneous proliferation of lymphoblasts which stain readily with pyronin. There is no evidence of lymphoid infiltration in the nerves or of perivascular cuffing in the cerebellum. In erythroblastosis, large numbers of erythroblasts can be found in smears of blood, liver and bone marrow and in sections of liver and spleen. In myeloblastosis, examination of liver and bone marrow sections shows the presence of numerous myeloblasts which are usually smaller and more acidophilic than lymphoblasts or erythroblasts.

The causative virus of the avian leukosis-sarcoma complex can be isolated from the blood and most of the soft organs of the affected carcase. In recent years, the use of susceptible chicks and embryonated hens' eggs for virus isolation has largely been superseded by cell cultures, despite the fact that the methods, e.g. the RIF test for non-cytocidal leukosis viruses, are not suitable for all members of the avian leukosis complex.

For the RIF test, material suspected of containing an avian leukosis virus is inoculated into susceptible chick embryo fibroblasts which are later tested for their susceptibility to Rous sarcoma virus. The presence of leukosis virus in these infected cultures is indicated by a ten-fold or greater reduction in the number of foci produced by a standard strain of Rous sarcoma virus.

The COFAL reaction is dependent on the presence of the group-specific protein antigen of avian leukosis virus in the cells of infected cultures. Infected chicken embryo fibroblasts are harvested and the fluids used as an antigen in the complement-fixation test. Samples which fix complement in the presence of a known antiserum are considered to be positive.

In the non-producer activation test, chick embryo fibroblasts infected with a defective Rous sarcoma virus are mixed with healthy susceptible chick embryo fibroblasts and inoculated with the suspect material. After 5–10 days of incubation, the tissue culture fluids are tested for infectious extracellular Rous sarcoma virus released by the activator leukosis virus in the test material.

Direct and indirect fluorescent antibody staining techniques have also proved useful for identifying avian leukosis viral antigen in infected chick embryo fibroblasts.

Serum neutralization tests in cell cultures can also be used to detect current or past infections with an avian leukosis or sarcoma virus.

Control

There are no vaccines available for the control of avian leukosis and all attempts to produce attenuated strains which do not produce disease have failed. Thus, control of the disease is only possible by suitable methods of flock management and, wherever possible, by the use of genetically resistant stock. Replacement birds should always be purchased from flocks with an absence or low incidence of the disease.

The widespread use of live attenuated avian virus vaccines prepared from non-leukosis-free eggs has undoubtedly played a major role in the spread of the disease and there can be no doubt that all such vaccines should be produced in leukosis-free eggs or, in the future, in susceptible chicken cell cultures.

Rous sarcoma virus

Historical

In 1910, Peyton Rous investigated the nature of a spindle-cell carcinoma found in a barred Plymouth Rock hen, and carried out several successful transplantations of this solid tumour in young and mature chickens. In a later study he showed that the tumour could also be transmitted by inoculating cell-free filtrates into young fowls of the same breed in which the tumour originally occurred. Several additional chicken tumours were subsequently studied by Rous and his colleagues and it soon became apparent that other tumours of the fowl were also caused by filterable agents.

At present, the RNA avian tumour viruses are included in the leukovirus group which consists of a large number of different viruses capable of inducing leukaemia and similar diseases in a variety of avian and mammalian species. Other members of the leukovirus group include viruses capable of produc-

ing solid tumours, e.g. the Rous sarcoma virus (RSV), the mouse sarcoma virus (MSV) and the mouse mammary tumour virus of Bittner (MTV).

Morphology and development

For all practical purposes, the spherical particles observed in Rous chicken sarcomas are indistinguishable from those found in lymphoid leukosis, myeloblastosis and erythroblastosis of chickens. Virus particles are to be found extracellularly or in very large numbers on the surface of infected cells. The virions are also present in the cytoplasm and within cytoplasmic vacuoles but they do not occur within the nuclei.

There is a striking relationship between the number of virus particles present and the ability of the preparation to induce tumours. This suggests that the virus particles seen in electron micrographs of Rous sarcoma cells are actually those of Rous sarcoma virus. It is emphasised that virus particles morphologically identical to those observed in Rous sarcomas can, occasionally, be found in cells of clinically healthy chickens and the possibility cannot be excluded that these represent virus particles which are responsible for such 'spontaneous' neoplastic diseases of poultry as leukosis or sarcomas.

However, it is not always easy to demonstrate virus particles even in active tumours, and large numbers of cells may have to be examined before the presence of the virus can be confirmed. A recent survey suggests that particles may be detected in as few as one in 50 tumour cells examined, but that they are more abundant in young actively growing sarcomas.

In general, the mature virus particles are released slowly from the surface of the plasma membrane and there is evidence that the tumour cells are in some form of equilibrium with the virus and, indeed, that certain strains of Rous sarcoma virus are defective. Thus, the Bryan strain of Rous sarcoma may grow and produce oncogenic effects in susceptible avian cells, but it cannot infect other cells unless 'rescued' by one or other of a small group of avirulent related viruses, the so-called Rous associated viruses (RAV).

Physicochemical properties

Although Rous sarcoma virus undoubtedly contains RNA (M.W. 9.6×10^6), its growth is suppressed by inhibitors of DNA, and there is clear evidence that one stage of its replicative cycle is dependent on cellular DNA activity. It has been known for some time that Rous sarcoma and other oncogenic RNA viruses can exist in a provirus state as virus-specific double-stranded DNA integrated into the chromosome DNA of the host cell; and recent reports suggest that the establishment of this provirus state occurs through a process of reverse transcription of the viral RNA to virus specific DNA. This RNA to DNA transcription is probably catalysed by an RNA-directed DNA polymerase ('reverse transcriptase') which is located internal to the lipoprotein envelope of the virus, and is a component of its nucleocapsid. The polymerase has antigenic determinants which may be shared by other mammalian oncornaviruses.

Rous sarcoma virus is inactivated when heated to 55°C. for only 15 minutes, and autolyzing tumour tissue held at the chicken's body temperature (41°C) remains active for less than 48 hours. The virus is rapidly destroyed *in vitro* by 20 per cent ether and antiseptic solutions such as 0·5 per cent phenol, but can be preserved for many years when dried from the frozen state (lyophilized) or stored in sealed ampoules at −70°C.

Strains of Rous sarcoma virus are remarkably resistant to x-ray irradiation and are 10 times more resistant to ultra-violet light than Newcastle disease virus, although both viruses are very similar in size, structure and RNA content.

Haemagglutination

Despite the obvious fringe of radiating projections on the surface of the mature virion as viewed by electron microscopy, there is no evidence of haemagglutinating activity by any of the sarcoma viruses.

Antigenic properties

Chickens affected with slow-growing sarcomas develop neutralizing antibodies in their serum, and these may also be produced by immunizing other species including geese, rabbits and goats. Rous sarcoma virus, like all other members of the avian leukovirus group, has a common group specific (gs) antigen associated with the internal component or nucleoid of the virion. This antigen can be detected by complement-fixation, agar gel diffusion and immunofluorescence tests. A second antigen which is detectable by its neutralizing activity is associated with the viral envelope, and is type specific.

The antigenic relationship between strains of RNA tumour viruses is complex and the problem has been further complicated by recent findings of antigenic heterogeneity in several strains previously thought to be homogeneous.

There are a number of different antigenic types of Rous sarcoma virus but the three strains mostly used in experimental studies are the Carr-Zibler strain, the Prague strain and the Schmidt-Ruppin strain. Among other well-known strains of Rous sarcoma virus, but with less pronounced oncogenic potential for mammals, are the Bryan strain, the Harris strain and the Mill Hill strain.

Although there have been a number of original isolations of avian tumour viruses from spontaneous chicken tumours, the above strains of Rous sarcoma virus are interrelated and probably were derived from the original strain that was isolated by Rous, in 1911, from his chicken Tumour No. 1. As a result of many serial passages in chickens in several laboratories throughout the world, these viruses have undergone variations in potency and antigenic properties. For example, the Harris strain is now only remotely related to the Bryan strain, and the Schmidt-Ruppin strain is also antigenically distinct from the Bryan strain. Nevertheless, there is some cross-neutralization between the Schmidt-Ruppin Rous sarcoma virus and avian myeloblastosis virus, and reciprocal-neutralization has been demonstrated between other Rous sarcoma viruses and avian lymphoid leukosis virus, but not erythroblastosis virus. The Bryan high-titre strain of Rous sarcoma virus itself shows immunological heterogeneity and consists of at least three antigenic variants. Similar observations have been made with the Schmidt-Ruppin strain of Rous sarcoma virus as well as with the myeloblastosis virus of avian leukosis.

Cultivation

Rous sarcoma virus can usually be propagated on the chorioallantoic membrane of developing hens' eggs, giving rise to foci of ectodermal proliferation. Some workers believe that a single infectious particle is sufficient to induce the formation of a tumour. Many chick embryos do not permit the growth of Rous sarcoma virus due to a genetically determined host resistance against the virus. Furthermore, resistance to inoculation with Rous sarcoma virus may also be due to congenital infection of the embryo with a field strain of avian lymphoid leukosis virus in a viraemic but clinically healthy laying hen. This sensitivity to specific interference by other avian leukosis viruses is governed by the protein coat in which the Rous sarcoma viral genome is enclosed.

Rous sarcoma virus grows well in monolayer cultures of leukosis-free chicken fibroblasts and produces foci of transformed cells which are clearly visible in stained and unstained preparations. The normally elongated spindle-shaped fibroblasts become rounded and vacuolated, and are seen as refractile clumps of sarcoma cells with an abundance of basophilic-staining material in the perinuclear zone. Entry of the virus into a susceptible host cell is followed by an eclipse phase lasting for 10–12 hours, during which no new virus is produced. By the fourteenth hour, free and cell-associated virus can be demonstrated in a few infected cells until, after 3 to 4 days of incubation, the majority of cells are involved and the amount of free virus exceeds that of the cell-associated virus. This is in marked con-

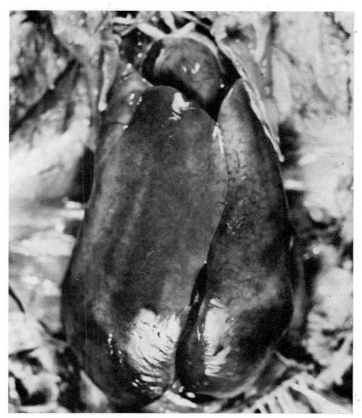

46.5 Diffuse form of avian lymphoid leucosis (avian lymphocytoma), showing gross enlargement of the liver which overlaps the abdominal cavity. Although not visible, the spleen is usually enlarged also.

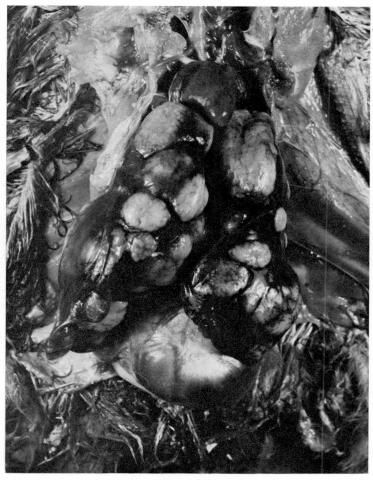

46.6 Discrete form of avian lymphoid leucosis, showing enlargement of the liver and multiple tumour nodules.

trast to the low escape-rate of virus from naturally occurring chicken sarcomas. Fluorescent antibody staining shows that viral antigen first appears within the cytoplasm and migrates to the cell surface in the form of small granules, whilst electron microscopy reveals the presence of large numbers of spherical particles on plasma membranes and within cytoplasmic vacuoles. As in leukovirus infections, the mature virions of Rous sarcoma virus are released by a process of budding. Other morphological features observed in infected cells are enlargement of the nucleoli and hypertrophy of the endoplasmic reticulum in the form of zones of densely packed lamellae which stain basophilically.

In cell cultures of mammalian origin, Rous sarcoma virus induces cellular transformation similar to that seen in chick fibroblast cultures. The effect is most pronounced with those strains that are also pathogenic for animals. Transformed mammalian cells contain the group antigen but fail to release infectious virus. This defective Rous sarcoma viral genome can be released from avian non-productive cells by superinfection with any avian leukosis virus, and virus can be recovered from most transformed mammalian cells by inoculating them into chickens.

Pathogenicity

Sarcomas occur sporadically amongst fowls but, unlike other diseases of the avian leukosis complex, horizontal transmission is highly inefficient and few birds in a flock are affected. Certain field strains of sarcoma virus have an extended host range and tumours have been transmitted to unrelated species of birds including ducks, pheasants, pigeons, turkeys and Japanese quail, and some strains have been adopted to grow preferentially in them.

Several types of 'spontaneously' occurring neoplasms have been described. These include spindle-cell sarcomas of different histological patterns, endotheliomas, fibrosarcomas, osteochondrosarcomas and myxosarcomas. In general the filterable chicken tumours are either rapidly growing soft growths containing mucinous material mixed with blood pigments or slow growing tumours that are firm and white in appearance. The tumours are usually progressive and fatal but they occasionally regress and may disappear completely.

The genetic constitution and the age of the chickens used for experimental transmission of tumour filtrates are of considerable importance. Certain breeds or strains of chickens are relatively resistant to infection while others, including the New Hampshire breed, White Leghorns and the Edinburgh strain of the Brown Leghorn breed are very susceptible. Younger birds are more susceptible than adults

and chickens ranging in age from 1–7 days are especially susceptible.

In newly hatched chickens the virus frequently causes haemorrhagic lesions and early death without evidence of neoplasia.

Serially passaged cell-free suspensions of certain strains of Rous sarcoma virus can induce tumours in 100 per cent of inoculated chickens even when dilutions of up to 10^{-4} are used. High multiplicities of virus inoculated into 2 to 6-week-old susceptible chickens show histological evidence of neoplasia as early as the 3rd or 4th day, while visible tumours may appear within 5 or 6 days after inoculation.

An important development in experimental cancer research was the observation that Rous sarcoma virus can also induce tumours in rats, mice, hamsters, guinea-pigs, rabbits and monkeys. In rats, the same tumour-inducing strain can produce either metastasizing sarcomas or multiple cysts and haemorrhagic lesions in the lungs, abdominal cavity, mesentery and other organs. In rodents, the induced tumours are usually undifferentiated sarcomas but in some instances rhabdomyosarcomas are produced in hamsters and fibrosarcomas in rabbits.

Although the induction of mammalian tumours by the avian Rous sarcoma virus has mostly been studied in experimentally infected rodents, the successful induction of sarcomas in newborn rhesus monkeys suggests that the Rous sarcoma virus has a much wider host range than hitherto suspected. Little information is available regarding the oncogenic potential of the virus in humans although it is known that inoculation of Rous sarcoma virus into a human volunteer in 1939 has not resulted in any pathological effects more than 30 years later. It is interesting to note that the virus strain used in this 'experiment' may have been identical to the one that was later found to be capable of inducing sarcomas in monkeys.

Ecology

Very little information is available about the natural methods of spread of Rous sarcoma viruses but contact transmission between artificially inoculated and uninoculated White Leghorn chicks has been reported. In one such experiment over 90 per cent of 9-day-old chicks inoculated by the subcutaneous route developed tumours about 14 days later and no fewer than 78 per cent of the non-inoculated birds of the same age, introduced into the same enclosure, developed tumours after 37–128 days. Most of the infected in-contact birds developed multiple tumours in the skin and subcutaneous tissues of the head, neck, wings, breast and legs but others produced sarcomas only in the lungs, mesentery, liver, spleen and kidneys.

Leukaemias in animals

In 1936, the host range of RNA virus-induced tumours was extended to mice as a result of the classical experiments of Bittner who clearly showed that a spontaneously occurring mouse adenocarcinoma was caused by an agent, later identified as the mouse mammary tumour virus, transmitted from mother to offspring through the milk. Some fifteen years later a number of other RNA containing viruses were isolated from various transplanted tumours in rodents and several of these were subsequently shown to induce leukaemia in mice; the most intensively studied being the Gross, Friend, Moloney and Rauscher strains. Within the past few years, RNA viruses have been shown to be associated with naturally occurring leukaemias in other animal hosts including cats, dogs and, possibly, cattle.

Apart from the mouse mammary tumour virus, all members of the leukosis or oncorna group of viruses are morphologically very similar to each other when viewed in electron micrographs of ultrathin sections of infected cells. The virions appear as C-type particles and mature by budding at the surface of the cell or on the membrane lining the intracytoplasmic vacuoles. In contrast, the Bittner virus is a B-type particle with an eccentric nucleoid surrounded by an envelope with more prominent surface spikes than the C-type particles. (Plate 46.4 facing p. 585).

Murine leukaemias
The first murine leukaemia virus was discovered by Gross who, in 1951, reported that leukaemia could be induced in certain inbred strains of mice by the inoculation of cell-free extracts of liver, spleen and mesenteric tumours from mice with either spontaneous or transplanted leukaemia. Following this discovery, some fourteen different leukaemogenic RNA murine viruses have been isolated from a variety of mice. Most were obtained by injecting filtrates of transplantable tumours into unweaned mice but the leukaemias produced do not usually correspond to any commonly occurring natural tumour. Thus, the majority of laboratory strains of murine leukaemia viruses probably do not bear any aetiological relationship to the tumour from which they were derived. For example, Graffi's virus was obtained from a type of myeloid leukaemia induced in newborn mice inoculated with cell-free extracts of transplantable carcinomas and sarcomas; Friend's leukaemia virus originated from an adult mouse inoculated shortly after birth with a cell-free extract of an Ehrlich ascites tumour; and the Moloney strain, which causes lymphocytic leukaemia, was derived from sarcoma 37.

In certain circumstances Gross's virus may give rise to almost all known types of leukaemia including lymphatic, stem-cell, myeloid and monocytic leukaemia, erythroblastosis, lymphosarcoma and reticulum cell sarcoma. Most murine leukaemia viruses produce leukaemia in rats and one of them, the Moloney strain, does so in hamsters as well.

Several different viruses have been described which produce either lymphoma or erythroid diseases of mice. All appear to share two common complement-fixing antigens. The first, which is demonstrable with sera obtained from rats bearing solid tumours induced by Rauscher virus, is a component of the viral envelope or capsid. The second is a soluble antigen released from purified virus particles by ether treatment and demonstrable by gel diffusion or complement-fixation tests.

Large amounts of infectious virus and of C-type particles are regularly observed in plasma or tissue extracts of mice rendered leukaemic by injection of some strains of leukaemia virus. Evidence of viral replication is obtained from electron microscopy showing virus particles budding from the cytoplasmic membranes of infected cells. It is difficult to find a strain of mice entirely free from leukaemia and, even in mice of strains having a low incidence of spontaneous tumours, there is evidence that lymphosarcomas or generalized leukaemia can frequently be induced by total body X-ray irradiation, by the application of oestrogenic hormones or by certain chemical carcinogens.

There are no differences between the various viruses as regards morphology, chemical composition or physicochemical characters, and most viruses can be readily propagated in cell cultures of mouse and rat cells. There is usually no cytopathic effect but virus is released continuously into the tissue culture fluid. Some members of the group, notably the Friend and Rauscher strains, are difficult to cultivate *in vitro*, but growth may occur in certain continuous mouse cell-lines with a cytopathic effect and, occasionally, cellular transformation.

Mouse (murine) sarcoma viruses
In the course of routine passage of mouse leukaemia virus in rats, it was observed that newborn mice inoculated with plasma from leukaemic rats developed solid tumours (sarcomas), instead of leukaemia, in the subcutaneous tissues and in the peritoneum near the site of injection. The affected animals showed splenomegaly and many died from splenic rupture. When the virus was passaged in newborn mice, rats or hamsters, tumours developed, usually at the site of inoculation within 3 weeks. However, some of the experimental animals did not develop early lesions and survived for at least 8 weeks, but some later developed lymphocytic leukaemia.

The murine sarcoma virus can readily be recovered

from the solid tumours and blood plasma of animals in which sarcomas had been artificially induced. It can also be propagated in tumour cell lines. Extracts from mouse sarcomas and also from the liver, spleen or salivary glands of virus-infected tumour bearing mice produce focal lesions of cellular transformation within 5 days; and the transformed cells continuously release virus into the medium.

Recent studies have revealed a marked similarity between the mouse sarcoma virus and the defective Bryan 'high-titre' strain of Rous sarcoma virus. It seems likely, therefore, that mouse sarcoma viruses and Rous sarcoma virus of chickens are very similar, as are the viruses of avian leukaemia and murine leukaemia.

The murine sarcoma-leukaemia viruses resemble their avian counterparts in having an internal group-specific (gs) antigen and also a type-specific antigen associated with the viral envelope. The 'gs' antigen, however, is distinct from that of the avian complex.

Murine mammary tumour virus

It has been known for many years that mammary tumours may occur spontaneously in adult female mice and that it is possible to develop inbred lines with either a very high or a very low incidence of cancer. These differences were believed to be genetical until Bittner showed that a tumour-inducing factor (the 'milk-factor') was transmitted to the young by the mother's milk. Subsequently, the milk factor was shown to possess virus characteristics including the ability to pass bacterial filters and to stimulate an antibody response. The Bittner virus is found naturally in 'high cancer' lines of mice even when such mice do not develop tumours until middle age. It multiplies in the mammary glands and is present in large quantities in the milk.

Although adult female mice may carry the virus for long periods of time, the incidence of mammary carcinoma depends on the strain of mice, not all being equally susceptible, and on hormonal stimulation of the mammary tissue by either artificial or natural means. The virus is present in male mice of the carrier lines and can be passed from them via the sperm to susceptible female mice which will, in turn, transmit it to their progeny. Transmission by cage contact is uncommon.

The virus induces carcinomas of the mammary glands only, following a latent period of 6–12 months. Unweaned mice can readily be infected by the oral, subcutaneous and intraperitoneal routes but adult animals are much more resistant. Irregular results are sometimes obtained and the suggestion has been made that in mice of 'low-cancer' strains there exists a second, related, 'nodule-inducing virus' with low oncogenic potential, that is capable of interfering with the mammary tumour virus. Infection occurs when baby mice ingest milk from mothers of a 'high-cancer' strain such as C3H. Fetuses are not usually infected *in utero* and if removed by caesarean section and suckled on mothers of a 'low-cancer' strain, they develop few if any tumours. Conversely, 'high-cancer' strains can arise from 'low-cancer' strains if the newborn are isolated from their mothers after birth and nursed by females of 'high-cancer' lines.

Although the Bittner virus has been extensively studied over a long period of time, no satisfactory means has been found of propagating it *in vitro*. Nevertheless, it has been found to survive in the yolk sac of fertile hens' eggs and in organ cultures of mouse mammary tissue, but multiplication has not been proved.

Virus particles in milk or extracts of infected mouse tissues are inactivated by trypsin and by heating at 56°C. for 30 minutes. The virus may be preserved by freeze-drying or by storage at –70°C.

Electron microscopical investigations have revealed the presence of two particles: a smaller type A particle, measuring about 70 nm in diameter, found in the cell cytoplasm in the region of the Golgi apparatus, and a large type B particle, measuring 100–110 nm found extracellularly. Recent studies of ultrathin sections of tumour tissues suggest that the B particles, with their eccentric nucleoids, represent the mature form of the virus.

No antibody against the virus has been found in mouse serum, but sera from guinea-pigs, rabbits and rats immunized with mammary tumour virus and mixed with the virus prior to injection into susceptible mice inhibit the development of mammary adenocarcinomas.

Feline leukaemia

In 1964, Jarrett and his colleagues clearly demonstrated that feline leukaemia (lymphosarcoma) could be transmitted with cell-free extracts of tumour tissue from a naturally occurring case of the disease. They have also shown that the causative agent has morphological and physical characteristics similar to those of the murine and avian leukoviruses. The importance of these observations is underlined by the fact that this is the first malignant disease of domestic mammals which has been proved to be caused by a virus.

Definition

The term 'leukaemia' is used to describe a wide range of cytologically distinct malignant diseases involving cells of the lymphoid and haemopoietic tissues of the body. In the cat, the most frequently observed form is lymphosarcoma.

Incidence

Several surveys have shown that leukaemia is undoubtedly the most common malignant neoplasm of the cat and it has been estimated that leukaemia-related tumours represent about 9–15 per cent of all malignant tumours in cats. In a recent report from California, the incidence was found to be 440 cases per million which is about twice that in dogs and cattle, and about 4 times the incidence in humans.

Aetiology

Electron microscopic studies of ultrathin sections of tumour tissues of induced and spontaneous cases of feline lymphosarcoma show the presence of leukaemogenic-type virions resembling the characteristic C-type particles found in murine and avian leukaemias. They are circular or oval in shape with an external diameter of about 100–110 nm. Most particles have two concentric electron-dense outer membranes separated from each other by an intermediate less opaque zone. The nucleoid is located in the centre of the particle and may be electron-lucent or electron-opaque: its average diameter is 50–65 nm.

The virus particles have been observed (1) extracellularly, (2) within the cisternae of the endoplasmic reticulum and (3) budding from the plasmalemma and cisternal membranes into the extracellular spaces. Incomplete particles are especially frequent at the surface of the plasma membrane. The early budding forms are semicircular in shape and show continuity of the plasmalemma of the cell with the limiting membrane of the emerging virus particle. In due course, the buds form a villiform elongation or 'stalk' of the surface membrane which eventually constricts and allows the mature particle to become detached from the cell. In certain tissues, particularly in the megakaryocytes, the C-type particles may be found in large clusters within the cytoplasmic vacuoles. Cells filled with virus particles may eventually undergo total destruction, thereby releasing large numbers of mature virus particles into the intercellular spaces; but in many instances the particles are assembled and liberated without any apparent damage to the cell.

C-type particles have been observed in a variety of tissues including lymph nodes, bone marrow, thymus and blood platelets, and a viraemia in which C particles were present in the plasma of kittens with induced lymphosarcomas has also been described.

Cultivation

The feline leukaemia virus (FeLv) is similar in many respects to leukaemogenic viruses in other animal species, and replication of the virus can be observed in cells before evidence of tumour growth is present.

Cell cultures derived from tumour tissues of cats with induced lymphosarcoma contain C-type particles, and suspended cell cultures of lymphoid cells can produce virus for at least 7 months. The virus can be propagated in normal embryonic feline cell cultures inoculated with extracts of tumour tissues, and the virus is produced extensively in these cells and is released into the culture fluid by a process of budding. Feline leukaemia virus can also infect and reproduce in cultured cells derived from canine, porcine and human sources, but fails to replicate in tissue cultures of chicken or bovine origin. It also induces leukaemia in experimentally infected puppies. There is recent evidence that feline leukaemia virus can activate defective mouse sarcoma viruses which replicate thereafter and produce foci of transformed cells in cat but not mouse cells. This 'rescued hybrid' will, in turn, produce sarcomas in experimentally infected kittens.

Antigenicity

An immunological relationship exists between the feline and murine viruses, and their 'gs' antigens have a component in common. The type-specific antigen of feline leukaemia virus is present in the envelope and is ether-sensitive. There are also 2 group-specific, ether-resistant antigens [gs] of which the 'gs-1' virion protein is specific for the species and common within the species, whereas the 'gs-3' antigen is shared by all C-type viruses of mice, hamsters, rats, cats and, possibly, of cattle. It has also been suggested that the group-specific antigen is present in human leukaemic cells. The 'gs' antigens are detected by complement-fixation, immunodiffusion and immunofluorescence tests. It should also be noted that non-virion cellular antigens associated with infected tissue cells include cell surface antigens and transplantation antigens, both of which may be specific.

Pathogenicity

The great majority of cases of feline leukaemia fall into three main types: multicentric, thymic and alimentary-mesenteric. The alimentary type is the most common and occurs in about 30 per cent of cases. It is characterized by sudden onset and is accompanied by inappetance, diarrhoea and progressive loss of bodily condition. A firm painless abdominal mass is palpable in most cases. Tumours are usually present in the mesenteric lymph nodes but the superficial lymph nodes are not affected. The spleen is not usually grossly enlarged.

In the multicentric type which may account for up to 20 per cent of cases, there is marked involvement of many of the lymph nodes of the body. The superficial lymph nodes are grossly enlarged and there is usually enlargement of the spleen and infiltration of the liver, kidneys and other organs. The onset may be either gradual or sudden.

The most striking change seen in the thymic form of feline lymphosarcoma is the presence of the main tumour mass in the anterior mediastinum. The thymic form is generally accompanied by some degree of generalization. The onset is usually sudden and the cat is in good bodily condition. There is respiratory distress, and dyspnoea is most marked when dehydration is also present.

In general, feline lymphosarcoma is a fatal disease of relatively short duration. About 40 per cent of cases die within 4 weeks of the onset of symptoms. More than 70 per cent die within 8 weeks and fewer than 10 per cent survive for periods longer than 4 months. There is no particular breed, age or sex incidence.

Feline lymphosarcoma can be readily transmitted by cell-free centrifuged extracts of spontaneous and induced tumour tissues, to kittens of less than 12 hours old. In one such experiment a spontaneous lymphosarcoma was transmitted to 56 per cent of 68 inoculated kittens through seven serial cell-free passages. The latent periods ranged from 30–139 days with a median of 53 days. Virus particles identical with those known to cause murine and avian leukaemia were seen in electron micrographs of thin sections of lymph node and other tissues taken from these experimentally infected kittens. They were predominantly of the mature type C form, but immature particles were also present.

Transmission

It is generally believed that feline leukaemia is transmitted vertically from an infected mother to her offspring *in utero*. However, recent reports from America indicate that the virus is present in the salivary glands, and there is increasing evidence that horizontal transmission can occur from cat to cat by biting and scratching.

Diagnosis

In a number of cases of feline leukaemia a provisional diagnosis can be made after a careful physical examination of the animal. For example, in the thymic form of feline lymphosarcoma the presence of the main tumour mass can be identified by radiography after removal of fluid from the thoracic cavity; and the presence of malignant lymphocytes in the fluid confirms the diagnosis. In most instances, a confirmatory diagnosis is based on the appearance and distribution of the lesions at autopsy supported by histological, immunological and electron microscopical examinations of affected tissues. Agar gel diffusion tests are particularly suitable for detecting viral antigen in the solid tumour mass of cases of lymphosarcoma, and immunofluorescence micro-scopy is of value for demonstrating either antigen in infected cell cultures or antibodies to sarcoma virus antigen in cat sera. Indirect haemagglutination-inhibition and serum neutralizing tests can also be used to detect specific antibody and are generally more sensitive than complement-fixation tests.

Control

Most feline leukaemia infections are transmitted vertically and no specific prophylaxis is at present possible. Effective control, in the future, may be achieved by immunotherapy or vaccination.

Leukaemia in other animals

Neoplasia of the lymphoid system is one of the most common malignancies of cattle, sheep and pigs. The aetiology of these conditions is unknown and, with the possible exception of bovine leukaemia, none has been successfully transmitted by means of cell-free extracts of lymphosarcoma cells. It is relatively easy to find characteristic virions in leukaemias and lymphosarcomas of hens, cats, mice and rats but it is surprisingly difficult to demonstrate viral particles in electron micrographs of ultrathin sections of leukaemic tissues from other species. However, these difficulties do not imply that neoplasia in cattle and other animals are not caused by a virus because there are many examples of virus-induced tumours which do not show the causative virus when examined under the electron microscope.

It is of interest that virus-like particles have recently been discovered in blood lymphocyte cultures obtained from cows with lymphosarcomas and that most of these 'successful' cultures were first stimulated with phytohaemagglutinin.

There is also a recent report that a virus resembling a leukovirus has been isolated from cattle with lymphosarcomas, and also from normal cattle. It produces syncytia in the baby hamster kidney cell line (BHK-21) and has been named bovine syncytial virus.

Human leukaemia

There is, as yet, no conclusive proof that human cancers are caused by viruses, but the finding of viral 'reverse transcriptase' in oncogenic RNA viruses of animals is proving of value in investigations of suspected leukovirus infections in man. In this connection the recent discovery that lymphocytes of human patients suffering from leukaemia contain an RNA-directed DNA polymerase suggests that it may be possible to purify the reverse transcriptase and produce a specific antiserum which could be used as an indicator system for detecting the presence of the enzyme in patients with cancer. Alternatively, the purified enzyme could be used as a screen for

possible chemotherapeutic substances that will
inhibit the RNA-directed DNA polymerase but leave
the normal cellular DNA-dependent DNA polymerase unharmed.

Simian foamy virus

Perhaps the commonest contaminant of 'normal'
monkey-kidney cultures is the monkey foamy virus
which has properties similar to those of the murine
mammary-tumour virus. The virions are pleomorphic structures varying in size from 110–120 nm
with a nucleoid (35 nm) surrounded by two shells 60
and 90 nm in diameter. The outer envelope carries
a fringe of short radially projecting surface spikes
12–15 nm long arranged in hexagonal patterns.
In some negatively-stained preparations there is an
inner helical component 10–12 nm across. The virus
matures by budding mainly at the plasma membrane, it is inactivated in 15 minutes at 50°C and is
ether-sensitive. So far, seven serotypes have been
described.

Primary and secondary cultures of monkey kidney
tissue carrying the virus show spontaneous degeneration characterized by the formation of multinucleate giant cells which subsequently become vacuolated and assume a lace-like or foamy appearance.
Cytopathic changes may also occur in HeLa, HEp2
and other primate cells, but infected cultures do not
haemabsorb guinea-pig, human group O, monkey or
chick erythrocytes. The virus has also been propagated in rabbit kidney cell cultures.

Monkey foamy virus has been isolated from 40–65
per cent of kidneys of rhesus and cynomolgus
monkeys, but not from patas or Malayan cristatus
monkeys. There is no evidence that this virus is
pathogenic for monkeys or other animals.

Although simian foamy agents closely resemble
RNA tumour-forming viruses in morphology and
morphogenesis, the type of nucleic acid they possess
has not been unequivocally determined and so an
attempt at classification is premature.

The contagious venereal dog sarcoma

The contagious venereal dog sarcoma is of interest
because it is one of the few naturally transmissible,
contagious tumours known. The growths usually
occur on the penis of the dog or in the vulva or
vagina of the bitch. They grow progressively and
may eventually disseminate, producing metastatic
nodules in the liver, spleen or other organs. The
tumours are generally firm, greyish-white structures
composed of round cells containing vesicular nuclei.
Although the microscopic appearance is similar to
that of a highly malignant neoplasm, cases of
venereal canine tumours are generally quite benign.

Type-C particles have been observed budding from
cell surfaces but the condition has not yet been
shown to have a viral cause.

Dogs in which venereal tumours regress spontaneously appear to be immune to reinoculation,
but the mechanisms involved are not known.

Further reading

BEARD J.W. (1957) Etiology of avian leukosis.
Annals of the New York Academy of Sciences, **68**,
473.

BEARD J.W., SHARP D.G. AND ECKERT E.A. (1955)
Tumour viruses. *Advances in Virus Research*. **3**, 149.

BIGGS P.M. AND PAYNE L.N. (1967) The avian
leucosis complex. *Veterinary Record*, **80**. suppl.
No. 7.

BLACK P.H. (1968) The oncogenic DNA viruses:
A review of *in vitro* transformation studies. *Annual
Review of Microbiology*, **22**, 391.

BURMESTER B.R. AND WITTER R.L. (1966) *An Outline
of the Diseases of the Avian Leukosis Complex.*
Production Research Report No. 94, Agriculture
Research Service, Washington: U.S. Department
of Agriculture.

CASTO, B.C. AND DiPAOLO, J.A. (1973) Viruses,
chemicals and cancer. *Progress in Medical Virology*, **16**, 1.

CRAWFORD L.V. (1969) Nucleic acids of tumor
viruses. *Advances in Virus Research*, **14**, 89.

DALTON A.J., MELNICK J.L., BAUER H., BEAUDREAU
G., BENTVELZEN P., BOLOGNESI D., GALLO R.,
GRAFFI A., HAGUENAU F., HESTON W., HUEBNER
R., TODARO G. AND HEINE U.I. (1974) The case
for a family of reverse transcriptase viruses:
Retraviridae. *Intervirology*, **4**, 201.

DULBECCO R. (1967) The induction of cancer by
viruses. *Scientific American* **216**, No. 4, 28.

DULBECCO R. (1969) Cell transformation by viruses.
Science, **166**, 962.

GROSS L. (1970) *Oncogenic Viruses*, 2nd Edition.
New York: Pergamon Press.

HABEL K. (1969) Antigens of virus-induced tumors.
Advances in Immunology, **10**, 229.

HOWATSON A.F. (1971) Oncogenic viruses: a survey
of their properties. In *Comparative Virology* Eds.
K. Maramorosch and E. Kurstak, p. 510. London:
Academic Press.

HUEBNER R.J. (1967) The murine leukemia-sarcoma
virus complex. *Proceedings of the National
Academy of Sciences*, **58**, 835.

HUEBNER, R.J. AND TODARO, G.J. (1969) Oncogenes
of RNA tumour virus as determinants of cancer.
Proceedings of the National Academy of Sciences,
64, 1087.

JARRETT W.F.H. (1966) Experimental studies of
feline and bovine leukaemia. *Proceedings of the
Royal Society of Medicine*, **59**, 661.

JARRETT W.F.H., CRAWFORD E.M., MARTIN W.B. AND DAVIE F. (1964) Leukemia in the cat: A virus-like particle associated with leukemia (lymphosarcoma). *Nature*, **202**, 567.

JARRETT W.F.H., CRIGHTON G.W. AND DALTON R.G. (1966) Leukaemia and lymphosarcoma in animals and man. I. Lymphosarcoma or leukaemia in the domestic animals. *Veterinary Record*, **79**, 693.

LAIRD H.M., JARRETT O., CRIGHTON G.W. AND JARRETT W.F.H. (1968) An electron microscopic study of virus particles in spontaneous leukemia in the cat. *Journal of the National Cancer Institute*, **41**, 867.

LAIRD H.M., JARRETT O., CRIGHTON G.W., JARRETT W.F.H. AND HAY D. (1968) Replication of leukemogenic-type virus in cats inoculated with feline lymphosarcoma extracts. *Journal of the National Cancer Institute*, **41**, 879.

LAIRD H.M., JARRETT W.F.H. JARRETT J.O. AND CRIGHTON G.W. (1967) Virus-like particles in three field cases of feline lymphosarcoma. *Veterinary Record*, **80**, 606.

LUCKE B. (1938) Carcinoma in the leopard frog: its probable causation by a virus. *Journal of Experimental Medicine* **68**, 457.

MACPHERSON I. (1967) Recent advances in the study of viral oncogenesis. *British Medical Bulletin*, **23**, 144.

MACPHERSON I. AND STOKER M. (1962) Polyoma transformation of hamster cell clones – an investigation of genetic factors affecting cell competence. *Virology*, **16**, 147.

MCALLISTER, R.M. (1973) Viruses in human carcinogenesis. *Progress in Medical Virology*, **16**, 48.

NAZERIAN K., DUTCHER R.M., LARKIN E.P., TUMILOWICZ J.J. AND EUSEBIO C.P. (1968) Electron microscopy of virus-like particles found in bovine leukemia. *American Journal of Veterinary Research*, **29**, 387.

RICH M.A. AND SIEGLER R. (1967) Virus leukemia in the mouse. *Annual Review of Microbiology*, **21**, 529.

ROUS P. (1911) A sarcoma of the fowl transmissible by an agent separable from the tumour cells. *Journal of Experimental Medicine*, **13**, 397.

RUBIN H. (1960) A virus in chick embryos which induces resistance *in vitro* to infection with Rous sarcoma virus. *Proceedings of the National Academy of Sciences of the United States of America*, **46**, 1105.

RUBIN H. (1962) Response of cell and organism to infection with avian tumor viruses. *Bacteriological Reviews*, **26**, 1.

SVOBODA J., MACHALA O. AND DEOZANEK T. (1968) Rescue of Rous sarcoma virus in mixed cultures of virogenic mammalian and chicken cells treated and untreated with Sendai virus and detected by focus assay. *Journal of General Virology*, **2**, 261.

TEMIN, H. (1970) Formation and activation of the provirus of RNA sarcoma virus. In *The biology of large RNA viruses* Eds. R.D. Barry and B.W.J. Mahy, p. 233. New York: Academic Press.

TEMIN, H. (1971) Mechanism of cell transformation by RNA tumour viruses. *Annual Review of Microbiology*, **25**, 609.

VIGIER P. (1970) RNA oncogenic viruses: structure, replication and oncogenicity. *Progress in Medical Virology*, **12**, 240.

VOGT P.K. (1965) Avian tumor viruses. *Advances in Virus Research*, **11**, 293.

VOGT P. (1971) RNA tumour viruses: The problem of viral defectiveness. In *Viruses Affecting Man and Animals*, Eds. M. Sanders and M. Schaeffer, p. 175. St. Louis: Warren H. Green.

WHO Scientific Group on viruses and cancer (1965) *Viruses and Cancer*. World Health Organization Technical Report Series No. 295, 1–60. Geneva: World Health Organization.

WOLSTENHOLME G.E.W. AND O'CONNER M. (1962) *Tumour Viruses of Murine Origin*. CIBA Foundation Symposium. London: Churchill.

CHAPTER 47

PICORNAVIRUSES

Picornaviruses

Definition

The name 'picornavirus' was introduced in 1962 to describe a group of very small (pico), ether-resistant RNA-containing viruses. The group includes the enteroviruses, a term used to designate poliomyelitis, coxsackie and echoviruses as well as a wide range of similar viruses derived from animal and avian sources including Teschen and Talfan of pigs, avian encephalomyelitis of poultry and duck hepatitis. The term also covers the rhinovirus sub-group which includes the human common cold viruses and the virus of foot-and-mouth disease. A third subgroup, calicivirus, has recently been proposed to include vesicular exanthema virus of pigs and a number of feline viruses formerly referred to as 'feline picornaviruses.'

Virus properties

Picornaviruses are very small spheres, 20–40 nm in diameter with perhaps 32, 42 or 60 regularly arranged surface capsomeres (Plate 47.1a–c, facing p. 606). The virions consist of a naked isometric capsid, probably with icosahedral symmetry, containing single-stranded RNA with a molecular weight of approximately 2.5×10^6 daltons. They are free of essential lipids and are very resistant to the action of ether, chloroform and bile-salts; in fact, they are remarkably stable to inactivation by most agents.

Most picornaviruses grow well in cell cultures producing a marked cytopathic effect which is usually characterized by granularity and rounding-up of the affected cells and complete destruction within 48–72 hours. Virus synthesis and maturation occur in the cytoplasm with occasional formation of crystalline arrays of viral particles. For practical purposes, picornaviruses are mostly cultivated in cells derived from kidneys of the animal species from which the virus was isolated. Polioviruses have an extremely narrow host range and require primate cells for propagation, whereas other picornaviruses such as foot-and-mouth disease virus have a much wider host range and grow well in a variety of cell types including primary and secondary pig or ox kidney cultures and the BHK-21 line of baby hamster kidney cells.

Most picornaviruses inhabit the intestinal tract and commonly cause no clinical illness. Some, however, may spread from the gut and cause destructive lesions in the central nervous system (polioviruses) while others parasitize the upper respiratory tract rather than the alimentary tract (rhinoviruses). Thus, the clinical syndromes resulting from infections with picornaviruses are extremely variable. For example, poliomyelitis of man and Teschen disease of pigs are characterized by paralytic disease, aseptic meningitis or other CNS disturbances; rhinoviruses cause acute upper respiratory tract infections or vesicular disease such as foot-and-mouth disease in ruminants; whereas, at the other extreme, the great majority of strains cause only mild or inapparent infections.

There are no serological relationships between the enterovirus (poliovirus, coxsackievirus, echovirus) and rhinovirus groups, nor between most of the serotypes within each group.

The classification of human and animal picornaviruses into the three genera, Enterovirus, Rhinovirus and Calicivirus, is shown in Table 38.1, page 412.

HUMAN ENTEROVIRUSES

Polioviruses

Polioviruses are frequently present in the intestinal tract of healthy humans and are excreted in the faeces, so that most children become infected at an early age. Fortunately, very few develop the clinical disease but those who do are frequently affected with paralysis, hence the term 'infantile paralysis'. In countries with higher standards of hygiene, fewer people are infected and the disease occurs later in life when the paralytic syndrome is generally more serious. Until a few years ago, poliomyelitis was one of the most feared of all human viral diseases but today, due almost entirely to the widespread use of the Salk and Sabin vaccines, cases of poliomyelitis are rare indeed.

There is still considerable doubt regarding the sequence of events leading to CNS involvement but most workers are agreed that the primary site of multiplication of the virus is either in the lymphoid tissues or in the oropharyngeal and intestinal mucosa. There are both virulent and avirulent strains of poliovirus but both may pass through the intestinal wall and reach the blood stream, giving rise to a viraemia. However, the presence of a viraemia does not invariably result in CNS involvement and many cases do not progress beyond that of a non-specific febrile illness. The incubation period in cases involving the CNS is from 4–35 days, with an average of 10 days.

There is good evidence that stress plays an important part in potentiating the clinical illness. Trauma associated with intramuscular injections enhances the possibility of an individual developing paralysis, particularly of the inoculated muscle, and tonsillectomy is also believed to predispose a patient to the paralytic disease. In paralytic poliomyelitis the main lesions are associated with destruction of the neurones, particularly those in the anterior horns of the spinal cord. If large numbers of neurones are destroyed death occurs.

Although the viral aetiology of poliomyelitis was discovered in 1909, very little was known about its biological and physicochemical characteristics until 1949 when Enders, Weller and Robbins, in the U.S.A., showed that the virus would grow readily in cultures of non-neural cells of human origin. This important and fundamental discovery led to a simple method of isolating, identifying and typing strains of poliovirus, of detecting antibody titres in patients' sera, and of propagating large quantities of virus for the production of inactivated and attenuated vaccines.

All three serotypes of poliovirus (I, II and III) grow well in primary and secondary cell cultures of human and primate origin, as well as on HeLa and other human cell lines. In general, they do not grow readily, if at all, in non-primate tissues. The rapid and destructive type of cytopathic effect of poliovirus lends itself well to plaque assay methods as well as to a colorimetric neutralization test which depends on the rapid cessation of metabolism in infected cell suspensions and, consequently, lack of acidity and colour (pH) change as seen in control tubes of actively growing non-infected cells.

Following natural infection, neutralizing and precipitating antibodies develop rapidly (5–7 days) and are generally present when symptoms become noticeable. Complement-fixing antibodies develop more slowly (6–8 weeks) and do not persist for long periods. Neutralizing antibodies reach their peak within 4–6 weeks and the resulting immunity is probably lifelong.

Antibody developed following the use of inactivated vaccine (e.g. Salk's formalised virus) is believed to prevent invasion of the CNS by poliovirus, whereas the more effective live attenuated virus vaccines (e.g. Sabin) produce a humoral antibody response and also increase the patient's resistance to gut infection.

Coxsackieviruses

The name coxsackie virus is derived from a village in New York state where an outbreak resembling poliomyelitis was being investigated and the causative agent was isolated, unexpectedly, in unweaned mice and differed from the recognised poliovirus type.

It is now known that coxsackieviruses are frequently present during the summer and autumn months in the alimentary tract of children, particularly those living in conditions of poor hygiene. The virus is harboured for only a very short period, about a week, during which time it may be excreted in the urine and faeces. Coxsackieviruses may give rise to inapparent infections, a mild non-specific type of illness involving the intestinal or respiratory tracts or, on rare occasions, sporadic cases of severe illness with or without paralysis and death. Many strains cause rash-like illnesses and some are associated with vesicular-ulcerative lesions of the pharynx and an exanthema of the extremities — the so-called 'hand, foot and mouth disease of man'. Other strains may be responsible for cases of acute respiratory disease, myocarditis or severe thoracic and abdominal pain with orchitis as in Bornholm disease.

Coxsackieviruses are divided into two groups, A and B, on the basis of their biological characters; their physicochemical properties are very similar. There are numerous serological types in each group, as shown by neutralization, complement-fixation and gel-diffusion tests, and some agglutinate fowl or human group 'O' red blood cells.

Type B strains grow well in monkey kidney cell cultures and produce a marked destructive effect similar to that of poliovirus. Several type A strains also grow well on primate cell cultures but the majority do not readily do so. A few type A strains have been adapted to growth in the yolk sac or chorioallantoic membrane of embryonated hens' eggs.

All coxsackieviruses readily multiply in unweaned mice when injected by various routes but the intracerebral method is preferred for type B viruses. Type A strains cause flaccid paralysis and generalised degeneration of the striated muscles whereas type B strains produce spastic paralysis and tremors with extensive necrosis of the neurones of the cerebral hemispheres. Muscular involvement, if present, is localised rather than extensive and there are clearly visible areas of congestion of the fat pads (brown fat) in the interscapular spaces of affected mice.

Unweaned mice provide a useful method of isolating type A coxsackievirus which, unlike type B strains, mostly do not grow on cell cultures. Otherwise the methods of isolating and identifying coxsackieviruses are similar to those employed for other picornaviruses

Echoviruses

The third sub-group of human picornaviruses are the Echoviruses. The name stands for 'Enteric Cytopathic Human Orphan viruses' because they were originally thought not to be associated with human disease. However, it is now known that many members of the group may cause aseptic meningitis and other illnesses, so the term 'orphan' is not always relevant.

Echoviruses were first discovered when monkey kidney cell cultures were introduced in the search for polioviruses and numerous isolates were not neutralized by antisera to the three types of polioviruses. Since then, more than thirty distinct serotypes have been described and their association with encephalitis, paralysis, gastroenteritis, colds and other respiratory tract infections has been firmly established.

All echoviruses grow well in primary and continuous cell cultures of primate tissues and produce marked cytopathic effects. The plaques induced by echoviruses on monolayer cultures are small, irregular in shape and have ill-defined edges which help to distinguish them from the large plaques of polioviruses.

Newly isolated strains are identified by neutralization of their cytopathic effects by specific antisera. A number of virus types haemagglutinate human group 'O' red blood cells and this may be used in their identification.

There is no growth in embryonated hens' eggs and they rarely cause disease in experimental animals.

ENTEROVIRUSES FROM ANIMAL SOURCES

Monkey enteroviruses

Many ECMO (enteric cytopathic monkey orphan) viruses have been isolated from intestinal contents of rhesus or cynomolgus monkeys and some have been found as latent viruses in monkey-kidney cultures. These have been given numbers in an SV (simian virus) series and several antigenic types have been identified.

Bovine enteroviruses

The term ECBO (enteric cytopathic bovine orphan) viruses has been suggested for those agents recovered from cattle faeces having properties in keeping with enteroviruses. Many strains have been isolated from intestinal contents of clinically healthy cattle while others have been obtained from herds with histories of respiratory disease and abortion.

Neutralization tests in cell culture reveal that there are numerous serotypes and these can be classified into two broadly reacting groups. Possible antigenic relationships between human and bovine enteroviruses have been described and several bovine strains are believed to share an antigen with poliovirus type II.

Some strains agglutinate bovine red blood cells at 5°C whilst others agglutinate horse, sheep, guinea-pig, or rhesus monkey erythrocytes, or none at all.

All strains grow well in calf kidney cell cultures producing a marked cytopathic effect, and some also grow in cells derived from other animal sources (Plate 47.3c, facing p. 607). Strains have differing abilities to grow in fertile eggs but some can multiply in the allantoic cavity or yolk sac while others may form pocks on the chorioallantoic membrane.

None of the bovine enteroviruses are naturally pathogenic for cattle but some may cause abortion in pregnant experimental guinea-pigs or produce lesions in unweaned mice and hamsters similar to those caused by coxsackie A viruses.

TESCHEN DISEASE VIRUS AND OTHER PORCINE ENTEROVIRUSES

There are numerous reports of the isolation in tissue culture of cytopathic agents from the alimentary tract of pigs and most of these agents have the characteristics of enteroviruses. Although viruses of the Teschen (Tésin) group can cause polioencephalitis in pigs, and other species of enteroviruses have frequently been associated with outbreaks of diarrhoea in swine, most infections are inapparent and there is no clear evidence that ECSO (enteric cytopathic swine orphan) viruses are responsible for natural disease in pigs.

Synonyms

Infectious porcine encephalomyelitis: pig poliomyelitis: Teschen (Tésin) disease: Talfan disease:

Austeckende: Schweinelahmung: ECSO (ECPO) viruses — enteric cytopathic swine (porcine) orphans.

Hosts affected
Domestic and wild-living swine are the only species that are susceptible to Teschen and other porcine enteroviruses.

History and distribution
The first member of the porcine enterovirus group to be recognized was the virus causing Teschen disease or poliomyelitis of swine. The name is derived from the region of Teschen in Czechoslovakia where the first outbreaks were observed in 1929–30 although it is possible that cases of the disease had occurred in Moravia in 1913. Since that time, severe outbreaks of Teschen disease have been reported in many countries of central and western Europe and it has also been observed in Madagascar and other parts of Africa. Typical outbreaks causing serious losses in the swine population have not been recognized in the western hemisphere.

Much milder forms of paralysis were described in 1955–57 in Denmark and England, and the causative agent (Talfan) was later proved to be a less virulent strain of Teschen disease virus. There is recent evidence that mild strains may also be present in Canada, the United States and Australia. Since 1958, several serologically separable groups of non-pathogenic porcine enteroviruses have been isolated from the intestines and faeces of pigs and it seems likely that they have a world-wide distribution.

Virus properties
Teschen and other porcine enteroviruses are small (25–30 nm in diameter), approximately spherical, non-enveloped particles having an isometric capsid consisting of 32 capsomeres (Plate 47.1b, facing p. 606). The central core contains single-stranded RNA with a molecular weight of approximately 2.5×10^6 daltons. They are ether- and chloroform-resistant, survive well at $-70°C$ in 50 per cent glycerol and at $4°C$ but readily lose infectivity if preserved by freeze-drying. Many strains resist heating to $60°C$ for 15 minutes but all are inactivated after 30 minutes at this temperature. Changes in pH have little effect on porcine enteroviruses and most strains are stable between pH 3 and pH 9 at $4°C$ for 24 hours. All are readily inactivated by UV radiation, by formalin and many other substances, and oxidising agents are said to be particularly effective.

Haemagglutination
There is no evidence, as yet, that porcine enteroviruses possess the properties of haemagglutination or haemadsorption.

Antigenic properties
It is generally agreed that porcine enteroviruses fall into several serologically distinct groups and that one of them contains all known strains associated with Teschen disease. It has further been suggested that the Teschen group of viruses can be subdivided into three subtypes, the first to include the Konratice and Bozen strains, the second to include the Talfan and Tyrol strains and the third to include the Reporyje strain. It is emphasised that there is no correlation between the serological subtype and virulence since the Talfan virus of subtype 2 produces only a mild disease whereas the Tyrol strain of the same subtype is highly virulent. Subtypes may also occur within some of the other main serological groups.

Cultivation
All strains can be readily cultivated in pig kidney cell cultures causing cytopathic effects similar to those of other enteroviruses. In general, they cannot be propagated in cultures from other species of animals. Some strains including the Teschen group produce rounding-up and necrosis of the affected cells (T-type) whereas others induce nodular or stellate protrusions around the periphery of the affected cells (V-type) (Plates 47.2a, b and 47.3a, b between pp. 606, & 607). Most strains produce plaque formation in Petri dish cultures of pig kidney cells. There is no evidence that porcine enteroviruses are pathogenic for small laboratory animals or chick embryos.

Pathogenicity
Most naturally occurring infections associated with Teschen virus are inapparent or of a sporadic nature affecting only individual animals on the same farm. At other times it affects nearly all swine, one case quickly following another until the entire herd is ill. Thus, there are several forms of the disease — inapparent, subacute, acute and chronic.

The incubation period of the natural disease is not known but after experimental exposure to the virus by intracerebral, intranasal or oral routes the period appears to vary from 4–28 days, or longer, depending on the dose and potency of the virus, and the resistance of the individual animal.

In field cases associated with virulent strains of virus the onset of the disease is usually accompanied by fever, $(40–41°C$ or higher), anorexia and depression. This is followed within 1–3 days by tremors and incoordination, particularly of the hind legs, nystagmus and stiffness of the extremities. In severe cases there are violent clonic convulsions, prostration, coma and death. The stage of excitement appears to result from inflammation of the central nervous system. Residual posterior paralysis occurs in animals which survive but convalescence is prolonged (1–3 months).

The pathogenesis of Teschen disease is very similar to that of poliomyelitis of man in that there are three stages of the disease: (1) multiplication of the virus in the alimentary tract and associated lymph nodes, (2) viraemia and (3) infection of the nervous system followed by destruction of the neurones.

Cases of Talfan disease in Britain are usually mild and affected animals show ataxia rather than paralysis.

Other porcine enteroviruses have been isolated from outbreaks of enteritis but there is little evidence that they can cause clinical illness in naturally infected pigs. Strains such as T-80 type viruses isolated from the tonsils and faeces of clinically healthy pigs have been shown to produce polioencephalitis when inoculated into new-born pigs deprived of colostrum but they do not cause clinical disease in the field.

The histological picture of Teschen and Talfan diseases is that of a diffuse encephalomyelitis which is more widespread than in human poliomyelitis. The lesions are most pronounced in the grey matter and include degeneration of neurones and perivascular cuffing. Cytoplasmic acidophilic masses have been observed in the affected nerve cells and fatty infiltration in the myocardium has also been reported.

Transmission

Porcine enteroviruses are comparatively resistant to the physical environment and their presence in mouth secretions and faeces for several weeks after infection undoubtedly facilitates transmission by direct and indirect contact. Viruses can be isolated with increasing frequency in pigs up to 8–10 weeks of age but are seldom found in piglets during the first month of life, due presumably to the presence of colostral antibodies. It is not known where the virus persists between outbreaks but it may be maintained by adult carrier swine. There is good evidence that the infection can be spread from farm to farm by infected materials as well as by infected sows. Susceptible pigs probably acquire the infection by ingestion or inhalation.

Diagnosis

Teschen disease cannot be diagnosed from the clinical symptoms alone, but the disease should be suspected when adult pigs show central nervous symptoms associated with high fever. Definitive diagnosis of Teschen and other porcine enterovirus infections is dependent upon laboratory investigations including isolation of the causative virus and its identification by cross-neutralization tests in pig kidney cell cultures.

Differential diagnosis

Confusion may arise, especially in the early stages of Teschen or Talfan diseases, with other swine infections including swine fever, rabies and Aujeszky's disease.

Control

Vaccines against Teschen disease are prepared from virus grown in porcine kidney cell cultures and are administered subcutaneously either as live attenuated or formalin inactivated vaccines. Both types induce the formation of neutralizing antibodies and give over 80 per cent protection.

Vaccination is not justified in the case of Talfan or other porcine enterovirus infections.

Swine vesicular disease

History and distribution

The first outbreak of a hitherto undescribed vesicular disease of swine occurred in Lombardy, Italy, in 1966. The condition was clinically indistinguishable from foot-and-mouth disease although the lesions healed within 2–3 days and only pigs were affected. In 1971, the disease was observed among swine in Hong Kong, both on farms on which the pigs had been recently vaccinated with the homologous type O strains of foot-and-mouth disease antigens and on neighbouring farms where the pigs had not been vaccinated. In 1972, swine vesicular disease was also diagnosed in two areas in Poland and further outbreaks were reported from Italy, Austria and France. In December of that year the disease was observed for the first time in the United Kingdom on a farm in Staffordshire and subsequently spread to other parts of the country. By February 1973 no fewer than 52 outbreaks had been reported in England.

Virus properties

The causative virus of swine vesicular disease is a small roughly spherical particle (30–32 nm in diameter) which is slightly larger than the virion of foot-and-mouth disease (20–25 nm). It consists of a naked capsid with isometric symmetry, containing a central core of single-stranded RNA. In negatively stained preparations the surface of the capsid is composed of a number of hollow cylindrical capsomeres. Unlike foot-and-mouth disease virus and other rhinoviruses, swine vesicular disease virus is stable at pH5 and is stabilized against thermal inactivation at 50°C by 1M $MgCl_2$. Its buoyant density is 1·34g/ml. compared with 1·43 g/ml for foot-and-mouth disease virus, and its sedimentation coefficient is 150 as opposed to 140 for foot-and-mouth disease virus. Both viruses are ether resistant. The virus of swine vesicular disease has not yet been fully characterized but there is general agreement among workers in this field that its properties are very similar to those of enteroviruses in the family *Picornaviridae*; and the English strain has been provisionally named Porcine Enterovirus England/72.

Antigenic properties

Comparative neutralization tests have revealed minor antigenic differences between strains of swine vesicular disease. For example, the Italy/66, Hong Kong/71 and France/73 viruses differ from each other, and from Italy/72, England/72, Austria/73 and Poland/73 group of viruses. It is emphasised, however, that there is no serological relationship between the viruses of swine vesicular disease and foot-and-mouth disease.

Haemagglutination

Haemagglutinins have not been described for the Italy/66, Hong Kong/71 or England/72 strains.

Cultivation

The virus can be readily propagated in cells cultivated *in vitro*. Vesicular fluids and extracts of vesicular epithelia from both naturally and experimentally infected pigs produce marked cellular degeneration in primary or secondary pig kidney cell cultures, as well as in the PK15 and IB-RS-2 lines of pig kidney cells. Unlike foot-and-mouth disease virus, there is no cytopathic effect in calf kidney, calf thyroid or the BHK21 line of baby hamster kidney cells. Cytopathic changes first appear approximately 20–24 hours after initial infection and mainly consist of cytoplasmic granulation and rounding-up of infected cells into small foci or microplaques. Extension of these plaques proceeds rapidly and usually results in complete disruption of the monolayer and dislodgement of the dead cells from the glass after 48 hours of incubation. Cellular changes have not been observed in tissue cultures prepared from the kidneys of horses, guinea-pigs or rabbits and there is no evidence that the virus can be cultivated in embryonated hens' eggs.

Pathogenicity

The clinical signs in spontaneous outbreaks of swine vesicular disease are indistinguishable from those of foot-and-mouth disease. These include high fever (41–42°C) and the development of vesicular lesions on the snout, coronary bands, bulbs of the heels and in the interdigital spaces. The vesicles are approximately 1–3 cm in diameter, and often coalesce and rupture after only 2–3 days of the clinical illness. Healing is rapid and affected animals generally make a complete and uneventful recovery. Vesicular fluids, vesicular epithelium and other infected tissues do not contain the foot-and-mouth disease complement-fixing antigen.

Subcutaneous or intradermal inoculation of infected tissue extracts into the bulbs of the heels of susceptible pigs produces severe vesicular lesions at or near the site of inoculation within 36 hours. Thereafter, the infection progresses rapidly and involves other parts of the body including the coronary bands, interdigital spaces, snout and tongue. In many cases, however, the artificially induced disease is not so severe as that observed in the field, but the majority of infected animals develop high levels of neutralizing antibodies which persist for at least 4–5 months.

The virus does not produce clinical illness when injected intralingually in horses, cattle, rabbits and chickens or following intradermal inoculation of the foot-pads of guinea-pigs or the abdominal skin of hamsters. However, intracerebral or intraperitoneal inoculation of one-day old mice with high doses of tissue culture virus (greater than $10^{3.5}$ p.f.u.) produces nervous symptoms leading to paralysis and death 5–10 days post inoculation. Seven-day-old mice, as used for propagating foot-and-mouth disease virus, are not susceptible.

Ecology

In the original outbreak in Italy, the disease appeared simultaneously on two farms both of which had recently introduced pigs from a common source. All of the newly purchased animals became ill but only a quarter of the other pigs developed vesicular lesions; and no fresh cases were observed after three weeks. The course of the illness was of short duration and the infection appeared to spread less rapidly than that of foot-and-mouth disease. This was also noted during the Hong Kong outbreak although the incidence rose to 70 per cent.

The source of infection in these three widely separated outbreaks of an apparently new vesicular disease of swine is not yet known but the information presently available suggests that most, if not all, cases have been associated with either direct contact with infected premises or feeding of uncooked swill.

Diagnosis

Because the symptoms and lesions of swine vesicular disease are clinically indistinguishable from those of foot-and-mouth disease, an accurate diagnosis can only be made in a suitably equipped laboratory. It is emphasised, however, that the disease occurs only in pigs and the lesions usually heal within 2–3 days.

The epithelium and fluid from vesicular lesions do not contain foot-and-mouth disease complement-fixing antigens of any of the seven known serotypes,

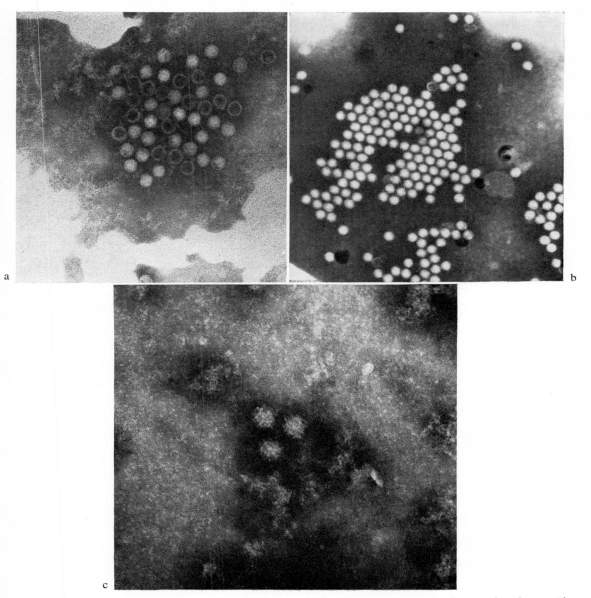

47.1a Porcine enterovirus; cell culture isolate showing penetrated and unpenetrated isometric virus particles, × 150 000. (Courtesy of Dr J. B. McFerran.)

47.1b Electron micrograph of enterovirus from cattle; cell culture isolate showing mainly unpenetrated particles, × 110 000. (Courtesy of Dr J. B. McFerran.)

47.1c Calicivirus. The feline picornavirus differs from other members of the group in being slightly larger and with an irregular, indistinct outline. In negatively stained preparations the capsid shows a number of large, dark, stain-penetrated cup-shaped structures from which the generic name calicivirus is derived, × 200 000. (Courtesy of Dr C. R. Madeley.)

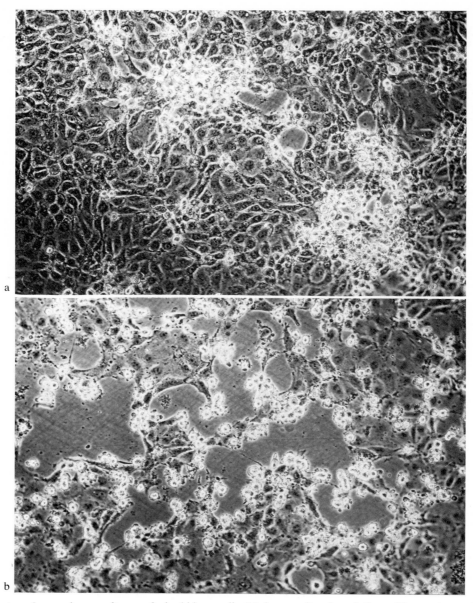

Micrographs of monolayer cultures of pig kidney cells 36 hours after inoculation with porcine enteroviruses. Unstained; phase contrast microscopy.

47.2a   The T-type strain produces rounding-up and necrosis of the affected cells, ×150.

47.2b   The V-type strain induces dark nodular or stellate protrusions around the periphery of the highly refractile infected cells, ×150.

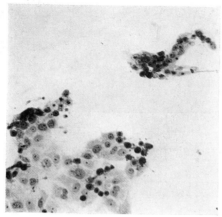

47.3a

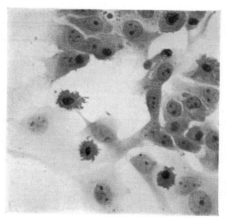

47.3b

Cytopathic changes in a line of pig kidney cells (PK15) infected with porcine enteroviruses.

47.3a After 72 hours' incubation the T-type strain causes marked cell retraction, rounding-up and necrosis of affected cells, followed by rapid lysis leaving a granular debris. Giemsa stain, × 170.

47.3b Cultures inoculated 48 hours previously with V-type virus show a cytopathic effect. Protrusions around the periphery of deeply stained infected cells give them a characteristic stellate appearance. Haematoxylin eosin stain, × 380.

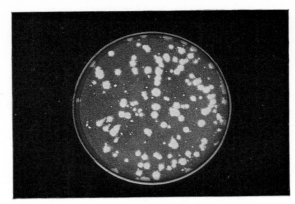

47.3c

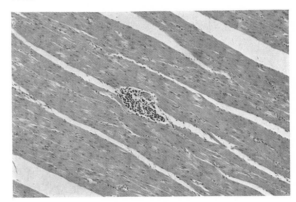

47.3d

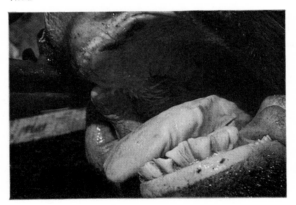

47.3e

47.3c Two plaque-type mutants of a bovine strain of enterovirus on a Petri dish culture of calf kidney cells. After 3 days' incubation in 10 per cent CO_2 the agar overlay is removed and the monolayer flooded with methylene blue. The dye stains the healthy growing cells, but individual areas of plaques of lysed affected cells remain unstained.

47.3d Section of myocardium from a chicken with epidemic tremor (infectious avian encephalomyelitis). Focal hyperplasia of lymphoid follicles in the musculature of the heart is diagnostic of the condition. Haematoxylin eosin stain, $\times 110$.

47.3e Early tongue lesions in a field case of bovine foot-and-mouth disease. Notice the pallor of the unruptured vesicles. (Courtesy of Mr I. S. Beattie.)

but they produce obvious cytopathic effects in primary, secondary or established monolayer cultures of pig kidney cells. Bovine tissue cultures are not affected. Identification of cell culture isolates can be readily obtained by comparative serum neutralization tests including virus plaque assays, and by complement-fixation tests with sera against known strains of vesicular disease virus.

Infected lesion material and cell culture fluids produce illness in pigs, particularly when injected intradermally or subcutaneously into the bulbs of the heels, but cause no apparent disease when inoculated into the tongue of horses, cattle, rabbits and chickens, or into the foot-pads of guinea-pigs or the abdominal skin of hamsters.

Electron microscopy and physicochemical studies can be used to confirm that the causal agent has the characteristics of a porcine enterovirus.

Differential diagnosis
Swine vesicular disease can be distinguished from foot-and-mouth disease and vesicular stomatitis by biological tests, but differentiation of vesicular exanthema is more difficult and may necessitate detailed ultrastructural and physicochemical investigations. Some of the methods used for the differential diagnosis of swine vesicular disease, foot-and-mouth disease, vesicular stomatitis and vesicular exanthema are outlined in Tables 44.2 and 47.1, on pages 553 and 620.

Control
There are no vaccines available at present for the immunization of pigs against swine vesicular disease. In the U.K., rigorous quarantine and slaughter policies and legislation prohibiting the feeding of uncooked swill to pigs are being enforced in an attempt to eradicate the disease.

Public health aspects
There is clear evidence that man is susceptible to infection with the virus of swine vesicular disease, particularly if exposed to large doses of virus in the laboratory. In human patients, swine vesicular disease virus produces symptoms of a mild feverish cold but, in a few cases, the illness is more serious and is accompanied by pain, loss of weight and aseptic meningitis.

Although swine vesicular disease virus is closely related to, but different from another enterovirus, Coxsackie B5, it is not related to Coxsackie A5 and A16 viruses which have been associated with a human illness characterised by fever and vesicular rash called hand, foot and mouth disease.

AVIAN ENTEROVIRUSES
Duck viral hepatitis
Definition
An acute, highly fatal and contagious viral infection of ducklings, characterized primarily by a short incubation period, sudden onset and the development of characteristic liver lesions.

Hosts affected
The disease is mostly confined to ducklings during the first 1–5 weeks of life. Thereafter they are refractory to the development of clinical symptoms. Infection has not been observed in other avian species.

History and distribution
Duck hepatitis was first recorded on Long Island, U.S.A., in the spring of 1949 and, by the autumn of that year, practically every farm in the area was affected. The disease was largely confined to Long Island until 1953 when an outbreak occurred on a farm in East Anglia, England. Since then, the disease has appeared in widely separated parts of the world including Canada, Holland, Germany and Egypt (1957), Hungary (1959) and Russia (1960). The infection is probably present also in France, Czechoslovakia, and other parts of Europe, in Brazil, Israel and India, parts of Africa, as well as in Thailand, Japan and other Far Eastern countries.

Virus properties
The causative agent was first isolated in 1950 and has recently been tentatively classified as a picornavirus. The virions are small, roughly spherical particles measuring between 20 and 40 nm in diameter, with a core of single-stranded RNA.

All strains resist treatment with ether, chloroform, and trypsin, and are stable at pH3.0 The virus is heat-stable and may remain active at 56°C. for 60 minutes, but some investigators consider that much of the virus is inactivated after 30 minutes at this temperature. Virus-infected embryonic fluids remain viable for 28 days at 25°C. and are still infective after as long as 9 years at –20°C. or 2 years at 4°C.

Duck hepatitis virus is very resistant to disinfectants and is not inactivated when exposed to 2 per cent lysol at 37°C. for 60 minutes, nor by 0.1 per cent formalin after 8 hours at the same temperature. It also resists adverse environmental conditions and may survive in uncleaned brooders for 10 weeks or longer, and in moist droppings for at least 5 weeks.

Cultivation

The virus can be propagated in the allantoic cavity of 9-day-old fertile hens' eggs, killing up to 60 per cent. of the embryos in 5–6 days. The affected embryos are stunted and oedematous and the virus, which is present in high titres in the allantoic fluids, becomes attenuated for ducklings after 20–30 serial passages in eggs. It is stressed, however, that the virulence of the chick embryo-passaged virus returns after passage through ducklings.

The virus may also be cultivated in cultures of chick-embryo tissues, without cytopathic effects, but no growth occurs in trypsinized chick embryo cells or mammalian cells. Some growth takes place in duck-embryo kidney cells after about the 8th passage and the cytopathic effects show focal areas of cellular degeneration and necrosis after 16 hours of incubation. The latent phase lasts approximately 2–4 hours, followed by release of the virus 4–8 hours post-infection which reaches its peak in about 24 hours.

Haemagglutination

None of the strains haemagglutinates chick, duck, horse, sheep, pig, rabbit, guinea-pig or mouse erythrocytes when tested at pH 6·8–7·4 and at temperatures of 4°, 22° and 37°C: but an indirect test using tannic acid-treated sheep red blood cells has been described.

Antigenic properties

All strains of duck hepatitis virus are immunologically similar although they vary widely in their pathogenicity. In a recent report, however, 2 serotypes have been described and antigens prepared from infected liver suspensions or cell cultures give 2 distinct lines of precipitation when diffused against immune duck sera.

Pathogenicity

The virus causes a severe disease of ducklings, particularly during the first week or two of life. The infection spreads very rapidly and mortality rates up to 90–95 per cent may occur on badly affected farms. Adult ducks, chickens and turkeys on infected premises do not show clinical symptoms of the disease but may harbour the infection for many weeks. In some outbreaks a number of chickens may also acquire an inapparent infection and pass the virus to other birds by direct contact.

In spontaneous outbreaks of the disease the incubation period is usually short, 18–24 hours, but may range from 1–5 days. This is followed by sudden onset of acute illness. Affected ducklings become lethargic, paddle spasmodically with their feet and die within a few minutes with typical opisthotonos. Practically all deaths occur within 3 days after the onset of the disease. In less acute cases, the affected ducklings appear drowsy, cease eating and drinking, and some may void fluid, green-coloured droppings.

The most conspicuous gross lesions are to be found in the liver which is markedly enlarged, oedematous and mottled with haemorrhages ranging from pin-point size to about 1 cm. in diameter. Microscopically, the affected hepatic cells show vacuolation within 24 hours of infection, followed by necrosis 1–2 days later. Other abnormalities include proliferation of the bile ducts with cellular infiltration and perivascular cuffing in the central nervous system.

Transmission

The virus usually spreads rapidly to all susceptible ducklings in the flock but at other times transmission of the infection appears to be very erratic. There is general agreement that egg transmission does not take place in duck hepatitis and that newly hatched ducklings are seldom responsible for introducing the virus on to clean premises. Thus, newly hatched birds from infected farms remain well when taken to premises where no ducks are kept.

Recovered or latently infected ducks may excrete virus in the faeces for up to 8 weeks after infection and there is evidence that wild birds may be mechanical carriers of the virus over short distances.

Diagnosis

A presumptive diagnosis may be based on the history and pathognomonic lesions since the sudden onset of a highly fatal and rapidly spreading disease of young ducklings with gross liver lesions is usually diagnostic.

For confirmatory diagnosis, the virus can be isolated by inoculating suspected liver suspensions or blood into the allantoic sac of 10-day-old embryonated hens' eggs. Infected embryos that die within 6 days are atrophied and show characteristic lesions including oedema, necrosis and enlargement of the liver. In many cases there is greenish discolouration of the embryonic fluids and yolk sacs which may first be detected when 'candling' the eggs. The liver of the embryos are generally greenish in colour and may have yellowish necrotic foci throughout its substance.

Serological tests are not commonly used for the diagnosis of duck hepatitis but virus neutralization and agar gel diffusion tests are of value in virus identification.

Control

Since ducklings hatched from eggs laid by immune birds are resistant to the infection, breeding stock may be immunized with live avirulent strains to ensure high levels of antibodies in the yolk of hatching eggs. In the absence of maternally derived antibodies, susceptible ducklings may themselves be actively immunized with attenuated strains of duck hepatitis virus. In both instances the vaccines mostly used are prepared from avirulent strains of virus propagated in embryonated hens' eggs.

On the other hand, many workers consider that serum therapy is the only effective practical method of control and that all ducklings should be inoculated intramuscularly with 0.5 ml. of antiserum. The serum is prepared from pooled blood samples collected at the time of slaughter from naturally recovered ducks, or ducks previously treated with antiserum, and held in storage until required. For best results, serum therapy should be initiated as soon as mortality is first seen in the flock.

Turkey hepatitis

In 1958, workers in Canada and the U.S.A. described an acute, highly contagious but frequently sub-clinical infection of turkeys which produces hepatic and pancreatic lesions. The causative agent of this condition is serologically related to duck hepatitis virus but is infectious only for turkeys. It multiplies readily in the yolk sac of 6–7-day-old fowl or turkey embryos and can be isolated without difficulty from the liver, pancreas and other tissues of turkey poults, but less easily from older birds. The virus is thermostable and resists exposure to ether, chloroform and phenol. It is susceptible to high but not low pH. Deaths occur only in poults and a second, more recently reported virus which causes hepatitis and mortality in goslings may or may not be related.

Gross lesions observed in turkey hepatitis include haemorrhage or congestion of the liver and focal areas of necrosis resembling "blackhead", but without caecal lesions.

The clinical disease mostly occurs in poults between 1–3 years of age and losses range from 2–20 per cent with an average of 5 per cent.

Recovered birds resist reinfection despite the apparent absence of circulating antibodies, and there are no vaccines available for immunizing birds against the disease.

Avian encephalomyelitis

Synonyms
Infectious avian encephalomyelitis: epidemic tremor.

Definition
An acute infectious viral disease of young chicks characterized by progressive ataxia of the leg muscles, tremors of the head and neck, and frequently terminating in death. The infection in mature birds is mild or inapparent.

Hosts affected
Avian encephalomyelitis has a limited host range and natural outbreaks have been observed only in chickens, pheasants and Japanese quail, but ducklings, turkey poults, young pigeons and guinea fowls may be infected experimentally.

History and distribution
A previously unknown disease causing tremors in a commercial flock of 2-week-old Rhode Island Red chicks was recognised in New England, U.S.A., in 1930. A year later similar outbreaks were observed in which both tremors and ataxia were present in affected chicks. The disease quickly spread to other parts of the U.S.A. and Canada, and was diagnosed for the first time in the U.K. in 1951. At the present time epidemic tremor of chicks probably exists in many other countries of the world where poultry are raised on a commercial basis.

Virus properties
The causative agent has similar properties to those of other enteroviruses in the family *Picornaviridae*. It resists exposure to ether, chloroform, pepsin, trypsin and deoxycholate and is protected against the effects of heat (50°C.) by divalent magnesium ions ($MgCl_2$).

Antigenic properties
No serological differences have been observed between the various strains of avian encephalomyelitis virus, and antigenically similar strains have been isolated on a number of occasions from rectal swabs of clinically healthy chicks. Other enteroviruses, falling into 15 or more distinct serotypes, have also been recovered from normal chicks and it has been suggested that avian encephalomyelitis virus is a particularly neurotropic member of a large group of avian enteroviruses.

Cultivation
The causative agent was first propagated in susceptible chicks by intracerebral inoculation in 1934. Since then, suspended cell cultures and monolayer cultures of chick embryo fibroblasts or chick kidney cells have been utilized for multiplication of the virus, and serial passage results in the production of large quantities of virus (10^{-8} ID_{50}/ml) but with concurrent decrease in its pathogenicity for chickens. Growth has also been described in cultures of monkey kidney cells. Infected chick kidney cell cultures show rounded cells, shrinking and cytoplasmic granulation.

The virus can also be adapted to growth in fertile hens' eggs by yolk sac, amniotic or allantoic inoculation, but care must be taken to select eggs from non-infected flocks since antibodies readily pass from immune hens into the yolk.

Several strains of field virus have been found to be non-pathogenic for chick embryos until they have become fully adapted to the embryo by rapid serial passage. One such virus, the van Roekel egg-adapted strain, is highly neurotropic and causes symptoms of the disease in chickens of all ages following parenteral inoculation.

Pathogenicity

Chicks experimentally infected by contact transmission, by oral administration or by various methods of inoculation have an incubation period of 6–10 days, or longer. In most cases, virus can be recovered from the brain and spinal cord of affected chicks and from various other tissues and organs. Virus is often present in the faeces and it has been suggested, therefore, that multiplication of the virus may occur in the intestinal tract of naturally infected birds.

Spontaneous cases of the disease mostly occur in young chicks between 2–3 weeks of age, but there are reports that baby chicks may appear lethargic and abnormally small before developing typical symptoms later.

The first recognisable signs of the disease are dullness of the eyes and weakness of the legs. As a result, affected chicks appear unsteady and often flop on to their hocks. As the disease progresses ataxia, general weakness and malaise become more evident, and may be accompanied by tremors. The muscular tremors may be so fine as to be appreciated only by holding affected birds in the hand, but usually they are clearly visible in the head and neck or the tail feathers. Severely affected chicks soon lose the use of their legs and are unable to reach the food and water troughs, and fall on their sides. Although the mortality rate in spontaneous outbreaks may be high, ailing birds frequently survive if they are removed and reared separately so that they can feed without being trampled on or asphyxiated by their healthy pen mates. Surviving chicks, even if reared to maturity, never fully recover from the damage to their nervous system. In adult flocks, the only signs of the disease may be loose droppings and a fall in egg-production.

At autopsy, there are no gross lesions attributable to the disease and only microscopical lesions are present. The principal histopathological changes are to be found in the central nervous system consisting of focal microgliosis, perivascular accumulations of lymphocytes and neuronal cell degeneration. Perivascular cuffing is usually pronounced throughout the entire brain. In the affected viscera there is hyperplasia of the lymphoid follicles occurring most frequently in the pancreas, in the musculature of the gizzard and proventriculus and, less commonly, in the heart, lung, liver, spleen and kidney. (Plate 47.3d facing page 607.)

Ecology

Although conclusive proof of embryo-transmission of the virus is lacking, many workers believe that the disease in young chicks is due to a transient, subclinical infection in laying hens during which the eggs become infected. It has also been suggested that the virus can be spread to susceptible chicks in incubators or under brooders through direct contact with a few egg-infected chicks.

Diagnosis

A tentative diagnosis of avian encephalomyelitis can usually be made when large numbers of young chicks show typical symptoms of ataxia and tremors. A confirmatory diagnosis is obtained by histopathological examinations or by the isolation and identification of the causative virus. Although the published reports concerning egg inoculation experiments are conflicting it is generally agreed that the virus can best be isolated in the yolk sac of 5–7-day-old embryonated hens' eggs. The embryos are allowed to hatch and are closely observed for symptoms of the disease during the first 10 days of life. Should clinical signs appear the brain, proventriculus and pancreas are examined for histopathological lesions. The virus may also be isolated by inoculating susceptible day-old chicks intracerebrally with brain material from spontaneous cases of the disease. Whichever method is utilized it is important to distinguish the virus from other avian enteroviruses either by neutralization tests in fertile eggs or tissue cultures, or by other serological methods. In some laboratories the van Roekel egg-adapted strain is used in eggs or cell cultures to determine the level of neutralizing antibodies in the sera of affected or recovered chickens.

Differential diagnosis

Avian encephalomyelitis must be differentiated from Newcastle disease, which also causes non-purulent encephalomyelitis, and from various other conditions of poultry including avian encephalomalacia, calcium deficiency, Marek's disease, mycotic encephalitis and brain abscesses of bacterial origin.

Control

In endemic areas, early immunization of breeder pullets of 8–20 weeks of age can be carried out by means of commercially available attenuated avianized virus vaccines. These may be administered parenterally or incorporated in the drinking water. Since chicks from vaccinated or naturally infected hens may retain maternal antibodies for 6–8 weeks, vaccination should not be attempted until they are 8–10 weeks old. Alternatively, adult birds may be vaccinated with live virus into the wing-web so that their offspring become resistant. In other areas, where the incidence of the disease is low, infected brain-tissue vaccines, inactivated with β-propio-lactone, are generally preferred. Effective immunization protects breeding birds against the disease and prevents the transmission of virus to the progeny via the egg-borne route.

RHINOVIRUSES

Introduction

The name rhinovirus was originally used for human strains associated with common colds but has more recently been extended to include viruses from other hosts including equine rhinoviruses, bovine rhinoviruses and the virus of foot-and-mouth disease.

Rhinoviruses are small spherical particles (20–30 nm in diameter) containing single-stranded RNA, with a molecular weight of about 2.8×10^6 daltons which is about the same as that of enteroviruses. All strains so far studied, are ether-stable and differ from enteroviruses in being rapidly inactivated at pH 5.3 and in not being effectively stabilized against inactivation at 50°C by 1M $MgCl_2$.

Neutralization tests carried out in tissue culture by plaque inhibition and other methods suggest that there are probably over 100 serotypes of human rhinoviruses but other types undoubtedly exist. So far as animal rhinoviruses are concerned there are 7 serological types of foot-and-mouth disease virus and numerous variants and subtypes exist within the main types. On the other hand, there appear to be only 2 or 3 serotypes of equine rhinoviruses whilst the few known strains of bovine rhinoviruses are serologically very similar.

Foot-and-mouth disease

Synonyms

Aphthous fever: epizootic aphthae: fièvre aphtheuse (Fr.): Maul-und Klauenseuche (Gr.): fiebre aftosa (Sp.).

Definition

An acute febrile highly contagious viral disease affecting almost exclusively cloven-footed animals. It is characterized by the formation of vesicles on the mucosa of the mouth, and sometimes of other parts of the alimentary tract and on the skin especially of the feet, teats and udder.

Distribution

The geographical distribution of foot-and-mouth disease is almost world-wide. At the present time the disease is endemic in continental Europe and continues to spread virtually unchecked and uncontrolled throughout large areas of Asia, Africa and parts of South America. It has not been reported from New Zealand at any time, and Australia had its last outbreak in 1872. Nine sporadic outbreaks have occurred in the U.S.A. prior to 1929, but it has not appeared since then. The disease had not occurred in Canada before its first and only outbreak in 1952. The comparative freedom of these countries is largely due to their favourable geographical position and to the stringency of their regulations to prevent the introduction of the disease.

Foot-and-mouth disease was first recorded in England in 1839 near Stratford, whence it spread rapidly through many counties to Scotland and Ireland. Thereafter, it continued to appear intermittently in the U.K. and the most serious outbreaks occurred in 1871, 1922–24, 1952 and 1967–68.

Hosts affected

The disease occurs naturally in cloven-hoofed animals, both domestic and wild-living. Cattle are most susceptible, followed by pigs but sheep and goats are generally considered to be least susceptible and are less severely affected. Wild game including many species of deer, buck and other ruminants may also be infected. Solipeds are completely resistant.

Although man is frequently exposed to the disease, only a few authenticated cases have been reported. Most human patients suffer only a mild illness with localized vesicles, usually on the hands. Guinea-pigs, baby mice and hamsters can be experimentally infected but other laboratory animals including dogs, cats, rats, rabbits and birds are only slightly susceptible to artificial infection. The European hedgehog may contract the disease naturally and spread the infection to other susceptible animals by direct and indirect contact.

Morphology

The causative agent of foot-and-mouth disease is one of the smallest animal viruses known. It has all the characteristics of a picornavirus and is now regarded as a member of the genus *Rhinovirus* The virion measures between 20–25 nm in diameter and is roughly spherical or hexagonal in shape. In negatively-stained preparations of purified virus the surface of the capsid appears to consist of approximately 32 short, hollow, cylindrical capsomeres which are rather larger than those of most other picornaviruses. Ultracentrifugation studies show that the virus contains 2 distinct particles measuring 25 nm and 7 nm, respectively. Both particles fix guinea-pig complement but it is the larger component that carries the infectivity properties of the virus.

Physicochemical characters

The virus particle contains single-stranded RNA with a molecular weight of 2.8×10^6 daltons. It is resistant to ether, chloroform, bile salts and detergents but is inactivated in 30 minutes at 56°C.

It is stable at pH 7·4–7·6 and at pH3. Because of its lability in the region of pH5 it has been classified with the rhinoviruses as an 'acid-labile picornavirus'.

Resistance

Although the observations of numerous investigators indicate that virus secreted in the saliva of affected animals may remain viable for up to 2 days at 37°C, 3 weeks at 26°C and for 5 weeks at 4°C, the resistance of the virus is closely related to environmental factors such as heat, moisture and pH. The virus is readily destroyed when exposed to direct sunlight and dessication, but may survive for several weeks in tissue fragments or on contaminated materials such as hay, straw, hair, hides, wood, etc. Virus in dried secretions and excretions on floors, walls, bedding, etc. inside contaminated buildings may remain infective for at least a month in summer and for 2 months or longer in winter.

The virus is readily inactivated by heat but some strains appear to have higher thermostable properties and withstand higher temperatures than others. In the laboratory, heat inactivation of the virus is promoted by molar $MgCl_2$. Most strains kept in an incubator at 37°C lose infectivity within 48 hours, but remain viable for many months at refrigeration temperatures (4–7°C) and can be preserved at low temperatures (–50 to –70°C) or by lyophilization for several years.

In general, the virus of foot-and-mouth disease is more resistant to many chemical substances which are popularly supposed to destroy it than are many other microorganisms. Phenolic-type disinfectants have little effect on the virus, especially when it is mixed with organic material, and various other substances have also proved unsatisfactory for practical use — notably alcohol, ether, chloroform, acetone, many other organic solvents and detergents such as sodium dodecylsulphate and Tween 80. Of the more commonly used 'disinfectants', sublimate of mercury, potassium permanganate, lactic acid, ethylene oxide, hypochlorite solution and formalin are usually effective within 30 minutes. Under field conditions, a solution containing 4 per cent sodium carbonate (washing soda) and soap has proved effective when speed of action is not important, whereas a 2·0 per cent solution of sodium hydroxide (caustic soda, lye) is more effective and destroys the virus in less than 2 minutes, but is very caustic. For the sterilization of infected bovine faeces, sulphuric acid (N/10) and caustic soda (N/1) are more effective than citric acid (0·2 per cent) or washing soda (4 per cent). It is stressed that the ability of chemical substances to penetrate tissue fragments and other organic substances is of great importance in determining their virucidal potency.

The viability of foot-and-mouth disease virus in milk and milk products depends to a large extent on the rate of acid formation as well as temperature. Thus, in fresh milk the virus is destroyed after exposure for 15 seconds at 70°C, 30 seconds at 65°C, 24 hours at 37°C, in 6 days at room temperature (18–22°C), and in 12 days at refrigeration temperature (4–7°C). Virus titres in milk are greatly reduced by pasteurization. Although it has been suggested that inactivation of the virus may be achieved by the souring of milk, either naturally or by the addition of suitable bacillary cultures, acid-resistant variants have been detected in several strains of foot-and-mouth disease virus. It has also been reported that virus may remain viable in unsalted butter for 8 days and in salted butter for 14 days.

In slaughtered animals the virus is rapidly inactivated in muscle tissues due to the formation of lactic acid in the normal process of *rigor mortis*. Lymph-nodes, liver, kidney and other tissues including bone-marrow are not affected and may remain infective for many weeks. The virus remains infective in vesicular epithelium for 2 months in the open during winter, or in bone-marrow, organs and offal for 2–3 months if held in a cold store.

The virus may survive in sewage and 'slurry' for several weeks. In liquid bovine faeces 0·1 per cent of the original infectivity of a field strain of virus was found to persist after 9 weeks at 4°C. Virus buried in solid manure at 34°C. loses its infectivity within 2 days but remains active for 4 days if kept on the surface at 24°C. On the other hand, virus may survive in liquid manure for 103 days during autumn and winter in temperate climates or, under laboratory conditions, for at least 6 weeks at pH 6·7 and 4°C.

Haemagglutination

Haemagglutinins have not been satisfactorily demonstrated and a claim that rat erythrocytes are agglutinated by the vesicular fluid of guinea-pigs infected with type O, A or C viruses awaits confirmation. However, a more recent report in 1973 describes direct haemagglutination of guinea-pig erythrocytes by strains of foot-and-mouth disease virus type SAT 2. The reaction, which is dependent on the presence of magnesium ions, is not obtained with the other 6 types of foot-and-mouth disease virus. As with ECHO viruses, type SAT 2 haemagglutinin activity is destroyed by incubation with trypsin but not with receptor destroying enzyme.

Antigenic properties

The virus of foot-and-mouth disease has several claims to a place in the history of virology. Not only was it the first animal virus to be discovered but it was also the first virus in which antigenic differences between strains were recognised. The existence of more than one antigenic type was discovered by

Vallée and Carré in 1922, when they observed that recovered cattle in France became reinfected when brought in contact with sick animals from Germany. In a series of carefully controlled experiments they failed to obtain cross-immunity between 2 groups of strains and the viruses were named O (Oise) and A (Allemagne), respectively, from their areas of origin. Four years later, a third type was described by Waldmann and Trautwein and designated type C. In the 1930s there was evidence that strains of virus isolated from outbreaks of typical foot-and-mouth disease in parts of Africa did not fit into the framework of the classification O, A and C and, in 1948, Galloway and his colleagues at Pirbright in England, confirmed the presence of 3 additional immunologically distinct sero-types by cross-immunity tests in cattle and pigs. These new strains of virus were isolated from regions of South Africa where types O, A and C did not seem to occur and were designated SAT (South Africa territories) 1, 2 and 3. In 1954 a further new type was identified by the Pirbright workers in material received from Pakistan and, subsequently, in samples from India, Thailand and Hong Kong. This strain, the seventh immunologically distinct sero-type of foot-and-mouth disease, was named ASIA 1.

At the present time, sero-types O, A and C are widespread in their distribution but ASIA 1 occurs only in Asiatic countries. Although SAT types 1, 2 and 3 are almost entirely confined to parts of Africa, one of them (SAT 1) escaped to the Middle East, thence to European Turkey, in 1962, but has not spread any further.

One or other of the O, A and C types has been isolated from all the affected areas of the world other than the southern regions of Africa, and recent surveys indicate that there is a tendency for type O strains to occur most frequently. On the other hand, SAT 3 has a very narrow geographical distribution and is almost entirely confined to Rhodesia.

In addition to the 7 main sero-types, immunological subtypes or variant strains are frequently encountered in natural outbreaks of the disease and give rise to difficulties in classification and immunization. The individual sub-types are indicated by a numerical subscript, A_1, A_2, A_3, etc. There are at least 11 sub-types within type O, 32 within type A, 5 within type C, 7 within type SAT 1, 3 within type SAT 2, 4 within type SAT 3 and 3 within ASIA type 1.

The different sero-types of foot-and-mouth disease virus can be distinguished by various serological techniques including neutralization tests in guinea-pigs, unweaned mice and cell cultures. Complement-fixation is mostly used to identify the 60 or more antigenically distinct variants and subtypes.

Newly isolated strains are apt to be antigenically unstable but there is no evidence that transformation can occur from one major type into another. Indeed, the degree of antigenic differences between the 7 main types is so great that instances have been recorded of animals becoming naturally infected with virus of 3 different types within 6 months, but in each type recovery results in a strong immunity to reinfection with virus of the homologous strain.

In the complement-fixation test, 2 antibodies are involved: the larger 25 nm virus particle combines with both while the smaller non-infective 7 nm component combines with only one. These 2 antigenic components produce 2 distinct precipitin lines when diffused against an homologous antiserum in agar gels.

Cultivation

Most strains of foot-and-mouth disease virus can readily be adapted to growth in a wide range of laboratory animals and, in 1921, it was first shown that guinea-pigs could be infected by scarification or by injecting the virus into the dermis of the hairless foot-pads. Not all strains, however, seem to be capable of infecting these animals. The clinical picture in artificially infected guinea-pigs is almost a counterpart of that in naturally occurring cases in cattle. Primary lesions develop at the site of inoculation within 24–48 hours and secondary lesions, in the form of vesicles on the mucous membranes of the mouth and uninoculated foot-pads, develop later (2–12 days) following generalised spread of the infection. Few animals die and complement-fixing antibody appears in the blood during convalescence. Since guinea-pigs are practically insusceptible to the natural disease, artificially induced infections do not spread spontaneously in guinea-pig colonies by direct contact. Rats, voles, squirrels, hamsters, young rabbits, dogs and cats can be infected artificially. Hedgehogs are not only highly susceptible experimental hosts but are generally believed to be capable of acquiring the infection spontaneously and of spreading the virus to other hedgehogs by contact, and to other animals including cattle.

In 1951 it was discovered that unweaned mice of between 7–9 days of age are highly susceptible to intraperitoneal injection of the virus and show signs of infection 2–3 days post inoculation. The main symptoms are of spastic muscular paralysis of the hindquarters and muscular weakness of the neck. Histopathological examination of affected mice reveals widespread necrosis of the skeletal musculature and some evidence of myocardial necrosis. Very high titres of virus are present in the affected tissues and young susceptible mice are more useful than cattle inoculated into the tongue for the titration of neutralizing antibody and for identifying subtypes of virus. Cross-infection by contact does not occur so that infected litters can be housed together and one litter can provide mice for more than one experiment.

Domestic poultry, including chickens, ducks, geese and turkeys can be experimentally infected by inoculation into the tongue or foot-pad but no evidence of spread of the disease by these birds has been obtained. Young chickens inoculated intravenously or intramuscularly develop characteristic tongue lesions which usually heal rapidly in 1–2 days. However, initial adaptation of the virus to chicken embryos is difficult and the first successful transfer of a cattle strain to the developing chick embryo was not reported until 1954. Intravenous inoculation of 14-day-old developing embryos is the most successful method and serial passage usually results in lowered pathogenicity for the host from which the virus was derived. Other strains have been adapted to growth on the chorioallantoic membrane of fertile hens' eggs and mouse-adapted strains can be readily propagated by a variety of routes.

In 1930–31, a number of workers reported that the virus of foot-and-mouth disease could be grown in living embryonic tissues derived from guinea-pigs, lambs or calves suspended in Tyrode's saline with added serum or plasma. Since then the virus has been shown to multiply in suspended tissue fragments of cattle tongue epithelium. In these suspended cell systems the time of appearance of free virus depends on the size of the initial inoculum but peak titres are usually obtained after 12–18 hours of incubation with a gradual decline thereafter. This method of cultivating the virus in Maitland-type suspensions of surviving epithelial cells is similar to that adopted by Frenkel in 1947, and has proved of value for fundamental research studies as well as for the provision of large quantities of virus for vaccines.

Most strains of virus multiply in and produce cytopathic effects in a number of trypsinized cell culture systems including bovine tongue epithelium, bovine thyroid, bovine embryonic skin-muscle, embryo rabbit lung, bovine, pig, lamb and goat kidney, as well as cell-lines of pig and hamster kidney. Calf thyroid cell monolayers are particularly susceptible and yield virus in exceptionally high titres; and are useful as a means of isolating virus from field specimens of affected tissues. The cytopathic effects of most strains are more marked in porcine than in bovine kidney cell cultures and are characterized by rounding-up of the infected cells which develop pycnotic nuclei. The rapid cellular degeneration enables the virus to be titrated either by the plaque assay method or by a metabolic plate test depending on the changes in pH and the colour of the growth medium.

Immunity

Animals that have recovered from an attack of foot-and-mouth disease are found to have varying degrees of immunity to the specific type of infecting virus. In cattle, the immunity does not usually persist for more than 1–2 years and in pigs and sheep the degree of immunity is even less, so that they can often be reinfected within a year with the same type of virus. The serum of recovered animals contains antibodies which can be measured in complement-fixation tests or in neutralization tests *in vivo* or *in vitro*. In endemic areas, most cases are caused by one distinct strain and subsequent outbreaks occurring a year or two later are generally due to another type of virus or another variant of the same type.

Passive immunity may be acquired as the result of transference of antibodies from an immune cow to her calf by means of the colostrum. It can also be produced artificially by injecting whole blood or plasma collected from convalescent cattle 2–4 weeks after the onset of the disease, or by the inoculation of hyperimmune serum. Immune sera were used extensively in Germany prior to 1938 in animals on farms surrounding an infected premises with a view to limiting the spread of the disease. Unfortunately, the volume of serum required per animal, up to 500 ml, the difficulties of preparing sufficiently large stocks of adequate potency against the different types of virus likely to be encountered, and the short period of protection (14 days) have rendered the method uneconomical.

Artificially acquired active immunity is similar to that which follows an attack of the natural disease and can be produced by the inoculation of live virus, given alone or in combination with specific antiserum, by modified live virus or by inactivated virus.

Virulent virus is still being used to some extent in certain endemic areas of Africa in an attempt to produce a zone of immunized animals, thereby preventing the disease spreading to other regions. In this method, which is referred to as aphthisation, all cattle in known infected areas are collected, inoculated with live virus and held in quarantine for a few weeks while the disease is spreading through the group. There are, however, many objections to aphthisation which is hazardous and has frequently resulted in the spread of the disease into neighbouring territories, with disastrous consequences.

The combined use of an immune serum and active virus has given inconsistent results due to the difficulty of adjusting the balance between the doses of serum and virus. Too much serum neutralizes the virus and prevents it stimulating the development of an active immunity, whereas too small a dose results in severe cases of foot-and-mouth disease in the inoculated animals.

Vaccines now in use are either inactivated virus vaccines or live attenuated virus vaccines. Most vaccines employed in recent years to control foot-and-mouth disease in continental Europe, Africa and South America belong to the former category and of the many methods that have been tried the two which have gained widest support are those developed by Waldmann and his colleagues in Germany in 1938–42 and by Frenkel in Holland in 1947–51.

In its original form the Schmidt-Waldmann vaccine-virus is obtained by inoculating susceptible cattle with diluted virus in many places over the surface of the tongue, the inoculum being deposited in the deeper layers of the epithelium. Within about 18 hours, large confluent vesicles develop, loosening practically the entire dorsal surface of the tongue. The animals are then slaughtered for food, the tongues collected, placed on scraping boards and the affected epithelium is removed. The mixture of vesicular fluid and epithelial tissues which contain very high titres of virus is homogenized and filtered to remove all but the finest particles. This constitutes the 'virus' which is adsorbed as a 1·5 per cent suspension on an aluminium hydroxide gel followed by inactivation with 0.1 per cent formalin at a temperature of 26°C for 2–4 days. After passing stringent safety and potency tests the vaccine is administered in 30 ml amounts by the subcutaneous route. In fully susceptible cattle the immune response reaches its peak in about 3 weeks and persists for 6–12 months. The Rosenbusch vaccine, which was largely instrumental in successfully controlling the outbreak in Mexico in 1946–51, is similar to the Waldmann vaccine except that it contains more virus (5 per cent) and is given in 2ml doses intradermally into the neck just behind the ears.

The Frenkel method which is suitable for producing high-titre virus (10^5–10^6/ml) is still being used in many countries and the results compare very favourably with those of other inactivated vaccines. The method of producing the vaccine consists of the collection of tongue epithelium from healthy cattle slaughtered for meat. The outer surface of the tongue is thoroughly cleansed and the epithelium removed in thin slices by a rotating knife, care being taken to discard the underlying muscle tissues because the sarcolactic acid would interfere with the growth of the virus. The epithelium is finely chopped and used as suspended cell cultures which are infected with the virus. After 24 hours of incubation in a synthetic growth medium aerated with 95 per cent O_2 and 5 per cent CO_2, the virus is harvested, inactivated with formalin and adsorbed on to aluminium hydroxide. Apart from formalin, a number of other substances may be used to inactivate the vaccine-virus, e.g. acetylethyleneimine which is just as effective as formaldehyde and perhaps more certain in its action. According to some workers the addition of saponin is said to increase the potency of the vaccines. Immunity develops after 7–14 days but does not reach its peak until 21 days, and lasts for about 4–6 months or longer.

Other methods of preparing inactivated virus vaccines have been described, including that in which the blood of infected cattle is treated with 0·05 per cent crystal violet for 6–8 days at 37°C.

More recently, the virulence of the virus of foot-and-mouth disease has been greatly reduced by repeated passage in embryonated hens' eggs, chickens, young rabbits or unweaned mice, and the adapted virus gives a satisfactory degree of immunity in cattle. Several cell culture systems have been used for the production of large quantities of live attenuated vaccine-virus and those most commonly used include pig or calf kidney cells and a line of baby hamster kidney cells (BHK-21). Live attenuated virus vaccines are administered intramuscularly and induce a satisfactory immunity with no evidence of spread to susceptible contacts. They are mostly used in regions where foot-and mouth disease is endemic whereas in most other areas inactivated vaccines are generally preferred.

Foot-and-mouth virus vaccines are produced as monovalent preparations but may be mixed before use to provide bivalent or trivalent vaccines depending upon the types of virus against which protection is desired. However, there is evidence that certain serotypes may interfere with each other and, therefore, trivalent virus vaccines are less effective than bivalent vaccines.

Pathogenicity

Naturally infected cattle usually develop symptoms within 2–5 days but the incubation period may be extended, according to the degree and duration of contact, and periods of up to 2–3 weeks have been recorded.

The first indication of the presence of the disease is a rise of temperature, which is particularly well marked in young animals, and is associated with dullness, inappetance and a sudden drop in milk production. This is followed within a few hours by the appearance of vesicles on the mucous membrane of the mouth (tongue, lips, cheeks, gums and dental pad) and on the skin of the interdigital space, on the coronary bands of the feet, at the bulbs of the heels and on the teats and udder. As the vesicles develop there is characteristic smacking of the lips, copious stringy salivation, difficulty in chewing and marked lameness. The vesicles usually rupture in 2–3 days' time leaving raw, eroded, red areas; the temperature drops rapidly and the affected animal appears to gain some relief. (Plate 47.3e, facing page 607).

The clinical symptoms in sheep, goats and pigs are similar to those in cattle except that salivation may not be very noticeable and the most obvious signs include sudden and acute lameness and marked disinclination to rise. In sheep the infection may be so mild that the mouth lesions are very small and heal rapidly, and the disease may pass unrecognized.

Foot-and-mouth disease is generally a mild affection of adult cattle but in-calf cows may abort and calves may die without showing any apparent lesions of the disease. In uncomplicated cases the lesions in the mouth heal completely within about a week but foot lesions tend to persist, especially when secondary infection has occurred. In cases where there is extensive involvement of the feet, separation of the horn from the skin and underlying tissues of the coronet may take place. When this occurs new horn is formed and gradually grows down the claw, replacing the old horn which is eventually shed. This process is often referred to as 'thimbling', and the extent of the growth of new horn is a valuable guide to the age of the lesions.

Affected animals usually lose condition very rapidly and may become emaciated if recovery is delayed. Although the morbidity is extremely high the mortality rate in typical outbreaks seldom exceeds 2 per cent. An exception to this general rule is a malignant form of the disease which sometimes occurs in Continental Europe, killing 50–70 per cent of young animals that are attacked.

The importance of foot-and-mouth disease lies not so much in the deaths to which it gives rise as in the disastrous economic losses which result from the marked fall in milk and meat production, together with the severe restrictions imposed on the movements of livestock and on the trade in animals and animal products derived from infected areas.

Although cattle, sheep and pigs are susceptible to foot-and-mouth disease it has long been known that natural adaptation of the virus can occur and that certain strains infective for pigs may fail to spread to cattle; conversely, strains naturally adapted to cattle may not always produce clinical disease in pigs. Thus, strains showing different degrees of adaptation range from almost exclusively cattle strains to almost exclusively pig strains.

Following the introduction of infection, the virus multiplies rapidly in susceptible animals and is present in high concentration in most of the tissue fluids during the acute, viraemic phase of the disease, and is readily voided in secretions and excretions. The greatest concentration of virus occurs in the vesicle fluids and in the overlying epithelium and, at the height of infection, viral titres may exceed $10^{9 \cdot 0}$ ID_{50}/ml. Although leakage or rupture of the vesicles causes contamination of the saliva there are a number of reports that virus may be present in the saliva due to its replication in the salivary glands before lesions appear in the mouth. On the other hand, virus is seldom detectable in the tissues of affected cattle later than 1–3 weeks after the end of the acute phase of the illness with the exception of the soft palate, tonsils and pharynx where it may remain 'dormant' in low concentration for up to 15 months or longer. Tonsillar and pharyngeal carriers have also been described among sheep 1–5 months after infection.

The first evidence of the development of vesicles is blanching and under-running of the epithelium. The affected areas quickly fill with lymph giving rise to the typical well-defined and often prominent vesicle or 'blister'. The lesions vary considerably in size, tend to coalesce and are easily ruptured with the release of clear or straw-coloured fluid. In many cases the covering epithelium is quickly shed leaving raw, red areas which soon begin to heal if uncomplicated by secondary bacterial infection.

Histological examination shows that the primary lesions are degenerative in type, consisting mostly of focal hydropic change of the affected cells in the stratum germinativum of the epidermis. As the infection progresses the cells undergo necrosis and release fluid which, combined with a moderate degree of inflammatory oedema, gives rise to small vesicles in the deeper layers of the stratum germinativum. The small vesicles coalesce and form large 'blisters' which may be up to 3 inches in diameter.

The susceptibility of man to clinical infection with the virus of foot-and-mouth disease has been debated for many years, but there is a growing volume of evidence that true infection resulting in active secretion of the virus, may occur in children drinking infected milk or in adults exposed to natural cases of disease in animals. Clinical manifestations of human infections are usually, but not invariably, of a mild nature with a short febrile course. Occasionally, during severe epidemics in animals, human contacts may develop vesicles on the lips, mouth, tongue, pharynx and conjunctiva as well as in the stomach and intestines. In most cases, however, the lesions heal rapidly and completely following rupture of the vesicles.

Ecology

Foot-and-mouth disease is one of the most troublesome and infectious diseases of livestock which spreads with amazing rapidity both by direct and indirect means. Direct spread usually occurs from animal to animal by droplet infection or when the virus contacts the mucosa of the mouth, nose, conjunctiva or an abraded skin surface. Infection may be indirect through contact with contaminated objects.

After an incubation period of 2–8 days, large

quantities of virus appear in the vesicular fluid and vesicular epithelium. Virus is also present in the blood and in various internal organs and may be excreted in the saliva, milk, urine and faeces. Although the infectivity of these tissues and fluids soon diminishes and most animals are non-infective 5–6 days after lesions appear, there is recent evidence that cattle and sheep may harbour small amounts of virus in the tonsils, palate and pharynx for a considerable period after complete clinical recovery. Despite many unsuccessful attempts to transmit the virus from carrier to contact animals, it is widely believed that persistently infected cattle and sheep may account for the emergence of new viral subtypes, particularly where the disease is enzootic and vaccination is practised. On the other hand, it has frequently been shown that the secretions and excretions of diseased animals may be infective even before they show the characteristic symptoms of salivation and lameness.

The virus is capable of multiplying in the secretory cells of the mammary gland and it has been demonstrated in cows' milk 1 to 4 days before the onset of clinical signs. During the viraemic phase of the illness large quantities of blood-borne virus (about $10^{5.0}$ ID_{50}/ml) are secreted in the milk and, during the 1952 outbreak in England, infective milk fed to calves in transit led directly and indirectly to over 100 new outbreaks at points 150–300 miles apart.

Indirect infection is of great importance in the spread of foot-and-mouth disease and takes place mostly through the contamination of food, water, bedding and pastures by the infected discharges of diseased animals. There is a considerable amount of experimental evidence to show that the virus can survive for long periods on diverse materials such as shoes, harness, ropes, clothes, straw, hay, fodder, the hair and wool of animals and the feathers of birds. There can be no doubt that the capacity for virus survival outside the host is largely responsible for the spread of foot-and-mouth disease and, in the U.K., the great majority of primary outbreaks are due to the importation of meat and meat products from South America where the disease is endemic. As a result, several major outbreaks have occurred because infected meat and offal were fed in uncooked swill to pigs which contracted the disease and spread it to other susceptible animals.

Because of the proximity of continental Europe, several outbreaks in Britain have been attributed to migratory birds, particularly starlings, since it has been shown that starlings may harbour the virus for many hours on their feet and feathers, and that large epidemics in South East England often coincide with severe outbreaks on the Continent.

Surprisingly little information is available regarding the longevity of foot-and-mouth disease virus in the open air, or of the importance of air-borne infection. However, there are a number of accounts of the accidental release of virus from research institutes and there is strong circumstantial evidence that the outbreak of SAT 2 virus infection which occurred on a farm 2 miles downwind from the Pirbright Institute was carried for at least part of the distance by the wind. It is considered that the virus can be carried by wind, if the conditions are ideal, over distances of more than 60 miles; and there can be little doubt that the presence of high winds blowing towards an area heavily stocked with susceptible cattle was an important factor in the 1967–8 epizootic in Shropshire, England.

Biological products such as swine fever vaccines and hyperimmune sera have occasionally been found to be contaminated with the virus of foot-and-mouth disease, and it has been reported that an outbreak in England in 1939 was due to injection of a cow with an imported pituitary extract.

In Africa, the migrating habits of the larger species of wild game undoubtedly play an important role in the dissemination of foot-and-mouth disease. In large herds of infected animals a 'smouldering' type of infection can persist for long periods and the use of the same grazing grounds and water-holes by wild game and by domesticated cattle, sheep and goats may result in fresh outbreaks of the disease. Many species of game animals are susceptible to foot-and-mouth disease but the African buffalo is believed to be moderately resistant and may be a potential vector of the virus. It is also well known that there is a tendency among wild game to abandon their natural habitats and grazing areas when the disease appears and to travel great distances, spreading infection as they move.

Diagnosis

The highly contagious nature of the disease and the presence of typical raised vesicles with blanched covering epithelium and filled with a clear straw-coloured fluid is usually pathognomonic of foot-and-mouth disease: but in endemic areas where the animals are partially immune, diagnosis may be more difficult. It is emphasised, however, that any vesicular disease occurring in ruminants and swine which is associated with 'blisters' on the tongue and feet must be regarded as foot-and-mouth disease until the contrary is proven.

Laboratory investigations are essential for rapid and accurate diagnosis. For this purpose vesicle fluids (which contain high titres of virus) and epithelial fragments of recently developed vesicles are collected, preferably from lesions on the tongue, palate or lips of individually affected animals and kept separate. Wherever possible, specimens should contain at least one gram ($2. \times 2$ cm) of material and these should be placed in a solution of M/25 phosphate buffered saline, pH 7·5–7·6, containing equal parts of pure glycerine with 0·001 per cent phenol red added as an indicator. The outside of the container is thoroughly disinfected with 4 per cent sodium carbonate or 0·2 per cent citric acid solution, the tightly-fitting screw-cap sealed with adhesive tape and the specimen labelled with full identification particulars. The container is then carefully wrapped in cotton wool or other absorbent material, placed in a sealed fluid-tight container, packed in a strong outer box of wood or reinforced cardboard and securely wrapped. The parcel must be despatched immediately by air or by the quickest means available, notifying the reference laboratory by cable or telephone of its despatch. The parcel should be labelled "FRAGILE — WITH CARE. Perishable biological material. DO NOT OPEN. No commercial value." The World Reference Laboratory in England is the Animal Virus Research Institute, Pirbright, Woking, Surrey, and the telegraphic address is Worreflab Research, Pirbright.

The laboratory procedures for identifying and typing foot-and-mouth viruses are based on complement-fixation tests, neutralization tests and cross-immunity tests in animals. In the serological tests adequate controls incorporating standard antisera and the appropriate virus types must be included.

Complement-fixation

The complement-fixation reaction is the most important and most commonly used test for identifying the type of virus in specimens obtained from suspected cases of foot-and-mouth disease in the field. A suspension of the original material is used as antigen and tested against specific hyperimmune antisera prepared in guinea-pigs. If the specimen fixes complement with one of the standard antisera the tissue contains virus and the animal is declared to be suffering from the disease. By this method a positive result can be obtained in about 2–3 hours after receipt of the specimen. Where necessary, the precise antigenic type of the causative virus is ascertained by cross-immunity tests.

Cell culture studies

In cases where the complement-fixation test is negative, the suspect material is inoculated into monolayer tube cultures of bovine thyroid and Roux flasks containing pig kidney cells. At an incubation temperature of 37°C, virus activity usually produces a marked degenerative type of cytopathic effect within 24–48 hours and the agent is identified as foot-and-mouth virus by applying a complement-fixation test to the culture fluids. In the absence of visible cellular degeneration, the cultures are passaged through a further one or two cycles in fresh cell cultures and re-examined by complement-fixation for the presence of virus.

Mouse inoculation

No matter how valuable the direct complement-fixation and cell culture tests may be, their success largely depends on the presence of sufficiently large amounts of virus in the original material to fix guinea-pig complement, and on the absence of contamination which may produce non-specific cellular changes in the cultured monolayers. Thus, final interpretation may depend upon the results obtained with experimentally infected animals. For this purpose susceptible cattle are by far the most important test animal but these are seldom used for routine investigations because of the expense involved and the difficulties of keeping individual animals in strict isolation.

Fortunately, unweaned mice from 6–8 days old are highly susceptible to artificial infection and can be used instead of cattle for primary isolation of virus from field specimens. The suspected material is inoculated into all the animals in a litter and, if any mice die within 1–7 days, their carcases are used as antigen in direct complement-fixation tests. If a negative result is obtained the carcase material is passaged through two further litters and these are later examined for the ability of their tissues to fix complement in the presence of specific antisera. The mouse test is not as sensitive as either of the cell culture methods but is less affected by bacterial contamination.

Cross-immunity tests

In special circumstances accurate identification of the virus can be obtained by inoculation of small groups of suceptible and immune cattle. Thus, if the suspected field material contains type A virus, only the 'A'-immune animals will resist the infection and complement-fixation tests on material obtained from the reacting animals in the remaining (e.g. O and C) immune groups will fix complement with a known type A hyperimmune serum.

Complement-fixation and cross-immunity tests are also useful for distinguishing between foot-and-mouth disease, vesicular stomatitis, vesicular exanthema and swine vesicular disease.

Neutralization tests

Virus and serum neutralization tests may be used to detect specific antibodies in the sera of recovered animals or for identification of the causative virus with known hyperimmune sera. The tests may be performed either in cell cultures or in animals.

Indirect complement-fixation

In most cases of foot-and-mouth disease, sera from

convalescent or recovered cattle do not sufficiently deflect the complement in the standard complement-fixation test to be of value in diagnosis. This difficulty is largely overcome by means of the indirect complement-fixation test which is based on the fact that the antibodies in a convalescent serum can partially or wholly engage known titrated foot-and-mouth disease antigen to the extent that the antigen is no longer capable of maximum fixation of complement in the presence of a known titrated hyperimmune serum. (See also page 382).

Gel diffusion
Precipitin tests in agar gel diffusion plates may also be of use in identifying unknown strains of virus in samples of vesicle fluid and vesicle fragments obtained early in the disease. The method is not very sensitive but in a positive test two narrow but well-defined lines of precipitation appear between the wells containing the test material and a known type of hyperimmune serum.

Differential diagnosis
In Africa and other overseas territories where foot-and-mouth disease may be endemic, the mouth lesions must be differentiated from those produced in rinderpest and mucosal disease. In the American continent the most difficult diseases to differentiate from foot-and-mouth disease are vesicular stomatitis and vesicular exanthema, although neither spreads so rapidly as foot-and-mouth disease. The clinical picture of vesicular stomatitis does not usually involve foot lesions in cattle and the host range of vesicular exanthema is mostly limited to swine. Differential diagnosis of these 3 vesicular diseases can best be made by complement-fixation and other serological tests or by studies of the host-range of the virus involved. In Europe and the Far East, foot-and-mouth disease in swine must be differentiated from swine vesicular disease. (Table 47.1, facing page 620).

Other conditions which are at times suggestive of foot-and-mouth disease include foot-rot and blue-tongue of sheep.

Control
Methods for dealing with an outbreak of foot-and-mouth disease vary in different countries. In Britain, where the disease occurs sporadically, a rigorous policy of stamping-out the disease by slaughter and disinfection is practised. Because of its favourable geographical position, the slaughter policy in Britain is said to afford more efficient control than would vaccination with the presently available vaccines, and the total cost is much less. Moreover, since most primary outbreaks of foot-and-mouth disease in Britain are thought to be due to the importation of meat from abroad, there seems to be little doubt that restriction of the importation of animal products and prevention of the feeding of uncooked swill to pigs are of the utmost importance in preventing the introduction of the virus.

To be effective, the stamping-out policy must be adequately supported by the following measures. Rapid and accurate identification of the virus and its subtype characteristics, control of the movement of livestock and persons on affected premises and in peripheral areas, prompt destruction of infected and in-contact susceptible species, effective disposal of carcases, fodder and other contaminated materials, thorough disinfection and cleansing of premises, adequate methods of tracing direct and indirect contacts, and early notification of outbreaks to neighbouring counties and countries.

In continental Europe and other countries where foot-and-mouth disease is endemic, the infection may be controlled by setting up a wide buffer-zone of immunized animals around fresh outbreaks. For this purpose, polyvalent antiserum prepared in cattle has been used prophylactically and therapeutically but its value is limited and the cost is often prohibitive. At the present time inactivated vaccines are widely used but the method largely depends on repeated vaccination and having sufficient vaccine available of the same type as the infecting virus. The value of the immunization policy is difficult to assess, while the incidence of recovered carriers of the virus and their danger to other in-contact animals is uncertain.

Equine rhinoviruses

In 1962, an equine respiratory virus with enterovirus properties was isolated in monkey-kidney cell cultures from the faeces of a number of horses in a research laboratory in England. The virus was found to occur commonly among horses and to reproduce in the pharynx of artificially infected horses causing a mucopurulent reaction, accompanied by a nasal discharge. The virus was later shown to resemble human rhinoviruses and to grow with a cytopathic effect in cell cultures prepared from horse, man, rabbit and other species. It differed, however, from many human rhinoviruses in that the requirements of low bicarbonate and low temperature were not necessary for growth of equine strains.

Since that time, numerous isolates have been reported from the U.K., Germany, Canada and the U.S.A., and it seems likely that the virus is world-wide in its distribution.

Three, and possibly more, serotypes of equine rhinoviruses have been identified but it appears that type 1 is the commonest and over 60 per cent of adult horses have neutralizing antibodies against it.

TABLE 47.1. The differential diagnosis of foot-and-mouth disease, vesicular stomatitis, vesicular exanthema and swine vesicular disease.

	FMD	VS	VE	SVD
Virus group	Rhinovirus	Rhabdovirus	Calicivirus	Enterovirus
Size [nm]	24	175×65	35–40	30–32
Morphology	Roughly spherical	Bullet-shaped	Roughly spherical [with dark capsomeres]	Roughly spherical
Lipid solvents	Resistant	Sensitive	Resistant	Resistant
Stability at pH5	Labile	Stable	Stable but susceptible to low pH[< 3] & high pH[> 12]	Stable
Stabilised by 1M $MgCl_2$	No	. . .	No	Stabilised
Sedimentation coefficient	140	625	160–170	150
Growth in cell cultures				
HeLa	−	+	−−	?
Pig kidney	+	+	+	+
BHK–21	+	+	?	−
Ox tissues	+	+	−*	−
Lesions in laboratory animals	+	+	−**	−***
Lesions in other animals				
Intralingual, horse	−	+	−/+	−
ox	+	+	−	−
pig	+	+	+	+
Intradermal, guinea-pig	+	+	−	−

FMD — foot-and-mouth disease
VS — vesicular stomatitis
VE — vesicular exanthema
SVD — swine vesicular disease
* = but growth may occur in cells of horse, dog or cat.
** = but lesions may be produced in dogs, guinea-pigs or hamsters.
*** = but one-day-old mice are susceptible to high doses of virus.

The incubation period after experimental infection is 3–7 days and is followed by pyrexia and viraemia lasting 4–5 days. Rabbits, guinea-pigs, monkeys and man can also be infected experimentally. High antibody titres have been demonstrated in stable workers and a human volunteer developed fever and viraemia.

Spontaneous outbreaks are characterized by acute upper respiratory tract infection with fever (39–41°C), serous rhinitis and pharyngitis similar to the common cold in man. In the later stages of the illness there may be anorexia, copious mucoid or mucopurulent nasal exudate, cough and submaxillary lymphadenitis. Uncomplicated cases usually recover spontaneously in 7–10 days but horses that develop secondary bacterial infections may require a period of convalescence of 4–6 weeks.

The infection spreads readily in stables by both direct and indirect means, and there are reports that the virus may persist in pharyngeal secretions for up to 1 month.

CALICIVIRUSES

Members of the calicivirus genus are distinguished from other picornaviruses by their stability at pH5 but not at pH3, and by the fact that the surface of their capsid is composed of a number of dark hollow cup-shaped structures from which the generic name is derived. (Plate 47.1c, facing page 606). Moreover, the virions are slightly larger than other picornaviruses (30–40 nm in diameter) and are seen in negatively-stained preparations as isometric particles, probably with icosahedral symmetry and 32 capsomeres. All strains are ether-resistant. Virus synthesis and maturation occur in the cytoplasm with occasional formation of crystalline arrays of particles. There is no evidence of replication in the nucleus.

Members of the calicivirus sub-group include the virus of vesicular exanthema of swine, San Miguel sea-lion virus and a number of feline viruses formerly classified as rhinoviruses.

Vesicular exanthema

Synonyms
California disease of swine: Blaschenausschlag (Ger.).

Definition
An acute highly infectious viral disease of swine which is characterized by the formation of vesicles on the mouth (lips, gums, tongue, palate), snout and feet (coronary band, accessory digits and toes).

Hosts affected
The only natural host is the domestic pig but horses and dogs are irregularly susceptible to artificial infection.

History and distribution
The disease was originally described in California in 1932 when an illness affecting only swine, and which was clinically indistinguishable from foot-and-mouth disease, occurred on a farm feeding uncooked swill. The outbreak was quickly stamped out within 10 days by a slaughter policy involving the destruction of more than 18 000 animals. Despite these drastic measures, together with the introduction of stringent quarantine regulations, a second outbreak occurred in California in the following year. Because the agent did not cause spontaneous disease in cattle and horses and was not transmissible to experimentally infected guinea-pigs, the condition was recognised as a new disease entity and was named vesicular exanthema of swine. Since then outbreaks occurred every year, apart from the period 1936–39, and all were confined to the state of California. However, in 1952, the virus escaped to Nebraska, thence to at least 19 other states in the U.S.A. within the short space of 6 weeks. By the middle of 1953 no fewer than 42 states were involved. A remarkable feature of this 'new' disease was that the introduction of legislation prohibiting the feeding of uncooked garbage was followed by a spectacular decrease in the number of new outbreaks. The last incident was reported in 1956, and in 1959 the whole of the U.S.A. was officially declared free of the disease. Apart from isolated outbreaks in swine *en route* to Honolulu in 1948 and again in 1949, the only other outbreak to occur outside the U.S.A. was reported in Iceland in 1955 on a farm that utilized uncooked swill from a nearby U.S. military base.

In 1973, a calicivirus indistinguishable from that of vesicular exanthema of swine, was isolated from sea-lions, and has been named San Miguel virus. The fact that it produces lesions in experimentally infected pigs characteristic of vesicular exanthema and has infected feral pigs on islands off the coast of Southern California, suggests the possibility of future spread to swine herds on the mainland.

Properties of the virus
Virus particles are roughly spherical in shape and measure between 30 and 40 nm in diameter. In ultrathin negatively-stained sections of infected cells, mature virions are seen within the cytoplasm and are frequently grouped in crystalline arrays. Mature virus contains single-stranded RNA with a molecular weight of about 2.3×10^6 daltons. All strains are resistant to ether, chloroform, deoxycholate and 0.3 per cent Tween 80, but are readily inactivated by 2 per cent sodium hydroxide. They are not stabilized by 1M $MgCl_2$ against thermal inactivation at 50°C. All strains are susceptible to either very low ($<$pH3) or very high ($>$pH12) hydrogen ion concentration. The virus may be preserved in the form of vesicular fragments in 50 per cent glycerol-saline (pH 7.4) at 4°C for several years and will even survive at 37°C for 24 hours or longer.

Antigenic properties
Vesicular exanthema virus shows a marked plurality of immunological types and cross-immunity tests in pigs indicate that each virus confers a specific immunity to itself but not to the others. Neutralization, complement-fixation, agar gel diffusion and cross-immunity tests conducted by workers both in America and England suggest that there are at least 13 immunologically distinct serotypes of the virus, and these have been named alphabetically in order of their isolation followed by 2 numerals each representing the year when the isolation was made (e.g. A48, B51, C52, D53, etc.). It is of interest that all but 3 of the serotypes have occurred only in California.

Cultivation
All known strains multiply readily and produce cytopathic effects in monolayer cultures of pig kidney, lung, liver, testis and amnion cells, and to a variable degree in cell cultures prepared from other hosts, e.g. horses, dogs and cats. There is a marked variation in the morphology of the plaques produced on monolayer cultures of pig kidney cells and, in general, virulent strains produce large clear plaques whereas less virulent strains produce very small opaque plaques. The viruses in different plaques are antigenically indistinguishable despite their marked differences in virulence.

There is no evidence that the virus can be adapted to growth in chickens or embryonated hens' eggs.

Repeated attempts to initiate infection in cattle, sheep, goats, mice, rats, guinea-pigs and hedgehogs have failed but some of these hosts are partially susceptible under certain conditions. For example, horses may develop fever and small local lesions when inoculated intradermally into the tongue with some strains but not with others. The lesions are sharply cirumscribed, flat, blanched areas of desquamation (5–8 cm in diameter) with little tendency to coalesce.

Dogs are irregularly susceptible to intradermal inoculation of the tongue and lesions, when present, show separation of the epithelium from the underlying corium, with a tendency to coalesce.

In hamsters, however, intradermal inoculation on the abdomen may produce circumscribed, vesicle-like lesions about 5–8 cm in diameter with a blackened covering, but lesions are not reproducible after 4–6 serial passages.

In most cases, guinea-pigs are refractory to inoculation by scarification or intradermal inoculation of the hairless foot-pads. However, several workers have described lesions in the tarsal pads and it has been suggested that reproduction of lesions in guinea-pigs depends on a symbiotic relationship between the virus and certain bacterial contaminants, e.g. *Alcaligenes*.

Pathogenicity

Vesicular exanthema is largely a disease of swine but cattle, sheep, goats and other domestic animals appear to be resistant to the disease. Although the mortality rates in spontaneous outbreaks of vesicular exanthema are usually less than 5 per cent, and recovery is generally complete, the disease is of importance not only because of the weight loss in affected animals and abortions in sows but also because of the difficulty in distinguishing the clinical illness from foot-and-mouth disease, swine vesicular disease or vesicular stomatitis.

The incubation period in both natural and experimental infections is usually between 24 and 96 hours, but periods up to 12 days have occasionally been observed.

The disease is characterized initially by a febrile reaction (40–42°C), disinclination to eat and the sudden onset of lameness due to the development of vesicles on the skin between the toes, the interdigital spaces, the coronary band and the sole of the foot. Lesions also appear on the snout, tongue, lips or other parts of the mouth and, as the fever subsides, the vesicles rupture revealing raw eroded areas. The typical raised vesicles, with their clear fluid contents and blanched epithelial covering, vary in size from 5–33 mm in diameter and are indistinguishable from the 'blisters' of foot-and-mouth disease. In uncomplicated infections the lesions usually heal within 5–7 days.

The mortality rate amongst adult pigs may be negligible but pregnant sows frequently abort and high losses can occur in young piglets. Many affected pigs show a marked loss of body weight but in uncomplicated cases complete recovery from the disease usually occurs within a week.

Histologically, the lesions of vesicular exanthema closely resemble those of vesicular stomatitis and foot-and-mouth disease. The main tissue changes associated with replication of the virus in the Malpighian layers of the epidermis include marked swelling and hydropic degeneration of the infected stratified squamous epithelial cells, followed by cellular necrosis, dissolution and considerable intercellular oedema. This results in separation of the overlying layer of the epidermis from the dermis and the formation of the characteristic vesicle.

Transmission

Vesicular exanthema is found almost exclusively on premises feeding uncooked garbage to pigs and particularly if the swill contains scraps of infected pork. Within an outbreak the infection is transmitted by direct contact from pig to pig and in many cases the disease spreads with amazing rapidity and involves most pigs in the herd. Virus is present in almost all tissues of infected swine and small amounts may be shed in the urine and faeces.

Diagnosis

Since the clinical signs of pyrexia, vesicle formation and lameness in affected pigs are indistinguishable from those of foot-and-mouth disease and vesicular stomatitis, a presumptive diagnosis must be confirmed as soon as possible by adequate laboratory investigations.

Fresh epithelial fragments of fluid from unruptured vesicles should be collected in glycerol saline and despatched, together with acute and convalescent phase sera, to the reference laboratory in suitable containers and by the quickest means possible.

In the laboratory, the specimen may be inoculated into healthy pigs, cattle, horses and guinea-pigs as a preliminary screen to eliminate the possibility of other vesicular diseases; and virus isolation can be attempted in various cell culture systems (Table 47.1). The paired sera are examined by neutralization and complement-fixation tests against known positive antigens.

Control

There are no vaccines available for the immunization of pigs against vesicular exanthema. Rigorous quarantine and slaughter policies were not entirely successful in controlling previous outbreaks of the disease and there can be no doubt that final eradication was largely due to the introduction, in 1953–58, of legislation prohibiting the feeding of uncooked swill to pigs.

Feline caliciviruses

In recent years, there have been a number of reports of the isolation of picornaviruses from cats with respiratory illness and symptoms of panleucopenia. Several serologically distinct groups have been identified amongst the large number of feline respiratory isolates (FRI), feline conjunctivitis viruses (FCV), feline respiratory viruses (FRV), feline stomatitis viruses and feline enteritis isolates so far studied. However, little is yet known about the antigenic relationships between the various groups and amongst individual viruses.

In many instances the properties of the feline isolates are very similar to those of other picornaviruses, but some more closely resemble caliciviruses in not being stabilized against thermal inactivation by divalent cations, and because they are less stable at pH3 than enteroviruses, but more stable than rhinoviruses. In addition, the surface structure of these viruses, as seen by electron microscopy, appears to resemble that of vesicular exanthema virus.

Feline caliciviruses can be propagated in feline kidney cell cultures and it is claimed that they grow more readily in stationary tube cultures than do rhinoviruses.

Further reading

ARMSTRONG R., DAVIE J. AND HEDGER R.S. (1967) Foot-and-mouth disease in man. *British Medical Journal*, **4**, 529.

ASPLIN F.D. AND McLAUCHLAN J.D. (1954) Duck virus hepatitis. *Veterinary Record*, **66**, 456.

ASPLIN F.D. (1961) Notes on epidemiology and vaccination for virus hepatitis of ducks. *Bulletin de l'office International des Epizooties*, **56**, 793.

BACHRACH H.L. (1968) Foot-and-mouth disease. *Annual Review of Microbiology*, **22**, 201.

BANKOWSKI R.A. (1965) Vesicular exanthema. *Advances in Veterinary Science*, **10**, 23.

BETTS A.O., Lamont P.H. and Kelly D.F. (1962) Porcine enteroviruses other than the virus of Teschen disease. *Annals of the New York Academy of Sciences*, **101**, 428.

BRADISH C.J., HENDERSON W.M. AND KIRKHAM J.B. (1960) Concentration and electron microscopy of the characteristic particle of foot-and-mouth disease. *Journal of General Microbiology*, **22** 379.

BROOKSBY J.B. (1958) The virus of foot-and-mouth disease. *Advances in Virus Research*, **5**, 1.

BROOKSBY J.B. (1967) Foot-and-mouth disease — a world problem. *Nature*, **213**, 120.

BURKI F. (1965) Picornaviruses of cats. *Archiv für die gesamte Virusforschung*, **15**, 690.

BURROUGHS, J.N. AND BROWN, F. (1974) Physicochemical evidence for the re-classification of the Caliciviruses. *Journal of General Virology*, **22**, 281.

BURROWS R. (1970) Proceedings of the Second International Conference on Infectious Diseases, Paris, p. 154. Basel: Karger.

COTTRAL G.E. (1969) Persistence of foot-and-mouth disease virus in animals, their products and the environment. *Bulletin de l'office International des Epizooties*, **71**, 549.

CRANDELL R.A. (1967) A description of eight feline picornaviruses and an attempt to classify them. *Proceedings of the Society for Experimental Biology and Medicine*, **126**, 240.

CRANDELL R.A. AND YORK C.J. (1966) New feline viruses: a review of their designations and significance. *Canadian Journal of Comparative Medicine and Veterinary Science*, **30**, 256.

DITCHFIELD J. AND MACPHERSON L.W. (1965) The properties and classification of two new rhinoviruses recovered from horses in Toronto, Canada. *Cornell Veterinarian*, **55**, 181.

HAMRE D. (1968) Rhinoviruses. In, Monographs in Virology. Basel: Karger.

HYSLOP N. ST. G. (1965) Secretion of foot-and-mouth disease virus and antibody in the saliva of infected and immunized cattle. *Journal of Comparative Pathology and Therapeutics*, **75**, 111.

HYSLOP N. ST. G. (1970) The epizootiology and epidemiology of foot-and-mouth disease. *Advances in Veterinary Science*, **14**, 261.

INTERNATIONAL COMMITTEE (1963) International Enterovirus Study Group. Picornavirus group. *Virology*, **19**, 114

LEVINE P.P. (1965) Duck virus hepatitis. In, Diseases of Poultry, 5th Edition, Eds. H.E. Biester and L.W. Schwarte, p. 838. Ames: Iowa State University Press.

MADIN S.H. AND TRAUM J. (1955) Vesicular exanthema of swine. *Bacteriological Reviews*, **19**, 6.

MANCINI L.O. AND YATES V.J. (1968) Cultivation of avian encephalomyelitis virus *in vitro*. 2. In chick embryo fibroblastic cell cultures. *Avian Diseases*, **12**, 278.

MARTIN S.J., JOHNSTON M.D. AND CLEMENTS J.B. (1970) Purification and characterization of bovine enteroviruses. *Journal of General Virology*, **7**, 103.

MAYOR H.D. (1964) Picornavirus symmetry. *Virology*, **22**, 156.

MELNICK J.L. AND WENNER H.A. (1969) Enteroviruses. In, Diagnostic Procedures for Viral and Rickettsial Infections, 4th Edition. Eds. E.H. Lennette and N.J. Schmidt, p. 529. New York: American Public Health Association Inc.

METHODS OF TYPING AND CULTIVATION OF FOOT-AND-MOUTH DISEASE VIRUSES (1957) O.E.E.C. Project No. 208. Paris: Organization for European economic co-operation.

McFERRAN J.B. (1962) Bovine enteroviruses. *Annals of the New York Academy of Sciences*, **101**, 436.

McFERRAN J.B., CLARKE J.K. AND CONNOR T.J. (1971) The size of some mammalian picornaviruses. *Journal of General Virology*, **10**, 279.

McFERRAN J.B., NELSON R., McCRACKEN J.M. AND ROSS J.G. (1969) Viruses isolated from sheep. *Nature*, **221**, 194.

MOWAT G.N., DARBYSHIRE J.H. AND HUNTLEY J.F. (1972) Differentiation of a vesicular disease of pigs in Hong Kong from foot-and-mouth disease. *Veterinary Record*, **90**, 618.

NARDELLI L., LODETTI E., GUALANDI G., BURROWS R., GOODRIDGE D., BROWN F. AND CARTWRIGHT B. (1968) A foot and mouth disease syndrome in pigs caused by an enterovirus. *Nature*, **219**, 1275.

PLATT H. (1956) A study of the pathological changes produced in young mice by the virus of foot-and-mouth disease. *Journal of Pathology and Bacteriology*, **72**, 299.

PLUMMER G. (1965) The picornaviruses of man and animals: a comparative review. *Progress in Medical Virology*, **7**, 326.

POVEY R.C. (1969) Viral respiratory disease. *Veterinary Record*, **85**, 335.

PRYDIE J. (1966) Viral diseases of cats. *Veterinary Record*, **79**, 729.

RICHTER W.R., ROZOK E.J. AND MOIZE S.M. (1964) Electron microscopy of viruslike particles associated with duck viral hepatitis. *Virology*, **24**, 114.

ROSEN L. (1965) Subclassification of picornaviruses. *Bacteriological Reviews*, **29**, 173.

SAHAN M.S. (1962) The virus of foot-and-mouth disease. *Annals of the New York Academy of Sciences*, **101**, 444.

SELLERS R.F., BURT L.M., CUMMING A. AND STEWART D.L. (1960). The behaviour of strains of the virus of foot-and-mouth disease in pig, calf, ox and lamb kidney tissue cultures. *Archiv für die gesamte Virusforschung*, **9**, 637.

SMITH A.W., ACKERS T.G., MADIN S.H. AND VEDROS N.A. (1973) San Miguel sea lion virus isolation, preliminary characterization and relationship to vesicular exanthema of swine virus. *Nature (Lond.)*, **244**, 108.

SMITH L.P. AND HUGH-JONES M.E. (1969) The weather factor in foot and mouth disease epidemics. *Nature*, **223**, 712.

SUTMOLLER P. (1971) Persistent foot-and-mouth disease virus infections. In, Viruses Affecting Man and Animals, eds. M. Sanders and M. Schaeffer, p. 295. St. Louis: Warren H. Green.

TYRRELL D.A.J. (1968) Rhinoviruses. *Virology Monographs*, **2**, 67.

TZIANABOS T. AND SNOEYENBOS G.H. (1965) Clinical, immunological and serological observations on turkey virus hepatitis. *Avian Diseases*, **9**, 578.

ZWILLENBERG L.O. AND BURKI F. (1966) On the capsid structure of small feline and bovine RNA viruses. *Archiv für die gesamte Virusforschung*, **19**, 373.

CHAPTER 48

REOVIRUSES
(AND OTHER DIPLORNAVIRUSES)

Reoviruses (and other diplornaviruses)

REOVIRUSES

Definition

The term 'reovirus' was introduced in 1959 as a group name for a number of viruses which were previously classified as ECHO type 10. The reasons for classifying reoviruses (*Respiratory-Enteric-Or-phan* viruses) separately from ECHO viruses (enteric-cytopathic-human-orphan viruses) were as follows: the virus particles are much larger than the other ECHO viruses, their genomes consist of double-stranded RNA, they produce a different type of cytopathic effect from that of all known enteroviruses and they have a complement-fixing antigen different from that of ECHO viruses.

Distribution and hosts affected

Reoviruses have a broad host range spectrum and are widespread amongst man, cattle and guinea-pigs. Serological studies indicate that antibody to reoviruses occurs naturally in a wide variety of animal species including cattle, sheep, camels, pigs, horses, dogs, cats, hares, guinea-pigs, monkeys, bats, birds and trout. Although the term 'reovirus' suggests an association with respiratory and enteric disease, very few strains of human or animal origin have been proved with certainty to cause disease.

Morphology

The reovirus particle measures 60–75 nm in diameter, with a central core or nucleoid, 40 to 45 nm across, consisting of several (generally 10–12) segments of double-stranded RNA. The total genome weighs 14–15×10^6 daltons. The virion is cubical, unenveloped, roughly hexagonal in shape and possesses an inner and outer capsid which renders it very stable. Although the exact arrangement of the capsid structure is still in doubt, it seems likely that the outer shell is composed of 80 hexagonal and 12 pentagonal (92) elongated hollow capsomeres measuring 10 nm long and 8 nm wide with a hole about 4 nm in diameter; arranged

in the form of an icosahedron and showing 5:3:2 symmetry. An alternative suggestion is that the outer capsid is composed of 180 solid capsomeres arranged in such a manner that 12 of the 92 holes on the surface of the shell are surrounded by 5 structural subunits and the remaining 80 by 6 subunits. The inner capsid, which measures approximately 45 nm in diameter may be constructed of 42 capsomeres. Whichever of these proposed structures is correct, there can be no doubt that in all strains of reovirus there is a clearly-defined inner layer between the nucleic acid core of the virus particle and the outer protein shell. The core possesses 12 spikes situated as if on the vertices of an icosahedron. (Plate 48.1a, facing p. 636.)

Chemical composition

The absence of DNA in reoviruses is indicated by the negative reaction of their inclusions when stained with Feulgen stain and by the lack of inhibition of replication by 5-fluoro-2′ -deoxyuridine (FUDR) and 5-bromo-2′ -deoxyuridine (BUDR) which inhibit the growth of DNA but not RNA viruses. The total molecular weight of the RNA component is about 15×10^6 daltons.

Reoviruses are unusual in that they belong to a small group of animal viruses that possess double-stranded ribonucleic acid. Consequently, the intracytoplasmic inclusions in infected cell cultures show an apple-green fluorescence when stained with acridine-orange. At a later stage in the developmental cycle an increasing number of inclusions stain a yellow-red colour which suggests that single-stranded RNA may also be present in older cultures (Table 48.1).

Physicochemical characters

Reoviruses are highly resistant to the action of sodium deoxycholate, diethyl ether and chloroform, indicating that there is probably a lack of essential lipid in the virus particle. Typical members of the group are also very resistant to heat and viral

Table 48.1. Identification of viral nucleic acids with acridine orange.

Virus smear (Alcohol fixed)	Colour reaction with 0·01% acridine orange at pH 4·0	Pepsin susceptibility
Double-stranded DNA animal virus	Yellow-green	+
Double-stranded DNA phage	Yellow-green	−
Single-stranded DNA phage	Orange-red	−
Single-stranded RNA virus	Orange-red	−
Double-stranded RNA virus	Yellow-green	+

infectivity survives heating to 56°C for 2 hours or 60°C for 30 minutes, but is rapidly inactivated thereafter and is completely destroyed in 2–3 hours. Reoviruses are stable in buffers over a wide pH range, between pH 2·2 and 8·0, and survive for at least one hour at room temperature in 1·0 per cent H_2O_2, 1·0 per cent phenol, 3·0 per cent formaldehyde or 20 per cent lysol. They are inactivated by 70 per cent ethanol at room temperature for one hour and by 3·0 per cent formaldehyde at 56°C for 30 minutes. Heating at temperatures of 50–55°C for 5–15 minutes in the presence of high concentrations of magnesium chloride results in an increase in infectivity, whereas the presence of magnesium ions at sub-zero temperatures (–20 to –40°C.) almost completely destroys the infectivity titre of the virus. Increased infectivity by these methods is unique to the reoviruses and is considered to be due to the removal or alteration of the outer layer of the viral double coat. An increase in infectivity can also be obtained by treatment with the proteolytic enzymes chymotrypsin and pancreatin.

Haemagglutination
Most strains of all 3 mammalian types, (*vide infra*), agglutinate human Group A, and to a lesser degree human Group O red blood cells, at various temperatures (4°, 25° and 37°C). Strains of type-3, but not types 1 and 2, agglutinate ox red cells at 4°C. Receptor destroying enzyme (RDE) renders ox cells inagglutinable to type-3 strains but does not have this effect on human erythrocytes which are agglutinable by all three types of reoviruses. There is also some evidence that the cell-receptors of ox cells are distinct from those involved in haemagglutination by myxoviruses. Pig strains agglutinate human and pig erythrocytes at 4°, 25° and 37°C but do not agglutinate chicken, rabbit or guinea-pig red blood cells. Studies of reoviruses by sucrose density gradient techniques reveal 2 types of haemagglutinin; the first is found in the heavier fractions and is associated with infectivity, while the second is found in the light top fraction and is not associated with infectivity. Ether treatment does not affect haemagglutinating activity nor infectivity, but chloroform destroys the haemagglutinin but not the infectivity. The haemagglutinins are associated with the virus particle and their production is generally enhanced if the virus is grown in roller tube cultures.

Antigenic properties
Mammalian reoviruses have been separated into 3 serological types (1, 2 and 3) by neutralization and haemagglutination-inhibition tests, and all 3 have been isolated from man and cattle. In addition, one or more types have been isolated from monkeys, dogs, cats, pigs, sheep, mice and turkeys. Neutralization tests, using unweaned mice or tissue culture, are superior to haemagglutination-inhibition tests for typing of the strains but complement-fixation tests are unsuitable because all types of reovirus possess a group specific complement-fixing antigen. The type-2 human strains have been divided into a number of sub-types, while 5 distinct serotypes of avian origin have also been described. A bovine strain, which was originally thought to be a new type of reovirus, is probably a member of the heterogeneous type-2.

An unusual feature of the reovirus group is that they share an antigenic component with a pathogenic, arthropod-borne plant virus, the wound-tumour virus, which is morphologically identical with the reovirus and also contains double-stranded RNA. This relationship is of particular interest since it is the first that has been reported between plant and mammalian virus pathogens; and provides a basis for new speculation concerning the ecology, reservoirs and biological potential of mammalian viruses.

Cultivation
Reoviruses have been propagated in many different hosts such as chicken embryos (by the chorioallantoic and allantoic routes) and have been adapted to monkeys, cattle, dogs, guinea-pigs, ferrets, hamsters and unweaned mice. They also grow well in a remarkably wide range of primary cell cultures of human and animal origin, as well as in HeLa cells and some other cell line cultures. The cytopathic effect, which may take from 7 to 14 days to develop, is different from that of ECHO and other types of enteroviruses and is characterized by the formation of Feulgen-negative RNA-containing intracytoplasmic inclusions which completely surround the nucleus. Studies of the replication cycle show that development is essentially in the cytoplasm and is

closely associated with the mitotic apparatus and, in particular, the spindle tubules. Maturation takes place within clearly defined granular cytoplasmic matrices and there is no evidence, as in togaviruses, of budding through the plasma or cytoplasmic membranes. Under normal circumstances the release of virus from the cell is mostly effected by complete dissolution of the cytoplasm.

Pathogenicity

There is very little evidence to show that reoviruses are responsible for any human illness but they are frequently isolated from the faeces of mild cases of diarrhoea and fever, and their presence has also been confirmed in patients with a hepatitis-encephalitis-respiratory syndrome. Serological tests have shown that human infections with each of the three serotypes are widespread and it is believed that they are mostly acquired early in childhood. Nearly all human isolates have been made from children but typical reoviruses have often been isolated from raw sewage and water.

Antibody to reovirus types-1, 2 or 3 occurs naturally in a wide variety of animal species, both domestic and wild, and it seems that in some species, notably pigs, sheep and poultry, infection with one type of reovirus is favoured.

The first bovine strain of reovirus was isolated from the faeces of normal calves in America, and at least 50 strains of all the three serotypes (1, 2 and 3) have been identified. As in man and other animals, inapparent infection is widespread in cattle and all calves are thought to be infected with at least one serotype by the time they are one year old. Outbreaks of respiratory disease of cattle in the United Kingdom are frequently associated with significant increases in the antibody titre. However, experimentally infected calves rarely elicit a clinical response, despite the fact that the virus can usually be recovered in high titre from the lungs and other tissues, and antibodies can be detected in the circulation. Very small pneumonic lesions may be present in the lungs of experimentally infected colostrum-deprived calves but they do not contain the kind of intracytoplasmic inclusions that are seen characteristically in reovirus-infected cell cultures. A report that a more severe reaction is obtained in experimentally infected calves with reovirus combined with psittacosis-type organisms is yet another example of the synergistic effects that mixed viruses, or viruses plus bacteria, may play in the aetiology of respiratory diseases in general.

In unweaned mice, reovirus type-3 gives rise to jaundice, diarrhoea, alopecia and death, and in the acute phase of the illness the virus produces lesions in the liver, spleen and other organs. About 1 per cent of mice suffering from the acute form of the disease survive for more than 30 days. Reovirus type-3 can also cause a neonatal infection in mice, followed by a chronic virus-free immunological disease which eventually leads to a runting syndrome with the characters of an autoimmune disease. There is also evidence that it may give rise occasionally to a murine lymphoma having many similarities to Burkitt's lymphoma. Although strains of type-3 reovirus have frequently been isolated from cases of Burkitt's African lymphoma, it has not been possible to assess the aetiological significance of these observations because of the broad distribution of reovirus in nature. There is also a report of the isolation of reovirus type-1 from a dog with a severe respiratory infection and it is interesting to note that the virus was pathogenic for experimentally infected puppies and produced a clear mucoid nasal discharge, cough and fever. Intranasal inoculation of 6-week-old pigs with the porcine PH strain gives rise to a febrile reaction and a fourfold and greater increase of haemagglutination-inhibiting antibody.

Diagnosis

Virus isolations can be obtained from samples of faeces from cases of gastroenteritis, from the lungs of patients showing respiratory involvement and, occasionally, from other infected organs. The virus can be propagated in kidney cell cultures from different animal species and produces a slow but characteristic cytopathic effect with perinuclear intracytoplasmic inclusions. In many cases, blind passages should be carried out because of the late development of the characteristic tissue changes in cultures infected with small amounts of virus.

Once an isolate has been placed in the reovirus group by means of the complement-fixation test other serological methods, particularly neutralization and haemagglutination-inhibition, should be employed for identifying the serotype and for detecting rising antibody titres in outbreaks of the disease.

OTHER DOUBLE-STRANDED RNA VIRUSES

Reoviruses are unusual in that they possess a genome consisting of several segments of double-stranded RNA. Thus, considerable interest was aroused when it was discovered that the wound tumour virus (WTV) of plants also contained double-stranded RNA, and that its structure was very similar to that of reovirus. Since then, more than 60 viruses from vertebrate, invertebrate, bacterial, higher plant and fungal hosts that are distinct in morphology and biological characteristics have been found to contain double-stranded RNA and, in 1968, Verwoerd proposed that these should constitute a new taxonomic group with the descriptive name 'Diplornavirus'. In contrast to reoviruses whose hosts are vertebrates, almost all members of this proposed group are transmitted by arthropod vectors or are associated with insects, but they differ from togaviruses on physicochemical and serological grounds. Important members of this newly proposed group include bluetongue virus of sheep, African horse sickness virus, epizootic haemorrhagic disease of deer virus, equine encephalosis virus, epizootic mouse diarrhoea virus, Colorado tick fever virus of man, rice dwarf virus of the rice plant, wound tumour virus of sweet clover and cytoplasmic polyhedrosis virus of the silkworm.

In 1971, Borden and his colleagues proposed the name Orbivirus (latin, *orbis* = ring or circle) for the 'bluetongue-like' viruses because of the large, distinctive doughnut-shaped capsomeres seen on the surface of the virion in negatively-stained preparations. They further suggested that the term Diplornavirus should be elevated to a higher taxon than at present and that the names reovirus and orbivirus should be accorded (generic) rank of equal taxonomic status. Should this scheme of classification be adopted officially, all double-stranded RNA viruses (whether arthropod-transmitted or not) could be sub-divided into 3 main taxonomic groups: (1) reoviruses, (2) orbiviruses and (3) other double-stranded RNA viruses with cubic symmetry. The first, with reovirus as its prototype, contains all acid stable (pH 3·0) strains whose nucleic acid core is surrounded by a double-layered capsid with 92 capsomeres in the outer layer. The second, with bluetongue virus as type species, includes all acid labile members whose core is surrounded by a distinct inner protein shell composed of 32 capso-

meres and a diffuse, structureless outer coat which is removed following exposure to caesium chloride. It should be noted also that reovirus-like particles found in the faeces of young children with acute gastroenteritis, as well as the virus causing diarrhoea in neonatal calves, differ morphologically both from reo- and orbiviruses, and have been provisionally designated rotaviruses.

Differences between members of the two main diplornavirus sub-groups and those of typical togaviruses are summarised in Table 48.2.

ROTAVIRUSES

In 1966, a virus was discovered which appeared to play an important role in many cases of calf diarrhoea. It was named the neonatal calf diarrhoea reovirus-like agent [NCDR] because of its morphological similarity to reoviruses. More recently, it has been reported that reovirus-like particles present in the faeces of infants with acute gastroenteritis and the virus causing acute diarrhoea in newborn calves are indistinguishable from each other in size and shape and, because they contain double-stranded RNA, they have been provisionally classified in the diplornavirus group. However, since there is now clear evidence that these viruses differ morphologically from reo- and orbiviruses, a third sub-group named rotavirus [Latin, *rota*, a wheel] has been suggested for them. (Plate 48.1c.)

In electron micrographs, the intact rotavirus particles possess a quasi-spherical capsid [60–66 nm in diameter], which exhibits cubic symmetry. The central core measures 36–38 nm in diameter and is surrounded by a membrane from which short

TABLE 48.2. Differences between reo-, orbi- and togaviruses.

| | REOVIRIDAE (Diplornaviruses) | | TOGAVIRIDAE |
	REOVIRUS	ORBIVIRUS e.g. bluetongue	
RNA genome	Double-stranded	Double-stranded	Single-stranded
Capsid	Core surrounded by 2 distinct protein shells	Core surrounded by a distinct protein shell & a diffuse featureless outer coat, removed by CsCl	Electron-lucent core component, surrounded by delicate non-rigid coat
Capsomeres	92 (180)	32	32
Symmetry	Cubic	Cubic	Mostly cubic
Envelope	Naked	Mostly naked	Mostly enveloped
Diameter (nm)			
Capsid	60–75	53– (68) –80	30–90
Nucleocapsid	40–45	54–60	20–40
Lipid solvents	Absolutely resistant	Relatively resistant	Sensitive
Acid pH (3.0)	Stable	Very labile	Labile
Heat	Resistant	Sensitive in absence of extraneous protein	Sensitive
Arthropod-borne	No	Mostly	Mostly

cylindrical capsomeres radiate outwards. An additional outer layer of capsomeres is attached to the ends of these capsomeres and gives the appearance of a sharply defined rim attached to short spokes upon a wide hub. The calf and human gastroenteritis viruses probably possess a serologically similar internal capsid protein, but they are antigenically unrelated to reo- and orbiviruses.

Rotaviruses are extremely difficult to cultivate but infection of cell cultures can readily be detected by means of immunofluorescent staining with antisera prepared in rabbits or gnotobiotic calves. A few strains of virus have been adapted to grow in bovine cell cultures with cytopathic effects, but without evidence of haemadsorption or haemagglutinin activity.

Infection can be diagnosed by the demonstration of very large numbers of virus particles, with characteristic morphology, in the faeces or small intestinal contents by electron microscopy. Although neutralizing antibodies are present in sera of affected calves, repeated infection and excretion of virus in immune animals probably occurs. The virus is resistant to heat and will survive at 60°C for 30 minutes, but is inactivated by pasteurization. Rotaviruses are also associated with enteritis in piglets, and calf strains are readily infectious to pigs, but attempts to infect calves with human strains have been unsuccessful.

Both inactivated and live cell-culture attenuated virus vaccines have been developed in the U.S.A. and are said to be effective in reducing the incidence of diarrhoea on affected farms.

ORBIVIRUSES

Bluetongue

Synonyms
Sore mouth: Sore muzzle: Ovine catarrhal fever: Vail Bek: Bekziekte: Lengua azul (Sp.): Blauzunge (Gr.).

Definition
Bluetongue is an acute arthropod-borne virus disease primarily of sheep, characterised by severe catarrhal inflammation of the mucous membranes of the buccal mucosa and gastro-intestinal tract. The lesions frequently involve the udder, the coronary band and the sensitive laminae of the hoof. There is epithelial desquamation but no vesicle formation.

Hosts affected
Sheep of all ages and breeds are highly susceptible but goats, cattle and wild ruminants suffer much milder symptoms and may act as non-clinical carriers of the infection. Horses, dogs, cats, ferrets, rabbits and guinea-pigs are not susceptible to the natural disease.

History and distribution
The disease has been recognised in South, East and West Africa since the latter part of the nineteenth century but there is an early report, dated 1652, of an acute febrile disease resembling bluetongue in Merino and other European breeds of sheep imported into Cape Colony. Bluetongue appeared outside the African continent for the first time in 1943 in Cyprus, and 3 years later it spread to a number of other Eastern European countries including Palestine, Israel, Syria and Turkey. The disease was diagnosed in California in 1952 but there is evidence that it may have existed earlier in Texas, and was known as 'sore muzzle'. In 1956, bluetongue was recorded in Spain and Portugal, and 3 years later a virus closely resembling that of bluetongue was isolated from a severe epizootic in cattle in Japan. There are unconfirmed reports that the disease occurred in West Pakistan in 1959 and in India in 1964.

Morphology
Although early reports suggested that the virus of bluetongue had a diameter of about 100–130 nm and possessed icosahedral symmetry with 92 capsomeres, more recent studies have shown that the virus particles are much smaller, 53–60 nm, and that the viral capsid consists of 32 hollow capsomeres. Details of the ultrastructure of bluetongue virus are frequently obscured by the presence of fine hair-like structures that seem to extend from the capsomeres. In some instances, a thick overlay of fibrillar material increases the overall diameter of viral particles in negatively stained preparations to 70–80 nm. Mature virions are frequently surrounded by a thick outer envelope and, occasionally, groups of as many as 30–40 virus particles are observed within a membrane-bound sac. These envelope-like structures which may consist merely of portions of cellular material, can be removed by treatment with ether or Tween 80 without appreciable loss of virus activity. Electron micrographs do not show a distinct double-layered capsid as is seen in the case of most reoviruses. (Plate 48.1a, facing p. 636. Plate 48.2a, b, facing p. 637.)

Chemical composition
The nucleic acid component contains RNA, and acridine-orange staining generally shows orange-red inclusions in the cytoplasm of infected cells. In early infections, however, the RNA genome is double-stranded with a total molecular weight of 15×10^6 daltons.

Physicochemical characters

Bluetongue virus differs from togaviruses and other arboviruses in a number of important respects. It is much more resistant and will remain viable in decomposed blood for many years. It is resistant to 20 per cent diethyl ether and 0·1 per cent sodium desoxycholate, but is inactivated by 3 per cent formalin and 70 per cent alcohol. It also survives drying in air and will retain its infectivity in serum, defibrinated blood and in a glycerol-oxalate-phenol mixture for 25 years at room temperature, but slow freezing at −10° or −20°C has a deleterious effect on its infectivity. Virus titres are maintained by storage in a medium containing 1 per cent of added neutral peptone and buffered at pH 7·4. Bluetongue virus is stable in a pH range between 5·6 and 8·0 but a fall of pH to below 5·6 or heating at 60°C for 30 minutes results in a marked loss of infectivity. Thus, survival of the virus in carcase meat is dependent on the degree of post-mortem pH change. Its marked sensitivity to acid consitutes an important difference between bluetongue virus and the acid-resistant reoviruses. The thermostability of purified virus preparations in the absence of extraneous protein material, can be enhanced by the addition of one per cent albumin, serum, peptone or other protein-derived substances.

Haemagglutination

In contrast to reoviruses and African horse sickness virus, the bluetongue virus does not possess hae-magglutinin activity, nor does it show haemadsorption in infected cell cultures.

Antigenic properties

Serum neutralization tests in cell cultures and other host systems reveal that there are at least 16 immu-nological types of bluetongue virus involving 4 major antigenic groups, but the origin of the multiplicity of types remains obscure. In South Africa, all but one of the 16 antigenic types have been identified, the single exception being the type 16 strain which occurs in West Pakistan and has recently been isolated from *Culicoides* species in South West Nigeria. On the other hand, only a single or limited number of serotypes exist in any one country in other parts of the world. In the U.S.A. and Portugal all recent outbreaks of bluetongue in sheep have been due to type 10 virus, while in Egypt types 1, 4 and 12 predominate.

Fluorescent antibody and gel precipitation techniques have shown that there is a group antigen which is shared by most, if not all, of the strains. Any single strain produces an immunity only against the homologous strain but, unfortunately, the immunity elicited by any one type may not be sufficient to provide protection against the other types and vaccinated animals are liable to react when exposed to infection with a heterologous strain. A suggestion that the virus is antigenically unstable awaits confirmation.

Cultivation

The bluetongue virus can be readily isolated from infected sheep during the febrile or early post-febrile phase of the illness. Growth is obtained in 6-day-old embryonated hens' eggs by the yolk sac route of inoculation provided the temperature of incubation is about 33·5°C i.e., at a temperature below the optimum for the development of the chick embryo. The virus can also be grown on the chorio-allantoic membrane when it produces specific mortality within 4–8 days, accompanied by extensive haemorrhages of the developing embryo. Intravenous inoculation is up to 100 times more sensitive than the yolk sac route. Virulent strains have been attenuated for sheep, without loss of antigenicity, by serial passage in fertile eggs but adaptation and attenuation of the virus takes place more rapidly at temperatures below 37·5°C. Bluetongue virus has also been adapted to growth in the brains of unweaned mice and hamsters. Infected animals show signs of encephalitis followed by death in about 3–7 days post-inoculation. Adult mice inoculated intracerebrally do not develop clinical symptoms although the virus replicates and may persist in their brains for short periods.

In 1956, egg adapted strains of bluetongue virus were first grown in primary monolayer cultures of lamb kidney cells. After 24–72 hours of incubation, cytopathic changes were observed in the form of a few foci of enlarged and refractile cells. The effect progressed rapidly until, within a few days, all the cells of the monolayer were involved and became detached from the glass. Since then, both egg-adapted and virulent strains of the virus have been propagated in many other types of cell cultures including primary cultures of calf kidney, adrenal and testis or in cell lines such as Chang liver, HeLa and baby hamster kidney (BHK–21). A plaque assay in mouse L cells has also been described. Cultures of kidney cells derived from dogs, cats and pigs do not, apparently, support the growth of the virus.

Studies of the growth cycle of bluetongue virus show that adsorption and penetration occur within the first 5–10 minutes with the virion entering the cell by means of a pinocytotic vesicle. Electron microscopical examination of ultra-thin sections of infected cell cultures shows dense inclusions and masses of fine filaments or microtubules within the cytoplasm. The mature virions leave the cell by budding through the cytoplasmic membrane or into the cytoplasmic vesicles, during which it acquires a well-developed outer membrane of host-cell origin.

Direct fluorescent antibody staining shows that intracytoplasmic inclusion bodies contain specific viral antigen while acridine orange staining indicates that some of the inclusions are RNA positive and some are RNA negative.

Tissue culture virus provides a satisfactory antigen for the complement-fixation and serum neutralization tests, the latter having the narrower specificity.

Pathogenicity

The incubation period following natural exposure is unknown but is believed to be about a week. Prolonged incubation periods up to 131 days have been recorded following experimental exposure. Affected animals show marked depression, anorexia, pyrexia (up to 42°C), copious salivation and the development of an excessive serous or mucous nasal discharge which dries and forms crusts around the nose. Hyperaemia, petechiation and swelling of the buccal mucosa, dental pads and tongue occur in the early stages of the disease. Later, the visible areas of hyperaemia may become cyanotic and purplish-blue in colour, and the appearance of the tongue gives rise to the popular description of the disease. Examination of the mouth almost a week after the first rise in temperature reveals multiple mucosal erosions, while the development of a blood-stained diarrhoea is indicative of involvement of the intestinal mucosa and may prove fatal. Oedema of the head, ears, intermandibular tissues, throat and brisket is frequently recognised and there may be involvement of the sensitive laminae of the feet. (Plate 48.1b, facing p. 636.) An additional feature of the disease in sheep is breaking of the wool fibres, and a badly affected animal may cast its entire fleece. In sheep that survive the febrile stage, there may be lameness, torticollis and muscular weakness, and badly affected animals may even walk on their knees. While heavy mortality (20–30 per cent) may occur in the earlier stages of the disease, chronically affected animals become thin and emaciated. The state of debility may persist for weeks and the economic losses in mutton and wool may be considerable. Additional economic losses include abortions of pregnant ewes and the loss of an entire breeding season. While the morbidity may be 50 per cent or higher, the mortality rates vary greatly depending on the strain of virus involved and the breed susceptibility of the hosts. In Africa and Europe the disease is particularly severe and up to 90 per cent of the animals in an infected flock may die whereas in America it is much milder and the mortality rates seldom exceed 1–7 per cent. Young animals, Merino sheep and certain British breeds are particularly susceptible.

Although cattle and goats may also be severely affected, and clinical signs and post-mortem changes closely resemble those seen in sheep, they mostly suffer milder symptoms and have prolonged viraemia. Natural infections of white-tail deer and other wild-living ruminants have been described in the U.S.A.

Pathological changes include congestion of the lungs, oedema and haemorrhages of the muscles and connective tissues as well as lesions of the mouth and coronet. In many cases there is diffuse, cloudy swelling and focal degeneration of the myocardium and skeletal musculature. Inclusion bodies have not been described in histological preparations.

The disease is readily transmitted experimentally by the inoculation of susceptible sheep with virulent blood, serum or macerated tissues. Young mice and unweaned hamsters are readily infected by the intracerebral route.

Spread and transmission

All domestic ruminants including cattle and goats are susceptible to the virus of bluetongue and it is probable that antelopes and other species of game animals may harbour the virus without showing clinical symptoms of the disease. There is no evidence that the infection is transmitted by direct contact although sheep may become infected by repeated oral administration of the virus. Cattle kept under insect-proof conditions have been shown to harbour the virus for at least 11 weeks. It has been realised for many years that the natural disease is transmitted by at least one of the 22 species of *Culicoides* in Africa, and by *Culicoides variipennis* in the U.S.A. Numerous experiments have been described in which pools of wild-caught *Culicoides*, emulsified and injected into susceptible animals, produce clinical evidence of bluetongue; and recent results suggest that the virus can multiply in the salivary glands of *C. variipennis*. There are also reports that the sheep ked *Melophagus ovinus* can also harbour the virus. Since *Culicoides* are active long before the onset of outbreaks in the latter part of the summer, it is likely that wild animal reservoir hosts, e.g. Blesbuck, play an important role in maintaining and perpetuating the infection during inter-epizootic periods.

Diagnosis

A tentative diagnosis of bluetongue may be based on the clinical signs and the nature and distribution of the lesions; but only when characteristic changes are present in highly susceptible sheep. Confirmation depends on positive transmission to susceptible sheep or the isolation of the virus in unweaned mice, susceptible primary cell cultures or, preferably, embryonated hens' eggs. Suitable material can be obtained from the blood or spleen of animals during the febrile or early post-febrile stages of the illness. The virus is identified by means of the complement-fixation test or, when type-specific results are necessary, by serum neutralization tests in tissue culture. In order to demonstrate a rising antibody titre in the convalescent serum of sheep, collected between the 30th and 45th days following recovery, antigens for the complement-fixation test are usually prepared from infected chorioallantoic membranes, tissue culture fluids or, preferably, brain and cord tissues of infected baby mice. Agar gel diffusion tests are being used more extensively not only because the procedure is simple and economic but because it is group-specific. Unlike complement-fixing antibodies, precipitating antibodies tend to persist for long periods and micro agar gel precipitation is useful in detecting the prevalence of the disease. The fluorescent antibody staining technique is also being used for the rapid diagnosis of bluetongue since both the indirect and direct methods are of value for detecting bluetongue viral antigen in infected tissues.

Differential diagnosis

In Africa, bluetongue in sheep must be differentiated from Rift Valley fever, Wesselsbron and heartwater, and in cattle, from foot-and-mouth disease and sweating sickness or ephemeral fever.

Control

Theiler and du Toit's original sheep-adapted virus vaccines were prepared by passing a mild field strain of the virus through 12 successive generations in sheep. Unfortunately, the virus was not sufficiently attenuated and produced severe systemic reactions in some sheep and failed to protect in others. In 1948, the use of these vaccines was abandoned in favour of live attenuated avianized vaccines. They have been widely used as freeze-dried monovalent vaccines in the U.S.A. and a quadravalent vaccine proved highly successful in controlling the spread of bluetongue through the Iberian Peninsula. In the enzootic regions of Africa, where numerous antigenic types of virus may be involved, polyvalent avianized vaccines must be used. The duration of the artificially induced immunity is unknown but it probably lasts for at least 12 months. Unfortunately, the efficacy of multiple egg vaccines may be hampered by interference between the virus strains, differences in their immunizing potency and by marked differences in the response of individual animals. It is stressed that modified live virus vaccines may produce viraemia in sheep of sufficient titre to infect the insect vectors feeding on the vaccinated animal and, following an appropriate extrinsic incubation period, these insects may be capable of transmitting the infection to susceptible animals.

Attenuated avianized vaccines should not be used in pregnant sheep because cerebral and other lesions may occur in lambs born from vaccinated ewes. Live vaccines may also interfere with oestrus. Sheep are normally vaccinated annually, several weeks before service and before the start of the rainy season. Passive immunity is acquired by the young through the ingestion of colostral antibodies from the immune dam. Because of this, lambs are not vaccinated until they are at least 3 months of age, when active immunity develops within 10 days.

African horse sickness

Synonyms

Perdesiekte; pestis equorum; pferdesterbe (Ger.).

Definition

An acute or subacute, febrile, arthropod-borne disease of solipeds that is characterized by oedema of the subcutaneous tissues and lungs, haemorrhages of internal organs and accumulations of serous fluids in the body cavities.

Hosts affected

Horses of all breeds are highly susceptible to natural infection, mules and zebras less so, but donkeys are generally resistant. In some parts of the Near East, donkeys are believed to be susceptible.

Distribution

The disease occurs principally in Southern, Eastern and Central Africa. It is also prevalent in most adjoining territories and as far north as the Nile valley. For many years horse sickness was considered to be enzootic only in certain areas of Africa but, in 1944 and subsequently, it spread to Syria, the Lebanon, Israel and other parts of the Middle East. In 1959–61 it appeared in Afghanistan and West Pakistan, and spread over a wide area to include Turkey, Iraq and India.

It is a seasonal disease, occurring mostly in the late summer in warm humid low-lying marshy districts. The incidence is often highest during unusually wet seasons and in some regions the infection is so severe that not a single susceptible horse survives.

Properties of the virus

Virions seen in negatively-stained preparations are very similar in morphology to those of bluetongue virus. The capsids, which are about 55 nm in diameter, show icosahedral symmetry probably with 32 capsomeres. Clusters of virus particles are occasionally seen within a thick-layered envelope which is generally considered to be derived from host cell membranes and is not an essential part of the virus.

Physicochemical characters

Horse sickness virus contains double-stranded RNA and is stable between pH 6 and 10, but is rapidly inactivated at pH 3·0. Infective blood remains viable for years when added to an equal volume of a glycerol-oxalate-phenol mixture. Infectivity remains unaltered for at least 6 months at 4°C in 10 per cent serum-saline and virulence is retained in putrid blood for 2 years or longer. The virus is inactivated in 15 minutes at 60°C, and by 1/1000 formalin in 48 hours at 22°C. Strains of horse sickness virus, unlike togaviruses and most other arboviruses, are ether-, deoxycholate- and trypsin-resistant.

Haemagglutination

Horse red blood cells are agglutinated by extracts of infected mouse brains, preferably at pH 6·4 and 37°C for about 2 hours.

Antigenic properties

Complement-fixation shows that strains of horse sickness virus possess a common group-specific antigen, but virus neutralization and haemagglutination-inhibition tests are type-specific. Many serotypes have been described, and experience of immunity in natural cases of the disease indicates that the virus is antigenically labile. Differences between strains are not clear-cut and it is possible that strains of horse sickness virus possess the same antigenic components but in widely different proportions. In Africa, nine distinct serotypes are recognized and considerable variation in virulence exists amongst individual strains within each immunological type. On the other hand, only a single antigenic type was involved in the Asian outbreak in 1961.

Cultivation

The virus infects mice, rats, guinea-pigs and other species of laboratory rodents when administered by the intracerebral route. Viscerotropic field strains can be converted into neurotropic strains by serial intracerebral passage in mice, and the adapted virus becomes attenuated for horses without losing its antigenic properties.

Dogs can be infected by intravenous or subcutaneous injections, and also by feeding on the flesh of infected horses. However, serological studies in enzootic areas suggest that dogs are very rarely infected through natural transmission and do not constitute a danger as reservoir hosts in the spread of the infection.

Ferrets can be infected by the intravenous route and pantropic strains of virus generally induce a febrile reaction within 4–7 days post-inoculation. The disease is otherwise inapparent and no distinct clinical symptoms have been observed. Ferrets appear to be particularly useful animals for isolating virus from horses whose immunity has broken down during a natural exposure. Rabbits, cattle and sheep cannot be infected.

Neurotropic mouse-adapted virus can be grown successfully on the chorioallantoic membrane of embryonated hens' eggs and multiplies readily in the chick embryo brain. Almost all strains will grow in the yolk sac of fertile eggs.

Horse sickness virus can be propagated in cell cultures of many different types. In South Africa, all 9 serological types of virus have been adapted to growth on stable lines of baby hamster kidney (BHK-21) and, more recently, on rhesus and African green monkey (Vero) cell-line cultures. It is claimed that the monkey lines are the most susceptible to horse sickness virus, so far reported, and both yield virus of high titre. In rhesus kidney cultures, the cytopathic effect consists of rounding and shrinkage of infected cells which remain attached to the glass unless vigorously shaken. Infected Vero cells are irregular in shape and detach from the glass in ones and twos. Acridine orange staining shows large perinuclear RNA-type inclusions in Vero cells, but not in rhesus monkey kidney cells. However, in both types of monkey cell-line cultures the colour of the nucleus gradually changes from green to greenish-yellow as the infection progresses. In most other tissue culture systems large cytoplasmic inclusions containing RNA and virus antigen appear, but protein inclusions free of RNA have also been described.

Pathogenicity

The incubation period in natural outbreaks of horse sickness is generally about 6–9 days, but in experimentally infected animals it varies from only 2 days to as long as 21 days.

Four different clinical forms of the illness are recognised:

(1) a very mild form of horse sickness fever which is frequently overlooked, although the temperature may reach 41°C, or higher; (2) the acute or pulmonary form (dunkop horse sickness) in which there is severe dyspnoea, pyrexia and coughing with an abundant frothy discharge from the nostrils. This form is commonly seen in virulent outbreaks of the disease and most affected horses die; (3) the subacute or cardiac form (dikkop horse sickness) which is characterized by remarkable swellings of the head, neck and supraorbital fossa associated with cardiac dyspnoea. Dikkop usually appears in horses whose immunity has been broken down by a natural infection or in animals inoculated with a mild strain of the virus. It is much milder than dunkop and many affected animals recover, and (4) the mixed form of horse sickness, which is

probably a combination of the pulmonary and cardiac forms and is rarely diagnosed during life except when a case of dikkop develops the clinical symptoms of dunkop which soon leads to the death of the animal.

In general, the mortality varies considerably under different conditions. In some outbreaks of the virulent form of the disease the mortality rate may be as high as 90 per cent in horses but lower in mules, whereas in milder outbreaks barely 25 per cent of affected horses will die.

The post-mortem findings vary considerably depending on the severity of the case. In the acute pulmonary form there is extensive oedema of the lungs and the thorax may contain several litres of fluid. The interlobular lung tissue is generally separated from the alveolar portions by infiltrations of a yellowish fluid. The more chronic cardiac form is usually associated with oedematous infiltrations of the subcutaneous, subserosal and other tissues, together with gross accumulations of fluid in the pericardial sac. Despite the presence of hydropericardium, the lungs and pleural cavity are rarely involved or show only moderate oedema.

Immunity

Experimental evidence indicates that the virus undergoes a profound antigenic change during serial passage from horse to horse, and that an animal immunized against a particular strain may break down when challenged with the homologous strain at a different passage level. Foals of immune dams are highly resistant as a result of having ingested antibodies in the colostrum, but immunity is lost after about 5 or 6 months. Horses and mules that have recovered from a natural attack of horse sickness are generally more resistant to disease than other equines and are known as 'salted', as are animals that have survived for a number of years in badly infected areas without ever showing obvious signs of the disease. The sera of horses that have recovered from the disease have little protective value whereas the sera of hyperimmunized animals may afford a considerable degree of protection. The rise in serum antibodies of a horse after immunization is slow and with the attenuated neurotropic mouse-passaged virus the peak may not be reached until the 200th day. With the viscerotropic virus-serum mixture the peak is usually reached by the 100th day. In general, the immunity produced by either the viscerotropic or neurotropic virus is solid and long-lasting against the homologous virus of the same passage level. However, strains of virus showing only minor antigenic differences from the vaccine strains may sometimes cause a severe and fatal breakdown in immunity.

Transmission

Horse sickness is not directly contagious and the possibility that the causative agent is carried by biting insects was first suggested by Theiler and others, in 1903, when they discovered that horses in mosquito-proof enclosures were protected against the infection. Various nocturnal biting insects, including mosquitoes, were incriminated, but definite evidence regarding a particular arthropod was not obtained until 1944 when horse sickness virus was isolated from a pool of *Culicoides*. There can be no doubt that these nocturnal insects are the most important vectors of the infection in Africa, but whether all or only some of the 22 species of *Culicoides* transmit the virus is not yet known. *Tabanidae* and *Stomoxys* have been incriminated in outbreaks in Turkey. Although recently recovered horses may act as reservoirs of infection for periods of up to 90 days, it has not been established how the virus survives during the 6 months of the year when horse sickness does not normally occur. Most workers believe that the virus is maintained in an unknown wild reservoir host from which *Culicoides* and some other vectors acquire the infection.

Although there is scientific evidence that the virus undergoes an antigenic change when passaged serially through horses there is no proof that such changes can occur in wild reservoir hosts or insect vectors.

Diagnosis

Typical outbreaks of African horse sickness can usually be diagnosed on the basis of the clinical symptoms and post-mortem findings. In many other instances, and especially in endemic areas where immunization is practised, it may be necessary to isolate the virus by transmitting the infection to other horses. The virus can then be identified by cross-protection or serum neutralization tests in white mice. Blood for this purpose should be collected during the early febrile phase of the disease because the viraemic phase in horse sickness is generally of short duration. Whole blood collected in an anticoagulant, or macerated spleen tissue is injected into unweaned mice by the intracerebral route. Deaths usually take place between 5 and 15 days postinoculation. Infective mouse brain is used as a source of antigen in the group-specific complement-fixation test which is particularly useful for primary identification. The antigenic type of the causative virus can be ascertained by serum neutralization and haemagglutination-inhibition tests using type-specific hyperimmune sera produced in rabbits or guinea-pigs. Heterologous antibodies present in the serum of vaccinated horses that have suffered a breakdown are capable of protecting mice against infection, but passage in ferrets usually overcomes this difficulty and ensures successful isolation of virus from an immunized horse. Tissue culture techniques are now being used in studies of horse sickness and should prove helpful in diagnosis.

Control

Several methods of immunization have been used in the past to control African horse sickness ranging from Theiler's intravenous virus-hyperimmune serum technique to formalised tissue vaccines administered subcutaneously. More recently, freeze-dried, live, attenuated neurotropic mouse brain virus vaccines have proved useful and polyvalent vaccines prepared from 7 or 8 antigenically distinct serotypes appear to be safe and highly effective against all field strains. The response of individual horses to the use of polyvalent vaccines varies considerably and antibodies against all 7 or 8 strains cannot always be detected subsequently by serological tests. For this reason, regular annual immunization is advocated and it has been estimated that in South Africa about 20 per cent of the total horse population are in fact, vaccinated annually. Tissue culture-adapted virus is believed to be greatly attenuated for horses, and hamster and monkey kidney culture vaccines are now widely used in Africa and the Middle East. Whatever vaccination procedures are adopted, horses in enzootic areas during an outbreak of horse sickness should be removed from low lying areas before sunset and stabled overnight in fly-proof quarters.

Other diseases possibly associated with diplornaviruses

Other diseases caused by or associated with double-stranded RNA viruses resembling reoviruses include epidemic diarrhoea of infant mice, epizootic haemorrhagic disease of deer, infectious pancreatic necrosis in trout, blue comb of turkeys and pullets, Gumboro disease or avian nephrosis, and infectious myocarditis of goslings.

Blue comb

Blue comb disease, pullet disease, avian monocytosis or avian infectious diarrhoea was first recognised in 1929 in the U.S.A. and has been reported later from other parts of the world where young turkeys and pullets are reared under intensive methods of husbandry. It occurs mostly when laying birds are reaching maturity and seldom affects birds under 4 months of age. Turkeys of all ages may be affected and birds that survive may remain carriers of the infection. The disease has not been observed in ducks and geese.

The aetiology of this condition remains uncertain but a filterable agent, unaffected by antibiotics, has frequently been propagated in 8-day-old chicken embryos, killing them in 36–72 hours. Strains resembling reoviruses in morphology and in physicochemical properties have been described in association with this disease but viruses differing from reoviruses have also been isolated from the tissues of affected birds.

The disease is highly contagious and can be reproduced by feeding filtrates of intestinal contents. The onset of the disease is sudden and is characterized by anorexia, depression, severe drop in egg-production, watery and frothy foetid diarrhoea and cyanosis of the comb and wattles. The incubation period is short (48–72 hours) and deaths may begin 2–3 days after the onset of clinical signs. The mortality rate is very variable and ranges from 1–50 per cent. At autopsy, the breast muscles are dehydrated, the liver may be fatty and congested, and the kidneys may be enlarged and contain mild to marked urate deposits. The feathers around the vent are frequently soiled with faecal and urate material.

Gumboro disease (Infectious bursal disease)

Gumboro disease of poultry, which is named after the locality in which the earliest outbreaks occurred, was first recognized in the U.S.A. in the autumn of 1957, and England in 1962. A similar condition known as infectious avian nephrosis has existed in Australia for several years.

Gumboro disease is a lymphoproliferative condition of young chickens which specifically affects the bursa of Fabricius, initially causing severe oedema followed by atrophy. The bursa often shows necrotic foci and may have haemorrhages on the serosal surface. Histological lesions may also be present in the bursa, spleen, thymus and caecal tonsil. The disease is of interest immunologically since young chickens affected by the disease are unable to deal satisfactorily with other infections because of the depression of bursa-derived lymphocytes.

The causative agent has been described as a reovirus but recent reports, based on immune electron microscopy, suggest that the disease has associated with it a virus-satellite system similar to that found with adenoviruses. The two viruses in this unusual system have surface antigens in common, but are morphologically distinct. The larger particle has a single-layered hexagonal capsid, 55–66 nm in diameter, resembling the diplornavirus of trout pancreatic necrosis virus [vide infra] while the second is much smaller [16–22 nm in diameter] and has the appearance of a parvovirus such as the adeno-satellite virus.

The disease occurs throughout the year and is especially prevalent in large broiler-producing areas of the U.S.A., Canada, Europe and Australia. Birds between 3 and 4 weeks of age are most commonly affected but outbreaks have occurred in chickens over 3 months old. Affected birds become dull and listless with ruffled feathers and watery diarrhoea. Some may show incoordination of gait and prostration. Trembling is a prominent feature in some outbreaks and, in Australia, respiratory distress is commonly seen particularly during the early stages of the disease. The mortality rate is generally higher in younger age groups and ranges between 5–15 per cent.

The carcases of affected birds are in good condition but dehydration may be severe and haemorrhages are frequently present in the leg muscles. In many cases, urates are present in the kidney tubules and ureters, and urate deposits may be found on the surface of the pericardium and liver. The bursa of Fabricius is markedly enlarged and contains large quantities of exudate or caseous material. The virus may persist for long periods in the environment and the infection is probably transmitted by means of contaminated feed or water.

Infectious pancreatic necrosis in trout

Pancreatic necrosis is an acute and highly contagious virus disease of young brook trout, rainbow trout and cut-throat trout. Salmon are probably resistant. The causative virus contains double-stranded RNA and measures about 65 nm in diameter. In ultra-thin sections, hexagonal virions are observed in the cytoplasm of infected cells frequently in association with microtubules 45 nm in diameter. Virus particles seen in negatively-stained preparations have naked icosahedral capsids with 92 capsomeres. The virus is ether-resistant but is readily inactivated at pH 3·0 It survives $2\frac{1}{2}$ years at 4°C in 50 per cent glycerol and some of its infectivity persists after 1 hour at 60°C. No evidence of haemagglutination or haemadsorption has been found. The virus, which was the first to be isolated from fish, grows readily at 23°C and produces a cytopathic effect in trout tissue cultures; growth has not been described in cultures of various mammalian or amphibian cells.

The onset of the disease is sudden, following an incubation period of about 6–10 days. Infected fish appear grossly normal but swim erratically in a whirling or corkscrewing manner. Others tend to lie on the bottom and respire feebly. Death usually ensues within an hour or two. Little is known about the disease in nature but mortality rates up to 80 per cent have occurred in hatcheries. Affected fish frequently develop exophthalmia, abdominal distension, petechial haemorrhages around the pyloric caeca and a digestive tract devoid of food. The presence of thick clear or milky mucous in the stomach and anterior intestines is a very reliable symptom of the disease.

Histologically, the disease is characterized by the destruction of pancreatic tissues and occasionally by necrosis of adjacent adipose tissue. In degenerating pancreatic tissue, round or oval cytoplasmic inclusion bodies are seen in the acinar cells and are often surrounded by a clear halo. The nature of these inclusions and their relationship to the growth cycle of the virus is uncertain but most workers consider that they are signs of necrosis rather than specific stages in viral development.

The disease has been transmitted experimentally by inoculation, by contact and by feeding infectious materials. Following outbreaks of spontaneous disease in hatcheries, some recovered adult trout may remain symptomless carriers of the virus.

Further reading

ALMEIDA, J.D. AND MORRIS, R. (1973) Antigenically-related viruses associated with infectious bursal disease. *Journal of General Virology*, **20**, 369

ANDERSON N. AND DOANE F.W. (1966) An electron-microscope study of reovirus type 2 in L cells. *Journal of Pathology and Bacteriology* **92**, 433.

BOWNE J.G. (1971) Bluetongue disease. *Advances in Veterinary Science*, **15**, 1.

BOWNE J.G. AND JOCHIM M.M. (1967) Cytopathic changes and development of inclusion bodies in cultured cells infected with bluetongue virus. *American Journal of Veterinary Research*, **28**, 1091.

CERINI C.P. AND MALSBERGER R.G. (1965) Morphology of infectious pancreatic necrosis virus. *Annals of the New York Academy of Sciences*, **126**, 315.

COHEN, J., POINSARD, A. AND SCHERRER, R. (1973) Physico-chemical and morphological features of infectious pancreatic necrosis virus. *Journal of General Virology*, **21**, 485.

COX H.R. (1954) Bluetongue. *Bacteriological Reviews*, **18**, 239.

FENNER, F., PEREIRA, H.G., PORTERFIELD, J.S., JOKLIK, W.K. AND DOWNIE, A.W. (1974) Family and generic names for viruses approved by the International Committee on Taxonomy of Viruses, June 1974. *Intervirology*, **3**, 193.

FERNANDES M.V. (1959) Isolation and propagation of bluetongue virus in tissue culture. *American Journal of Veterinary Research*, **20**, 398.

HAIG D.A., McKERCHER D.G. AND ALEXANDER R.A. (1956). The cytopathogenic action of blue-tongue virus on tissue cultures and its application to the detection of antibodies in the serum of sheep. *Onderstepoort Journal of Veterinary Research*, **27**, 171.

HIRAI K. AND SHIMAKURA S. (1974) Structure of infectious bursal disease virus. *Journal of Virology*, **14**, 957.

HOWELL P.G. (1962) The isolation and identification of further antigenic types of African horse sickness virus. *Onderstepoort Journal of Veterinary Research*, **29**, 139.

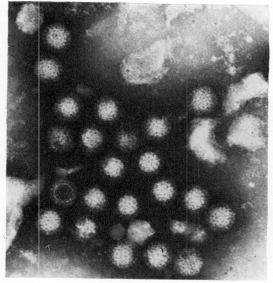

48.1a

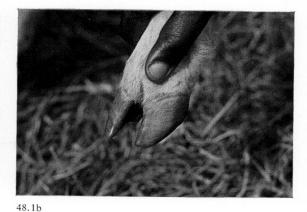

48.1b

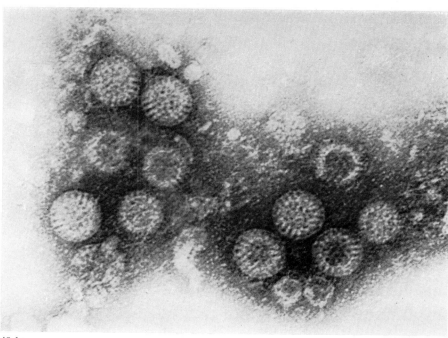

48.1c

48.1a Electron micrograph of a sheep strain of reovirus; cell culture isolate. The inner capsid is clearly visible as an arrangement of hexagonal and pentagonal capsomeres each with a dark hollow core. The outer shell is poorly defined and appears as a fringe of elongated hollow projections, ×100 000. (Courtesy of Dr J. B. McFerran.)

48.1b The lesions of bluetongue of sheep frequently involve the coronary band and the sensitive laminae of the hoof. (Courtesy of Dr W. B. Martin.)

48.1c Rotavirus in lamb faeces. Notice that the larger particles show an additional outer capsid layer giving the appearance of a sharply defined rim attached to short spokes upon a wide hub, ×200 000. (Courtesy of Dr D. R. Snodgrass.)

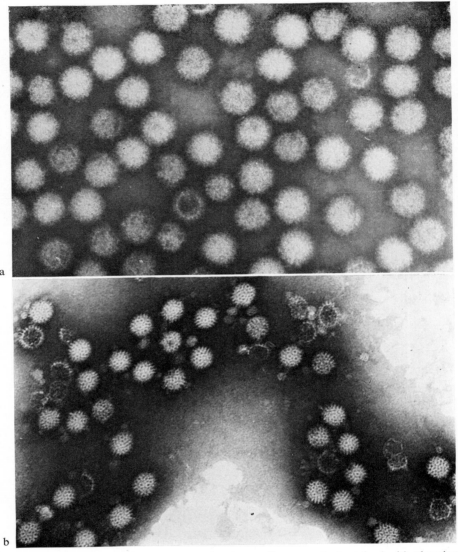

48.2a   Complete particles of bluetongue virus from sucrose gradient, negatively stained with phosphotungstic acid. Notice diffuse appearance of the virions, 68 nm in diameter. (Courtesy of Dr D. W. Verwoerd.)

48.2b   Particles of bluetongue virus from CsCl gradient, pH 6, showing more surface details. The inner capsid (diam. 55 nm) consists of a single layer of regularly arranged morphological units or capsomeres, ×125 000. (Courtesy of Dr D. W. Verwoerd.)

HOWELL P.G. (1966) Some aspects of the epizootiology of bluetongue. *Bulletin de l'office International des Epizooties*, **66**, 341.

HOWELL P.G. AND VERWOERD D.W. (1971) Bluetongue virus. *Virology Monographs*, **9**, 35.

KASZA L. (1970) Isolation and characterization of a reovirus from pigs. *Veterinary Record*, **87**, 681.

KAWAMURA H., SHIMIZU F., MAEDA M. AND TSUBAHARA H. (1965). Avian reovirus. Its properties and serological classification. *National Institute of Animal Health Quarterly*, **5**, 115.

KUROGI H., INABA Y., TAKAHASHI E., SATO K., GOTO Y., OMORI T. AND MATUMOTO M. (1974) New serotypes of reoviruses isolated from cattle. *Archiv für die gesamte Virusforschung*, **45**, 157.

LEE V.H., CAUSEY O.R. AND MOORE D.L. (1974) Bluetongue and related viruses in Ibadan, Nigeria: isolation and preliminary identification of viruses. *Journal of American Veterinary Research*, **35**, 1105.

LUEDKE A.J., BOWNE J.G., JOCHIM M.M. AND DOYLE C. (1964). Clinical and pathologic features of bluetongue in sheep. *American Journal of Veterinary Research*, **25**, 963.

MACRAE A.D. (1962) Reoviruses of man. *Annals of the New York Academy of Sciences*, **101**, 455.

MAURER F.D. (1961) African horse-sickness. *Journal of the American Veterinary Medical Association*, **138**, 15.

MAYOR H.D., JAMISON R.M., JORDAN L.E. AND VAN MITCHELL M. (1965) Reoviruses II. Structure and composition of the virion. *Journal of Bacteriology*, **89**, 1548.

MCINTOSH B.M. (1958) Immunological types of horse sickness virus and their significance in immunization. *Onderstepoort Journal of Veterinary Research*, **27**, 465.

MILLWARD S. AND GRAHAM A.F. (1971) Structure and transcription of the genomes of double-stranded RNA viruses. In Comparative Virology, eds. K. Maramorosch and E. Kurstak, p. 389. London: Academic Press.

OWEN N.C., DU TOIT R.M. AND HOWELL P.G. (1965) Bluetongue in cattle: typing of viruses isolated from cattle exposed to natural infections. *Onderstepoort Journal of Veterinary Research*, **32**, 3.

ROSEN L. (1962) Reoviruses. in animals other than man. *Annals of the New York Academy of Sciences*, **104**, 461.

ROSEN L. (1968) Reoviruses. *Virology Monographs*, **1**, 73.

SHOPE R.E., MACNAMARA L.G. AND MANGOLD R. (1960) Epizootic haemorrhagic disease of deer. *Journal of Experimental Medicine*, **111**, 155.

STANLEY N.F. (1967) Reoviruses. *British Medical Bulletin*, **23**, 150.

Symposium on bluetongue. (1975) *Australian Veterinary Journal*, **51**, No. 4, 165.

THEILER A. (1921) African Horse Sickness. Union of South Africa, Department of Agriculture Science Bulletin, No. 19.

TSAI K-S AND KARSTAD L. (1970) Epizootic hemorrhagic disease virus of deer: an electron microscopic study. *Canadian Journal of Microbiology*, **16**, 427.

VERWOERD D.W. (1970) Diplornaviruses: a newly recognized group of double-stranded RNA viruses. *Progress in Medical Virology*, **12**, 192.

VERWOERD D.W., LOUW H. AND OELLERMANN R.A. (1970) Characterization of the bluetongue virus ribonucleic acid. *Journal of Virology*, **5**, 1.

WILHELM A.R. AND TRAINOR D.O. (1967) A comparison of several viruses of epizootic hemorrhagic disease of deer. *Journal of Infectious Diseases*, **117**, 48.

WOLF K. (1966) The fish viruses. *Advances in Virus Research*, **12**, 35.

WOODE, G.N. AND BRIDGER, J.C. (1975) Viral enteritis of calves. *Veterinary Record*, **96**, 85.

CHAPTER 49

TOGAVIRUSES

Togaviruses

ARthropod-BOrne viruses (arboviruses) are maintained in nature by infection cycles that involve a vertebrate host and a haematophagus or blood-sucking arthropod as a vector. They are mostly to be found in tropical and subtropical rain forest countries or in temperate zones during the warmer, wetter seasons of the year when the insects are most active, and where they are able to live in close and intimate contact with large populations of wild and domestic animals. Thus, the term 'arbovirus' is used in a purely biological sense and is endowed with ecological but not with structural significance.

During the last few years a considerable volume of evidence has been accumulating concerning the properties and mode of multiplication of these agents and, in 1970, the name 'togavirus' (latin, *toga* = cloak) was introduced to cover arboviruses having taxonomic characters like those of Casals' serological groups A and B. These are now known as alpha- and flaviviruses, respectively. It is emphasised that arthropod transmission is not confined to togaviruses, and certain members of other structural groups e.g. picorna-, reo- and rhabdo- viruses can also be transmitted by this means. Nevertheless, the properties of togaviruses are sufficiently different from those of arthropod-borne members of other virus groups to justify this classification. Togaviruses are widely distributed in nature and recent studies of unclassified and newly isolated strains of virus indicate that some members are not transmitted through the agency of arthropod vectors and these have been provisionally designated as non-arthropod-borne (nonarbo) viruses of the family *Togaviridae*: candidate members include rubella virus of man, lactic dehydrogenase virus of mice, the causative viruses of equine arteritis, bovine viral diarrhoea-mucosal disease, swine fever (hog cholera) and, possibly, the virus of border disease of lambs.

Arthropod-borne togavirus infections are characterized by fever and viraemia in the early phase of the illness and it is only during this period when there are high concentrations of virus in the blood stream that the arthropod acquires the virus when it takes a blood meal from its animal host. During the following 10–14 days the ingested virus penetrates the gut wall, multiplies in the tissues of the arthropod and finally reaches the salivary glands and the saliva. Only after the completion of this 'extrinsic incubation period' is the vector capable of transmitting

the infection to another host. The arthropod is not harmed by the virus and usually remains infected for life. One of the rare exceptions to this general rule is that of the human body louse (*Pediculus corporis*) which is killed by *R. prowazekii* of typhus fever. Although most blood-sucking insects remain infective for life, it is extremely unlikely that the virus is transmitted through the egg to future generations; but in ticks, transovarial transmission may occur and infected ticks become permanent reservoirs of infection.

Should the virus not survive in the biological vector from one season to another, the infection may be conserved in various reservoir hosts such as game animals, wild-living rodents and birds, particularly if these reservoir hosts suffer only a mild or sub-clinical illness. Birds or animals with a short life-span constitute the main vertebrate re-reservoirs of infection rather than larger animals which often succumb to the disease. Thus, arthropod-borne togavirus infections are characterised by 2 biological cycles: one occurring in arthropods and the other in animals.

Transmission of infection from one vertebrate to the next may depend on more than one arthropod species, and several animals may be infected by the bite of the vector. On the other hand, some viruses are spread by only one primary vector, such as *Ixodes* in louping ill of sheep, whilst others, including African horse sickness, may be spread by several species of *Culex*, *Anopheles* or tabanids. An excellent example of 'vector specificity' is shown by *Aëdes aegypti* which is the vector in Western equine encephalomyelitis but cannot transmit the related Eastern equine encephalomyelitis virus.

The chain of infection may simply be vector-vertebrate host-vector, as in bluetongue of sheep (Fig. 49.1)

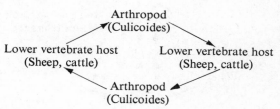

FIG. 49.1. The infection chain of bluetongue. (Orbivirus)

or it may be more complex, as in Rift Valley fever, where the vertebrate-arthropod cycle may be associated with tangential infection of man (Fig. 49.2).

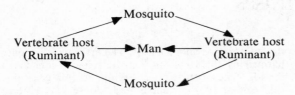

FIG. 49.2.   The infection chain of Rift Valley fever. (Togavirus)

In cases where the agent is transmitted from the adult arthropod to its offspring by transovarial passage, the cycle may continue with or without the intervention of a vertebrate host (Fig. 49·3).

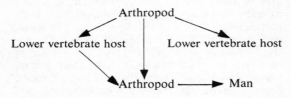

FIG. 49.3.   The infection chain of Colorado tick fever. (Diplornavirus)

Direct spread from vertebrate to vertebrate hosts may occasionally occur as in the transfer of Russian spring summer encephalitis virus by means of infected milk, or as an occupational hazard in butchers, farmers, veterinary surgeons and laboratory workers handling carcases or infected cultures; for example, Rift Valley fever and louping ill. In Japanese B encephalitis, the causal virus is probably a parasite primarily of wild birds but domestic pigs, which are regularly infected, may maintain the virus in a secondary role. Man, horses and other animals are only infected incidentally. (Fig. 49.4)

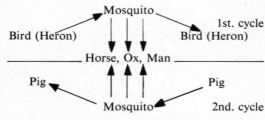

FIG. 49.4.   The infection chain of Japanese B. encephalitis. (Togavirus)

It should be noted that natural transmission of arbovirus infections differs from that of other virus diseases including swine pox, fowl pox and myxomatosis where biting lice, fleas or other arthropods may transmit the infection directly from one animal to another by mechanical means; there being no 'extrinsic period' or developmental cycle of the virus within the arthropod.

More than 260 members of the togavirus family have been recognised to date and all contain single-stranded RNA. The virions so far studied by electron microscopy are small, spherical particles surrounded by a non-rigid and delicate lipoprotein envelope. In most alpha-and flavi- viruses the envelope carries a number of radially arranged projections whereas in nonarbo togaviruses it displays a smooth surface. The central core contains between 32 and 92 capsomeres and shows hexagonal contours indicating an icosahedral rather than a helical architecture. Within the nucleocapsid is an electron-lucent centre giving a ring-shaped appearance to the densely stained core. The genome is infectious and consists of a single-stranded polyribonucleotide with a molecular weight of $3-4 \times 10^6$. Thus, togaviruses are the only enveloped riboviruses which yield infectious RNA. They are also the smallest lipid containing animal viruses so far described, the alphaviruses measuring 30–40 nm and the flaviviruses 20–30 nm in diameter. (Plate 49.1, facing p. 650).

Alpha- and flavi- viruses agglutinate red blood cells of a number of animal species in a definite pH range but the only nonarbo togavirus with haemagglutinating activity is rubella virus. In most instances the reactions between the haemagglutinin and the red blood cell is irreversible and the virus does not elute from the cells. This suggests that the mature virion is deficient in neuraminidase.

Togaviruses are unstable at room temperature but will survive for a few months at –20°C. They are best preserved at –70°C with stabilizer in the form of added protein, such as rabbit serum or bovine albumin. They are readily inactivated by low concentrations of formalin.

A wide range of animals may be infected with togaviruses and many different species of laboratory animals, including unweaned mice and hamsters, are highly susceptible. The viruses can be readily propagated in embryonated hens' eggs by the chorioallantoic membrane or yolk sac routes and most strains grow well and produce a marked cytopathic effect in primary and secondary cultures of chicken embryo or mouse embryo cells, as well as in a variety of stable cell lines, e.g. HeLa. Electron microscopic studies of infected cells suggest that alpha- and flavi -viruses differ with respect to their morphogenesis. Both are formed by budding, the former enveloping their nucleocapsids on the marginal membrane of the cell whereas the latter emerge from intracytoplasmic membranes.

The togaviruses have been classified into a number of major groups, according to their antigenic relationships, each consisting of viruses that share, to varying degrees, complement-fixing, haemagglutination-inhibiting and neutralizing antigens. Approximately 60 per cent fall into 7 major groups, 20 per cent are distributed in some 16 or so small groups and the remainder are, as yet, unclassified. Although most groups are antigenically distinct, subtle interrelationships between and within each genus are revealed by haemagglutination-inhibition, complement-fixation and virus neutralization tests.

Numerous arboviruses have been isolated from human patients with overt disease but comparatively few are of veterinary importance. Many isolates have been obtained only from mosquitoes or ticks, either directly or through infection of 'sentinel' animals, and are not known to be associated with disease. In general, pathogenic arthropod-borne togaviruses give rise to a relatively severe form of encephalitis or to visceral diseases such as yellow fever. The majority of infections are characterized by a variable incubation period of 4–21 days, sudden onset of fever, marked drowsiness, depression or stupor and a mortality rate of between 5 and 25 per cent or higher, depending on the nature of the virus.

ARTHROPOD-BORNE TOGAVIRUSES ALPHAVIRUSES

Diseases of man and animals caused by alphaviruses include Western equine, Eastern equine and Venezuelan equine encephalomyelitis (America), Semliki Forest disease, Chikungunya and O'nyong-nyong (Africa), Sindbis (Africa and India), Ross River fever (Australia) and Sagiyama virus disease (Japan).

Antigenic relationships within the genus are revealed most easily by haemagglutination-inhibition, less by complement-fixation and least by virus neutralization tests. Thus, the viruses of Western equine encephalomyelitis, Eastern equine encephalomyelitis and Venezuelan equine encephalomyelitis, which are related to each other and to other members of the group in haemagglutination-inhibition tests, are readily separable from each other as well as from the other alphaviruses by complement-fixation and neutralization tests. Moreover, plaque-inhibition tests have shown that Western equine encephalomyelitis virus is more closely related to Sindbis virus than to others of the group, whereas the Semliki-Mayaro-Chikungunya triad bear a close serological relationship with O'nyong-nyong and Sagiyama viruses. Many other members of the alphaviruses are probably separate from each other and from the rest (Table 49.1).

Alphaviruses, formerly designated group A arboviruses of Casals and Brown, are small, spherical, single-stranded RNA viruses, having a molecular weight of about 3×10^6 daltons. Mature alphavirus particles are generally larger (40–80 nm in diameter) than those of the flaviviruses (20–50 nm in diameter). In negatively-stained preparations, the virion has a membrane or envelope, surrounding a central nucleoid, about 25–30 nm in diameter, containing several fine tubular structures. The capsid shows isometric, probably icosahedral symmetry, and consists of 32 ring-like morphological sub-units. In addition to the antigenic and morphological differences between the two main togavirus genera, alphaviruses are resistant to the action of trypsin and sulfhydryl agents, whereas flaviviruses are not. Moreover, all alphaviruses have been proved to multiply in arthropod vectors and are serologically related.

Western equine, Eastern equine and Venezuelan equine encephalomyelitis

Definition
These are destructive diseases of horses caused by 3 related but distinct alphaviruses which occur naturally in other species of animals and have been found as the causative agents of serious diseases of man.

History and distribution
The different forms of equine encephalomyelitis have been known for many years in the U.S.A., Southern Canada and in South America as far south as Argentina. The Venezuelan form is enzootic in parts of South America but outbreaks have occurred in Mexico and Florida.

The causative virus of Western equine encephalomyelitis was first isolated from horse brain in 1930 during a severe epizootic in California. During the next few years, the incidence of encephalitis increased sharply in the Western States and spread quickly eastwards to the Middle West until no fewer than 184 662 cases were reported in the single year 1938. In 1933, a second type of virus was isolated in the Eastern States of America from cases of encephalitis of man and horses, and was designated Eastern equine encephalomyelitis virus. Coincident with the disease in horses, both viruses were isolated from cases of encephalitis in man and, in 1941, at least 3000 human cases were reported with mortality rates ranging between 8 and 15 per cent. The viruses have spread widely among wild and domestic animals, including birds, and there are now many reservoir host populations in most endemic areas. In 1938, a milder form of equine encephalomyelitis was reported in horses in Venezuela, due to a third distinct serotype named Venezuelan equine encephalomyelitis virus.

Properties of the viruses

The viruses are typical of the alphavirus group, having spherical nucleocapsids measuring between 40–80 nm in diameter and containing single-stranded RNA. Haemagglutination of red blood cells occurs at pH 6.1. Equine encephalomyelitis viruses grow well and produce marked cytopathic effects in tissue cultures derived from chick embryo, mouse, hamster, monkey, guinea-pig and other species. They can be propagated readily in embryonated chicken eggs causing haemorrhages and deaths of the embryos in 24–48 hours. Every member of the equine encephalomyelitis triad shows cross-reactions in the haemagglutination-inhibition test with one or more viruses in the alphavirus group, but are readily separable from the others and from themselves by complement-fixation and virus neutralization tests. Cross-protection tests and a plaque-inhibition test in cultures of chick fibroblasts are particularly useful in revealing differences between the Western, Eastern and Venezuelan viruses. Thus, immune sera prepared from a single strain will contain strain-specific as well as group-specific antibodies.

Pathogenicity

The clinical features of established cases of Western and Eastern equine encephalomyelitis are indistinguishable. Affected horses show fever, somnolence, paralysis of the lips and pharynx and incoordination of movement. Deaths may occur in 3–8 days after the onset of clinical signs. Horses infected with the Venezuelan virus become ill but not necessarily with encephalomyelitis. The 3 diseases are, in fact, diphasic. In the first stage of typical encephalomyelitis, the virus multiplies in the viscera giving rise to viraemia between the 2nd–5th days of the illness, i.e., 2–3 days before the first signs of CNS involvement. In the second phase, the virus multiplies in the central nervous system and causes nerve cell degeneration in many parts of the brain and spinal cord. Affected areas show mononuclear infiltration with perivascular cuffing. In the Eastern and Western forms of the disease, the main lesions are to be found in the brain stem, whereas in Venezuelan equine encephalomyelitis, the virus is viscerotropic rather than neurotropic and gives rise to necrotic foci in the spleen and lymph nodes. Mortality rates in Eastern equine encephalomyelitis may be as high as 90 per cent in horses, and up to 80 per cent in human patients. In Western equine encephalomyelitis they are usually between 20–30 per cent. and 5–15 per cent, respectively, whereas in Venezuelan equine encephalomyelitis the mortality rates are generally low. Laboratory infections occur most readily with the Venezuelan virus and are probably acquired by inhalation.

Many species of laboratory animals are readily infected by various routes, but with older animals intracerebral inoculation is usually necessary. The virus of Eastern equine encephalomyelitis is generally more invasive than that of Western equine encephalomyelitis, but the virus of Venezuelan equine encephalomyelitis is more virulent for laboratory rodents than either of the other two. Some strains given intracerebrally will produce meningoencephalitis in sheep, pigs, dogs or cats but few will induce infection in cattle.

Immunity

Complement-fixing and neutralizing antibodies appear in the sera of recovered animals and immunity is permanent after a single infection.

Spread and transmission

The viruses of Eastern and Western equine encephalomyelitis spread naturally in birds and normally produce harmless and symptomless infections. The main primary vectors are species of culicine mosquitoes, some of which may transmit the infection incidentally to horses and man after an extrinsic incubation period of from 3–12 days. Virus may spread directly amongst pheasants, infecting the viscera rather than the CNS, and small rodents which are known to harbour the virus during the winter months carry the virus in the respiratory tract and kidneys. Affected horses may shed virus in their nasal secretions, urine and milk, and direct contact infection from horse to horse can occur.

Diagnosis

Equine encephalomyelitides are diagnosed in the laboratory by serological methods or by recovery and identification of the causative virus. Neutralizing and haemagglutination-inhibiting antibodies are detectable within a week of the onset of clinical signs and may persist for years, if not for life; whereas complement-fixing antibodies develop later and may be lost within a few months. The haemagglutination-inhibition test is a simple and reliable diagnostic procedure but it has the disadvantage that it recognises group rather than type characters. The degree of specificity of neutralizing, complement-fixing and haemagglutination-inhibiting antibodies for the virus type, decreases in that order. Paired sera are required for the serological tests, the first sample being taken as soon after the onset of the illness as possible and the second about 3 or 4 weeks later. Isolation of virus can be attempted from blood taken during the early viraemic phase of the illness, usually before clinical signs develop. In fatal cases, virus can usually be isolated from brain and spinal cord by the inoculation of unweaned mice or hamsters. Alternatively, embryonated eggs and tissue cultures may be employed.

Control

Formalised vaccines prepared from infected chick embryos have been used successfully to control equine encephalomyelitis. They have also proved useful for protecting laboratory workers exposed to infection, but are not available commercially.

FLAVIVIRUSES

Flaviviruses, formerly called the B group of arboviruses, constitute at least 30 strains which are delineated mainly on immunological grounds. All show some degree of serological cross-reaction by means of haemagglutination-inhibition and complement-fixation tests but none shows an antigenic overlap with arboviruses in other groups. The degree of antigenic cross-reactivity is much more marked in flaviviruses than in alphaviruses but differences revealed by type-specific complement-fixation and virus-neutralization tests suggest that the former contains 4 distinct classes of viruses plus an additional 17 strains that are less closely related to each other. The 4 main classes are (1) yellow fever and related viruses, (2) dengue viruses, (3) encephalitis viruses, such as St. Louis, Japanese B, West Nile and Murray Valley encephalitis viruses and (4) viruses of the tick-borne encephalitis complex (Table 49.1).

Most flaviviruses are transmitted by *Culicoides* but the 9 species in the tick-borne encephalitis complex are transmitted exclusively by ixodid ticks and are unable to multiply in mosquitoes. Others have no known invertebrate hosts. All have certain properties in common and several are pathogenic for man and domestic animals, giving rise to acute encephalitis and even death. Many strains produce fatal encephalitis after intracerebral inoculation of unweaned mice and most can be readily propagated in eggs and in various tissue cultures usually with the production of a cytopathic effect Haemagglutinins obtained from infected mouse brains or, to lower titre, in various tissue culture systems, agglutinate the red blood cells of geese and newly hatched chickens. The optimum conditions for this reaction are pH 6·4–6·8, and 4°C or 22°C. Flavivirus haemagglutinins are generally active over a much broader pH and temperature range than those of alphaviruses. Dilutions of virus for experimental purposes are best stored in 10 per cent. normal serum or in 0.75 per cent bovine serum albumin at –60°C to –70°C, or in the lyophilized state. Members of the flavivirus group are ether- and deoxycholate-sensitive, and treatment with formalin or β-propiolactone reduces infectivity without undue loss of antigenicity.

Neutralizing and haemagglutination-inhibiting antibodies usually appear in animals about a week after infection and persist for many years, whereas complement-fixing antibodies appear after 2–4 weeks and persist usually for 1–3 years. Although the encephalitis group of flaviviruses such as St. Louis encephalitis can cause serious illnesses in man, they are rarely held to be responsible for clinical disease in domestic animals. Nevertheless, some strains, e.g. Japanese B virus gives rise to mild or inapparent infections in horses, sheep, goats, pigs and birds. On the other hand, most of the members of the tick-borne encephalitis complex are responsible for several serious diseases of veterinary and public health importance.

Yellow fever

Definition
Yellow fever is an enzootic virus infection occurring in the jungles and forests of tropical Africa and South America, with man as an incidental host.

Virus properties
The causative virus is the type species of the flavivirus group of togaviruses (*vide supra*).

Yellow fever virus multiplies in a variety of laboratory animals including monkeys, mice and guinea-pigs. Unweaned mice develop encephalitis following subcutaneous and intraperitoneal inoculation. It is readily cultivated in various cell culture systems and many isolates produce a cytopathic effect. Embryonated hens' eggs can be infected by chorioallantoic and yolk sac inoculation, usually only after adaptation of the virus to mice or cell cultures. All strains belong to one antigenic type and most haemagglutinate erythrocytes from day-old chicks or geese.

Pathogenicity
Yellow fever varies in its clinical features from a symptomless or mild feverish influenza-like disease, through a range of increasing degrees of severity to a fulminating and fatal infection. The overall mortality rate in clinically diagnosed cases is usually between 5 and 10 per cent. The incubation period in natural infections is 3 to 6 days.

In typical cases of classical yellow fever there is an acute onset with rapidly rising fever, shivering, headache and backache. Within 3 or 4 days, the patient becomes extremely ill, shows a jaundiced appearance and is likely to vomit. The vomitus may appear black as the result of the presence of altered blood. The mortality rate in this form of the disease is very high and death ensues 6 to 8 days after the patient becomes ill.

The principal findings at necropsy include profound jaundice, albuminuria, gastro-intestinal haemorrhage and severe mid-zonal necrosis of the

TABLE 49.1.   A list of togaviruses and unclassified arboviruses and their world distribution.

Alphaviruses:	Eastern equine encephalomyelitis	(Americas)
(20 members)	Venezuelan equine encephalomyelitis	(Americas)
	Western equine encephalomyelitis	(Americas)
	Sindbis	(Africa & India)
	Semliki Forest disease	(Africa)
	Mayaro	(Americas)
	Chikungunya	(Africa: S.E. Asia)
	O'nyong-nyong	(Uganda)
	Sagiyama	(Japan)
	Ross River	(Australia)
	Uruma	(Americas)
	Middleburg	(S. Africa)
	etc., etc.	
Flaviviruses:	Japanese encephalitis	(S.E. Asia)
(36 members)	St. Louis encephalitis	(America)
	Murray Valley fever	(Australia)
	West Nile fever	(Africa, India, France)
	Brazilian Bussuguara virus	(Americas)
	Bat salivary gland virus (U.S.)	(America)
	Dengue	(S.E. Asia, etc.)
	Yellow fever	(Africa & America)
	Uganda S	(Africa)
	Zika	(Africa)
	Ntaya	(Africa)
	Ilheus	(Americas)
	etc., etc.	
Tick-borne flaviviruses:	Far Eastern Russian encephalitis and Russian Spring-Summer enceph. (Eastern)	(U.S.S.R.)
	Central European TBF (RSSE-Western)	(Europe)
	Louping-ill	(UK & Europe)
	Negishi	(Japan)
	Omsk haemorrhagic fever	(U.S.S.R.)
	Kyasanur forest disease	(India)
	Powassan	(America)
	Langat	(Malaya)
Other flaviviruses:	Modoc	(Americas)
	Spondweni	(Africa)
	Wesselsbron	(Africa)
	Turkey meningo-encephalitis	(Israel)
	etc., etc.	

Other arboviruses:		
Group C.	(11 members)	
Bunyamwera group	(15 members)	
Phlebotomus (Sandfly fever) group	(10 members)	
Californian group	(11 members)	
Miscellaneous group	(16 small groups)	
Singleton or unrelated group:–	(52 viruses)	
Includes Rift Valley fever		(Africa)
Nairobi Sheep Disease		(Africa)

liver parenchyma. The contents of necrotic parenchymal cells fuse together to form irregular masses of acidophilic hyaline material called Councilman bodies. Granular acidophilic intranuclear inclusions (Torres bodies) are commonly found surrounding the nucleoli and their presence is of diagnostic value.

Neutralizing antibodies are present in human sera from the fifth day onwards, and haemagglutinin-inhibiting antibodies also develop rapidly in most cases. Complement-fixing antibodies are rarely found after mild infection or vaccination, but they appear later than the neutralizing antibodies in more severe infections, and disappear within a matter of months rather than years.

Ecology

Yellow fever is primarily an enzootic disease of monkeys and perhaps some other forest animals, and is transmitted from one host to another by various species of mosquitoes. It is only when man is bitten by these infected arthropods that he contracts the disease. Although the urban form of yellow fever has been brought under control in most areas by the eradication of *Aëdes aegypti* and the widespread use of vaccine, the infection still persists in jungles and forests of tropical Africa and South America. In African forests certain *Colobus* and *Cercopithecus* monkeys are involved and the vectors are principally *Aëdes africanus* and *A. simpsoni*, whereas in South America *Alouatta* (howler monkey) and *Ateles* (spider monkey) play the leading role, together with *Haemagogus* mosquitoes. The virus multiplies in mosquitoes, which are then infected for life, although no evidence of transovarial transmission of the virus has been found. There is an extrinsic incubation period of about 12 to 14 days before the arthropod can transmit the virus.

Control
A live virus vaccine developed in the U.S.A. in 1937 has been widely used for the protection of human beings. It is prepared in embryonated hens' eggs using a strain of yellow fever virus (17D) already partly attenuated by passage in mice and cell cultures. It is administered by subcutaneous inoculation and confers solid, long-lasting immunity. A booster dose is generally required 7 to 10 years after primary vaccination.

Japanese B encephalitis

Synonyms
Japanese B; Japanese encephalitis; Russian autumn encephalitis; summer encephalitis in man; infectious encephalitis in domestic animals.

Definition
An acute, infectious arthropod-borne virus disease that affects both man and animals.

History
First recognised as an encephalitis of man in 1871 and of horses in 1899, in Japan. The causative virus was isolated in mice from human cases and from the brains of 2 fatal equine infections in 1935. Virus was identified in cattle, pigs and goats during extensive epidemics in man and horses in 1948 and 1949, respectively.

Distribution
Japanese B encephalitis occurs all over the Far East, from Siberia to Malaya and South-east India.

Properties of the virus
The virus is a typical flavivirus. It contains a large amount of lipid and is sensitive to ether and deoxycholate. Most strains agglutinate red blood cells of geese, pigeons and newly-hatched chickens and the reaction is optimal at pH 6·5–6·8. Old laboratory strains may lose their agglutinins. The virus can be stored for at least 8 years at –70°C but is inactivated at 56°C after 30 minutes.

Japanese B virus has a wide natural host range and can infect a variety of laboratory animals. Experimentally infected monkeys, hamsters, guinea-pigs, rabbits and chickens usually show inapparent infections with viraemia. Young mice are particularly susceptible and most strains of virus produce encephalitis and deaths after intracerebral inoculation. The virus grows readily in various cell culture systems, sometimes without destructive effects, but most strains can be adapted to produce marked cytopathic changes, including plaques, on monolayers of chick fibroblasts and established lines of baby hamster and pig kidney cells. Growth also occurs in fertile eggs, and embryonic deaths following yolk sac inoculation are used as a basis for titration.

Antigenicity
There is some antigenic overlapping with other flaviviruses such as Murray Valley fever, St. Louis encephalitis and West Nile viruses; and minor antigenic differences exist between some of the Japanese B strains. Antigenic modifications have been described following serial passage through mice.

Virus neutralizing, complement-fixing and haemagglutination-inhibiting antibodies are produced in the host serum after infection. Neutralizing and haemagglutination-inhibiting antibodies appear within 7–14 days and may persist for many years, but complement-fixing antibodies appear much later and disappear sooner.

Pathogenicity
In mild infections of horses, there is fever and loss of appetite but most animals recover completely within a few days. Several cases in horses are characterized by encephalomyelitis, following an initial febrile phase. Clinical signs include restlessness and excitability, disturbances of vision, paralysis of the facial and ocular muscles with drooping of the lips and ears, difficulties in mastication and swallowing, and paralysis of the hind quarters. Deaths may occur 3–7 days after the onset of fever and in severe outbreaks mortality rates may be as high as 40–70 per cent.

Lesions in the brain may resemble those of other togavirus encephalitides but many cases show no definite changes other than oedema, congestion and small haemorrhages or, occasionally, an increase in the amount of cerebrospinal fluid.

There are reports that the virus can cause abortions in pigs. However, infected sows do not show clinical symptoms of disease during pregnancy or after parturition, and most give birth to healthy piglets at subsequent farrowings.

Ecology
Japanese B virus is probably a parasite primarily of wild birds, and many avian species (but especially those of the heron family) may play an important role in disseminating the virus. Night herons usually have a high incidence of antibodies in their serum and it is possible that they harbour the virus and, as reservoir hosts, provide the arthropod vector with a source of infection. The main vectors are culicine mosquitoes. Apart from herons and other species of wild birds, hibernating mosquitoes, bats and domestic pigs which are regularly infected, may maintain the virus in a secondary role. Man, horses and other species are only infected incidentally.

Diagnosis
In severe epizootics, Japanese B encephalitis can usually be diagnosed by the clinical symptoms and histological findings. However, these are by no means specific and a provisional diagnosis can only be confirmed by isolation of the virus in unweaned mice or other susceptible host systems. Isolates are identified by virus neutralization, complement-fixation and haemagglutination-inhibition tests; but in areas where other flavivirus infections exist detailed serological differentiation may be necessary.

Control
For prophylactic purposes, formalised mouse-brain or chicken embryo vaccines have been used successfully in horses and pigs. Vaccines have also been prepared from cultures in hamster and pig kidney cells. In man, attempts are being made to vaccinate individuals first with an avirulent flavivirus, e.g. West Nile, followed by a 'booster' dose of inactivated Japanese B virus.

Murray Valley encephalitis
Murray Valley encephalitis or Australian X-disease is widely distributed in Northern and Eastern territories of Australia, as well as in Papua and New Guinea. It is a serious illness of man and causes high mortality, particularly in young children.

The clinical picture is not distinctive but the pathological lesions closely resemble those of Japanese B encephalitis. Horses and other animals may become infected but do not show clinical signs of illness.

Murray Valley encephalitis virus is a member of the flavivirus group of togaviruses containing St. Louis, West Nile, Ilheus, Kunjin and Japanese B viruses; and haemagglutinin-inhibition tests suggest that it is more closely related to the last than to the others. It can be isolated from the central nervous system of fatal cases by inoculation of the chorioallantoic membrane of 10- to 11-day-old fertile hens' eggs, with the production of pocks and deaths of the embryos. It causes fatal encephalitis when inoculated intracerebrally in mice, hamsters, sheep and monkeys and, in contrast to Japanese B virus, it infects hamsters when injected by peripheral routes. The virus multiplies in various species of mosquitoes, but the most important vector is probably *Culex annulirostris*.

Complement-fixing, neutralizing and haemagglutinin-inhibiting antibodies appear in the sera of patients during the course of the disease, and their presence is of diagnostic value. Surveys carried out in Australia show that horses and other animals, including domestic and free-living birds, frequently have antibodies to Murray Valley encephalitis in their sera; and the presence of inapparent infections in these hosts is a potential danger to the human population in endemic areas.

TICK-BORNE ENCEPHALITIS COMPLEX

Flaviviruses include a small sub-group of some 8 or 9 members that are very closely related antigenically and are transmitted by ticks. These include Central European, Russian spring-summer and Far Eastern Russian encephalitis, Louping-ill, Omsk haemorrhagic fever, Kyasanur forest disease, Negishi, Powassan and Langat viruses. Of these, Russian spring-summer and Far Eastern Russian encephalitis are so similar antigenically as to be indistinguishable, for all practical purposes. Moreover, both are closely related to louping-ill and Negishi viruses and, to a lesser degree, to Omsk haemorrhagic fever and Kyasanur forest disease. In general, the tick-borne encephalitis group of flaviviruses can only be differentiated from each other with difficulty.

Members of the group are widely distributed throughout the northern hemisphere but some occur outwith the temperate zones. Most are responsible for infections of birds and mammals that are characterized in human and animal incidental hosts by fever and encephalitis.

General properties
The properties of the tick-borne flaviviruses are similar to those of other members of the group. All are capable of haemagglutinating red blood cells of geese, especially ganders, and of day-old chicks. They grow readily in embryonated hens' eggs by yolk sac inoculation, and some produce discrete pocks on infected chorioallantoic membranes. They can also be propagated on a variety of tissue culture systems, including stable cell lines, usually with

marked cytopathic effects. Young mice inoculated intracerebrally are particularly susceptible, and all but Omsk haemorrhagic fever virus will cause encephalitis and death. Most of them are pathogenic when inoculated into rhesus or cynomolgus monkeys by the intracerebral route.

Ecology

The viruses are normally transmitted by ticks and, as transovarial transmission has been definitively established, it is probable that ticks can also act as permanent reservoirs of the infection. In temperate zones, ticks are most active in the spring and early summer months of the year when the tick-borne diseases are most prevalent, but in tropical climates the highest incidence occurs during the dry season when the tick activity is greatest.

Louping-ill

Synonyms

Ovine encephalomyelitis: Infectious encephalomyelitis of sheep: Acute viral encephalitis of sheep: Trembling-ill: Spring-krankheit (Ger.).

Definition

An infectious, tick-borne, viral encephalomyelitis of sheep and cattle that is characterised chiefly by cerebellar ataxia. The word 'louping' is derived from an old Norse word meaning to leap, and refers to the peculiar gait of affected animals.

Hosts affected

Sheep are mostly affected but the disease can occasionally occur in dogs and cattle. Human infections have been reported among laboratory workers, butchers, veterinary surgeons, sheep farmers and shepherds.

History and distribution

Louping-ill of sheep has been recognised for nearly 2 centuries in Scotland. It was first transmitted experimentally to sheep in 1929 by inoculation, and by the bites of infected ticks. This latter experiment may be the first recorded transmission of a neurotropic virus disease by an arthropod vector. Louping-ill is prevalent in certain areas of Scotland, England, Wales and Ireland, as well as in Czechoslovakia and parts of West and East Russia. It occurs in early spring, commonly on farms where there is rough hill grazing, and is spread by the tick *Ixodes ricinus*.

Properties of the virus

The virus is a member of the tickborne encephalitis complex of the group B arboviruses or flaviviruses, and its properties are similar to those of other mem-

bers of the group. It retains its viability in 50 per cent glycerol-saline at room-temperature for at least 3 months, and in infected brain and spinal cord for several years at −70°C, but it may not survive for 14 days at 4°C. It is inactivated in 5 minutes at 60°C and within a few hours by 2 per cent phenol or 1 per cent formalin. A solution of 0·25 per cent formalin for 4 days at 4°C is sufficient to inactivate virus in tissue suspensions used for the production of vaccines.

Haemagglutination

A haemagglutinin is produced which agglutinates red blood cells of geese (ganders) and newly-hatched chicks.

Antigenic properties

Haemagglutination-inhibition tests show crossing with other flaviviruses and especially with other members of the tick-borne encephalitis complex. In particular, louping-ill is closely related to the Central European type of virus, whereas its relationship with Powassan and Langat viruses is more distant.

Cultivation

Louping-ill virus can be readily propagated in fertile hens' eggs, whether on the chorioallantoic membrane, where discrete pocks appear, or by the yolk-sac route. Growth also occurs in various primary and secondary tissue culture systems derived from primate, bovine, and sheep tissues, and in HeLa and other continuous cell lines. Pig kidney cultures are especially suitable and plaque production has been described on chicken tissues. Most isolates produce a marked cytopathic effect in susceptible monolayer culture. (Plate 49.2c, facing p. 651).

Pathogenicity

In sheep exposed to natural infection, a period of 6–18 days may elapse before the appearance of the first clinical symptoms. The disease has 2 phases, the first of which is characterized by fever, up to 42°C, and viraemia. In uncomplicated cases, the temperature falls within a day or two and the animal appears healthier. About 5 days later a second temperature rise occurs, the virus invades the CNS, and this is accompanied by inco-ordination and ataxia followed by progressive paralysis, coma and death, depending on the severity and location of the damage to the nerve cells. In some cases, the second phase of the illness may be absent and affected sheep recover after an almost symptomless illness. The most common signs of louping-ill in sheep are trembling of the head and limbs, ataxic movements with incoordination of gait and paresis. Recovered animals are solidly immune but those that develop nervous signs frequently die or, if they survive, show permanent sequelae in the form of torticollis and impairment of movement, usually of the hind limbs. The impaired locomotion and peculiar leaping gait gave rise to the colloquial name 'Louping-ill'.

The clinical signs in cattle are similar to those in sheep. Affected animals develop muscular twitching, ataxia and show the characteristic louping-ill gait with the fore-legs lifted high and the head tilted backwards. In man, louping-ill is a rare disease which takes the form usually of a diphasic influenza-like illness associated with serous meningitis and encephalitis, and eventual recovery. Compared with the Russian types of tick-borne encephalitis viruses, the louping-ill virus shows a decreased pathogenicity for man.

Louping-ill has a wide host range and, apart from sheep (and occasionally man), natural infection may occur in cattle, horses, deer, dogs, the common shrew, the woodmouse and the red grouse but usually without showing clinical signs of the disease. Mice, of all ages, and young mice in particular, are susceptible to the virus given by the intracerebral route, but adult mice are less readily infected when inoculated subcutaneously, intraperitoneally, intranasally or intraocularly. Adult rats inoculated intranasally may develop an inapparent infection. Many other species, including cattle, sheep, goats and pigs can be infected intracerebrally but rabbits and guinea-pigs are resistant. In experimentally infected monkeys there is usually cerebellar ataxia and tremors without paralysis.

Pathological lesions

There are no gross abnormalities at autopsy. Microscopically, there is a non-suppurative meningo-encephalomyelitis with severe damage to the Purkinje cells, the motor nuclei, the vestibular nuclei and the ventral horns, together with perivascular cuffing, neuronophagia and glial proliferation. (Plate 49.2a, facing p. 651.)

Ecology

The vector of louping-ill is the tick *Ixodes ricinus* which may also act as the reservoir of infection. Transovarial infection has been reported and tick larvae and nymphs may acquire the virus and transmit it to susceptible sheep at their next instar. Infected larvae also carry the virus to the adult stage. Thus, the incidence of the disease is seasonal and is related to the periods of maximum tick activity, i.e. in April, May and early June and again, perhaps, in September.

Virus isolation and antibody studies suggest that the virus may also be maintained in nature by certain mammals including red deer, hares, other rodents and, perhaps, by ground-living birds such as red grouse; but sheep may also serve as amplifying hosts.

Man and other animals may become infected by tick-bite but laboratory workers usually acquire the infection by the conjunctival or respiratory routes.

Diagnosis

Naturally occurring cases of louping-ill cannot readily be diagnosed on the basis of clinical signs only. For confirmatory diagnosis, attempts should be made to isolate the virus from freshly obtained brain or spinal cord during the latter stages of the illness. Suspect material may be inoculated intracerebrally into young mice or on pig kidney cultures and other susceptible cell systems. Identification of the virus is obtained by neutralization and other serological tests. Wherever possible, acute and convalescent phase sera should be obtained and examined for the presence of rising antibody titres. The serum neutralization or haemagglutination-inhibition tests are preferred for the diagnosis of louping-ill since complement-fixing antibodies appear in 2–6 weeks and may persist for only 3–4 weeks, whereas only half of the animals showing neutralizing or haemagglutination-inhibiting antibodies may have detectable levels of complement-fixing antibodies at the same time. Furthermore, neutralizing and haemagglutination-inhibiting antibodies appear sooner and persist for 6 months or longer in recovered animals. The former are usually identified by the intracerebral inoculation of mice or by means of susceptible cell culture systems.

Control

For many years, the use of formalised infected sheep brain, spinal cord and spleen vaccines successfully reduced the incidence of louping-ill in both sheep and cattle. In enzootic areas all sheep under one year of age were vaccinated before the tick season began in the early spring, as were all adult sheep and cattle newly introduced into an infected area. Lambs acquired a passive immunity from their dams and were not vaccinated under 4 months of age. Egg-adapted virus vaccines have also been used but these were subsequently withdrawn because of the danger to staff engaged in their manufacture. More recently, sheep kidney cell culture fluids precipitated with methanol or acetone have been developed and preliminary observations indicate that the serological response is equal to that which results from natural infection.

Wesselsbron disease

Definition

A mild but sometimes acute febrile arthropod-borne

disease giving rise to abortions among sheep and deaths of newborn lambs and pregnant ewes.

Hosts affected
Outbreaks are mostly confined to lambs and ewes in advanced stages of pregnancy, but abortions may occasionally occur in cattle. Inapparent infections frequently occur in horses, cattle and pigs. An influenza-like disease is produced in man, and laboratory workers are commonly infected.

History and distribution
The disease was first reported in the late summer of 1954 in Merino sheep in the Wesselsbron area of the Orange Free State, South Africa. It is probably enzootic in certain areas of South Africa, Rhodesia and Mozambique.

Properties of the virus
The causative virus contains RNA and is about 30 nm in diameter. It is antigenically related to the flaviviruses but is not particularly closely related to any other togavirus. It can be propagated readily in embryonated chicken eggs by the yolk-sac route, but the mortality rate is low and irregular. It grows in cell cultures of lamb kidney and produces intracytoplasmic inclusion bodies.

Pathogenicity
In naturally occurring cases, a short incubation period of 24–72 hours is followed by a febrile reaction which generally lasts for 2–3 days. Affected newborn lambs show symptoms of weakness, loss of appetite, encephalitis and lethargy, with death in 3–4 days. The mortality rates in lambs and pregnant ewes may be as high as 20–30 per cent. Jaundice is a characteristic feature of the disease in sheep.

The most striking lesions on post-mortem examination are those of diffuse necrosis and fatty infiltration of the liver. The gall-bladder is enlarged, blood-streaked and almost black in colour. In lambs, the spleen may be enlarged and the liver has a golden-yellow appearance; but in pregnant ewes, the liver is pale and resembles the changes seen in cases of pregnancy toxaemia.

The virus has a wide host range and many different species of animals, including laboratory animals, can be infected. Most strains of virus are pantropic with neurotropic tendencies and have a predilection for mammalian embryonic tissues. In experimental infections, pregnant ewes abort and lambs may die, but only a mild fever is produced in cattle, horses, pigs and non-pregnant sheep. Unweaned mice are highly susceptible to intraperitoneal, intracerebral and intramuscular inoculation, and usually die within 48 hours. Deaths may be induced in adult mice also, but only after intracerebral injection.

Experimentally infected guinea-pigs and rabbits show no clinical symptoms but pregnant animals abort or give birth to young which die within a few days.

Transmission
Wesselsbron virus is transmitted by mosquito-bite, the 2 important vectors being *Aëdes caballus* and *Aëdes circumluteolus*.

Diagnosis
Field cases of Wesselsbron disease cannot readily be diagnosed because the clinical symptoms and pathological features are very similar to those of Rift Valley fever which frequently occurs in the same locality. However, cross-serum neutralization tests and complement-fixation tests show that the causative viruses of Wesselsbron disease and Rift Valley fever are antigenically distinct from one another.

Confirmation of the diagnosis usually depends on the isolation and identification of the virus. For this purpose, lamb kidney cell cultures or unweaned mice are inoculated with serum collected at the height of fever, but liver and brain from aborted fetuses or liver and spleen from lambs which have died of the disease are also suitable sources of the virus. The isolates are identified by serum neutralization, complement-fixation and haemagglutination-inhibition tests.

Control
A freeze-dried vaccine prepared from the brain of infant mice injected with a neurotropic mouse-adapted strain of virus has been used successfully to control Wesselsbron disease. The immunity following natural recovery or vaccination is usually life-long.

UNCLASSIFIED 'ARBOVIRUSES'

Rift Valley fever

Synonym
Enzootic hepatitis.

Definition
Rift Valley fever is an acute, mild or sometimes inapparent infectious virus disease of sheep, cattle and other animals that is characterised by high abortion rates amongst pregnant ewes and cows and heavy mortality in young lambs and calves. The disease is arthropod-borne and normally runs a rapid course after a short incubation period.

Hosts affected
Rift Valley fever is primarily pathogenic for sheep

and other domestic animals such as goats and cattle, but certain wild rodents may also be affected. Horses and pigs are not susceptible. Man is secondarily infected by direct contact during the course of epizootics in the field, and infection among laboratory workers is common.

History and distribution
The disease was first described in Kenya in 1912 and the causative virus was identified in 1931 during investigations of an extremely virulent epizootic in young lambs and adult sheep on the shores of Lake Naivasha in the Rift Valley of Kenya. The losses in young lambs were considerable and there were about 200 human cases reported at this time. The first known epizootic of Rift Valley fever in South Africa was reported in 1950–51. It now seems that the disease is widespread in the Sudan and many parts of East and Equatorial Africa, occurring in a mild or inapparent form, causing only sporadic abortion in susceptible species.

Morphology
The spherical, mature virions of Rift Valley fever virus contain single-stranded RNA and measure 60–75 nm in diameter. The surface of the particle is covered with hollow cylinders looking like short spikes. Recent reports indicate that the size of the virion varies following serial passage in eggs and mice, and spheres 94 nm across with a 77 nm core surrounded by a distinct membrane have been observed in mouse tissues. There is also evidence of a translucent layer, 8 nm wide, between the core and capsid-like outer layer. These discrepancies in size may be due to the presence of the outer ring of hollow cylinders which sometimes appears to be detached from the more obvious dense central core of the virion.

Physicochemical characters
The virus survives well when frozen or lyophilized. In some circumstances it appears to be more stable than other 'arboviruses' since infective virus has been found to persist at –4°C in serum for 3 years and at room temperature for 3 months. It is pH-, ether- and deoxycholate-sensitive, is inactivated after 40 minutes at 56°C and by 1/1000 formalin, but withstands 0.5 per cent phenol for 6 months.

Haemagglutination
Red blood cells of newly hatched chickens are agglutinated, optimally at pH 6.5 and 25°C. The haemagglutinin will also act on mouse, guinea-pig and human Group A cells.

Antigenic properties
Although it is immunologically distinct from alpha-

and flaviviruses, and is more stable than most typical members of the group, the Rift Valley fever virus is regarded as a candidate for inclusion in the family *Togaviridae*, genus *Hylovirus*. Complement-fixation, agar gel diffusion, haemagglutination-inhibition and neutralization tests have all been used successfully for characterization of the virus. There is only one immunological type.

Cultivation
The virus grows readily in embryonated hens' eggs when inoculated via the yolk sac and chorioallantoic membrane routes. By the latter method there is thickening of the membrane but no macroscopic pocks. The virus, which is generally of a pantropic character with a high affinity for hepatic and renal parenchymal cells, may become neurotropic during serial intracerebral passage in mice or serial yolk sac passage in fertile eggs. The passaged virus is attenuated for sheep but not for man. It can be propagated readily in cell cultures of chicken, rat, mouse, hamster and other species. Infected lamb kidney cells contain multiple acidophilic intranuclear inclusions.

Pathogenicity
Rift Valley fever is a disease of sheep, goats and cattle causing abortions and, sometimes, high mortality in pregnant and new-born animals. African buffalo, antelopes, camels and humans are known to have contracted the natural infection. The incubation period in sheep and cattle is from 4–6 days but is very much shorter in experimentally infected animals. In the peracute form of the disease, new-born lambs may die without showing clinical symptoms, while young lambs of a few days old may collapse and die within 36 hours after infection. In such cases, the mortality rate may reach 90 per cent. The acute form is usually encountered in young stock but mild symptoms are shown in adult sheep, goats and cattle. Pregnant ruminants usually abort. Sick animals, particularly cattle, may show fever, anorexia, vomiting, greenish mucopurulent nasal discharge, profuse salivation, general weakness and haemorrhagic diarrhoea. The mortality rate in adult cattle seldom exceeds 10 per cent although it may be much higher in calves. In man, the incubation period is about a week but the disease is rarely fatal and the clinical features are similar to those of dengue fever with sudden onset followed by pyrexia, prostration, severe pain in the extremities and joints, tenderness of the abdomen and gastro-intestinal distress. There is also marked leukopenia but convalescence is short and recovery is generally complete. In South Africa, cases of retinitis with detachment of the retina have occasionally been reported.

Laboratory animals, including puppies, kittens,

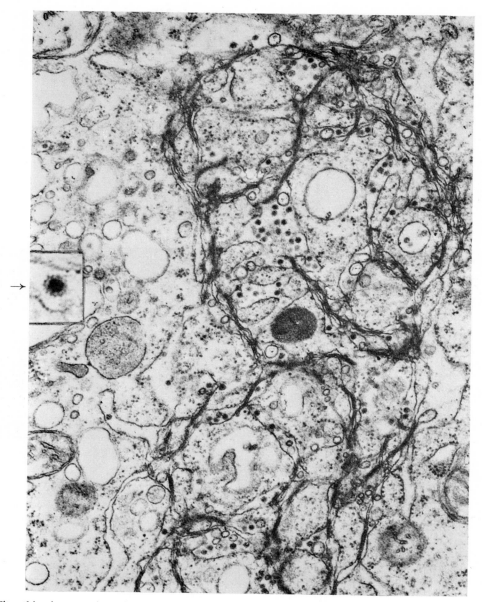

49.1　Ultra-thin tissue section of mouse cerebellum showing louping-ill virus in the cytoplasm of a Purkinje cell, ×45 000.

Inset (arrow): Louping-ill virus particle, ×180 000. (Courtesy of Mr W. Smith.)

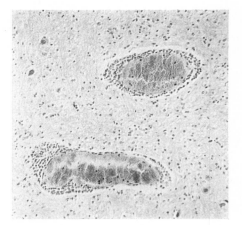

49.2a

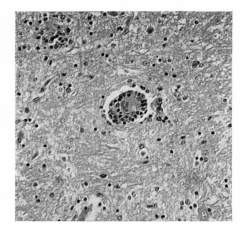

49.2b

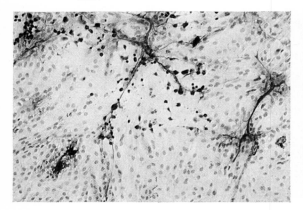

49.2c

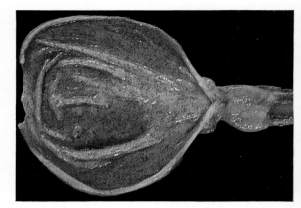

49.2d

49.2a Section of brain (medulla) from fatal case of louping-ill in a sheep, showing marked perivascular cuffing. Pyrrol blue eosin stain, × 100.

49.2c Early cytopathic effect of louping-ill virus on a primary culture of sheep kidney cells. Haematoxylin eosin stain, × 70.

49.2b Section of brain from a pig dying from swine fever. The presence of vasculo-endothelial proliferation is of diagnostic importance since swine fever is probably the only viral encephalomyelitis of pigs in which this type of lesion occurs. Haematoxylin eosin stain, × 170.

49.2d Petechial haemorrhages on the bladder wall of a piglet dying from acute swine fever. (Courtesy of Mr I. S. Beattie.)

rats, mice and hamsters, can be infected by various routes and they mostly die with hepatitis after 36–72 hours. Ferrets infected intranasally develop fever and lung consolidation, and infected guinea-pigs may abort. Horses, pigs, rabbits and birds are not susceptible.

Immunity
Complement-fixing, neutralizing and haemagglutination-inhibiting antibodies develop during convalescence and persist for many years.

Pathological lesions
In lambs, as in other animals, the primary lesion is a focal necrotic hepatitis. Affected animals show characteristic macroscopic liver lesions in the form of small white foci about 1·0 mm in diameter evenly distributed throughout the tissues. This granular appearance is more pronounced in young lambs, kids and calves than in adult animals. There may also be oedema and emphysema of the lungs, subserous petechiae and enlargement of the spleen. Acidophilic intranuclear inclusions (Daubney-Hudson-Garnham bodies) that resemble the Councilman bodies of yellow fever are present in affected livers. Blood lakes are also seen in the liver, and degenerative changes and perivascular cuffing may be present in the brain.

Spread and transmission
Transmission in the field is usually by mosquitoes and it appears that a variety of species can act as vectors. It is also possible that co-habitation between affected and susceptible animals may result in transmission and there is some evidence that carnivores may pick up the infection by ingestion. Intrauterine transmission is common. In Africa, forest rats and other wild animals may act as reservoir hosts. In man, Rift Valley fever is an occupational disease and numerous infections have resulted after contact with infected carcase material.

Diagnosis
Rift Valley fever should be suspected when there is a history of deaths among young lambs and abortion among adult sheep and cattle, especially when such an outbreak is associated with illness in people handling infected animals and carcases. Diagnosis is not always easy to obtain but the virus can be isolated by means of biological tests on susceptible ruminants and laboratory animals, e.g. mice and hamsters, which are susceptible at all ages to challenge by intracerebral and intraperitoneal inoculation. Confirmation of the diagnosis can be obtained by histological examination of the liver and by serum neutralization tests. Complement-fixation tests, using acetone-ether extracted antigen against standard antisera, are of diagnostic value, as are agar gel diffusion tests with unknown tissue suspensions. The disease must be differentiated from Wesselsbron disease, bluetongue, Nairobi sheep disease and heartwater fever.

Control
Control involves the protection of flocks and herds from infected mosquitoes, together with restrictions of movement in enzootic areas. Immunization has given satisfactory results and useful vaccines have been prepared from virus strains attenuated by serial passage in mice and embryonated eggs. Live neurotropic mouse-adapted virus vaccines have been used successfully on a large scale to immunize sheep but they should not be given to pregnant animals. Young lambs and kids may possess a passive immunity which persists for 3–6 months and they will not respond well to immunization during this period. Since the vaccination of males may result in a temporary sterility the immunization programme is usually planned for the Spring, a month before mating. Annual vaccination is recommended.

A formalised vaccine, which has been prepared from the pantropic virus grown in monkey tissue culture, has been used in man. It is safe to use, produces a good neutralizing-antibody response and an immunity which lasts for at least 18 months.

Nairobi sheep disease

Synonym
Congo Kisenyi sheep disease.

Definition
An acute, infectious disease of sheep characterised by a marked febrile reaction followed by severe haemorrhagic gastroenteritis.

Hosts affected
The natural hosts are sheep and goats. Cattle and other domestic animals are not susceptible.

History and distribution
Nairobi sheep disease was first reported in 1910 as a highly fatal infection of sheep in the Kikuyu country between Nairobi and Mount Kenya in East Africa. In recent years, it has been recognised in Uganda, Zaire, Mozambique, Lesotho and parts of South Africa.

Properties of the virus
It is generally agreed that the causative agent is a member of the 'arbovirus group' but it differs from all other viruses in neutralization tests. An early report that it is related immunologically to a number of group B arboviruses (flaviviruses) has not been

confirmed and it is presently ungrouped in the classification of Casals and Brown. (Table 49.1).

Electron micrographs of thin sections of baby hamster kidney cells infected with Nairobi sheep disease show aggregations of spherical and elongated virus particles within cytoplasmic vacuoles. The spherical particles measure about 70 nm in diameter while the elongated forms are about 60 nm in width and up to 500 nm in length. Particles, irrespective of their shape, consist of an electron dense nucleoid surrounded by a narrow zone of lesser density and an electron-dense outer layer. The nucleic acid core contains RNA.

The virus survives lyophilization and is resistant in infected blood or serum stored at 4°C. It withstands heating for an hour at 50°C but is inactivated after 5 minutes at 60°C. The virus is believed to survive for many months in the larval, nymph and adult forms of the tick *Rhipicephalus appendiculatus*.

The virus of Nairobi sheep disease cannot be propagated readily in embryonated hens' eggs but it grows well in cultures of lamb and goat tissues, and in a continuous line of hamster kidney cells. The cytopathic effect is associated with the presence of pleomorphic intracytoplasmic inclusions, some of which completely surround the nucleus.

Pathogenicity
The disease is essentially an ovine ailment but cases have occasionally been described in goats. The first sign of illness in sheep is an acute febrile reaction which appears about a week after exposure, and usually lasts for 7–9 days. The visible symptoms include mucopurulent nasal discharge, rapid and apparently painful respiration and haemorrhagic gastroenteritis. Affected sheep may show considerable pain and straining, and the evacuations are often discharged involuntarily In ewes, the vulva becomes swollen and congested and pregnant animals often abort. The mortality rate varies between 30–70 per cent, but severe epizootics may occur in fully susceptible sheep when up to 90 per cent may die within a month. Contrary to expectation, the mortality rate is lower in exogenous breeds of sheep.

At autopsy, the mucosa of the alimentary tract may be congested and haemorrhagic while the lymph nodes are generally enlarged and oedematous.

The disease is transmissible to laboratory animals and produces encephalitis and death in infant mice inoculated intracerebrally or intraperitoneally. Adult mice are only susceptible by the intracerebral route. Mouse adapted virus is attenuated for sheep and can be grown on chicken embryos.

Spread and transmission
As a result of Montgomery's report in 1917, Nairobi sheep disease is one of the first virus diseases of animals considered to be tick-transmitted. It is now known that several species of ticks are capable of spreading the disease, but the most efficient is undoubtedly *Rhipicephalus appendiculatus*. Pastures contaminated with infected ticks are considered to be a hazard for sheep for 18 months. The virus passes from the adult tick to the larval stage through the egg and all 3 stages of the tick (larval, nymphal and adult) can transmit the disease after becoming infected during a preceding instar. Since infected ticks can survive for 2 years without feeding, they act as complete reservoirs of the disease, but wild ruminants including the blue duiker (*Sylvicapra grimmi grimmi*) and certain rodents may be additional reservoir hosts.

The virus has not been isolated from the blood of recovering animals for more than 24 hours after the temperature reaction has subsided.

Diagnosis
The disease should be suspected from the clinical signs and the post-mortem lesions in sheep in enzootic areas where the vector *R. appendiculatus* is abundant. A confirmatory diagnosis can be obtained by the intracerebral inoculation of mice followed by serum neutralization tests in mice or cell cultures. Nairobi sheep disease may be confused with heartwater fever but the non-susceptibility of experimental cattle for Nairobi sheep disease virus, together with cross-immunity tests, should help to differentiate the two infections. The disease can be distinguished from Rift Valley fever by routine serological and virological methods and by the knowledge that Rift Valley fever virus has a wide host range.

Control
Recovered animals possess a solid long-lasting immunity and mouse attenuated virus is under trial as a vaccine.

NON-ARTHROPOD-BORNE TOGAVIRUSES

A number of unclassified viruses that have many characters in common with the togavirus family, but are not transmitted by insects, have been provisionally designated non-arthropod-borne or nonarbo-togaviruses. Candidates for inclusion in this recently proposed group include lactic dehydrogenase virus of mice and the causal agents of rubella (German measles) in man, bovine viral diarrhoea-mucosal disease, equine arteritis and swine fever (hog cholera).

Thus, the nonarbo-togaviruses are relatively small

($\leqslant$ 100 nm in diameter), isometric, enveloped particles whose genome nucleic acid consists of single-stranded RNA. The equine arteritis, lactic dehydrogenase and rubella viruses, together with most alphaviruses, show the greatest diameter (30–40 nm), whereas those of mucosal disease, swine fever and most members of the flavivirus group are slightly smaller (20–30 nm). With the exception of rubella, none of the nonarbo-togaviruses show hae-magglutinating activity; and it is of interest, therefore, that the rubella virion possesses surface projections similar to those of alpha- and flaviviruses, whereas equine arteritis, swine fever and other non-haemag-glutinating nonarbo-togaviruses have envelopes with a smooth surface.

An antigenic relationship between mucosal disease and swine fever has been repeatedly confirmed but, as yet, no relationship has been described among other members of the nonarbo-virus group. However, there is recent evidence from New Zealand, Australia, the U.K. and U.S.A. of a serological relationship between the causal agents of mucosal disease, swine fever [hog cholera] and border disease of lambs, and it is possible that the virus of border disease will be added to the list of candidate members for inclusion in the nonarbo-group of togaviruses.

Swine fever

Synonyms
Hog cholera; pestes porcine (Fr.); Schweinpest (Ger.).

Definition
A highly contagious viral disease of pigs character-ised in acute cases by sudden onset, marked haemorr-hages of the internal organs and high mortality.

Hosts affected
Swine are the only animals in which the disease is known to occur naturally, but the virus can be adapted to rabbits by alternating serial passage.

History and distribution
Swine fever was first described in Ohio, in 1833. It is probably indigenous to the U.S.A. and for many years was the most serious disease of pigs in both North and South America. An early claim that hog cholera was caused by *Salmonella choleraesuis* was refuted in 1903–04 when several workers clearly demonstrated that the causative agent was a 'filterable virus', and that the bacterium was only a secondary organism which caused non-specific changes in the tissues.

In Europe, swine fever was first observed in England in 1862 whence it appears to have been conveyed by breeding sows to Sweden in 1887 and then to Denmark later that year. Soon afterwards, outbreaks were recorded in France, Germany, Italy and Spain. Swine fever has been present in Africa since 1903, and has been reported in India, Australia, Japan and other parts of the Far East.

Morphology
Despite numerous attempts to define the virus morphologically, its ultrastructure has not yet been finally determined. At the present time, electron microscopy of negatively-stained preparations sug-gests that the virions are small spherical particles measuring about 40 nm in diameter with a core 20–30 nm across and a limiting membrane or envelope 6 nm thick. It has been suggested that the inner com-ponent consists of a tightly-wound filament of ribonucleoprotein, similar to that of myxoviruses, but more recent observations indicate that the nucleo-capsid possesses cubical (isometric) symmetry and closely resembles that of mucosal disease virus or equine arteritis virus.

Physicochemical characters
The virus is sensitive to ether and other lipid sol-vents, and is moderately sensitive to trypsin. It is a stable virus and virulent blood stored at 4°C will remain viable for a considerable period. Studies of its stability to pH change indicate that virus in defibrinated blood is more stable when held at pH 4·8–5·5 than at neutral pH. The virus is rapidly inactivated when dried in air under field conditions but when dried *in vacuo*, and stored in sealed glass ampoules, it may remain active at room temperature, or even at 37°C, for several years. Swine fever virus is relatively heat-stable and in defibrinated blood is only inactivated after 30 minutes at 69°C or 60 minutes at 66°C. It survives for 3 days at 50°C and for 7–14 days at 37°C. The virus keeps well in the cold when mixed with glycerol and there are reports that defibrinated infected blood preserved in 0·5 per cent phenol may retain its infectivity for 72–480 days when kept in cool surroundings.

Swine fever virus is very sensitive to putrefaction and loses infectivity within 3–4 days if the carcase is allowed to decompose, except in the bone marrow which may remain infectious for 15 days. On the other hand, the virus persists for long periods in infected pork and garbage, and in meat kept in cold storage. For example, the virus may survive in smoked ham for 1–2 weeks, in bacon for 4 weeks, in ham pickled in brine 5 weeks, in salted pork for 12 weeks and in frozen carcases for at least 4 years.

The virus is fairly resistant to most of the ordinary disinfectants and virulent serum is rendered inert only when exposed to the action of 5 per cent formalin for 2 hours. Five per cent cresol or 5 per cent sodium hydroxide (soda lye) destroys the virus in 1 hour but it is completely inactivated in 15 minutes by 5 per cent phenol or by a solution of hypochlorite containing 1·66 per cent available chlorine. Other chemicals have been used to inactivate the virus for use as a vaccine, the most successful being crystal violet in a final concentration of 1/2000.

Antigenic properties
Recovered pigs are permanently immune. There appears to be only one serological type of virus but a variant strain giving rise to 'break-downs' in the course of attempted immunization has been reported in the U.S.A. Although this strain is poorly neutralized by specific antisera, no distinct stable antigenic type has been confirmed, so far.

Agar gel diffusion tests reveal that swine fever virus has an antigenic component in common with mucosal disease virus of cattle.

Haemagglutination
Despite a report to the contrary, there is general agreement that all strains of swine fever virus do not agglutinate red blood cells.

Cultivation
For many years the only reliable method of propagating swine fever virus was by the inoculation of susceptible pigs. In 1959, however, the virus was adapted to growth in embryonic pig tissues embedded in chicken plasma, and in Maitland-type suspended cell cultures of minced pig spleen. Three years later, it was reported that a strain of virus of attenuated virulence would grow with a cytopathic effect on monolayer cultures of pig kidney cells and in embryonic skin-muscle cells. Since then, various cell culture systems derived from swine tissues have been used for primary isolations and for fundamental studies of the physical, chemical and biological properties of the virus. The tissues mostly used include kidney, spleen, bone-marrow, testicle, lymph-node and leucocytes. Although field strains of swine fever virus grow well in both primary and continuous cell cultures and can be readily demonstrated by immunofluorescence, there is usually no evidence of cytopathic effects, or only minimal ones, in the infected monolayers. However, in 1958, the interesting observation was made that the mild cytopathic effects of Newcastle disease virus on monolayers of pig testis cultures is enhanced by all strains of swine fever virus, and that the marked cellular degeneration that ensues is a reliable method for detecting the presence of swine fever virus in suspected swine tissues. For best results the suspected material is inoculated on to monolayer cultures of swine testis cells, incubated for 4–5 days at 37°C, superinfected with Newcastle disease virus, reincubated for a few more days and examined for marked cytopathic effects. A neutralization test for swine fever virus by means of this phenomenon of Enhancement of Newcastle Disease (END test) is based on the observation that swine fever immune serum specifically inhibits the exalting effects of swine fever virus on Newcastle disease virus. For this purpose, the serum-virus mixtures are incubated at 37°C for 60 minutes, or overnight at 4°C, and tested for infectivity by the END method.

Recently isolated strains of virus do not grow on embryonated hens' eggs but adaptation of the virus to duck embryos and to chick embryos has been reported. Replication of the virus in minced swine testicular tissue spread on the chorioallantoic membrane of the developing chicken embryo has been described.

Animals other than swine do not develop clinical symptoms of infection with swine fever virus, but several strains have been successfully grown by serial passage in cattle, sheep and goats with or without attenuation of the virus. Several groups of workers have shown that virus passaged directly through rabbits or by alternate passages between pigs and rabbits is modified and loses its virulence after 150–200 consecutive passages so that it can be used as a live attenuated virus-vaccine for pigs.

Pathogenicity
Domestic pigs of all breeds and ages, but especially young animals, are highly susceptible to swine fever. In a typical outbreak the first indication of the disease may be sudden death of an animal followed by illness in other pigs and fairly rapid spread to the rest of the herd. The incubation period varies considerably under different conditions but is usually from 3–8 days after natural exposure. The earliest signs of disease are dullness, listlessness and anorexia accompanied by a marked thermal response with temperatures usually around 41–42°C. The high temperature may persist until shortly before death when it falls suddenly to below normal. Most affected animals show an apparent weakness in the hindquarters which is manifested by an incoordination of movements and a staggering or swaying gait. In many cases there is conjunctivitis, vomiting and constipation, followed by diarrhoea. Red or purple haemorrhagic areas may appear on the skin of the abdomen or on the ears and snout, and there may be raised cutaneous necrotic areas. There is usually dyspnoea, bronchitis and coughing, while nervous symptoms resembling those of encephalomyelitis have also been described.

The course of the disease varies but is usually from 5–16 days although in extremely acute cases a number of pigs may be found dead in their sty overnight without having shown any signs of illness. Chronic cases may survive for 30 days or longer. The mortality rate is often extremely high and may be over 90 per cent. High mortality rates are usually associated with secondary bacterial infections of the lungs and intestines. In North America, the virus strains are mainly of high virulence whereas in Europe, strains tend to be of low virulence and a considerable number of chronic cases are encountered.

The virus enters the body either by ingestion or inhalation, and initial multiplication probably occurs in the lymphoid patches in the upper respiratory tract or tonsil. From these sites the virus is widely disseminated during the viraemic phase of the illness to other parts of the body, presumably by being carried in the leucocytes in the lymphatics or blood stream. Swine fever virus has a special affinity for tissues of mesodermal origin, particularly haemopoietic and vascular tissues, and damage to these cells leads to enlargement of the lymph nodes and widespread haemorrhages. Experimental evidence suggests that virus appears in the blood on about the third day and reaches its 'peak-titre' between the sixth and eighth days after infection. By the fifth day of the clinical illness most animals show a marked leucopenia, involving all types of circulating leucocytes; and a striking reduction in the number of circulating platelets. This thrombocytopenia probably plays an important role in the development of the haemorrhages.

Thus, the outstanding lesions of acute swine fever comprise degeneration of small blood vessels leading to haemorrhages in the kidney, bladder, skin and lymph-nodes. (Plate 49.2d, facing p. 651) Subcapsular splenic infarcts are also present as well as foci of infarction of the skin and mucosa of the alimentary tract and, significantly, extensive evidence of lymphoid necrosis. Because of secondary bacterial infection through breaks in the intestinal mucosa produced by viral activity, the initial lesions of lymphoid necrosis may be considerably enlarged and, in chronic cases of swine fever, give rise to the 'classical' circular or oval, raised 'button ulcers' which are most prevalent in the caecum and proximal portion of the colon.

In the U.K., the great majority of pigs dying from swine fever showed evidence of non-suppurative encephalitis. Several of the lesions were of a non-specific nature including necrosis, microgliosis and mononuclear perivascular cuffing, but the presence of vasculo-endothelial proliferation was usually considered to be of diagnostic importance since swine fever is probably the only viral encephalomyelitis of swine in which this type of lesion may be appreciated. (Plate 49.2b, facing p. 651).

Immunofluorescence studies indicate that the virus appears mainly in the cytoplasm in the earlier stages of infection but may occur in the nucleus later. A number of workers have described inclusion material in parenchymal liver cells and in cells of the reticulo-endothelial system in a number of animals examined at the seventh to the tenth days after infection, but the specificity of these abnormalities is in doubt.

Ecology

The infection is transmitted readily by direct and indirect contact. The virus is usually acquired by the respiratory route or by the ingestion of food and water contaminated with fresh discharges and secretions from infected pigs. The urine and nasal or ocular discharges are generally regarded as being the most infective.

In the U.K., about 50 per cent of outbreaks were caused by the movement of pigs through public markets and there was reliable evidence that the urine of infected animals played an important role in spreading the infection. There can be no doubt, however, that the most important cause of the great majority of initial outbreaks was the feeding of uncooked swill, with subsequent spread of infection by movements of the infected pigs.

The eradication policy of slaughter, introduced in the U.K. in 1963, has confirmed previous suspicions that apparently healthy recovered animals can act as carriers of the virus when introduced into clean herds. In pregnant sows the virus can cross the placental barrier and infect the fetuses leading to stillbirths of abnormal piglets or to piglets dying soon after farrowing. Although virus can readily be recovered from these piglets, healthy litter-mates born at the same time remain healthy and do not develop the disease. It has also been shown that virulent virus can be recovered from stillbirths born to crystal-violet vaccinated sows which had been exposed to swine fever virus during early pregnancy. Vaccination with virulent virus plus serum is still being used in a number of countries throughout the world and there is clear evidence that the indiscriminate use of these vaccines often leads to the spread of the disease.

Diagnosis

The diagnosis of swine fever is not easy since the incubation period may vary widely and the strain of virus causing the condition may be of low pathogenicity. Nevertheless, in typical cases of the disease a tentative diagnosis may be based on the high temperatures, high mortality and rapidly spreading nature of the infection, together with the presence of gross lesions which include purple discolouration of the skin on the ears, snout and abdomen, petechial haemorrhages of the kidney, lymph nodes, urinary bladder and other tissues, button ulcers in the intestines, infarcts in the spleen, tonsils and intestinal mucosa, and enlarged, oedematous and haemorrhagic lymph nodes. Of greater value is the presence of a leukopenia together with histopathological evidence of lymphoid necrosis and viral encephalomyelitis associated with vasculoendothelial proliferation.

A wide range of laboratory procedures may be utilized for obtaining a confirmatory diagnosis. These range from the inoculation of suspected material into groups of susceptible and immune pigs, to immunofluorescence and other serological tests.

Although conglutination-complement-absorption and complement-fixation tests have been described for the detection of specific antibody, there appears to be little evidence that they are of value for routine diagnosis. Perhaps the most accurate method of measuring antibody levels in suspected sera is by means of a neutralization test that was developed, following the report in 1963, that a strain of attenuated virulence could multiply in pig kidney tissue cultures in the presence of lamb serum, and produce a clearly visible cytopathic effect. Sera immune to all strains of swine fever virus so far tested, neutralize the cytopathic effect; and the neutralizing titres are believed to correlate well with resistance in the pig to infection with swine fever virus. The method can also be used for testing the susceptibility of pigs to infection and for determining the efficacy of vaccines.

In 1957, the Ouchterlony technique of double diffusion in agar gel was first used to demonstrate specific antigen-antibody precipitin reactions in swine fever, but the method is relatively insensitive and cannot be readily adapted to quantitative measurements. Nevertheless, the gel diffusion test was used successfully for a number of years for testing suspected tissues for the presence of specific swine fever precipitinogens. Various organs from affected swine contain soluble antigens which precipitate with hyperimmune serum but the pancreas was found to give a more marked reaction than other tissues. Unfortunately, the test is only of value after clinical symptoms have been present for at least 5 days so that further tests are required in all negative cases. The test can also be used to demonstrate antibody in serum or in the colostrum of carrier sows.

More recently, the fluorescent antibody-staining method has been adapted for the detection of swine fever antigen or antibody and is probably the most useful test for detecting virus both in field specimens and in infected cell culture systems, particularly where there are no obvious cytopathic changes in the infected monolayers. The test is extremely reliable provided a labelled antibody with high specificity and titre is used.

Control

There are 3 recognised methods of vaccination against swine fever, none of which has received unqualified approval.

(1) Simultaneous vaccination with virulent swine fever virus and high titre antiserum is still permitted in some countries, but there can be no doubt that the use of these virulent virus vaccines has contributed to the perpetuation of swine fever. It is emphasised that the serum must be administered in amounts sufficient to protect all animals in the herd against infection and that the amount required depends on the weight of the animals, and usually ranges from 20 to 80 ml. Although the method causes a severe reaction in some pigs, and sometimes death, the survivors are solidly immune.

(2) Attenuated live virus-vaccines modified by serial passage in rabbits, swine or tissue cultures are probably the most frequently used immunizing agents against swine fever. Although they are capable of inducing long-lasting immunity in susceptible animals there is strong circumstantial evidence to suggest that the modified virus not only replicates in the recipient host but is capable of spreading infection to other animals. In the U.K., for example, it was found that pigs injected with the modified lapinized virus spread the infection by contact with unvaccinated pigs and that the infection produced lesions which were indistinguishable from those found in typical swine fever. The infection also gave rise to specific precipitating antigen-antibody reactions. In countries where modified live virus-vaccines are used, only healthy pigs are vaccinated and the treated animals are held in strict isolation for 3–4 weeks. The vaccine should not be used in breeding sows or in young pigs prior to weaning. In piglets under 2 weeks of age, 2–5 ml of hyperimmune serum should be given followed by modified live-virus vaccine plus serum at weaning time. Although the rabbit-adapted virus-vaccine has frequently been given without the simultaneous use of serum, it is now generally agreed that antiserum should be employed with all live-virus vaccines.

(3) Inactivated virus-vaccines are safe to use and do not produce clinical disease. However, the immunity takes longer to develop and is not as strong, or as durable, as that induced by live modified or virulent virus-vaccines with serum. Thus, they are employed mainly in areas where the danger of exposure is not great.

Virus inactivated by crystal violet has been widely used for the past 30 years and was available in the U.K. from 1947 until the introduction of the eradication scheme in 1963. The extent of the demand for crystal violet vaccine in Britain at that time is underlined by the fact that over 8000 litres were issued in 1961. Two doses of 5–10 ml are usually administered subcutaneously, two weeks apart. Immunity develops in 2–3 weeks and lasts for about 8–12 months. The vaccine is safe to use and does not produce abnormal reactions, Moreover, there is no evidence of leukopenia, as found in animals vaccinated with live virus vaccines, and there is no dissemination of the virus. In Britain, all pigs were vaccinated at least once a year and the breeder was obliged not to sell any unvaccinated pigs, except piglets under 4 weeks of age sold with their vaccinated dam.

The use of mucosal disease virus as an immunizing agent against swine fever is being investigated and recent results show some promise.

Newborn piglets obtain antibody from the colostrum of an immune sow. Very little, if any, antibody crosses the placenta and the piglets are completely susceptible to swine fever virus until they have ingested and absorbed the colostrum. Passively derived antibody is lost at a fairly constant rate and piglets are usually susceptible to infection at 3–4 months of age. Hyperimmune sera can be used to give temporary protection when the disease appears in a herd, but the presence of this acquired passive immunity may interfere with the satisfactory development of active immunity following subsequent vaccination. Large doses of antiserum will protect animals in the early incubative stage of the disease and those newly exposed, but it has no therapeutic value in pigs showing clinical signs of the disease.

There can be no doubt that swill containing pork scraps from infected pigs is one of the commonest sources of infection and, for this reason, most countries now prohibit the feeding of uncooked garbage to pigs. In other countries or in circumstances where the feeding of uncooked swill cannot be satisfactorily controlled, it is imperative that all pigs should be effectively immunized.

In Britain, a Swine Fever Order was introduced in March, 1963, whereby all infected pigs and their contacts are slaughtered and their carcases cremated or buried. Consequently, the use of crystal violet and all other forms of swine fever vaccines was abandoned. In the first 9 months of the campaign for the eradication of swine fever there were more than 1000 confirmed outbreaks; in 1964 the number of outbreaks was just over 400, and in 1965 approximately 100. Since June 1966 only an occasional isolated outbreak has occurred and at the present time the disease is considered to have been eradicated. Thus, in 3 years, the slaughter-policy has virtually eliminated a disease which had been a serious problem in this country for more than 100 years, and which had defied vaccination and other methods that had been employed for its control.

The Virus Diarrhoea-Mucosal Disease Complex

Synonyms
Bovine virus diarrhoea: Mucosal disease: Schleimhaut krankheit (Ger.)

Definition
A group of viral diseases of cattle having similar clinical and pathological characters. The infection is mostly inapparent or mild, but acute cases are characterized by fever, anorexia, diarrhoea, nasal discharge and buccal ulceration.

Hosts affected
Cattle are principally affected but naturally occurring outbreaks have been reported in deer.

History and distribution
In 1946, an apparently new disease of cattle was described in New York State which was characterized by ulcerations of the alimentary tract and diarrhoea. Later, the disease was named virus diarrhoea. In 1953, a similar disease entity appeared among cattle in Iowa that closely resembled virus diarrhoea except that the clinical and pathological changes were more severe than those seen in the New York outbreaks, and many of the affected animals died from haemorrhagic gastroenteritis. This latter syndrome is known as mucosal disease.

A large number of strains of virus isolated from both types of disease in different parts of the world have been examined by immunological and serological methods and, during the period 1961–63, several groups of workers showed that the causative viruses are related antigenically, although they may give rise to a wide range of clinical manifestations.

At the present time, the virus diarrhoea-mucosal disease complex is widely distributed throughout the world and has been reported from other parts of the U.S.A., as well as from Canada, the U.K., Sweden, Germany and other countries in continental Europe, Africa, India, Australia and New Zealand.

Morphology
The agents of the virus diarrhoea-mucosal disease complex have not yet been adequately characterized but most reports of electron-microscopy and ultrafiltration experiments suggest that the virus particles are approximately spherical in shape, measuring between 40–65 nm in diameter, with a central core 24–30 nm across. However, during recent studies of electron-micrographs of virus diarrhoea isolates cultivated in primary bovine kidney cells, various particulate entities were observed which could be

classified into 3 distinct size ranges, (1) large (80 — > 100 nm) pleomorphic membrane-bound particles representing mature virions, (2) moderately sized (30–50 nm) particles of different types and (3) small (15–20 nm) virus-specific precursor particles considered to represent a 'ribosome-like' soluble antigen. It was further suggested that the ability of the large virus-diarrhoea virion to fragment into a number of smaller particles, which retain their infectivity, may be a characteristic feature of this and other members of the nonarbo-togavirus group.

The virus particle is surrounded by a sac-like envelope which is generally smooth and only rarely bears prominent surface projections. The nucleocapsid probably has cubical symmetry and the internal architecture of large mature particles may appear as a closely-knit meshwork of ring-like morphological subunits.

Physicochemical characters

Growth is not inhibited by 5-IUDR or 5-BUDR and it is suggested, therefore, that the virion contains RNA. A more recent report claims that the infectious RNA, which is sensitive to RNase, can be extracted by phenol from the virion. Mature virus particles are sensitive to ether, chloroform and other lipid solvents. They are sensitive to low pH (< 3·0) and are not stabilized at 50°C by $MgCl_2$. Heat inactivation studies indicate that the virus is readily inactivated at 56°C but most strains are stable at low temperatures and remain viable for years in the lyophilized state, or when stored at –70°C.

Haemagglutination

Many investigators have failed to demonstrate haemagglutinins, but others have shown that certain serotypes of virus are capable of haemagglutinating rhesus monkey, pig, sheep or chick red blood cells.

Antigenic properties

Comparisons of numerous isolates from various forms of clinical and experimental disease with standard virus suggest that virus diarrhoea and mucosal disease are caused by strains of viruses which are closely related on the basis of both serological and immunological reactions. In a British survey, 53 strains were classified into 7 serotypes of which a number were associated with clinical mucosal disease; and one serotype was isolated from 75 per cent of cattle with infertility. A more recent study, utilizing cytopathic isolates, has confirmed that virus diarrhoea and mucosal disease viruses are identical, or closely related antigenically, but serum neutralization tests combined with immunofluorescence suggest that the non-pathogenic strains are more closely related to one another than to the cytopathic strains.

Because the clinical and pathological manifestations of the virus diarrhoea-mucosal disease complex closely resemble rinderpest of cattle, it is emphasised that sera from calves recovered from mucosal disease do not neutralize rinderpest virus, nor are the calves resistant to challenge with rinderpest virus. Furthermore, reciprocal cross-protection tests in calves and reciprocal neutralization tests in cell cultures fail to show any immunological relationship between the two virus groups.

On the other hand, a close antigenic relationship undoubtedly exists between the viruses of mucosal disease and swine fever. This was first shown, in 1960, in agar gel diffusion tests when a line of precipitation was observed between a swine fever antigen and a mucosal disease antiserum. Not only has this relationship been confirmed by other workers but it has also been shown that inoculation of most strains of virus diarrhoea-mucosal disease viruses confer resistance to pigs when subsequently challenged with virulent swine fever virus.

Cultivation

Most investigators have failed to cultivate the virus diarrhoea-mucosal disease viruses in embryonated hens' eggs but a number of more recent reports indicate that certain serotypes can be grown in the yolk-sac while others multiply and produce pocks on the chorioallantoic membrane. The viruses have a narrow host spectrum and can readily infect cattle, sheep, goats and rabbits but do not grow in any other host.

Isolates from naturally occurring cases of both virus diarrhoea and mucosal disease can be propagated in cultures of bovine tissues and may or may not produce a cytopathic effect. The agent of virus diarrhoea has also been adapted to growth in pig kidney cultures. Cytopathic strains produce visible cellular changes, 2–5 days after inoculation, that are characterised by elongation and shrinkage of the affected cells, many of which assume bizarre forms. Most cytopathic strains produce translucent circular plaques in monolayer cultures, after 72 hours of incubation at 37°C, which are inhibited by specific antisera. Moreover, some produce virus titres of between $10^{5\cdot0-6\cdot5}$ $TCID_{50}$/ml in embryonic bovine skin or muscle cells, embryonic calf and lamb testicular cells, bovine kidney cells and human intestinal (Henle) cells.

Although immunofluorescence procedures can be used to demonstrate non-cytocidal strains in the cytoplasm of infected cells, it is of interest that their presence in embryonic kidney cultures can also be detected by their ability to inhibit the formation of 50 plaque forming units (p.f.u.) of a known cytopathic strain of virus diarrhoea or mucosal disease virus.

Evidence of virus multiplication of non-cytopathic strains can also be obtained by enhancement of the cytopathic effects of Newcastle disease virus in bovine testicular cell cultures, similar to the END test with swine fever virus.

Pathogenicity

Many workers consider that two distinct but similar forms of disease occur in cattle infected with virus diarrhoea-mucosal disease viruses. The main differences between them are the severity of the clinical signs and the environmental conditions under which they occur. The form known as virus diarrhoea is highly contagious and is characterized by mild clinical and pathological changes, with high morbidity but low mortality. Mucosal disease, on the other hand, is not highly contagious under field conditions but affected calves frequently show severe clinical signs and lesions; and many cases terminate fatally. Other investigators believe that virus diarrhoea and mucosal diseases are different manifestations of the same infection because they are very similar clinically and pathologically, and the numerous strains of virus isolated from naturally occurring cases are closely related immunologically.

There can be no doubt, however, that there is a marked variation in the severity of the clinical signs and that the morbidity and mortality rates vary greatly in the virus diarrhoea-mucosal disease complex. In mucosal disease, which is primarily a disease of young cattle (6–18 months old), the onset of the clinical signs is sudden, following an incubation period of 7–9 days, and are characterized by fever (40–42°C.), anorexia, serous nasal discharge, and some degree of depression. The initial temperature peak is accompanied by leukopenia which lasts for 1–6 days. This is followed by a slight leukocytosis and, then, by a recurrence of leukopenia. Within 2–3 days, superficial erosions may appear on the mucosa of the buccal cavity, the animals salivate profusely and the breath is extremely foetid. Diarrhoea occurs shortly after the appearance of severe mouth lesions and the faeces, which are initially watery in consistency, contain blood and mucus in the later stages of the illness. The course of the disease varies from a few days to about 1 month, the morbidity varies from 2–50 per cent or higher but the mortality rate in severely affected calves may exceed 90 per cent. On the other hand, the morbidity rate in a spontaneous outbreak may be very low while in some herds inapparent infections undoubtedly occur. In naturally occurring cases of virus diarrhoea the clinical signs are similar or of a more chronic form than those of mucosal disease, and the mortality rate of those affected seldom exceeds 5 per cent. Abortions may occur in pregnant cows and congenital abnormalities have been observed in calves.

The main pathological changes occur in the alimentary tract. These include hyperaemia, haemorrhage, oedema, erosion and ulceration of the squamous epithelium and mucosa of the entire alimentary canal and portions of the respiratory tract. Petechial haemorrhages are frequently present in the myocardium, especially along the coronary grooves and the endocardium of the ventricles. The lymphatic tissues are also affected and the lymph nodes and Peyer's patches may be enlarged and ulcerated. The nares, lips and buccal cavity may be hyperaemic and in severe cases there are shallow, circumscribed, dull or red-coloured ulcers on the muzzle or in the mouth. Occasionally, the mucosa of the buccal cavity and muzzle becomes completely eroded and in some animals inflammation and ulceration may extend to the pharynx and oesophagus. The lesions in the oesophagus are similar to those in the mouth but are generally more linear in shape.

Susceptible artificially infected calves develop a diphasic temperature reaction 2–4 days after inoculation but the illness is generally mild with few visible abnormalities other than reddening of the gums and an occasional discrete ulcer in the buccal cavity. However, the course of experimental infections with certain strains of mucosal disease virus is usually more prolonged than that produced by virus diarrhoea isolates and, in some cases, artificially infected calves show typical signs for 20–30 days. In those instances in which death ensues, the pathological lesions are similar to those observed in fatal field cases and include oedema, haemorrhage, erosion and ulceration of the alimentary tract and ulceration of the oral mucosa.

Immunity

Recovery from natural infection usually confers a solid, durable immunity to subsequent infection. Calves recovered from artificial infections resist reinfection for 12–16 months or longer.

Ecology

Infections caused by virus diarrhoea-mucosal disease agents spread from infected to susceptible cattle by direct and indirect contact. Although cattle are the primary host, naturally occurring outbreaks of the disease have occasionally been reported in deer. Goats and sheep can be infected experimentally and it is possible that these and other species of domestic and wild-living animals may serve as reservoirs of the infection or as a means of transmitting the disease from herd to herd.

Antibodies for mucosal disease-virus diarrhoea have been detected in the sera of pigs but there is no evidence that swine develop clinical disease or are capable of spreading the infection to cattle.

Diagnosis

In severe outbreaks, the history of the disease together with the clinical and pathological findings are strongly indicative of the virus diarrhoea-mucosal disease complex, but milder outbreaks may present difficulties. It is stressed that the clinical picture of virus diarrhoea and mucosal disease is similar to that of other bovine diseases such as malignant catarrhal fever, infectious bovine rhinotracheitis, vesicular stomatitis and foot-and-mouth disease, while the clinical signs and pathological changes are almost identical to those of rinderpest. For this reason it may be necessary to obtain a confirmatory diagnosis as quickly as possible by appropriate serological tests and, perhaps, by isolation and identification of the causative virus.

Blood samples for serological examination should be collected from a number of cattle that are in the early, acute stages of the disease and, where possible, from the same animals 3–4 weeks' later. The paired sera are examined for a four-fold or greater increase in antibody titre by neutralization tests against a standard strain of virus known to be cytopathic in bovine tissue cultures. Other serological procedures which may be used include immunofluorescence and complement-fixation tests. Agar gel diffusion is the standard test applied to tissues removed at autopsy. Mesenteric lymph nodes, mucous membrane of the intestinal tract, pancreas or almost any tissue showing ulceration are considered to be suitable sources of precipitinogens. The method is reliable and simple to perform, and several workers have found that about 60 per cent of affected cattle give positive results when portions of small intestinal tissue are diffused against a known positive antiserum.

The causative virus is readily isolated in cell cultures inoculated with clotted blood from affected animals since one of the features of this group of diseases is the long period of viraemia compared with that of some other viral infections. The typing of these isolates by neutralization tests in cell cultures is a useful means of establishing an association of the virus with the disease.

The histopathological features are not pathognomonic of the virus diarrhoea-mucosal disease complex but demonstration of leukopenia is usually of some diagnostic value when considered with the clinical and pathological changes.

Control

A number of strains of virus have been attenuated by serial passage in rabbits and these have been used to immunize cattle against the disease. Several cytopathic strains have been attenuated for calves after serial passage in tissue culture and are said to be effective for use in vaccines. The combined use of immune serum and live virus vaccines is also believed to confer protection. However, the efficacy of commercially available vaccines including a number containing other viruses, e.g. infectious bovine rhinotracheitis or parainfluenza-3 remains to be proved. At the present time encouraging results are being obtained in a number of laboratories throughout the world where swine fever virus is used to immunize calves against mucosal disease.

Umea disease

In 1960, an apparently new disease entity was reported among cattle in Sweden. The syndrome was characterised by marked respiratory and enteric signs, and the causative agents were found to be a mixed infection of mucosal disease and parainfluenza-3 viruses. The illness, which was named Umea disease from the district in Northern Sweden where it first occurred, has since been reported in Finland and Denmark. It spreads very rapidly and its incubation period is generally shorter (7–8 days) than for mucosal disease (9–11 days). A number of cytopathic strains isolated from outbreaks in Scandinavia are closely related immunologically to the standard strain (Oregon C24V) of mucosal disease virus.

Border disease of lambs

Border disease or 'hairy shaker' disease is a congenital condition of lambs characterized clinically by excessive hairiness of the birth-coat, poor growth and nervous abnormalities. The condition occurs in the U.K., New Zealand and Australia, but may also be present in a number of other countries including the U.S.A. and Eire.

The incidence of the disease is low and is usually first recognised at lambing time by the presence of a number of undersized lambs with abnormally hairy fleeces. A number show involuntary muscular tremors of the head and neck, sometimes involving the whole body, and most die before weaning. However, in the few that survive, the nervous signs gradually disappear within 3–4 months. Abortions can occur in affected flocks at all stages of pregnancy and there is evidence that an acute focal necrotising placentitis, involving principally the caruncular septa, develops about 10 days after maternal infection. Histological examination of affected tissues reveals defective myelination of the central nervous system and glial abnormalities.

The natural mode of transmission is not known, but the disease can be reproduced experimentally by the intraperitoneal or subcutaneous inoculation of ewes preferably before the 85th day of gestation, either with crude tissue suspensions of brain, spinal cord and spleen from affected lambs, or with cell-free inocula. Experimentally infected ewes develop anti-bodies and are immune to challenge in subsequent pregnancies. Affected lambs reared to maturity may bear affected offspring without further challenge and it is possible, therefore, that the infection may persist throughout adolescence. It has been reported that the presence of 7S gamma-globulin in the sera of affected lambs that have not ingested colostrum may provide additional evidence of an infectious disease.

The nature of the aetiological agent has not been established but present knowledge suggests that it is a small, isometric virus, approximately 27 nm in diameter, with an ether-sensitive envelope, and is inactivated by heating to 60°C for 90 minutes. Isolates obtained on ovine cell cultures are mildly cytopathic and form small foci of vacuolated and degenerate cells, but do not produce inclusion bodies. Haemagglutination and haemadsorption have not been described.

Although a specific agent has not been definitely identified, there is clear evidence that sera obtained from sheep with natural or experimental border disease contain precipitating and neutralizing anti-bodies to the viruses of mucosal disease and swine fever. Also, that cattle inoculated in the early months of pregnancy with tissues from lambs affected with border disease frequently abort, the fetuses show marked retardation of growth and the cows develop antibodies against mucosal disease virus. Abortions and neonatal deaths have also been reported in pregnant goats inoculated with border disease affected lamb tissues. Live kids born at full term may be clinical 'shakers' and some show hypomyelinogenesis at autopsy.

In view of these findings, and the fact that an immunological relationship exists between border disease of lambs, mucosal disease and swine fever, it is likely that the three diseases are caused by closely related viruses; and that the agent of border disease can be provisionally classified with mucosal disease and swine fever viruses as candidate members of the non-arthropod-borne group of toga-viruses.

Infectious arteritis of horses

Synonyms
Viral arteritis of horses: Equine viral arteritis: Epizootic cellulitis: Pink-eye: Pferdestaupe: Rot-laufseuche: formerly 'equine influenza'.

Definition
An acute infectious disease of horses characterized clinically by fever, depression, mucopurulent rhinitis, stiffness and oedema of the conjunctiva, trunk, limbs and external genitalia.

Hosts affected
Horses of all ages are affected but unweaned foals are particularly susceptible. Other species are not susceptible. Severe losses (50–70 per cent) may occur from abortions, especially in the later febrile or early convalescent period of the infection.

History and distribution
Isolation of a virus causing arteritis of horses was first reported in 1957 during investigations of an outbreak of abortions in horses accompanied by many of the symptoms described for equine influenza. Until this time, viral abortion in horses was con-sidered to be a manifestation of infection of pregnant mares by the equine influenza virus. It is now known, however, that the causative agents of equine abortion or equine rhinopneumonitis (herpesvirus), equine influenza (orthomyxovirus) and equine arteritis (unclassified togavirus) are unrelated viruses possess-ing distinctly different properties.

The name 'viral arteritis' was chosen for this hitherto unrecognized disease because the main pathological change is a hyaline necrosis in the tunica media of small muscular arteries.

Equine viral arteritis occurs sporadically in North America but its distribution in other parts of the world is not known. In Europe, up to 1970, the causative virus has only been isolated in Switzerland and Austria.

Morphology
Electron microscopy of purified preparations of equine arteritis virus reveals enveloped, spherical particles 50–70 nm in diameter with a core 30–40 nm across. No detailed structure of an internal com-ponent can be seen but mature virus particles with an architecture resembling that of mucosal disease virus have been described. More recently, a number of workers have observed tiny (3–5 nm in length), tail-like protrusions (blebs) on the surface of the virion, which suggests that some of the virus particles possess an osmotically-sensitive limiting membrane. In negatively-stained preparations, the envelope frequently shows ring-like structures about 12–14 nm in diameter.

Physicochemical characters
The viral nucleic acid is almost certainly RNA and the lipid nature of the outer envelope is suggested by its sensitivity to ether and chloroform. All strains are readily inactivated by molar $MgCl_2$ at 50°C and are sensitive to low pH, but resistant to the action of trypsin, They survive for 6 years at −20°C, 75 days at

4°C, 2 days at 37°C and for 20 minutes, but not 30 minutes, at 56°C.

Antigenic properties

Arteritis virus is distinct in its properties and serology from rhinopneumonitis, influenza, infectious anaemia and other equine viruses. Antibodies in sera from infected horses are demonstrable by virus neutralization and complement-fixation tests.

Haemagglutination

No haemagglutinin has been detected in any of the strains of virus so far studied.

Cultivation

There is no evidence that the virus can be adapted to growth in embryonated hens' eggs and attempts to establish the infection in laboratory animals have proved unsuccessful.

The virus can, however, be isolated and propagated in monolayer cultures of horse or rabbit kidney cells, and equine tissue-adapted strains can be grown in hamster kidney cell cultures with the production of clearly visible plaques, 2–4 mm in diameter. Growth in horse and rabbit kidney cells is characterized by a cytopathic effect 3 days after inoculation and, by the end of the sixth day, most of the cells in the infected cultures show cytoplasmic shrinkage and pycnosis, and readily detach from the glass. Intracytoplasmic or intranuclear inclusions have not been observed. Plaque assays of equine arteritis virus have been described in BHK-21, Vero, RK13 and equine kidney cell cultures.

Infected baby hamster kidney cells show extensive cytopathic changes 42 hours after inoculation, and electron microscopical examination of ultrathin sections suggests that the main release mechanism of virus particles from infected cells is by a process of budding from the cytoplasmic matrix into cisternae of the endoplasmic reticulum; the process probably starting in the vicinity of the Golgi apparatus. It has been suggested that liberation of the mature virions probably occurs as a result of fusion between the infected cisternae of the endoplasmic reticulum and the outer cellular membrane.

Pathogenicity

Following an incubation period of 5–10 days, the natural disease is initiated by a febrile response which persists for 4–9 days with temperatures ranging between 39–41°C. This is usually accompanied by leukopenia but the leukocyte count returns to normal as soon as the temperature reaction subsides.

The most consistent clinical symptoms of uncomplicated infection by arteritis virus are fever, conjunctivitis, excessive lachrymation, rhinitis, congested nasal mucosa, respiratory distress, anorexia, weakness and debility. Other frequently observed signs include palpebral oedema, enteritis, colitis, oedema of the trunk, legs, mammary gland or scrotum and sheath, depression, muscular weakness and prostration. Leukopenia, fever and other clinical symptoms are usually resolved in 7–14 days but recovery is often delayed in horses with severe enteric or pulmonary involvement.

In recent years, the mortality rate has been much lower than in earlier outbreaks, although a fatal outcome is likely in poorly nourished animals, and the heaviest losses are from abortion. Over 50 per cent of pregnant mares may abort, due to active infection of the fetus rather than to fever or general debility of the mare, and virus is readily isolated from the blood, liver, spleen and other tissues of aborted fetuses. It is emphasised that abortion induced by arteritis virus occurs 12–30 days after infection whereas that caused by rhinopneumonitis virus (herpesvirus –1 infection) occurs 1–4 months after exposure.

In experimentally infected horses, the virus is found in nasopharyngeal secretions, blood and plasma during the early febrile phase of the illness. It is also present in the spleen and other tissues of animals that succumb to the infection.

The main pathological lesions in fatal cases of the disease are palpebral oedema, congestion and haemorrhage of the upper respiratory tract, bronchopneumonia, oedema of the larynx and mediastinal tissues, petechial haemorrhages on the serous surfaces, gross effusion of fluid into the peritoneal and pleural cavities, catarrhal enteritis, haemorrhage and infarction of the spleen and degenerative changes in the liver and kidney. In pregnant mares there is usually submucosal oedema of the uterus and oedema of the broad ligaments. Infected fetuses, however, show no specific lesions and are readily distinguished from abortions caused by rhinopneumonitis virus which are invariably characterised by oedema of the lungs, excessive fluid in the pleural cavity, focal necrosis of the liver and the presence of Cowdry type A intranuclear inclusions.

The essential microscopical changes in naturally occurring cases of equine arteritis are those of medial necrosis of small muscular arteries. Parts of the affected arterial musculature lose their nuclei and become hyaline and acidophilic in appearance. Oedema is present in the adventitia of the artery and lymphocytic infiltration is evident in both the adventitia and the damaged media. It is generally believed that the endothelial arterial lesions are the underlying cause of the characteristic haemorrhages and oedema seen in many of the affected organs, including the infarctions of the lung, spleen and intestines.

Electron microscopical studies of infected tissues reveal changes in the cytoplasm of the endothelial cells. These abnormalities include crystalline arrays of dense ribosome-like particles within the cisternae of the endoplasmic reticulum, micro-tubule formation, aggregates of electron dense particles and virions about 60 nm in diameter; some with double membranes, situated within the cytoplasmic vacuoles.

Transmission

The causative virus of equine arteritis is extremely contagious and is readily transmitted, especially among foals, probably through the respiratory tract. Spontaneous outbreaks usually arise following movement of horses from premises where the disease is present. Recovered adult horses may be carriers and transmit the infection.

Diagnosis

Clinical diagnosis may not be possible in the case of mildly affected individual animals but in typical outbreaks of naturally occurring disease the clinical signs are generally characteristic of viral arteritis and readily differentiate it from other viral infections of horses. A confirmatory diagnosis can be obtained by demonstrating the characteristic lesions of medial necrosis of smaller arteries and by cross-protection tests in suitable horses. The causative virus may be isolated in horse, rabbit and baby hamster kidney cells from the nasal secretions, or from the spleens of horses that have died. Virus isolates are identified by neutralization of the cytopathic effects with specific antiserum.

Control

Antiviral vaccines for the prevention of equine arteritis are not yet available commercially, but preparations from virus attenuated in tissue culture are under development.

Lactic dehydrogenase virus

Lactic dehydrogenase virus (LDH-V), or Riley virus, is a non-pathogenic virus that is present in saliva, urine and faeces of apparently normal mice.

It has received a great deal of attention not only because it is perhaps the best known example of an infectious agent producing a persistant tolerant infection, but also because it is the first example known of a virus that stimulates an infected animal to produce an increase in enzymic activity in the peripheral circulation. This is apparently due to impaired clearance of lactic dehydrogenase and other enzymes when mice are infected, as a result of blockage of the reticulo-endothelial system by the action of the virus. The virus may persist in infected carrier mice for very long periods and, during early acute viraemia, titres may reach 10^{10} particles/ml

of plasma. The virus is widely distributed in mouse colonies and causes no clinical illness. Because of this, isolates of mouse tumour viruses are frequently contaminated with LDH-V.

Lactic dehydrogenase virus grows readily in cell cultures of mouse macrophages and mouse embryo cells, usually without an apparent cytopathic effect. Virus particles are spherical (40–57 nm in diameter), oblong (35 × 45 nm) or, sometimes, rod-shaped. A central featureless nucleoid (25–33 nm in diameter) is surrounded by a dense double membrane. The virus is sensitive to the action of ether, contains infectious RNA but does not form haemagglutinins.

Further reading

ACLAND, H.M., GARD, G.P. AND PLANT, J.W. (1972) Infection of sheep with a mucosal disease virus. *Australian Veterinary Journal*, **48**, 70.

Arboviruses and human disease (1967) WHO Technical Report Series, No. 369. Geneva: World Health Organization.

BAKER J.A. (1946) Serial passage of hog cholera virus in rabbits. *Proceedings of the Society for Experimental Biology and Medicine*, **63**, 183.

BARLOW, R.M. AND GARDINER, A.C. (1969) Experiments in border disease. I. Transmission, pathology and some serological aspects of the experimental disease. *Journal of Comparative Pathology and Therapeutics*, **79**, 397.

BROTHERSTON J.G. AND BOYCE J.B. (1970) A non-infective protective louping-ill antigen. *Journal of Comparative Pathology and Therapeutics*, **80**, 377.

BROTHERSTON J.G. AND SWANEPOEL R. (1965/6) Ovine encephalomyelitis (Louping-ill). In, Veterinary Annual, ed. W.A. Pool. Seventh issue, p. 133. Bristol: John Wright and Sons Ltd.

BÜRKI F. (1965) Eigenschaften des virus des equinen arteritis. *Pathologia et Microbiologia*, **28**, 939.

BÜRKI F. (1966) Further properties of equine arteritis virus. *Archiv für die gesamte Virusforschung*, **19**, 123.

CASALS J. (1971) Arboviruses: Incorporation in a general system of virus classification. In, Comparative Virology, eds. K. Maramorosch and E. Kurstak, pp. 307.

CASALS J. (1961) Procedures for identification of arthropod-borne viruses. *Bulletin of the World Health Organization*, **24**, 723.

CHAMBERLAIN R.W. (1968) Arboviruses, the arthropod-borne animal viruses. *Current Topics in Microbiology and Immunology*, **42**, 38.

CLARKE D.H. AND CASALS J. (1958) Techniques for haemagglutination and haemagglutination-inhibition with arthropod-borne viruses. *American Journal of Tropical Medicine and Hygiene*, **7**, 561.

DALLING T. (1949) Swine fever (hog cholera) crystal

violet vaccine. *Food and Agriculture Organization Studies*, **10**, 46.

DARBYSHIRE J.H. (1962) Agar gel diffusion studies with a mucosal disease of cattle. II. A Serological relationship between a mucosal disease and swine fever. *Research in Veterinary Science*, **3**, 125.

DEMADRID, A.T. AND PORTERFIELD, J.S. (1974) The flaviviruses [Group B arboviruses]: a cross-neutralization study. *Journal of General Virology*, **23**, 91.

DINTER Z. (1963) Relationship between bovine virus diarrhoea virus and hog cholera virus. *Zentralblatt für Bakteriologie. I. Abt. Originale*, **188**, 475.

DITCHFIELD J. AND DOANE F.W. (1964) The properties and classification of bovine viral diarrhea virus. *Canadian Journal of Comparative Medicine and Veterinary Science*, **28**, 148.

DOHERTY P.C. AND REID H.W. (1971) Louping-ill encephalomyelitis in the sheep. II. Distribution of virus and lesions in nervous tissue. *Journal of Comparative Pathology*, **81**, 531.

DOHERTY P.C., REID H.W. AND SMITH W. (1972) Louping-ill encephalomyelitis in the sheep. V. Histopathogenesis of the field disease. *Journal of Comparative Pathology*, **82**, 337.

DOLL E.R., BRYANS J.T., MCCOLLUM W.H. AND CROWE M.E.W. (1957) Isolation of a filterable agent causing arteritis of horses and abortion by mares. Its differentiation from the equine abortion (influenza) virus. *Cornell Veterinarian*, **47**, 3.

DOW C., JARRET W.F.H. AND MCINTYRE W.I.M. (1956) A disease of cattle in Britain resembling the viral diarrhoea-mucosal disease complex. *Veterinary Record*, **68**, 620.

DUNNE H.W. (1963) Field and laboratory diagnosis of hog cholera. *Veterinary Medicine*, **58**, 222.

EASTERDAY B.C. (1965) Rift Valley Fever. *Advances in Veterinary Science*, **10**, 65.

FERNELIUS A.L. AND LAMBERT G (1969) Detection of bovine viral diarrhea virus and antigen in tissues of experimentally infected calves by cell inoculation and fluorescent antibody techniques. *American Journal of Veterinary Research*, **30**, 1551.

GARDINER, A.C., BARLOW, R.M., RENNIE, J.C. AND KEIR, W.A. (1972) Experiments in border disease. V. Preliminary investigations on the nature of the agent. *Journal of Comparative Pathology and Therapeutics*, **82**, 159.

GLEISER C.A., GOCHENOUR W.S., BERGE T.O. AND TIGERTT W.D. (1962) The comparative pathology of experimental venezuelan equine encephalomyelitis infection in different animal hosts. *Journal of Infectious Diseases*, **110**, 80.

GORDON W.S., BROWNLEE A., WILSON D.R. AND MACLEOD J. (1962) The epizootology of louping-ill and tick borne fever with observations on the

control of these sheep diseases. Symposia of the Zoological Society of London, No. 6.

HAIG D.A. (1965) The arboviruses. *Veterinary Record*, **77**, 1428.

HARDING J.D., DONE J.T. AND DARBYSHIRE J.H. (1966) Congenital tremors in piglets and their relation to swine fever. *Veterinary Record*, **79**, 388.

HORZINEK, M.C. (1973) The structure of togaviruses. *Progress in Medical Virology*, **16**, 109.

HORZINEK M.C. (1973) Comparative aspects of togaviruses. *Journal of General Virology*, **20**, 87.

HUCK R.A. (1957) Mucosal disease complex. *Journal of Comparative Pathology and Therapeutics*, **67**, 267.

KISSLING R.E. (1957) Growth of several arthropod-borne viruses in tissue culture. *Proceedings of the Society for Experimental Biology and Medicine*, **96**, 290.

KUMAGAI T., SHIMIZU T., IKEDA S. AND MATUMOTO M. (1961) A new *in vitro* method (END) for detection and measurement of hog cholera virus and its antibody by means of effect of HC virus on Newcastle disease virus in swine tissue culture. I. Establishment of standard procedure. *Journal of Immunology*, **87**, 245.

LUGINBUHL R.E. SATRIANO S.F., HELMBOLDT C.F., LAMSON A.L. AND JUNGHERR E.L. (1958) Investigation of eastern equine encephalomyelitis. II. Outbreaks in Connecticut pheasants. *American Journal of Hygiene*, **67**, 4.

MENGELING W.L., GUTEKUNST D.E., FERNELIUS A.L. AND PIRTLE E.C. (1963) Demonstration of an antigenic relationship between hog cholera and bovine viral diarrhea viruses by immunofluorescence. *Canadian Journal of Comparative Medicine*, **27**, 162.

MENGELING W.L. AND TORREY J.P. (1967) Evaluation of the fluorescent antibody-cell culture test for hog cholera diagnosis. *American Journal of Veterinary Research*, **128**, 1653.

MILLS J.H.L., NIELSEN S.W. AND LUGINBUHL R.E. (1965) Current status of bovine mucosal disease. *Journal of the American Veterinary Medical Association*, **146**, 691.

PLANT, J.W., LITTLEJOHN, I.R., GARDINER, A.C., VANTSIS, J.T. AND HUCK, R.A. (1972) Immunological relationship between border disease, mucosal disease and swine fever. *Veterinary Record*, **92**, 455.

PRITCHARD W.R. (1963) The bovine viral diarrhoea-mucosal disease complex. *Advances in Veterinary Science*, **8**, 1.

REID H.W. (1975) Experimental infection of red grouse with louping-ill virus (Flavivirus group). I. The viraemia and antibody response. *Journal of Comparative Pathology*, **85**, 223.

REID H.W. AND BOYCE J.B. (1974) Louping-ill virus in red grouse in Scotland. *Veterinary Record*, **95**, 150.

SCHERRER R., AYNAUD J.M. COHEN J. AND BIC E. (1930) Etude en microscope électronique du virus de la peste porcine classique (hog cholera) dans des coupes ultra-fines de cellules infectées in vitro. *Comptes rendu hebdomadaires des séances de l'Académie des sciences*. Paris, D271, 620.

SHOPE R.E. (1959) The natural history of hog cholera. *Perspectives in Virology*. London; Chapman and Hall.

SLAVIN G. (1938) The resistance of the swine fever virus to physical agencies and chemical disinfectants. *Journal of Comparative Pathology and Therapeutics*, **51**, 213.

SMITH K.M. (1962) The arthropod viruses. *Advances in Virus Research*, **9**, 195.

SMITH C.E.G., MCMAHON D.A., O'REILLY K.J., WILSON A.L. AND ROBERTSON J.M. (1964) The epidemiology of louping ill in Ayrshire: the first year of studies in sheep. *Journal of Hygiene*, **62**, 53.

SPRADBROW P. (1966) Arbovirus infections of domestic animals. *Veterinary Bulletin*, **36**, 55.

STAIR E.L., RHODES M.B., AIKEN J.M., UNDERDAHL N.R. AND YOUNG G.A. (1963) A hog-cholera virus-fluorescent antibody system. Its potential use in the study of embryonic infection. *Proceedings of the Society for Experimental Biology and Medicine*, **113**, 656.

TEEBKEN D.L., AIKEN J.M. AND TWIEHAUS M.J. (1967) Differentiation of virulent, attenuated and inactivated hog cholera viruses by fluorescent-antibody technique. *Journal of the American Veterinary Medical Association*, **150**, 53.

THOMSON R.G. and SAVAN M. (1963) Studies on virus diarrhoea and mucosal disease of cattle. *Canadian Journal of Comparative Medicine and Veterinary Science*, **27**, 207.

WEISS K.E. (1957) Rift Valley Fever: a review. *Bulletin of Epizootic Diseases of Africa*, **5**, 431.

WEISS K.E. (1957) Wesselsbron virus disease. *Bulletin of Epizootic Diseases of Africa*, **5**, 459.

WEISS K.E., HAIG D.A. AND ALEXANDER R.A. (1956) Wesselsbron virus — A virus not previously described, associated with abortion in animals. *Onderstepoort Journal of Veterinary Research*, **27**, 183.

CHAPTER 50

ARENAVIRUSES

CHAPTER 50

Arenaviruses

The genus *Arenavirus* includes lymphocytic chorio-meningitis (LCM) virus and some other species that are responsible for severe illnesses of man, e.g. American haemorrhagic fever in Argentina and Lassa fever in West Africa. All are spherical, ovoid or pleomorphic RNA viruses measuring 85–100 nm in diameter, but larger forms reaching 350 nm in their longest dimension have been described. The virions are surrounded by a dense well-defined, outer envelope, covered with closely packed surface projections, although the interior of the particle appears unstructured and contains a variable number of electron dense granules (20–30 nm in diameter) giving a sandy appearance from which the name arenavirus is derived. (Latin, *arenosus* — sandy). Virions are synthesized within the cytoplasm and matured by budding from the marginal membranes. All arenaviruses are sensitive to lipid solvents and rapidly lose infectivity below pH 5.5 and above pH 8.5. They are also relatively heat sensitive. In the natural host, e.g. mice, hamsters and guinea-pigs, they frequently give rise to persistent symptomless infections. All strains share at least one group-specific antigen demonstrable by immunofluorescence, and are sensitive to lipid solvents.

Lymphocytic choriomeningitis

Synonyms
Pneumopathie des Cobayes. Humphreys' disease of guinea-pigs.

History and distribution
In the early 1930s it was observed that a virus, later named lymphocytic choriomeningitis (LCM) virus, was present as a latent infection in mice used during studies on St. Louis encephalitis and swine fever. Since then, naturally occurring inapparent LCM infections have been reported in various strains of laboratory and wild mice, as well as in guinea-pigs, hamsters, monkeys and man.

Hosts affected
LCM has a broad host range and susceptible species include mice, guinea-pigs, rats, dogs, pigs, monkeys and chimpanzees. There are no known reports of the virus affecting rabbits, chickens or horses. Man is susceptible and cases have been reported in laboratory workers handling latently infected mice, or even in people living in houses infested with mice.

Properties of the virus
Virus particles in ultra-thin sections are round, oval or pleomorphic and the majority measure approximately 50–60 nm in diameter; but larger forms, up to 200 nm, are frequently seen. The virion contains single-stranded RNA with a total molecular weight of 3.5×10^6 daltons. The symmetry of the capsid is not known. All strains are ether-sensitive and are extremely thermo-labile being readily inactivated by exposure to 56°C for 20 minutes. They are stable in 50 per cent glycerol and can be stored for long periods at –70°C, or when lyophilized, but they are unstable at acid or alkali pH. The virus is inactivated by 0.05 per cent formalin, or ultra-violet light, but not by 0.5 per cent phenol; and its infectivity titre is greatly reduced by treatment with 1/10 000 merthiolate. Replication occurs within the cytoplasm and nucleocapsid development is on the plasma membrane.

Haemagglutination
Although LCM particles are adsorbed to the surface of susceptible red blood cells there is no evidence, so far, that the virus contains haemagglutinins.

Antigenic properties
Soluble complement-fixing antigens can be prepared from infected animal tissues by extraction with ether-sucrose or with fluorocarbon, and are readily separable from the virus particles. They are heat-stable at 56°C and can be used in complement-fixation tests to measure the production of specific antibody. Precipitation in agar gel is also associated

667

with the presence of a soluble antigen. Neutralizing antibodies may not be formed by infected mice but they are invariably present in sera from recovered human patients and from most susceptible animal species in which they may persist for long periods. Immunofluorescence is a sensitive and specific method for detecting antibody.

Immunity of mice in infected colonies may be due to 'persistent tolerated infection' in unweaned mice, or to active immunity in adults.

Cultivation

The virus can be readily propagated on the chorio-allantoic membrane of developing hens' eggs but without the production of visible 'pocks'.

Most continuous cell lines of human origin as well as primary cell cultures derived from chicks, mice, monkeys, cattle and other species support the growth of LCM virus, but cytopathic changes may only be seen after adaptation. Nevertheless, cytopathic effects have been described in chicken embryo cell cultures, baby hamster kidney cells and in KB and HeLa human cell lines. Within 48–72 hours, infected cells develop cytoplasmic areas of aggregated particles indistinguishable from ribosomes. In the process of budding, one or more ribosome-like particles are incorporated into the maturing virion. Plaques are produced in chicken embryo cell cultures, but only after 12 days of incubation; and a plaque assay technique has been described. Immunofluorescent staining suggests that viral antigens are present in the cytoplasm of relatively few cells in an infected tissue.

Pathogenicity

Lymphocytic choriomeningitis virus is indigenous to mice which may harbour it for life and spread the infection transplacentally to succeeding generations. Strains of LCM virus differ in virulence and some will produce a rapidly fatal generalized infection when inoculated intracerebrally into adult mice from susceptible stocks. On the other hand, when mice become infected *in utero* or during the first few days after birth a generalised persistent infection usually develops without damage to the host. In this chronic type of infection the virus is present in high titres in all tissues and organs, and the mice remain resistant to reinfection. Although circulating antibody cannot be demonstrated by conventional serological methods, the mice do have neutralizing antibody to the virus. The disease is of particular interest immunologically because it provides a classical example of the phenomenon of immunological tolerance. After about 10 months of age, however, many of the carrier mice develop a fatal progressive disease involving the central nervous system accompanied by high levels of

LCM virus in the brain, blood and other tissues, together with the production of viral antibody. It has been shown recently that the antibody response results in a large accumulation of antigen-antibody complexes in the kidney which, in turn, leads to chronic glomerulonephritis and death. The renal lesions are similar to those seen in Aleutian disease of mink, systemic lupus erythematosus in man and a number of other disorders where there is a relationship between an autoimmune phenomenon and disease. The influence of immune mechanisms in the pathogenicity of LCM is underlined by the fact that virus meningitis may be produced in carrier mice of infected stocks by the intracerebral inoculation of sterile broth.

Experimentally, LCM virus will infect susceptible mice when introduced by various routes, the intracerebral being the most and the intranasal the next most effective. Mice of susceptible stocks develop signs of illness 5–12 days after intracerebral inoculation of the virus and death usually occurs 1–3 days after the onset of clonic convulsions. On the other hand, mice infected intranasally or subcutaneously show only slight clinical signs of illness but develop complement-fixing antibodies and are resistant to subsequent challenge with the virus.

Lesions associated with LCM infection include lymphocytic infiltration around blood vessels and in various other tissues. There may also be pleural and peritoneal effusions and some animals may show hepatitis with marked lobulation of the liver.

The human form of the disease ranges from a mild influenza-like fever to severe meningoencephalitis. The latter is sometimes fatal but fortunately rare.

Ecology

Although virus is excreted in the urine and faeces of infected mice, the most important method of intercolony transmission of recently introduced LCM virus is by infected nasal secretions. Later, as the infection establishes itself and many mice become symptomless carriers, the infection can be transmitted congenitally to their offspring who, in turn, will develop the carrier state for the rest of their lives.

Several reports suggest that arthropods may help to spread the infection and contaminated dust has also been suspected as a vehicle for infection.

Diagnosis

Latent LCM infection of mice can usually be diagnosed by the intracerebral challenge of suspected mice with a neurotropic strain of the virus. At least 90 per cent of susceptible mice will die whereas inapparent virus-carriers will survive. Alternatively, the virus may be isolated by inoculating suspect tissue suspensions intracerebrally into known susceptible mice or on to various cell culture systems. Infected mice usually succumb to the infection and the presence of specific viral antigen in cell cultures can be demonstrated by immunofluorescence. Fluorescent antibody staining methods of livers of suspected mice will reveal the presence of LCM viral antigen in the cytoplasm of infected parenchymal cells.

Although infected mice do not produce appreciable amounts of protective or neutralizing antibodies, neutralization tests can be carried out if the serum-virus mixture is first incubated for 24 hours at 37°C. Alternatively, a satisfactory neutralizing antiserum can readily be prepared in other species of susceptible animals. Complement-fixation tests can be carried out but the titres are relatively short-lived following the acute type of infection and are non-existent in chronic infections.

Control

It is very difficult to protect a clean colony completely from the accidental introduction of LCM virus. Mice should only be purchased from known LCM-free stocks and wild mice must be prevented from entering the mouse-room since they are probably the most likely natural reservoir host of the virus.

Lassa fever

Lassa fever is a serious, often fatal, illness of man which has recently been described in Nigeria and other parts of West Africa. The incubation period is 6–20 days. The disease is characterized by fever, headaches, sore throat, muscular pain, loss of appetite, vomiting and diarrhoea. Autopsy findings include pleural effusion, renal haemorrhage and mucosal oedema of the small intestine. Although the epidemiology of the disease remains unknown, recent isolations of Lassa virus from tissue suspensions from rodents suggests the existence of extra-human reservoirs and the possibility of arthropod vectors. Lassa virus has been isolated on Vero cells from throat washings, blood and urine of affected patients, and produces a cytopathic effect within 4 days. Infected cultures show basophilic, pleomorphic intracytoplasmic aggregates, and about half of the cells in the monolayer detach from the glass in 5–8 days. The virus is ether-sensitive and is antigenically related to lymphocytic choriomeningitis virus. On the basis of morphology, RNA content and sensitivity to lipid solvents, Lassa virus is provisionally included in the arenavirus group.

Further reading

CASALS, J. AND BUCKLEY, S.M. (1974) Lassa fever. *Progress in Medical Virology*, **18**, 111.

DALTON A.J., ROWE W.P., SMITH G.H., WILSNACK R.E. AND PUGH W.E. (1968) Morphological and cytochemical studies on lymphocytic choriomeningitis virus. *Journal of Virology*, **2**, 1465.

LEHMANN-GRUBE F. (1971) Lymphocytic choriomeningitis virus. *Virology Monographs*, **10**, 1.

MIMS C.A. AND WAINWRIGHT S. (1968) The immunodepressive action of lymphocytic choriomeningitis virus in mice. *Journal of Immunology*, **101**, 717.

MURPHY F.A., WEBB P.A., JOHNSON K.M., WHITFIELD S.G. AND CHAPPELL W.A. (1970). Arenaviruses in Vero cells: ultrastructural studies. *Journal of Virology*, **6**, 507.

PFAU, C.J. (1974) Biochemical and biophysical properties of the arenaviruses. *Progress in Medical Virology*, **18**, 64.

WILSNACK R.E. (1966) Lymphocytic choriomeningitis. In, Viruses of Laboratory Rodents. National Cancer Institute, Monogram 20, p. 77.

WILSNACK W.P. AND ROWE W.P. (1964) Immunofluorescent studies of the histopathogenesis of lymphocytic choriomeningitis virus infection. *Journal of Experimental Medicine*, **120**, 829.

CHAPTER 51

UNCLASSIFIED RNA VIRUSES

Unclassified RNA Viruses

Equine infectious anaemia

Synonyms
Swamp fever: Pernicious anaemia of horses: Ansteckende Blutarmut der Pferde.

Definition
An acute, sub-acute, chronic or symptomless infection of *Equidae*, characterized by viral persistence, intermittent fever, marked depression, petechiae in various organs, subcutaneous oedema, progressive debility, and frequently resulting in severe anaemia.

Hosts affected
Horses are the only animals which may become infected regularly but outbreaks in donkeys and mules have been recorded. Japanese workers claim that pigs may become infected occasionally. Man may also be susceptible and there are a number of unconfirmed reports of human infections characterized by anaemia, diarrhoea and skin eruptions. In one such case the patient's blood remained persistently infected for many weeks and was infective for horses.

History and distribution
Equine infectious anaemia was first described in France in 1843 and its viral aetiology recognized in 1904. By the end of the 19th century it had been reported in most countries in Continental Europe as well as in Japan, the U.S.A. and Canada. Outbreaks have also occurred in the U.S.S.R., parts of Africa, Central and South America, Australia, Korea, Viet-Nam and other Far Eastern countries. The disease is reported to exist in Pakistan, Burma and Malaya and was diagnosed in England in 1975. The prevalence of the disease is generally low and enzootics tend to be limited to fairly well-defined areas.

Morphology
In negatively-stained preparations of purified virus, the virions appear as spherical particles measuring 90–140 nm in diameter surrounded by an outer envelope. There is no clear evidence of a central component but in ultra-thin sections of infected cells the virus particles contain a pleomorphic nucleoid with a diameter of 40–63 nm.

In most electron micrographs the mature virus particles appear to be readily damaged during preparation of the specimens and spontaneous disruption of many of the virions is frequently observed. In most disrupted particles there is evidence of an unorganized meshwork of fine fibrillar material, or granular chains, comprising the inner region; but no distinct morphological pattern can be identified. All disrupted virions possess a well-defined outer envelope approximately 9 nm in thickness and in some of the particles the limiting membrane is partly covered with fine, short, radially-arranged projections not exceeding 5–6 nm in length.

Chemical composition.
Lack of inhibition by IUDR suggests that the viral nucleic acid is RNA. However, there is evidence of an early requirement for DNA synthesis after infection and it is suggested that the presence of an RNA-directed DNA polymerase is a necessary component for viral replication.

Physicochemical characters
The virus of equine infectious anaemia shows considerable resistance to heating, putrefaction, dessication and chemical disinfectants. Infected dried blood retains its virulence for several months provided it is protected from strong sunlight. Virus in serum or infected tissues remains infectious for one year when stored at $-20°C$ but loses its activity when heated at $60°C$ for 1 hour. Virus in serum is also inactivated in 1 hour by 2 per cent phenol but sera from infected horses retain their pathogenicity in 0·5 per cent phenol for 30 days at room temperature. Virus is readily inactivated when treated with 1/500 mercuric chloride for 30 minutes and by 4

per cent formalin in 5 minutes, but 0·1 per cent formalin takes up to 30 days to destroy the virus. It is also inactivated by 4 per cent NaOH in 15 minutes but hypochlorites, $KMnO_4$ and other oxidising agents are less effective. Recent reports indicate that the virus is ether-sensitive but trypsin-resistant.

Haemagglutination

A number of workers have reported that sera from infected horses agglutinate chicken, frog and human group O erythrocytes. In experimentally infected horses the highest haemagglutination titres are reached at 5–10 days after the rise in body temperature but are low in horses during the afebrile stage of the illness. On the other hand, recent investigations in America have failed to confirm the presence of either hot (37°C) or cold (4°C) haemagglutinins in sera of horses infected with equine infectious anaemia.

Antigenicity

The antigenicity of equine infectious anaemia virus has not been studied adequately, but most isolates appear to share a common group-specific antigen. Recent reports indicate that isolate-specific surface antigens may differ as a result of mutation of the agent *in vivo*.

Cultivation

Many attempts to propagate the virus of equine infectious anaemia on the chorioallantoic membrane, allantoic cavity and yolk sac of developing chicken embryos have failed but, in 1954, a group of workers claimed to have passaged the virus in eggs with consequent diminution of virulence for horses. However, negative results for the propagation of virus were indicated by haemagglutination tests and the validity of this report awaits confirmation.

Many unsuccessful attempts were also made to establish infection in plasma-clot and monolayer cell culture systems until it was discovered in 1960–61, that strains of equine infectious anaemia virus grow well in cultures of bone marrow cells or of leukocytes obtained from the circulating blood of horses, and produce cytopathic effects in both systems.

Electron micrographs of infected leukocyte cultures reveal that the viral particles are formed by budding and appear as clusters of mature virions within cytoplasmic vacuoles. The diameter of the virions is usually within the range of 90–150 nm, and each virus particle contains a distinct pleomorphic nucleoid.

Further studies on equine leukocyte cultures have shown that maximum inhibition of viral growth occurs when IUDR is added one hour after inoculation

of the virus, but the effect of the IUDR rapidly decreases and is almost ineffective when it is added 12 hours after inoculation. The fact that IUDR is effective only at the early stage of infection seems to suggest that DNA-mediated synthesis of RNA is a prerequisite of the formation of progeny virus. There is also evidence that the growth characters of equine infectious anaemia virus, including the reverse transcriptase enzyme, are similar to those of some RNA enveloped membrane-forming viruses, especially RNA-tumour viruses and members of the visna-maedi complex.

Pathogenicity

The disease is readily transmitted by the injection of infected blood, tissues or cell culture material by any parenteral route. The incubation period of the naturally occurring disease is usually 1–3 weeks but it may be longer, and periods of over 90 days have been recorded. The general condition of the animal and the severity of exposure appears to influence the period of incubation. The virus often persists for the life of the animal and the incidence of these latently infected horses is highest in areas where the disease is endemic.

In the acute form of the disease, which occurs most often when the infection has been recently introduced into a susceptible population, there is a sudden but fluctuating rise in temperature to 104–108°F (40–42°C). The main clinical signs are depression, anorexia, thirst, serous ocular and nasal discharge, and progressive weakness and debility. The visible mucous membranes appear congested and the presence of petechial haemorrhages, especially beneath the tongue, are considered to be characteristic of the disease. After a few days the fever may abate, giving the impression that the horse has recovered. Unfortunately, the animal usually remains a virus-carrier and renewed attacks of fever may occur at variable intervals thereafter. The acute illness lasts about 3–5 days and, if it does not terminate fatally, passes to the sub-acute or chronic form. In the sub-acute form, relapses of the febrile illness may occur at regular intervals of only 1–2 weeks, but the clinical signs are less severe. Oedematous swellings may develop in the lower trunk or limbs, and horses may die unexpectedly during a relapse. In the chronic form, attacks occur only at intervals of 1–3 months or longer, when signs of debility and anaemia develop. Few, if any, clinical signs are present in latently infected horses but severe attacks may be provoked at any time by intercurrent disease, bad weather, overwork, malnutrition or other adverse factors. Some horses may remain symptomless virus-carriers for very long periods (10–18 years) if not for life.

The disease spreads rapidly in highly susceptible

populations, particularly in areas where insect vectors are prevalent, and morbidity rates may approach 100 per cent in horses kept in crowded conditions. Mortality rates vary between 30–70 per cent, depending upon various environmental factors and the general condition of the animals, but figures of 50 per cent are not uncommon.

The only animals naturally susceptible are horses, asses and mules, but pigs may become affected occasionally. Several workers have reported successful transmission to sheep, goats, rabbits, mice and rats with few or no symptoms being produced, but other workers have been unsuccessful.

The most pronounced lesions in severe acute cases are numerous small haemorrhages in the mucous and serous membranes and on the surfaces of various internal organs and viscera. The subcutaneous tissues and other connective tissue structures are frequently infiltrated with gelatinous or serous fluids, and the abdominal lymph-nodes are swollen and haemorrhagic on section. There may also be enlargement of the liver, spleen, kidneys and heart, and the mucous membranes of the intestine and bladder may show haemorrhages. The bone marrow usually shows marked evidence of acute haemato-poiesis and there is replacement of yellow by red marrow in all the long bones.

Microscopical examination reveals marked erythrocytic destruction with lymphoid hyperplasia and reticulo-endothelial cell proliferation in the spleen and lymph nodes. The histological picture is characterized by extensive areas of necrosis accompanied by accumulations of macrophages and lymphocytes in the liver, kidneys, heart and other organs. In acute febrile cases, damage to the erythrocytes leads to the deposition of haemosiderin in the liver, spleen and lymph-nodes. Haemosiderin-containing cells can also be demonstrated in the circulation. These changes, together with characteristic nodule formation in the liver caused by reticulo-endothelial cell proliferation, are considered to be of diagnostic importance.

Ecology

Under natural conditions the disease spreads slowly and usually occurs in the sporadic form. However, severe epizootics may occur if conditions become favourable for the spread of the infection during the transportation and congregation of large numbers of horses, some of which are symptomless carriers. Equine infectious anaemia has a seasonal incidence and is most prevalent during late summer and autumn. Most outbreaks are established by the bite of blood-sucking insects. The commonest vectors are probably species of *Aëdes*, *Anopheles* and *Psorophora* but biting flies of the family *Tabanidae* and *Stomoxys calcitrans* may also play an important part in the spread of naturally occurring infections. There is no evidence, however, that the virus of equine infectious anaemia undergoes a replication cycle in the bodies of arthropod vectors and it is presumed that the virus is transmitted only mechanically by these insects. On the other hand, mechanical transmission has occurred as a result of the use of infected surgical instruments and syringe needles and it has been suggested that the disease became widely distributed in Africa from about 1904 onwards by the use of equine material for immunizing horses against African horse sickness. Other workers claim that infection may arise through open wounds, by droplet infection, or by the oral route. Vertical transmission also occurs, but not all foals from affected mares acquire the disease.

Diagnosis

Equine infectious anaemia is difficult to diagnose because of the wide range of its clinical and pathological manifestations and the present lack of simple and reliable laboratory tests. Intermittent fever, depression, progressive debility and oedema of the dependent parts are suggestive signs, and many field investigators consider that the presence of multiple sublingual haemorrhages is a reliable guide. Anaemia may be absent, transitory or progressive. Clinical, histological and pathological studies, when carried out separately, are of limited value but when combined with one another are often of considerable value in arriving at a diagnosis. In the past, the only reliable method of confirming a diagnosis was by inoculating 20 ml of whole blood or serum from an infected animal into young (8–12 months) healthy foals and observing whether characteristic symptoms developed. Unfortunately, these transmission experiments are expensive to perform and are generally handicapped by the frequency of latent infections in the test animals.

Complement-fixation tests have been extensively studied but they have not given consistent and reproducible results. Other serological procedures for the demonstration of specific viral antigen and antibody in the circulation have been described but these have also proved unreliable because of false positive reactions or failure to identify chronic cases of the disease. More recently, spleens from experimentally infected ponies, infected cell cultures or purified virus disrupted by ether treatment, have been used as antigen for detecting precipitating antibodies by the agar gel immunodiffusion (AGID) or Coggin's test. Preliminary observations suggest that the prospects for this method as a diagnostic test are good since almost all horses infected from 18 days to $5\frac{1}{2}$ years seem to have demonstrable precipitating antibodies in their sera. Complement-fixing antibodies appear 2–4 weeks post-infection, but the titres quickly fall and the sera become negative after several weeks.

It has recently been shown that labelled sera from clinically infected horses yield conjugates which give bright specific fluorescent staining of equine infectious anaemia antigen, and both direct and indirect immunofluorescence techniques have been developed and used for the demonstration of specific viral antigen. Studies of infected horse peripheral leukocyte cultures show that equine infectious anaemia viral antigen is present on the second day after inoculation, and appears as discrete dots or irregular clusters within the cytoplasm or as accumulations of material along the cell membrane.

Immunity

There is increasing evidence that a strong and lasting humoral antibody response is generated by the infected host and a number of serological tests have been used to show that specific antibodies probably co-exist with the virus in the circulation. Data regarding cellular immune responses are not available. It is generally believed that the lesions of equine infectious anaemia are immunologically mediated and that they are produced as a result of the formation of virus-antibody complexes which give rise to accumulations of sensitized lymphocytes in the tissues.

Control

No specific vaccination procedure is at present possible and none of the many experimental vaccines gives satisfactory results.

The symptomless carrier-animal probably constitutes the most serious source of infection and steps must be taken to prevent the introduction of carrier-horses into stables free from the disease. Thus, prompt and accurate diagnosis of clinically healthy and latently infected horses is essential. It is advisable, where possible, to slaughter all infected and suspected animals, and to dispose of the carcases by deep burial or cremation.

Borna disease

Synonyms

Meningoencephalomyelitis enzootica equorum: Seuchenhafte Gehirn-Rückenmarkentzündung der Pferde: Bornasche Krankheit: Koppkrankheit: Enfermedad de Borna: encéphalomyélite enzootique: maladie de Borna: Enzootic encephalomyelitis of horses: Near East equine encephalomyelitis.

Definition

An acute or sub-acute, non-purulent, often fatal viral encephalomyelitis of solipeds and occasionally of sheep.

Hosts affected

The disease mainly affects horses and sheep, but a number of unconfirmed reports of spontaneous outbreaks in cattle and roe deer have been recorded. Rabbits, rats, mice and guinea-pigs are susceptible to experimental infection. Human infections have not been reported.

History and distribution

The disease known as 'hot head' was first described in Würtemburg in 1813 but only a proportion of the cases reported were probably meningoencephalomyelitis enzootica equorum. Other outbreaks occurred in Europe during the years 1824–28 and were described as 'nerve fever'. In Saxony, typical cases of the disease developed with increasing frequency from 1878 onwards, and between 1894–96 an unusually severe epizootic affected horses in the district of Borna. The disease continues to occur in Germany and is responsible for heavy economic losses especially among horses engaged in agricultural work. The incidence of Borna disease in other countries is not known but sporadic cases have been observed in Poland, Rumania, Russia, Albania, Libya, Syria and Egypt. A virus causing equine encephalomyelitis in Nigeria and the Middle East may be the same.

Properties of the virus

Although the causative virus was first isolated in 1926, little information is available as to its morphological and physicochemical properties. The diameter of the virus particle has been estimated by filtration and ultraviolet microscopy to be between 85 and 140 nm, but a report in 1967 suggests that it is capable of passing 20 nm membrane filters.

The virus is highly resistant to drying and may survive for at least 300 days, or even for 3 years if protected from light. It is susceptible to high temperatures and is inactivated in 10 minutes by heating to 70°C. It retains its infectivity in tap water for 30 days and in sterilized cows' milk for over 100 days. The commonly used disinfectants do not readily destroy the virus and 1 per cent carbolic acid may take as long as 3–4 weeks to do so.

Antigenicity

There is only one antigenic type of Borna disease virus and all known strains are immunologically distinct from Eastern, Western and Venezuelan equine encephalitis, Japanese B-encephalitis, Murray Valley encephalitis and other viruses causing similar CNS infections of horses. Neutralizing and complement-fixing antibodies can be detected in the sera soon after the first clinical signs appear but the titres are generally very low or may be absent.

Cultivation

Recent reports indicate that Borna disease virus can be propagated on the chorioallantoic membrane of 11-day-old fertile hens' eggs incubated at 35°C, and on cell cultures of lamb testis and monkey kidney.

Monkey kidney (MS) cell monolayers inoculated with the Würtemburg strain of Borna virus and incubated at 31–32°C remain apparently normal for 4–5 days post-infection but, after a further 24 hours' incubation at 37°C, numerous pin-head plaques appear on the unstained monolayer. Continued incubation at 37°C results in enlargement and coalescence of the discrete plaques until eventually all the infected cells fall off the glass. In coverslip monolayer cultures stained by May-Grünwald Giemsa, the infected nuclei appear swollen and the nucleoplasm contains several brick-red, moderately defined inclusions. Also present within the nuclei are clumps of dense basophilic chromatin set in a pale or colourless background. Later, there is marginal massing of the chromatin giving the periphery of the nucleus a beaded appearance. Supernatant cell culture fluids produce typical Borna disease when inoculated into experimental animals.

Pathogenicity

The incubation period of the natural disease is about 30 days but in young experimental rabbits an encephalitis develops 15–20 days post-inoculation, followed by death in 5–17 days. Affected horses show slight fever (38°C), anorexia, excessive salivation, frequent yawning, lassitude and constipation. As the clinical picture develops there is gradually increasing drowsiness, followed by a period of restlessness, ill-temper, biting or kicking, attacks of giddiness and excitability. Reflex irritability is increased and the animal is easily startled and may fall into convulsions. Paralytic signs appear early in the disease and frequently take the form of generalized paresis. The virus may produce similar symptoms in sheep. In horses, the duration of the disease is usually 1–3 weeks and the prognosis is invariably unfavourable. In animals showing symptoms of encephalitis, the mortality rate averages 90 per cent or more and even in milder outbreaks it seldom falls below 75–80 per cent.

Rabbits up to 5 days old are very susceptible, and a highly fatal infection can be induced by intracerebral inoculation and by various other routes also. Monkeys, guinea-pigs and rats are also susceptible to experimental infection and develop symptoms of somnolence, salivation, paralysis, coma and death. Cats, dogs and ferrets are probably resistant, and human infections are unknown. In horses, virus is present in the saliva and nasal secretions during the acute illness, and serum from surviving horses may harbour the virus for 6 months after recovery.

Histologically, lesions of meningoencephalomyelitis are found in the central nervous system and characteristic Cowdry type B inclusions, the Joest-Degen intranuclear bodies, are present in the nerve cells particularly those of the hippocampus and olfactory lobes. In contrast to the development of Cowdry's type A inclusions, the nuclear changes associated with the formation of Joest-Degen type B inclusions are less dramatic. In the early stages, local accumulations of acidophilic material occur but the rest of the nucleus is unaffected. As the inclusion develops and enlarges, other nuclear structures tend to accumulate around the periphery of the nuclear membrane. In affected ganglion cells stained by Lentz's modification of Mann's method, the Joest-Degen inclusions are clearly visible as bright red, spherical or oval bodies of different sizes, each surrounded by a colourless halo against the bluish-violet background of the nucleus. They are quite distinct from the nucleoli which do not have a clear halo and stain a deep violet colour.

Ecology

In Europe, Borna disease tends to occur annually or at intervals of a few years, and usually only agricultural horses are affected. The outbreaks first appear in early Spring, reach a peak in warm, damp weather during May and June and usually disappear in the autumn.

In the natural disease, spread of infection is believed to result from contamination of food and water by virus shed in the saliva and nasal secretions during the acute illness. There is also evidence that the virus is excreted in the milk and urine. Nevertheless, the striking fall in the number of new cases during the months of August and September suggests that arthropod vectors may play an important part in the spread of infection. In recent years, Borna disease virus has been isolated from the brains of herons and other wild birds, as well as from ticks of the genera *Hyalomma*, *Dermacentor* and *Ornithodoros*. It has also been transmitted transovarially in *Hyalomma anatolicum*. It is possible, therefore, that the causative agent of Borna disease is an arthorpod-borne virus, but lack of information about its characteristics precludes it from being classified with togaviruses or other arboviruses.

Diagnosis

Accurate diagnosis is very difficult in the early stages of the disease, particularly in isolated cases in non-endemic areas. Even in fully developed cases, the disease can only be suspected from the clinical signs.

Specific laboratory tests are as yet unsatisfactory since the titres of neutralizing and complement-fixing antibodies in the sera of affected animals are generally low or absent. However, the presence of a complement-fixing antigen in the brains of infected rabbits may provide confirmation of the diagnosis. At present, the most reliable methods of diagnosis are the histological demonstration of Joest-Degen intranuclear inclusions in the large ganglion cells of Ammon's horn and the isolation of the causal virus from rabbits inoculated intracerebrally with brain emulsion from suspected cases. The recent successful propagation of Borna disease virus in cell culture should greatly facilitate confirmatory diagnosis in the future.

Control

Animals recovered from Borna disease are immune, but the duration of the immunity is not known. Thus, specific prophylaxis may be practised by active immunization of exposed animals using infected rabbit or horse brain tissues inactivated with phenol or phenol-glycerol. A single dose of vaccine administered subcutaneously during the autumn months is believed to provide protection for about a year. Vaccination has proved successful in sheep but there are differing opinions on its efficacy in horses.

In enzootic areas horses should not be fed and watered together in large numbers and should not be kept in contact with sheep or cattle.

Further reading

BOULANGER P., BANNISTER G.L. AND CARRIER S.P. (1972) Equine infectious anemia: preparation of a liquid antigen extract for the agar-gel immunodiffusion and complement-fixation tests. *Canadian Journal of Comparative Medicine*, **36**, 116.

COGGINS L., NORCROSS N.L. AND NUSBAUM S. (1972) Diagnosis of equine infectious anemia by immunodiffusion test. *American Journal of Veterinary Research*, **33**, 11.

DAUBNEY R. (1967) Viral encephalitis of equines and domestic ruminants in the Near East — Part II. *Research in Veterinary Science*, **8**, 419

DAUBNEY R. AND MAHLAU E.A. (1967) Viral encephalitis of equines and domestic ruminants in the Near East — Part I. *Research in Veterinary Science*, **8**, 375.

HENSON, J.B. AND McGUIRE, T.C. (1974) Equine infectious anaemia. *Progress in Medical Virology*, **18**, 143.

ISHII S. (1963) Equine infectious anaemia or swamp fever. *Advances in Veterinary Science*, **8**, 263.

ISHITANI R. (1970) Equine infectious anemia. *National Institute of Animal Health Quarterly*, **10**, Supplement 1–28.

Johnson A.W. (1966) Equine infectious anaemia: an annotation. *Veterinary Bulletin*, **36**, 465.

KOBAYASHI K. AND KONO Y. (1967) Propagation and titration of equine infectious anaemia virus in horse leukocyte culture. *National Institute of Animal Health Quarterly*, **7**, 8.

KONO Y. (1969) Viraemia and immunological responses in horses infected with equine infectious anaemia virus. *National Institute of Animal Health Quarterly*, **9**, 1.

MYERS W.L., SEGRE D AND EL-ZEIN A. (1969) Equine infectious anaemia. Reports of progress in research. *Journal of the American Veterinary Medical Association*, **155**, 352.

ROSSDALE P.D., HUNT M.D.N., PEACE C.K., HOPES R. AND RICKETTS S.W. (1975) A case of equine infectious anaemia in Newmarket. *Veterinary Record*, **97**, 207.

RYDEN L (1975) On equine infectious anemia (EIA): A serological and field study. Monograph, Royal Veterinary College, Stockholm.

STEIN C.D., MOTT L.O. AND GATES D.W. (1955). Some observations on carriers of equine infectious anaemia. *Journal of the American Veterinary Medical Association*, **126**, 277.

CHAPTER 52

POXVIRUSES

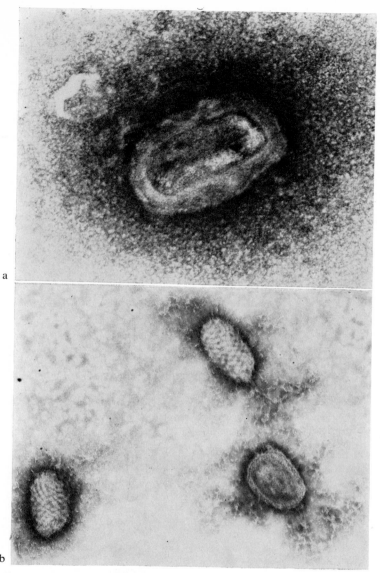

a

b

Electron micrographs of poxvirus particles stained with phosphotungstic acid.

52.1a Structure of intact cow pox virion showing the central nucleoid protected by a thick multilayered covering membrane, × 100 000.

52.1b Orf virus particles in specimen prepared from a lesion on the lips of a young lamb. Notice the criss-crossing arrangement of the nucleoprotein strands on the surfaces of two of the virus particles. In the case of the third virion (lower right) penetration of the stain has revealed the central nucleoid and the double layered covering membrane, but does not show the characteristic 'ball of wool' morphology of Orf and other parapoxviruses, × 50 000.

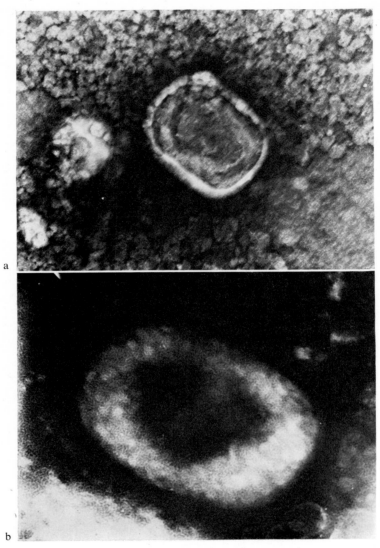

Negatively stained preparations of myxoma virus.

52.2a   The virions are usually brick-shaped, with a coiled inner component, × 130 000.

52.2b   Occasionally, the arrangement of the surface tubules gives the particle a beaded appearance, × 200 000.

CHAPTER 52

Poxviruses

The term 'pock' was originally applied to the pustular eruption of the skin associated with smallpox in man. The name smallpox was introduced in the 15th and 16th centuries to distinguish the disease from 'large pox' or syphilis.

Poxviruses are the largest of the 'true' viruses and are readily distinguished by their characteristic large, brick-shaped morphology, but some members are slightly smaller and more oval in appearance. All are related immunologically by a common internal antigen and can be divided into sub-groups or genera on the basis of their more specific antigens, their morphology and their natural hosts. They produce spontaneous disease in both man and animals, including birds although, surprisingly, they have not been identified in dogs and cats. Almost all mammals have their own specific types of poxviruses but some have become adapted to different hosts and, as a result, it is often extremely difficult to determine how many of them should be regarded as distinct entities.

In 1974, the International Committee on the Taxonomy of Viruses decided that the family *Poxviridae* would consist of a number of genera, namely *Orthopoxvirus* (formerly Subgenus A), *Parapoxvirus* (formerly Subgenus B), *Capripoxvirus* (formerly Subgenus C), *Avipoxvirus* (formerly Subgenus D) and *Leporipoxvirus* (formerly Subgenus E). Members of a sixth genus named *Entomopoxvirus*, are limited to arthropods and do not multiply in vertebrate hosts. It should be noted that some poxviruses including horse pox, swine pox, camel pox and molluscum contagiosum, cannot yet be placed in any recognized genus and, in the present text, are grouped as unclassified poxviruses. A classification of the animal poxviruses is shown in Table 38.1, pages 414–5.

Morphology

The mature viral particles, originally called elementary bodies, are somewhat rounded, oval or brick-shaped when seen in dried films under the electron microscope, but are ellipsoid when observed in ultrathin sections of infected cells. (Plates 37.4a, b, facing p. 431). The virions measure approximately 250–350 nm in length by 200–250 nm in width. They have a complex structure consisting of an electron-dense pepsin resistant central body (100–200 nm across) the nucleoid, surrounded by a highly convoluted double outer membrane (20–30 nm thick) of phospholipids, cholesterol and protein. The outer envelope of the poxvirus virion is an unique structure since it is assembled inside the viroplasmic matrix of the cytoplasm and not on the cell membrane. The nucleoid may appear in the form of a biconcave disc or dumb-bell with a rounded 'lateral body' occupying each concavity. In negatively-stained preparations the central body appears to contain dense filamentous material, often in the shape of the letter 'S'; but there is no helical or cubical nucleocapsid. Immediately surrounding the nucleoid is a wide, clear middle zone showing a palisaded structure in the form of a fringe of fine, short, regularly arranged spikes. The surface of the outer membrane contains large numbers of tubular protein threads formed from loops of filaments 8–15 nm wide. The arrangement of the threads may differ in the various subgroups giving the virions a mulberry-like surface, a ball of wool appearance, etc. (Plates 52.1b, 52.2b, facing pp. 676b–677). However in many negatively-stained preparations the surface components may not be clearly visible due to the deep penetration and masking effects of the stain. The structural components of a poxvirus are shown diagrammatically in Fig. 52.1 p. 678.

Physicochemical characters

The chemical composition of a poxvirus resembles that of a bacterium in that it contains protein, DNA, phospholipid, neutral fat, carbohydrate, copper, flavin and biotin. Estimates of extractable lipid range from 5 per cent in vaccinia to 27 per cent in fowl pox virus, but much of this is not 'essential' lipid and the members vary in their sensitivity to

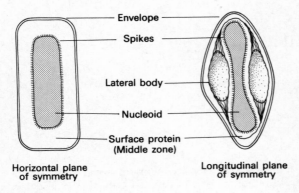

Horizontal plane
of symmetry

Longitudinal plane
of symmetry

Fig. 52.1 Diagrammatical illustration of the structural
components of a poxvirus.

ether. For example, ortho- and most avipoxviruses
are ether-resistant but para-, capri- and lepori-
poxviruses are ether sensitive. The bulk of the
nucleic acid is double stranded DNA having a
very high molecular weight ($120-240 \times 10^6$ daltons),
sufficient to code for several hundred proteins.
Within the central core are four enzymes including
a DNA-dependent RNA polymerase (transcriptase),
a nucleotide phosphohydrolase and two DNases.
The transcriptase catalyses the synthesis of early
mRNA in the intact core, even before the DNA
genome is released or uncoated. Thus, poxviruses,
like other DNA viruses induce DNA-dependent
DNA polymerase, but they resemble many RNA
viruses in that they carry their own DNA-dependent
RNA polymerase.

Poxviruses may withstand drying for months,
even when held at room temperature, and they can be
stored at $-70°C$. for many years. They are relatively
resistant to heat and in the dry state can withstand
$100°C$. for 5–10 minutes, but are destroyed in the
moist state at $60°C$. for 10 minutes. They are also
fairly resistant to common disinfectants but 50 per
cent alcohol or 0.01 per cent $KMnO_4$ inactivates
the virus within one hour at room temperature.

Haemagglutination

Extracts of cells infected with smallpox, vaccinia,
mousepox (ectromelia) and cowpox viruses agglutinate red blood cells from turkeys and some but
not all fowls. The haemagglutinin is a lipoprotein
complex that is separable from the virions by
centrifugation and, therefore, does not occur in
purified preparations of the virus. It has a diameter
of about 65 nm, withstands boiling but is inactivated
by lecithin. It does not elute spontaneously from
agglutinated erythrocytes, and antibodies that

inhibit poxvirus haemagglutination do not neutralize
infectious virus.

Antigenic properties

The antigenic structure of poxviruses is complex and
numerous viral antigens can be revealed by complement-fixation, virus neutralization, haemagglutination-inhibition and precipitation tests. For
example, up to 20 antigens capable of forming
precipitin lines with antiviral sera can be detected in
the vaccinia-variola (orthopox) group and in the
myxoma-fibroma (leporipox) group of viruses.
Moreover, members of the orthopox group of
viruses are very similar antigenically and differ
by not more than one antigen by this test.
Studies of the antigenic relationships among poxviruses have revealed two major groups of antigens:
1) an antigen that is found in extracts of infected
cells or dissociates spontaneously from viral particles, called the LS antigen, and 2) an antigenic
fraction which can be released from the core of the
viral particle by weak alkaline digestion and is
termed the nucleoprotein (NP) antigen. The LS
antigen contains two immunogenic groups on a
common structure: a heat-labile (L) antigen which
is inactivated at $60°C$. and a heat-stable (S) antigen
which withstands even $90-100°C$. The L and S
components occur combined in solution and constitute part of the surface of the viral particle,
but antisera prepared against both antigenic groups
do not neutralize viral infectivity. The NP antigen
on the other hand, contains a group-reacting component common to at least one member of each
genus and is situated in the core of the virion,
together with a subgroup-specific component located
on the surface of the virus which induces the
formation of neutralizing antibody.

Cultivation

Most but not all poxviruses grow readily in
embryonated hens' eggs and produce 'pocks' or
nodular focal lesions on the chorioallantoic membrane. (Plates 42.3a, d, facing p. 480). The
pocks vary in size, shape and colour according to the
nature of the infecting virus, and their appearance
can be useful for the rapid identification of a virus
in clinical specimens. Some poxviruses including
variola and myxoma form small, discrete, gray-white
pocks whereas others such as cowpox and neurovaccinia show a tendency to invade the underlying
blood vessels and produce haemorrhagic necrotic
pocks. Stained sections of infected membranes
show ballooning degeneration of the affected cells
and round or oval acidophilic cytoplasmic inclusions.

Poxviruses can be propagated in cultured cells of
many different types and from a number of animal
species, e.g. bovine kidney, rabbit kidney, HeLa

cells and chick embryo fibroblasts. Cytopathic effects are not always obvious but infected cells may haemadsorb, and stained monolayer preparations usually contain cytoplasmic and nuclear inclusions. (Plate 42.10d, facing p. 481 and plate 52.5a, facing p. 708).

Pathogenicity

Poxviruses are pathogenic for man and many species of animals including birds, but some of the viruses differ widely in the range of host species they infect. For example, myxoma affects rabbits only, whereas cowpox can develop in several species. Poxviruses tend to generalise in the animal body and the consequent viraemia may give rise to widespread skin eruptions (papules, vesicles, pustules and scabs) and foci of necrosis in the viscera. The viruses of orf and fowl pox are essentially proliferative rather than pustular and produce marked hyperplasia of the dermis whereas others, such as fibroma virus of rabbits, produce benign tumours in cells of connective tissue origin.

Most poxvirus infections are characterized by the formation of multiple, round or oval, Feulgen positive (DNA-containing), intracytoplasmic inclusions corresponding to the classical Guarnieri bodies of variola and vaccinia. In Giemsa stained methanol fixed preparations, the inclusions appear reddish purple in colour whereas in cells fixed with Bouin's solution and stained with haematoxylin-eosin they assume a haematoxylinophilic tinge. They contain large amounts of virus-specific antigen when examined by fluorescent antibody staining, and have recently been named Kato B-type poxvirus inclusions. In addition to the B-type inclusions, cowpox, fowl pox, ectromelia and some other poxviruses produce a larger, more spherical cytoplasmic body which stains pale blue with Giemsa and an intense bright red colour surrounded by a clear halo with haematoxylin-eosin. They are Feulgen negative, do not show any antigenicity when stained by immunofluorescence techniques and are termed Kato A-type poxvirus inclusions. Development of these A-type inclusions is always subsequent to B-type formation, and they are never produced in the absence of B-type inclusions. It should be noted that basophilic intracytoplasmic and intranuclear inclusions are found from time to time in myxoma, swine pox and some other poxvirus infections but their significance is obscure.

Because of their well recognized characteristics, poxviruses are very suitable for genetic studies and when 2 closely related poxviruses are grown in eggs, cell cultures or animals, hybrids or recombinant forms having the properties of both 'parents' may be formed. It is reasonable to suppose that this may be one method by which new strains of virus arise naturally.

Certain strains of poxviruses may also be used to illustrate the phenomenon of reactivation whereby strains inactivated by heat or 6 M urea may have their activity restored within cells in which another poxvirus is growing. Thus, rabbits inoculated with a mixture of heat-inactivated myxomavirus and live fibromavirus develop myxomatosis and die from frank clinical disease. Reactivation, which is confined to poxviruses, can be produced by members of the same or different sub-groups but will not take place if the DNA of the inactivated virus has been destroyed. It seems, therefore, that heat or urea treatment alters the nature of the protein coat protecting the nucleic acid core, and that the live reactivating viral particles initiate the enzymic process of uncoating the inactivated virus. In this way, the intact DNA is liberated from the denatured viral coat permitting initiation of replication and the production of infectious progeny virus. Reactivation, unlike recombination, is not a true genetic phenomenon since it involves the protein coat and not the DNA genetic core. However, genetic recombination may also ensue when reactivation is induced by members of the same immunological group (homeoreactivation), but not when it is accomplished by a virus from a different immunological group (heteroactivation).

Transmission

Spread of infection is commonly by the respiratory route as in human smallpox, or through skin abrasions as in orf of sheep. Swine pox, however, is known to be transmitted mechanically by arthropods although a developmental cycle in these vectors is thought to be unlikely.

Diagnosis

Many poxvirus infections can be rapidly diagnosed by direct demonstration of virus particles in scrapings from maculopapules, vesicle fluid or crusts when viewed under the electron microscope. (Plates 52.1a, b, between pp. 676b–677).

The common pox group antigen is demonstrable when the patient's lesions are used as antigen and tested for complement-fixation with suitably prepared antisera, or for lines of precipitation by agar gel diffusion.

In a high percentage of cases the causative virus can be isolated on the chorioallantoic membrane of chick embryos and observed for the development of 'pocks' (paravaccinia and orf viruses are notable exceptions) or on susceptible cell culture systems and examined for the presence of cytoplasmic inclusions or other cellular changes. (Plates 42.3a, d, facing p. 480 and Plates 42.10c, d, facing p. 481).

The specificity of the reaction can also be confirmed by immunofluorescence. In other instances it may be necessary to inoculate the suspected material into susceptible experimental animals. (Plate 52.5d, facing p. 708).

Serum antibody can be detected by various serological tests including complement-fixation, neutralization, haemagglutination-inhibition and immunodiffusion, where applicable.

Control

Both live unmodified and live attenuated virus vaccines are useful for the control of many poxvirus infections.

ORTHOPOXVIRUS

Smallpox

Definition

Smallpox (variola major) is an acute infectious viral disease characterized by severe systemic involvement and an extensive, often confluent, rash affecting the face and extremities more than the trunk (centrifugal distribution). The case mortality rate varies from 5 per cent (discrete rash) to over 40 per cent (confluent rash).

A mild form of smallpox, Alastrim (variola minor) also occurs, but the rash is less extensive and the lesions are shallower or more superficial. The mortality rate is low and seldom exceeds 0.5 per cent.

History and distribution

Severe epidemics of smallpox have been recorded from the earliest times and an eighteenth century writer claimed that one-tenth of all mankind was killed, crippled or disfigured by the disease. In recent years, smallpox has been rare in Europe and North America but epidemics have been reported in Central and South America, Africa and Asia, with India and Pakistan being the most severely involved. At the present time, 1976, very few pockets of infection are known to exist and, as a result of the World Health Organization's massive international immunization programme, there is reason to believe that the disease will soon cease to exist.

Properties of the virus

Variola virus is a member of the sub-group which includes vaccinia, cowpox, buffalo pox, rabbit pox, monkey pox and mouse pox (ectromelia). It is very stable and withstands drying for months, and has survived in skin crusts kept at room temperature for over a year. Vesicle fluid remains active for years if stored in sealed ampoules in the cold. The virus resists most common disinfectants, is moderately resistant to phenol, but is very susceptible to $KMnO_4$ (0.01 per cent) and other oxidising agents. It is not readily inactivated by ether.

Haemagglutination

The haemagglutinin is not an integral part of the virion and can be obtained free from the virus particles. Agglutination of fowl red blood cells can be inhibited by convalescent smallpox serum.

Cultivation

The virus grows well on the chorioallantoic membrane of 7 to 13-day-old embryonated eggs and produces small non-haemorrhagic 'pocks' which are dome-shaped but less necrotic than those of vaccinia. Growth is also possible by the yolk-sac and amniotic routes but allantoic inoculation is unsuccessful. Variola major (smallpox) produces pocks in eggs incubated at 38°–38.5°C., unlike variola minor (alastrim) which will only do so below 38°C.

Smallpox virus can be grown in a wide range of cell culture systems giving rise to slowly developing cellular changes which become maximal in 5–8 days. The cytopathic effects include syncytial formation, lengthening of cytoplasmic processes and 'ballooning'. Many of the infected cells contain basophilic and eosinophilic intracytoplasmic inclusions. Some of the effects may be due to a 'toxic' action for which living virus is not necessary. Infected cells may haemadsorb erythrocytes from about 50 per cent of fowls.

The natural host range of variola virus is restricted to man and monkeys. Although it cannot be propagated serially in rabbits it can initiate local skin lesions; and the production of keratitis and Guarnieri inclusion bodies in the eyes of inoculated rabbits (Paul's test) was formerly used in diagnosis. Unweaned mice are uniformly susceptible and fatal infections can be induced by the intranasal, intraperitoneal and intracerebral routes.

Pathogenicity

The incubation period of smallpox is usually about 12 days, with limits of 9–15 days. The disease is sudden in onset and is characterized by fever, headache, pain in the back and limbs, vomiting and prostration. The extensive, often confluent rash appears about the 3rd to 5th day of the illness; the skin lesions passing through the typical macular, papular, vesicular and pustular stages. Scabbing occurs about the 12th day and crusts begin to separate after approximately 3 weeks.

Virus is present in the upper respiratory tract of the patient and infection is probably airborne from the mouth and nose early in the disease (i.e. from the 11th or 12th day after contact and just before the onset of symptoms), and later from dried crusts and contaminated bed linen. Patients remain contagious until convalescence but immune persons who develop only a few lesions and scarcely feel ill are highly infectious to others.

Diagnosis

The laboratory diagnosis of smallpox includes direct electron and light microscopy of specimens taken in the papular and vesicular stages of the illness. The presence of large brick-shaped virus particles readily distinguishes smallpox virus from chickenpox and other herpesviruses. Gutstein's or Nicolau's stains may be used to show the small, even-sized elementary particles, and small multiple cytoplasmic inclusions (Guarnieri bodies) are present in the epithelial cells.

Viral antigens can be demonstrated in suspected material by complement-fixation, immunodiffusion and immunofluorescence tests; but these only detect common pox group antigens.

To distinguish between variola and vaccinia the virus should be isolated on the chorioallantoic membrane of embryonated hens' eggs and observed in 2–3 days for small white pocks which grow at 38–38.5°C. Alastrim does not grow at this temperature and vaccinia produces large grey fluffy pocks with necrotic centres. Cell cultures can also be employed to differentiate variola from other poxviruses, such as vaccinia and cowpox, since neither variola major nor variola minor are able to form plaques on monolayers of chick embryo fibroblasts.

Control

Vaccination is carried out with living vaccinia virus propagated on the skin of the abdominal wall of calves or sheep and is administered by scarification or multiple pressure. The 'lymph' collected from the resulting vesicles is usually preserved in glycerol (to prevent bacterial contamination) but freeze-dried vaccines with better keeping properties are available.

A vesicle appears at the 7th–8th day and the reaction reaches maximal intensity at the 12th day. Since there is a close immunological relationship between vaccinia and variola viruses, vaccination confers a solid immunity against smallpox which lasts for about 3 years, but declines at a variable rate over the next 7–10 years.

Unfortunately, vaccination is not without risk and encephalitis or post-infectious encephalomyelitis may result in about one per 100,000 vaccinates. A second form of complication is generalized vaccinia, in which the virus causes lesions outside the vaccinated area, and is seen mainly in infants. Although serious complications are rare they have, nevertheless, aroused doubts about the wisdom of continuing the policy of routine vaccination of young children in Britain and certain other countries free from the disease.

Vaccination is only of value therapeutically if administered in the early days of the incubation period but recent results suggest that thiosemicarbazones may prevent smallpox even if given late in the incubation period.

Vaccinia

There is considerable doubt as to the origin of the vaccinia strain used for vaccination against smallpox in man. Variola virus modified by repeated passage through rabbits and calves has been suggested, but an alternative claim that it originated from cow pox is, perhaps, more likely. It is even possible that Jenner's original coxpox strain that was used to confer immunity in human patients became contaminated with smallpox and that vaccinia is, in fact, a stable recombinant of both types of virus. Detailed studies of the antigenic structure of poxviruses seem to indicate that standard vaccinia virus is more closely related antigenically to smallpox than to cowpox virus.

Properties of the virus

Vaccinia or, as it is sometimes called, *Poxvirus officinale* does not occur in nature but is known to exist in the laboratory in 2 forms. The first of these is dermo-vaccinia, which produces a nodule on intradermal inoculation into rabbits, does not grow well if injected intracerebrally, and is used for producing vaccine 'lymph' in the skin of the abdomen of calves, sheep and rabbits. The second is neuro-vaccinia which is neurotropic and gives rise to fatal encephalitis when inoculated intracerebrally into rabbits.

The elementary bodies or mature viral particles, sometimes called Paschen bodies, were first described by Buist of Edinburgh in 1887, and are visible in carefully prepared Giemsa-stained films of vesicular fluid by light microscopy.

The morphology, chemical composition and physicochemical characteristics of vaccinia are similar to those of most other poxviruses.

Antigenic properties

The viruses of vaccinia, variola, cowpox and ectromelia are very closely related serologically but differences can be detected by neutralization tests on the chorioallantoic membranes, agar gel diffusion and indirect complement-fixation.

The virus particle contains heat-labile (L) and heat-stable (S) surface antigens as well as a nucleoprotein (NP) antigen in the central core: but adsorption of immune serum with all 3 antigens fails to remove its neutralizing antibody.

Haemagglutination

After incubation for an hour at 37°C., preparations of vaccinia virus agglutinate the red blood cells of turkeys and about 50 per cent of fowls. The haemagglutinin is a heat-stable lipoprotein complex, which is distinct from the LS surface antigens but does not exhibit receptor destroying (neuraminidase) activity.

Cultivation

Vaccinia virus grows well on the chorioallantoic membrane of embryonated hens' eggs and 'pocks' develop up to a temperature of 40.5°C. Different strains of virus produce different types of pocks: most are large, white or greyish-white in colour with necrotic centres but those produced by neurovaccinia may be haemorrhagic. The yolk sac, amniotic and allantoic cavities may also be used but these are less sensitive than the chorioallantoic membrane.

Vaccinia grows readily in a variety of cell culture systems including primate cells, chick embryo, bovine embryo and kidney, rabbit kidney, HeLa cells and other types of cell-lines. Growth occurs more rapidly and in a wider range of animal cells than does variola virus. The cytopathic effects of vaccinia virus appear 18–24 hours post inoculation and include syncytial formation, reticulum formation due to lengthening of the cytoplasmic processes, 'ballooning' degeneration and the development of both basophilic and acidophilic inclusions in the cytoplasm of the infected cells. (Plate 42.10d facing p. 481).

The replicative cycle of vaccinia virus presents the unusual situation that mRNA and DNA are synthesized in the cytoplasm instead of the nucleus (Chapter 31). Indeed, poxviruses are the only DNA-containing viruses to replicate solely within the cytoplasm.

Many animals, including man, are susceptible to vaccinia; particularly rabbits, calves and sheep.

Pathogenicity

Generalized vaccinia may occur in children following vaccination and an even rarer condition, progressive vaccinia, has been described in hypogammaglobulinaemic patients and is usually fatal. Infection may be accidentally acquired by laboratory workers or transmitted by recently vaccinated persons to susceptible human contacts or, possibly, by farmworkers to milking cows.

Control

Laboratory workers should be vaccinated before handling the virus.

A number of substances have proved active against vaccinia infections including methisazone and other thiosemicarbazones, rifampicin and even IUDR (5-iodo-2′-deoxyuridine).

Cowpox

Definition

A benign disease of cattle affecting principally the skin of the udder and teats.

Hosts affected

The disease occurs naturally in milking cows but the virus, like vaccinia, has a wide host range both in the field and in laboratory animals. It is an occupational disease of man.

History and distribution

Until the middle of the 19th century, cowpox appears to have been a common disease which frequently spread from the teats of infected cows to man by direct contact during milking. Conversely, infection occasionally originated in cattle from contact with milkers who had been recently vaccinated against smallpox. These outbreaks caused by vaccinia virus were clinically indistinguishable from natural cases of cowpox.

The disease is now rare and little is known about its geographical distribution. However, sporadic cases still occur in the U.K. and other European countries and possibly in North America.

Properties of the virus

The morphological, chemical and physicochemical characteristics of cowpox virus are very similar to those of vaccinia. (Plate 52.2 a facing p. 677).

Haemagglutination

As with vaccinia, the haemagglutinins of cowpox virus clump turkey and fowl red blood cells, but to lower titres.

Antigenic properties

Cowpox virus is closely related immunologically to vaccinia and smallpox viruses. The minor antigenic differences are distinguishable by complement-fixation, agar gel diffusion and antibody-adsorption tests.

Cultivation

Cowpox virus grows well in several types of cell culture systems and produces plaques on monolayers of chick embryo cells as well as human and bovine kidney cells.

The biological properties of cowpox and vaccinia viruses are very similar, but the following host reactions to cowpox virus are distinctive: 1) pocks are formed more slowly on the chorioallantoic membrane and rather less haemagglutinin is produced, 2) the virus tends to invade mesodermal tissues involving the capillary endothelium causing large, deep red haemorrhagic pocks (Plate 42.3d, facing p. 480), but not at temperatures above 40°C. Occasionally, variant strains have been isolated, producing white pocks, 3) the intracytoplasmic inclusions in infected cells are larger and more intensely acidophilic than the Guarnieri bodies of vaccinia and variola (Plate 42.10d, facing p. 481) and 4) in contrast to vaccinia, there is less rapid epithelial necrosis in experimentally infected animals; keratitis is produced more slowly in rabbits and the lesions on the cornea are smaller.

Pathogenicity

After an incubation period of 3–7 days, affected cattle may show slight fever and anorexia, but in many cases these prodromal symptoms pass unnoticed. During milking the udder may be sensitive to the touch and the teats swollen and warmer than usual. Small congested spots (roseola stage) appear on the teats or adjacent areas of the udder and quickly develop into the papular stage with small oval or circular lesions about the size of a lentil or pea. By the seventh day, flattened vesicles appear in the centre of the dark red papules. These contain clear lymph and are red, blue or yellow-brown in colour. After a few days, the vesicles show a central depression with a raised firm edge (umbilication) unless ruptured earlier as a result of trauma during milking. This is quickly followed by suppuration and the formation of dry crusts. The swelling and induration slowly subside and the crusts fall off after about a fortnight, leaving white depressed cicatrices in the skin. The number of vesicles varies from 1 or 2 up to about 15 or 20, and they appear in crops at intervals of a few days, the later vesicles being smaller than the earlier ones. The vesicles are generally discrete but they may coalesce giving rise to large moist areas of denuded skin that are very painful to the touch. In the male animal, cowpox virus may affect the cutaneous tissue of the scrotum. In dairy cows, secondary bacterial infections may give rise to mastitis but, apart from such complications, the disease is generally mild and is rarely associated with systemic upset.

Recovery from the natural disease usually results in an active immunity, but little definite information is available concerning the duration of the immunity since some animals suffer from a second or third attack. In general, herds in which an outbreak has occurred are not likely to suffer again from cowpox for several years. Calves born of immune dams acquire passive protection through the ingestion of antibodies in the colostrum, but the duration of this protection is not known.

In man, cowpox infection usually runs a benign course and is self-limiting, but in unvaccinated adults the resulting illness may be severe, with lymphadenitis and fever. A fatal case was described in 1951 in a human patient where death occurred due to meningo-encephalitis. In man, the vesicular inflammatory lesions of cowpox are usually confined to the hands but sometimes the forearms and face are affected.

Transmission

Once cowpox is introduced into a herd it tends to spread rapidly until practically all cows are affected. The infection is probably spread during the process of milking, either by the hands of dairy men or by contaminated teat cups of milking machines. There is little evidence that air-borne infection occurs or that insects play a part in transmission of the disease.

Diagnosis

The diagnosis of cowpox is based on the appearance of firm, dark-red circular or oval lesions with raised edges and a depressed centre on the skin of the teats or udder, together with the fact that the infection tends to spread rapidly through the herd. A confirmatory diagnosis can be obtained by isolation of the virus from the lesions and by serological methods for its identification. Direct electron microscopy of material from a lesion is helpful in distinguishing cowpox virus from the causative agents of Milker's node (parapoxvirus), foot-and-mouth disease (rhinovirus), bovine mammillitis (herpesvirus) or teat papilloma (papovavirus). The appearance of bright red, haemorrhagic pocks on the chorioallantoic membrane of embryonated hens' eggs is also of diagnostic value.

Control

Although cattle can be actively immunized by vaccination with smallpox vaccine, cowpox is not a sufficiently common condition to justify this procedure. There is no specific method of treatment.

Monkey Pox

Definition

A generalized infection of monkeys and apes characterized by fever and the development of a cutaneous eruption of varying severity over the trunk, buttocks and extremities. The disease resembles naturally occurring variola (smallpox) in man and experimental variola in monkeys.

History and distribution

There are very few accounts of naturally occurring

poxvirus infections in non-human primate populations. Indeed, prior to 1950 only seven such episodes had been described and only three occurred during the present century. The first description of monkey pox as a specific agent in the group of poxvirus diseases was recorded by Danish workers in 1959, following their investigations of a spontaneous non-fatal pox-like disease in captive *Cynomolgus* monkeys. Since then, six outbreaks of monkey pox have been reported in animal colonies in the U.S.A. (1959–66), two in the Netherlands (1964–65) and one in France (1968).

Hosts affected
Only monkeys and apes are naturally affected, but recent reports suggest that man may acquire the infection and develop a rash resembling smallpox.

Properties of the virus
Monkey pox virus belongs to the orthopox group of viruses and its properties are intermediate between those of variola and vaccinia. It is resistant to ether, moderately resistant to dessication but is readily inactivated by chloroform, methanol, formalin and by heating at 56°C for 20 minutes. Repeated thawing and freezing has little effect on the infectivity titre of the virus. It stores well at 4°C and −70°C, but at −20°C the loss of infectious virus is more than 4 $\log_{10}$ after 15 months.

Haemagglutination
All strains agglutinate chicken red blood cells at 37°C and the haemagglutinin is present in both cell-free and cell-associated fractions of infected tissues. The titre is generally higher in extracts from infected chorioallantoic membranes than from cell culture fluids. Other species of erythrocytes including horse, sheep, guinea-pig, mouse, hamster, dog, cat and human group O cells are not agglutinated.

Antigenicity
The mature virion has a complex antigenic structure and shares with other orthopoxviruses common structural and soluble antigens. All monkey pox isolates so far studied are homogeneous and no qualitative differences have been observed between monkey pox, variola and vaccinia viruses in agar gel precipitation tests.

Cultivation
All strains grow well in embryonated hens' eggs when incubated at 37°C. The chorioallantoic membranes are oedematous and whitish pocks are produced which are similar in appearance to those produced by variola but appreciably smaller than those of vaccinia. The ceiling growth temperature for monkey pox and mouse pox (ectromelia) viruses

is 39°C compared with 38.5°C for variola, 40°C for cowpox and 41°C for vaccinia and rabbit pox viruses. This feature is frequently used as a means of distinguishing members of the orthopox group of viruses.

Monkey pox virus can be propagated on a variety of primary, secondary and continuous kidney cell cultures derived from monkey, rabbit, ox, guinea-pig and mouse, as well as some of human origin. In most cell culture systems it produces a marked cytopathic effect which is characterized by rounding-up, degeneration and, finally, detachment of cells from the glass, leaving visible holes or plaques in the remaining portions of the monolayer. Unlike variola virus, monkey pox and vaccinia viruses also produce plaques on chicken embryo fibroblasts. Progeny virus particles are mostly associated with the cells but are readily released by ultrasonic treatment. Infected cells invariably contain a number of small, spherical or oval, acidophilic intracytoplasmic inclusions resembling the Guarnieri bodies of smallpox and vaccinia. Sometimes intranuclear inclusions are seen but never concurrently in a cell with cytoplasmic inclusion bodies.

Pathogenicity
The disease in both naturally occurring and experimental infections is characterized by sudden fever, generalized lymphadenopathy and the appearance of a rash of varying severity depending on the species of animal affected. *Cynomolgus* monkeys and baboons are particularly susceptible and express the disease more intensely than rhesus and other species of primates. The cutaneous eruption generally appears by about the 7th. to 14th. day of the clinical illness and consists of multiple, discrete, blanched, shot-like papules varying in diameter from less than 1 mm to approximately 4 mm. The lesions are usually seen on the face (which may be oedematous), oral mucosae, trunk, buttocks and extremities; and are particularly abundant on the palms of the hands and on the soles of the feet. The cutaneous lesions rapidly pass through the stages of papule, vesicle, pustule and crust. The pustules, which last about 2 days, contain grayish, viscid, purulent material and frequently become umbilicated. Later, they become covered with reddish-brown crusts which fall off in 7–10 days, leaving a small scar. In fatal cases the skin eruptions have a tendency to become haemorrhagic. Lesions involving the skin and mucous membranes show epithelial degeneration, reticulation, endothelial proliferation and inflammatory cell infiltration. Small intracytoplasmic inclusions can be found which are most numerous in the epidermal cells along the margins of the lesions. They are generally acidophilic but basophilic structures can sometimes be seen in the cytoplasm and nuclei.

The mortality rate of monkey pox varies from less than 3 per cent to about 50 per cent, depending on species susceptibility and the presence or absence of concurrent bacterial infection.

In experimental infections, serum neutralizing and haemagglutinin-inhibiting antibodies develop within approximately 10 days, reach peak titre by the third week and remain at a constant level for many months. In contrast, complement-fixing antibodies appear 2–3 weeks after infection and tend to decline slowly over a period of 90 days or longer. Monkey pox has a wider host range than smallpox, and susceptible non-human primates include cynomolgus, rhesus, macaque, African green, marmoset and squirrel monkeys as well as orangutan, gorilla, chimpanzee and other species of apes. All can be infected by intradermal, subcutaneous, intramuscular or intranasal inoculation. It is also of interest that variola infections have been induced in rhesus and macaque monkeys, and the clinical picture closely resembles that of monkey pox. In rabbits, intradermal inoculation of monkey pox virus produces haemorrhagic lesions progressing to necrotic ulceration, in which respect it is quite different from vaccinia. On the other hand, monkey pox virus can be passed serially through rabbits by the intradermal route without difficulty, but variola virus cannot. Unweaned mice are susceptible to intracerebral inoculation, and a fatal meningoencephalitis develops within 4 days.

Ecology

During spontaneous outbreaks of the disease in captive monkeys and in colonies of experimentally infected monkeys, clinical and sub-clinical infections can occur in uninoculated companion monkeys held in separate cages. This suggests that the natural method of spread is probably by the respiratory route although transmission by ingestion of infective particles is also possible. The sporadic appearance of monkey pox and the isolation of the causative agent from uninoculated monkey kidney cell cultures also suggests that the virus may exist as a silent infection in wild and captive monkey populations; but whether these carrier animals are capable of shedding the virus and spreading the infection to other animals including man has not been clearly established.

Diagnosis

The presence of a vesicular eruptive disease in primates, together with the nature and distribution of the lesions, is suggestive of monkey pox, especially in large colonies of captive animals. The development of serum neutralizing, haemagglutinin-inhibiting and complement-fixing antibodies and the presence of small, acidophilic Guarnieri-like intracytoplasmic inclusions in epidermal cells are of diagnostic value. The pocks produced on the chorioallantoic membrane are smaller than those of vaccinia and the virus, unlike variola, induces a fatal meningoencephalitis when injected intracerebrally into unweaned mice.

Control

Rhesus and cynomolgus monkeys have been protected against monkey pox by inoculation with vaccinia virus. Thus, smallpox vaccination of all newly purchased primates combined with quarantine for about 4–6 weeks is recommended as a preventive measure.

Public health aspects

In the 10 recognised outbreaks of monkey pox in captive primate colonies, no human infection was observed despite the close contact of animal attendants with the infected animals. Quite unexpectedly, however, a number of human patients with illnesses at first indistinguishable from smallpox were discovered in 1970 in smallpox-free forest areas of West and Central Africa where monkeys are frequently eaten and their skins processed. All of the patients showed a diffuse vesiculopustular eruption on the skin; some were seriously ill but recovered. The causative agent was isolated from the cutaneous lesions and identified later as monkey pox virus. No secondary cases occurred, nor was man-to-man transmission reported. Serological surveys for antibodies to poxviruses in West African primate populations have so far failed to detect any significant source of monkey pox infection. Although the presence of a non-human reservoir of smallpox is possible the likelihood of this on present evidence seems remote.

Rabbit Pox

Synonym
Rabbit plague.

Definition
An acute, generalized highly fatal viral disease of laboratory rabbits characterized by nasal and conjunctival discharge and skin rash.

History and distribution
In 1930, and again in 1932, epidemics of a disease presenting many of the characteristic features of smallpox in man appeared in colonies of experimental rabbits in America. In 1933 the causative agent of the disease was identified as a virus of the pox group which was clearly related to vaccinia but not identical with either the neurotropic or dermatropic forms. The disease has also been

reported among laboratory rabbits in Holland but it has not been recognised in wild rabbits.

Properties of the virus

The causative virus is closely related to vaccinia and since it is now known that some of the early outbreaks occurred in rabbits that had been inoculated previously with vaccinia, and that in some instances neurovaccinia had been used, the agent may well be a laboratory 'sport' from vaccinia. It is also well known that infection with vaccinia virus is readily transmissible from one rabbit to another by contact.

Rabbit pox virus grows well in fertile hens' eggs and produces surface pocks on the chorioallantoic membrane which are often haemorrhagic, but large opaque white vaccinial forms and small forms may also be seen. In 1967 a strain of rabbit pox was described which grows in embryonated chicken eggs but does not produce surface pocks. Histological examination of infected membranes shows the presence of intracytoplasmic inclusions which are diffuse in character compared with the large circumscribed inclusions of cowpox virus. Reports that the virus is resistant to ether have been disputed by some workers. The white-pock mutants of rabbit pox virus agglutinate fowl red blood cells but other strains do not.

Rabbit pox virus grows readily in cell cultures producing acidophilic intracytoplasmic inclusions and nuclear changes. It is pathogenic to rabbits by all routes of inoculation, to calves by scarification and to mice intracerebrally.

Pathogenicity

During the early stages of a new epidemic the incubation period may be as short as 3–5 days but, as the outbreak progresses, the period is usually between 1–2 weeks. In typical cases the earliest symptoms include marked pyrexia (41°C.), anorexia, diarrhoea, laboured respiration, extreme weakness and photophobia. The nervous system is frequently involved and affected animals show incoordination, nystagmus and paralysis. One of the first signs of illness is enlargement of the lymph nodes of the popliteal, inguinal and other regions. Lymphadenitis usually persists throughout the illness and in some cases is the only sign of infection. Mostly, however, swelling of the lymph nodes is accompanied by a macular rash, giving rise to papules which eventually become umbilicated, dry and covered with crusts. The skin lesions are usually scattered irregularly over the body but are almost always present on the ears, lips, eyebrows, trunk and scrotum. Papules are also found about the anus, vulva and prepuce. Eye involvement is an almost constant occurrence

and the lesions commonly include diffuse keratitis with corneal ulceration. In some animals, the skin eruption is the main clinical picture while in others lymphadenitis, orchitis or ophthalmia is the only external manifestation of the disease. Although the mortality rate varies with different breeds, it is usually about 10–20 per cent in adults, but over 70 per cent in young rabbits less than 8 weeks of age. Death is apparently due to a terminal bronchopneumonia but many badly affected animals may recover and the lesions undergo slow resolution over a period of many weeks. Most recovered rabbits bear permanent scars or disfigurements but there is no evidence that they are persistent carriers of the infection.

The most distinctive macroscopic lesions of rabbit pox are the small nodules and papules consisting of mononuclear infiltrations accompanied, in some cases, by oedema, haemorrhage and extensive necrosis of the affected tissues. In fatal cases of infection the pleural and pericardial cavities usually contain an excess of clear fluid and the lungs may show small miliary translucent or pearl-white nodules. The popliteal and many other lymph nodes are swollen, oedematous and show focal lesions. The liver and spleen are usually enlarged, and numerous translucent white or grey nodules about 1 mm in diameter are scattered over the surface and distributed throughout the tissue.

Following exposure to aerosols of vaccinia, variola or rabbit pox infective particles, primary lesions develop at two distinct sites in the lower respiratory tract (bronchioles and alveoli). Rabbit pox produces a fatal generalised infection characterized by high titres of virus in the adrenals and gonads: whereas the other two viruses produce a milder reaction and faster resolution. Rabbit pox also differs from the other two viruses in its ability to spread by aerial routes to other rabbits, probably by infected oculonasal discharges.

Immunity

Rabbits recovered from experimental or spontaneous rabbit pox develop a solid immunity but are susceptible to inoculation with herpesvirus III of rabbits and myxoma virus. On the other hand, they are completely refractory to inoculation with dermovaccinia, but vaccinia recovered rabbits are not completely refractory to inoculation with rabbit pox virus. Moreover, rabbit pox recovered rabbits are partially refractory to inoculation with neurovaccinia, and neurovaccinia recovered rabbits are partially refractory to inoculation with rabbit pox virus. These, and other findings, suggest that the relationship between rabbit pox virus and neurovaccinia virus is closer than that between rabbit pox and dermovaccinia.

Transmission

Spread of infection throughout an animal-house is very rapid and the virus is probably transmitted to other animals by droplet infection or by indirect contact with equipment contaminated by infected oculo-nasal discharges or skin lesions.

Diagnosis

A provisional diagnosis of rabbit pox depends on the occurrence of the characteristic skin lesions. The most distinctive sign of infection is the pock-like eruption which is often widespread over the body. The causative virus may be isolated in susceptible rabbits or in embryonated hens' eggs and identified by serological and cross-immunity tests.

Control

Vaccines for the control of rabbit pox are not available commercially but rabbits inoculated with smallpox vaccine (vaccinia) are partially immune to rabbit pox.

Infectious Ectromelia

Synonyms

Mouse-pox: ectromelia of mice.

Definition

Ectromelia is a highly contagious, often fatal, generalised infection that can be carried in a latent form by individual mice and is readily activated by experimental procedures and various other stress factors.

Hosts affected and distribution

The infection occurs in laboratory mice in many parts of the world but has rarely been recorded in wild mice. Other hosts are not naturally susceptible.

Properties of the virus

The causative agent is a poxvirus which is classified in the subgroup of viruses related to vaccinia. Morphologically it is indistinguishable from vaccinia virus, measures about 230 x 170 nm and contains double-stranded DNA. It is resistant to ether and bile salts and will withstand 1 per cent phenol for 50 days. It is inactivated by 0.01 per cent formalin in 48 hours but can be preserved in glycerol, by lyophilization or by storage at $-70°C$. There is a very close antigenic relationship with vaccinia virus from which it may be distinguished by indirect complement-fixation, antibody-adsorption and gel diffusion tests. Haemagglutinins are produced as for vaccinia, and anti-haemagglutinins may or may not be present in the sera of latently infected mice.

Cultivation

Ectromelia virus grows well on developing hens' eggs and produces small white 'pocks' on the chorio-allantoic membrane. It can also be propagated in mouse fibroblasts, chicken embryo and other types of cell cultures as well as on continuous lines of HeLa and L cells. There is evidence in monolayer cultures of cell-to-cell transmission of infection and of giant-cell formation.

Pathogenicity

The infection may be latent in colonies of laboratory mice and produce no signs of disease. However, the introduction of virus into susceptible colonies usually results in high mortality, especially in young mice. Affected mice show early lesions on the lips, feet and tail in the form of oedematous swellings which become vesicles and later scabs. The primary lesion on the lips or on a hind foot is generally followed some 10 days later by a secondary eruption of vesicles, involving the face, the other feet or the tail, and occasionally by the loss of a limb. Mice developing extensive lesions usually die, but less severely affected animals may recover and will be solidly immune. The mortality rate in susceptible stocks may be as high as 80 to 90 per cent. Peracute infections with deaths in a few hours may take place where there is little or no evidence of skin lesions. At necropsy, peracute cases show an increase in pericardial and pleural fluids with necrotic areas or mottling of the liver and spleen. White spots may also be present in the peritoneum due to fat necrosis following pancreatic damage. Histological examination shows the presence of numerous intracytoplasmic inclusions in the epithelial cells of many organs. The incubation period in experimental infections is about 5 days. Following inoculation into the foot-pad of susceptible mice, the virus spreads within a matter of a few hours to the regional lymph nodes draining the site of its entry, and replication takes place within the cells of this primary focus. After 24–48 hours, the virus is released into the blood stream and this stage of early viraemia is followed by localization and multiplication in certain internal organs, usually liver, spleen or bone marrow. All of these developmental changes take place during the incubation period and there is little evidence of clinical illness until internal replication produces a sufficiently high titre of virus. When this occurs, the agent re-enters the blood stream in very large amounts (secondary viraemia) whence it is taken up by the phagocytic cells in various organs and transported to other sites. This leads to further foci of infection that may include the endothelium of dermal capillaries or the skin epithelium itself, giving rise to the characteristic rash or eruption of vesicles. With virulent strains of ectromelia virus generalization follows with focal necrosis of the liver and spleen, whereas with less virulent strains, although a viraemia occurs, lesions are only seen locally. In other laboratory animals, such as rabbits and guinea-pigs, local lesions may be produced in the skin but serial transmission has not been reported.

Ecology
Ectromelia may be introduced into a mouse colony by food contaminated by infected mice, or by the introduction of symptomless carriers. The virus may be shed in the urine and faeces for several months after recovery from clinical infection, and transmission probably occurs by direct contact from skin lesions and via the respiratory tract.

Diagnosis
The disease is readily diagnosed in healthy laboratory stocks when there is sudden onset of illness and high mortality associated with skin lesions on the lips and extremities and necrotic foci in the liver and spleen. Confirmatory diagnosis, especially among symptomless carriers, can be made by isolating the virus in embryonated eggs or cell cultures, whilst the presence of cytoplasmic inclusions in stained sections is also helpful. Specific antibodies can be demonstrated in sera from recovered mice and in many asymptomatic chronically infected mice.

Control
The mortality rate in an outbreak can be greatly reduced by scarifying the tail or foot pad with vaccine prepared from vaccinia virus. Immunization can also be carried out intra-nasally but neither method is wholly effective as a prophylactic. Although isatin-β-thiosemicarbazone is effective against vaccinia in mice but not against ectromelia, several derivatives of the drug act against ectromelia but not vaccinia. As none of these procedures will reliably eliminate infection from a colony, the destruction of all affected and in-contact animals together with thorough disinfection is advisable. Because of the risk of introducing symptomless carriers, the mixing of mice from different colonies must be avoided and healthy mice must be rigorously isolated.

PARAPOXVIRUS

Pseudo-cowpox

Synonyms
Milkers' nodules: milkers' nodes: paravaccinia: vaccine rouge (Fr.).

Definition
Pseudo-cowpox is a benign disease causing proliferative lesions on the udder and teats of lactating cows. It is probably the commonest viral infection of the udder and teats of cattle and is much more prevalent today than is true cowpox, with which it is often confused.

Hosts affected
Milking cows are the commonest natural host of pseudo-cowpox, but man commonly acquires the infection (milkers' nodes).

History and distribution
Pseudo-cowpox was recognised as a distinct entity by Jenner as long ago as the late 18th century. It is still a common infection of dairy cattle in Britain and continental Europe as well as in Australia, New Zealand, Japan and the U.S.A.

Properties of the virus
Under the electron microscope, the virus particles of pseudo-cowpox are oval or cylindrical in shape and somewhat narrower than those of vaccinia and cowpox, measuring about 290 x 170 nm in diameter. A dense central core is usually seen after treatment with pepsin. The fine structure of the cytoplasm surrounding the central core of nucleic acid consists of a criss-cross pattern of concentric smooth walled tubular 'threads' which gives the virus particle the appearance of a ball of wool. Other viruses showing this characteristic spiral structure include orf and bovine papular stomatitis. (Plate 37.4b, facing p. 431).

Physicochemical characters
There is little definite information about the chemical composition of pseudo-cowpox virus except that the dense central core contains DNA and is surrounded by an outer covering of protein. The virus is moderately sensitive to ether and its activity is destroyed by exposure to chloroform for 10 minutes. It survives freezing and can be stored at −70°C for months without significant drop in titre. No haemagglutinin has been described.

Antigenic properties
There is no cross-immunity between pseudo-cowpox virus and cowpox or vaccinia, and recent work suggests that it is difficult to distinguish this virus on serological grounds from that of orf and bovine papular stomatitis.

Cultivation
Pseudo-cowpox, unlike cowpox virus, has a strictly limited experimental host range, and it has not yet been propagated in rabbits, mice, guinea- pigs

or chicken embryos. In contrast to vaccinia virus, it does not infect young chickens by feather follicle inoculation, nor will it produce pocks on the chorioallantoic membrane of developing hens' eggs. Freshly isolated strains of pseudo-cowpox virus will grow well on primary cell cultures of bovine testis, sheep testis and human amnion, and especially if the monolayers consist of rapidly growing cells. Foci of rounded cells produced after 6–8 days are mostly the 'closed plaque' type consisting of groups or clumps of rounded poorly refractile cells which become detached from the glass in the later stages of the infection as the cytopathic effect progresses. Occasionally, 'open plaques' are seen where the infected cells regularly detach from the glass to become a clear central area surrounded by degenerating cells in the early stages of infection. Basophilic juxtanuclear cytoplasmic inclusions are seen in stained preparations of infected cells and the nuclei, which sometimes contain inclusions, are somewhat elongated, distorted or twisted. Highly refractile and sometimes very conspicuous acidophilic granules of varying sizes, are commonly present in the cytoplasm. There are no cellular abnormalities in continuous cultures of hamster kidney, mouse L cells or human KB cells.

Pathogenesis
The disease is usually confined to milking cows and most frequently appears during lactation. After an incubation period of 7–8 days, mild erythema of the teat is quickly followed by the formation of small cherry-red papules that develop within the next 2–3 days into dark red raised scabs of about 1 cm in diameter. In more acute cases an erythematous eruption of the teat develops into microscopic vesicles or pustules which rupture within 48 hours and later form scabs, some of which are very large. Scabs are shed after about 12 days or can be manually removed without pain to the animal, leaving a red crescentic area with a characteristic horse-shoe-shaped ring of minute scabs at its circumference. A wart-like granuloma is left which may persist for many months. In most cases of pseudo-cowpox in cows, vesication is rarely observed. The lesions are raised, firm, mottled, red-blue in colour, and often painless to the touch and the scabs are dry with no exudation. In man, the incubation period is about 5 days and the lesion, which is one of endothelial proliferation, takes the form of hemispherical dark red papules similar to the lesions of orf. They are relatively painless but frequently cause an itching sensation. Apart from slight swelling of the axillary lymph nodes, there is little evidence of generalization and the lesions disappear after 4–6 weeks. In histological sections large acidophilic inclusions are seen in the cytoplasm adjacent to the nucleus and, more rarely, within the nucleus.

The experimental inoculation of non-milking heifers with recent isolates of pseudo-cowpox virus is followed by transient small firm red nodules which regress by 11 days. However, in cows in their second lactation, subcutaneous or intradermal inoculation of the teats gives rise to dry raised scabs which may persist for as long as 23 days. When the scabs are shed, they leave a red moist crescentic area, and adjacent secondary lesions develop 11–14 days after infection. Material from a milkers' nodule lesion in man inoculated by scarification into a cow's teat produces lesions similar to natural cases of pseudo-cowpox. The clinical picture of the disease and the frequency of successive crops of lesions that commonly follows primary infection suggests that cattle build up little, if any, immunity to pseudo-cowpox virus. In human infections, complement-fixing antibodies are produced a few weeks after the nodules develop but the titres decline fairly rapidly.

Ecology
Primary infection among cattle probably occurs as a result of mechanical spread either on the hands of milkers or on the teat-cups of milking machines.

Diagnosis
Pseudo-cowpox is probably the commonest viral infection of the udder and teats of cattle and a presumptive diagnosis can usually be obtained in milking cows from the appearance of the lesions. In most animals they are usually small multiple, 2–10 per teat, and cause little apparent discomfort. The presence of raised scabs and the horse-shoe-shaped lesions with secondary foci, is characteristic of the disease. In cowpox, on the other hand, the lesions are fewer in number, smaller but with more intense local reaction. They also develop more quickly, are more painful to the touch and heal more rapidly. For confirmatory diagnosis, the viruses of pseudo-cowpox and cowpox may be rapidly and accurately differentiated by electron microscopy of material obtained from 'clean' lesions on the teat, by observing the nature of the cytopathic effect produced on cell cultures and by the ability of most strains of cowpox, but not pseudo-cowpox, to produce haemorrhagic pocks on the chorioallantoic membrane of fertile hens' eggs. The presence of lesions on the hands of dairymen vaccinated against smallpox helps to distinguish pseudo-cowpox from true cowpox.

Control
No specific methods of treatment are known.

Orf

Synonyms

Contagious pustular dermatitis (of sheep): CPD: Contagious ecthyma of sheep: Sore mouth: Scabby mouth: Infectious labial dermatitis: Echthyma contagieux (Fr.): Austeckende pustolose Hautentzundung (Ger.).

Definition

A contagious dermatitis of sheep and goats, affecting primarily the lips of young animals. Man may also become infected. The natural disease is not known to occur in other domestic species. An infection described in Chamois is thought to be due to orf.

History and distribution

Orf has been recognised as a contagious disease of sheep in Europe since about the middle of the 18th century. Today, the disease has a world-wide distribution and appears wherever sheep and goat husbandry is practised. Outbreaks develop wherever and whenever there is a highly susceptible population at risk and the highest incidence occurs amongst lambs of 4–6 months of age or younger.

Morphology

Mature elementary bodies of orf and of bovine papular stomatitis resemble those of milkers' node (pseudo-cowpox) and differ morphologically from the normal appearance of poxviruses. They are slightly smaller (290 x 160 nm) and more oval in outline having an axis ratio of about 1:6 compared with 1:3 for vaccinia. Each particle consists of a thick outer wall and an electron-dense centrally placed core or inner body. In negatively-stained preparations the arrangement of the tubular thread component gives the virion its characteristic ball of wool appearance. Examination of the fine structure of the upper and lower surfaces of the virus particle shows that the surface filament is in the form of a left-hand spiral coil of a single strand which measures about 12 nm in diameter. The criss-cross pattern is probably achieved by the crossing of 2 sets of parallel threads; which is due to superimposition of the images of threads that run at different angles in the upper and lower surfaces, as seen in an X-ray photograph. (Plate 37.4b, facing p. 431 and plate 52.1b, facing p. 676b).

When penetration of the virus by heavy metal salts is achieved, the limiting membrane, the peripheral protein layer and the inner body become visible. The inner component is very similar to that of vaccinia, and consists usually of 2 or 3 tubular strands of material arranged as an S-shaped structure. Thus, the structural elements of orf and vaccinia viruses are very similar, the differences being produced by the manner in which they are arranged.

Chemical composition

The inner component probably contains the nucleic acid which consists of double-stranded DNA.

Physicochemical characters

The virus is very resistant to dessication and can survive outside the body for many months or even years in dried scabs, or at room temperature in the laboratory for upwards of 15 years. It is inactivated by chloroform and by a temperature of 60°C for 30 minutes, but will withstand heating for 30 minutes at 55°C. It is only slightly sensitive to ether.

Haemagglutination

Haemagglutinins have not been described in orf nor in any other member of the parapox group of viruses.

Antigenic properties

Sera from immunized sheep and rabbits precipitate a soluble antigen and fix complement specifically, but the levels of the neutralizing antibodies are variable and generally not significant. Although it has been reported that antigenic cross-reactions can be demonstrated by gel diffusion and complement-fixation between orf and some of the true pox viruses, there is a much closer relationship between this virus and other members of the parapox group of viruses, namely, pseudo-cowpox (milkers' nodule) and bovine papular stomatitis.

Cultivation

Orf virus has not been grown in fertile hens' eggs, but can be propagated serially with some difficulty in rabbits. Other laboratory animals are not susceptible. Growth occurs with a cytopathic effect in various cell culture systems including embryonic sheep skin, sheep and bovine testis, embryonic sheep, calf and goat kidney cells and human amnion. Testis cell cultures are particularly suitable and the cytopathic changes seen in stained preparations include the formation of multiple compact, granular cytoplasmic inclusions consisting of an acidophilic paranuclear mass and an irregular shaped basophilic peripheral area. Similar cytopathic effects are produced by bovine papular stomatitis and pseudo-cowpox viruses.

Pathogenicity

The disease mainly affects lambs and kids since most adults are either vaccinated or have developed an immunity through previous contact with the infection. The morbidity is generally very high and may reach 100 per cent but the mortality rate is low except among very young lambs. Lesions are mainly confined to those parts of the skin free from wool, especially the lips and mouth and occasionally the periorbital region of the face, and the interdigital region and coronet of the feet. Genital infections may occur at mating times and ewes nursing infected lambs may develop lesions on the udder. Uncomplicated lesions pass through the stages of erythema and vesication followed by papules, pustules and ulcers 3–4 days later. In many cases, coalescence of numerous discrete lesions leads to the formation of large proliferative wart-like masses which become covered with a hard keratinized crust or scab. Healing usually takes place after 10 days to 4 weeks depending on the site involved, the age of the animal and the nature and extent of secondary bacterial contamination. In contrast to infected cell cultures, parasitized cells in stained sections of affected tissues seldom contain cytoplasmic inclusions. Animals, including man, can be readily infected by scarification, the lesions appearing in 3–4 days. Recent evidence suggests that calves are susceptible to experimental inoculation with material from lesions in sheep as well as cell culture adapted virus, but other workers have failed to confirm this. There is also a report that dogs have been infected after eating unskinned sheep carcases. In man, papular lesions slowly increase in size until they appear as firm, painless, bluish-red nodules generally without vesication. Lymphadenitis may be present. Generally, the lesions heal spontaneously and disappear without scar formation after 2 or 3 weeks.

Ecology
The portal of entry of the virus in natural cases is through small wounds or abrasions of the skin. Infection is probably by direct contact with infected scabs, soil, posts, utensils or infected animals. The persistence of the virus and the contagious nature of the disease accounts for the very high incidence of infection that occurs in older animals kept in conditions of intensive husbandry.

Diagnosis
The rapid spread of infection, particularly in young lambs, and the characteristic appearance and distribution of the proliferative type of lesion in the absence of a systemic reaction is indicative of orf. Confirmation is obtained in the laboratory by the demonstration of typical 'ball of wool' virus particles in lesions by electron microscopy, and by isolating the virus in cell culture. The presence of viral antigen in the lesions is demonstrable by agar gel diffusion and complement-fixation tests, the latter being the more sensitive method. In man, biopsy material is preferable to swabs and scrapings. Transmission of the infection to healthy susceptible lambs by scarification is also useful.

Control
The scarification of a living virus vaccine, consisting of finely powdered dried infected scabs suspended as a 1 per cent concentration in 50 per cent glycerol, will generally produce a satisfactory level of immunity in lambs and kids. The usual sites for vaccination are inside the thigh or, in the case of adult animals, behind the shoulder several weeks before the lambing period. Lambs are usually vaccinated at about 1 month of age and, for best results, are revaccinated 2–3 months later. A reaction shows within 7 days and vaccinated animals are said to be immune for at least 8 months, and in some cases up to 28 months. Sheep in endemic areas should be revaccinated annually. The vaccine should be handled with caution to prevent infections of the finger, and used containers must be carefully disposed of to prevent contamination of the soil with this resistant virus.

Bovine Papular Stomatitis

Synonyms
Stomatitis papulosa of cattle. Occasionally referred to as 'infectious ulcerative', 'erosive', 'proliferative' or 'pseudo-aphthous' stomatitis of cattle.

Definition
Bovine papular stomatitis is generally a benign, non-febrile disease occurring mostly in young cattle and which is characterized by the presence of lesions in the epithelial cells of the oral mucosa, muzzle and external nares.

Hosts affected
The virus has a very narrow host range and, apart from cattle, transmission to other species of domestic or laboratory animals has not yet been confirmed.

History and distribution
Papular stomatitis, which was first described in Germany, has been recognised as a disease of cattle for nearly 100 years, and its viral aetiology was first reported about 60 years ago. The disease is widespread in Europe and has been confirmed in Great Britain. It also occurs in North America, Africa and Australasia.

Classification
Recent evidence suggests that the causative virus of bovine papular stomatitis is very similar, if not identical, to that of pseudo-cowpox or milkers' nodule. These two viruses, together with that of

contagious pustular dermatitis (orf) of sheep, have recently been classified in the genus *Parapoxvirus*.

Morphology

Compared with orthopoxviruses, the particles of bovine papular stomatitis virus are smaller, more elongated and ovoid and measure about 250 x 125 nm. Under the electron microscope, negative-staining techniques show the structure of the virions to have the spiral 'ball of wool' appearance as for orf and pseudo-cowpox.

Physical characters

The virus survives freeze-drying well but, unlike orthopoxviruses, is only partially ether-resistant.

Antigenic properties

Except for the common poxvirus nucleoprotein antigen, the bovine papular stomatitis virus does not cross react with the viral or soluble antigens of cow-pox or other poxviruses outwith the parapox group of viruses. There is, however, a close serological relationship with orf and pseudo-cowpox.

Cultivation

There is now general agreement that the virus of bovine papular stomatitis does not grow in fertile hens' eggs but it does produce cytopathic effects on some cell culture systems. On primary sheep testis, bovine testis and human amnion cells, it induces a cytopathic effect after 5 days which is essentially similar to that of pseudo-cowpox virus. Both 'closed' plaques of clusters of infected cells and, less commonly, 'open' plaques with clear central areas of detached cells are produced. In some preparations of established calf testis mono-layers, infected cells contain large intracytoplasmic inclusion bodies. These inclusions are characterized by a paranuclear acidophilic zone which is partly surrounded by a separate outer arc or horse-shoe-shaped mass of more basophilic material. The nuclei of affected cells are often irregular in shape and shrunken. Bovine testis cells are considered to be slightly inferior to sheep testis cells for the growth of bovine papular stomatitis and pseudo-cowpox viruses.

Pathogenicity

Following a short incubation period of about 4 to 7 days, lesions appear in the mouth and sometimes on the muzzle. In natural cases of the disease, the early lesions are small rounded areas of intense congestion measuring 1.5–2 cm in diameter and, in pigmented skin, they appear as raised roughened areas with a greyish necrotic centre. In many cases pathognomonic ring-shaped sores appear, due to peripheral extension of the lesions forming concentric rings of alternate brownish coloured necrosis and cherry-red congestion. Lesions on the muzzle and around the external nares are usually in the form of raised, roughened, brownish plaques about 1 cm. in diameter. Fresh lesions may arise at any time during the course of the disease.

Ecology

The virus of bovine papular stomatitis is present in the saliva, nasal secretions and other lesions of affected animals, and transmission may occur both by direct and by indirect contact. Calves probably acquire the infection early in life from infected adults which may act as 'carriers', since recurrence of infection can take place in recovered animals many weeks or months after initial infection. The stability of the virus at room temperature suggests that it may persist for several days on clothing, feeding utensils and the like.

Diagnosis

The distribution of the lesions and their characteristic appearance are often sufficiently typical of the disease to enable a provisional diagnosis to be made. The absence of vesicles or diarrhoea and other systemic reactions is helpful in differentiating bovine papular stomatitis from foot-and-mouth disease, vesicular stomatitis, rinderpest and mucosal disease. For confirmation, the assistance of the laboratory is necessary. Histological examination of biopsy and post-mortem material taken from lesions will reveal typical tissue changes including ballooning, degeneration and intracytoplasmic in-clusions in affected cells, mostly within the stratum spinosum of the epithelium. Tissue culture methods using primary cultures of bovine testis cells can be used for isolation and identification of the virus, and electron microscopy of specimens obtained from lesions may show the characteristic 'ball of wool' structure of a parapoxvirus.

Control

There is no specific method of treatment and no vaccines are available. Bovine papular stomatitis is generally a mild illness of little economic im-portance and most cases make an uncomplicated recovery, although complete resolution of the lesions may take several weeks.

AVIPOXVIRUS

Fowl Pox

Synonyms

Avian pox: Contagious epithelioma: Bird pox: Bor-reliota avium: *Poxvirus avium*: Avian diphtheria: Geflugelpocken (Ger.).

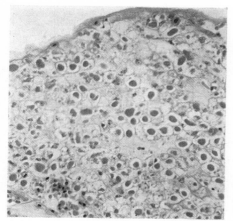

52.3a

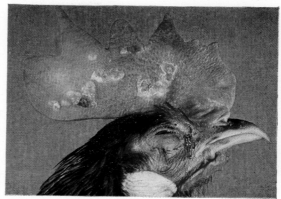

52.3b

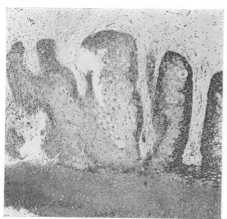

52.3c

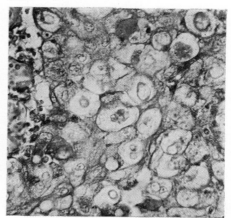

52.3d

52.3a Section of the chorioallantoic membrane of a developing chick embryo inoculated 4 days previously with cow pox virus, showing the presence of numerous, large, regularly shaped acidophilic intracytoplasmic inclusions (Bollinger bodies). Haematoxylin eosin stain, ×280.

52.3c Section through one of the cutaneous lesions shown in Plate 52.3b. Marked proliferation of the surface epithelium, ballooning or hydropic degeneration of affected cells and the formation of large acidophilic intracytoplasmic inclusions are characteristic of fowl pox. Haematoxylin eosin stain, ×44.

52.3b Cockerel artificially infected with fowl pox virus by scarification. Extensive proliferation of the epithelial cells at the sites of inoculation has given rise to wart-like lesions on the comb.

52.3d Section prepared from the same tissue shown in Plate 52.3c but photographed at higher magnification. The large, irregularly shaped red masses within the vacuolated cells are intracytoplasmic inclusions. The nuclei are smaller and stain blue. Mann's stain, ×350.

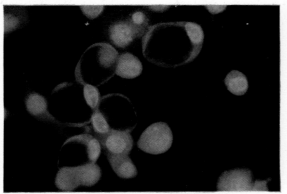

52.4a

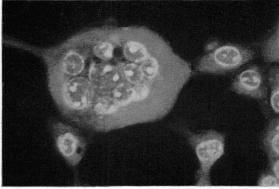

52.4b

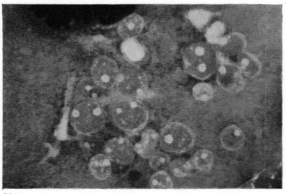

52.4c

52.4a The **MDBK** line of bovine kidney cells inoculated 48 hours previously with a recently isolated strain of myxoma virus, showing hydropic change and displacement of nuclei towards the periphery of affected cells. Acridine orange stain, × 420.

52.4b Multinucleate syncytium formed in the PK15 line of pig kidney cells infected with myxoma virus. Acridine orange stain, × 420.

52.4c Detail of a syncytium in PK15 cells infected with myxoma virus, showing increased nuclear fluorescence (top) and an elongated mass of yellow-green fluorescence in the cytoplasm (left). Acridine orange stain, × 480.

Definition

Fowl pox occurs mainly in two forms. Most commonly it is a cutaneous infection of epithelial tissues of the non-feathered portions of the skin characterised by the formation of wart-like nodules on the comb, wattles, oral commissures, eyelids, feet and legs of chickens. Alternatively, it appears as an infection of the mucous membranes of the mouth, nose and eyes giving rise to diphtheritic pseudo-membranes in the mouth, pharynx and larynx, and sometimes referred to as avian diphtheria. Both forms are due to the same virus but the diphtheritic type is mostly responsible for the mortality associated with the disease.

Hosts affected

The disease chiefly affects poultry, i.e. chickens, turkeys, guinea fowl, peacocks, domestic and feral pigeons and, very occasionally, water-fowl, pheasants, other game birds, canaries and sparrows. It is generally accepted that there are 4 main strains of the virus, namely fowl pox, turkey pox, pigeon pox and canary pox, and, while each affects and is usually more pathogenic for its own host, some are undoubtedly capable of infecting birds of various families. Although all avian poxviruses are closely related immunologically, most show a considerable degree of host-modification. For example, fowl pox virus can be transmitted to pigeons by parenteral inoculation only with difficulty, and pigeon pox virus, which is only slightly pathogenic for domestic poultry, immunizes chickens against fowl pox and constitutes a good vaccine for this purpose.

It is seldom possible to establish infection in mammals with an avian poxvirus, or *vice versa*. It should also be noted that the disease in man commonly known as chickenpox is not a poxvirus infection but is caused by varicella virus which is a member of the herpesvirus group. (Chapter 56).

History and distribution

Fowl pox has been recognised as a serious illness of birds for a very long time and it occurs in all countries of the world where poultry are kept in large numbers. The disease appears most frequently in early spring and late autumn. The widespread use of vaccines has greatly reduced the incidence of the disease until it is now no longer the cause of very severe economic losses in the poultry industry.

Morphology

The elementary bodies, or Borrel bodies as they are sometimes called, closely resemble other pox viruses and appear as minute blue-coloured spherical particles within infected cells in smear preparations stained by Giemsa. They are about 330 x 280 nm in size.

Under the electron microscope each has a centrally placed electron dense pepsin-resistant core, or nucleoid, which contains DNA (MW 200–240×10^6 daltons). The appearance of thinly sectioned fowl pox virus often resembles that of vaccinia virus with 2 or 3 outer membranes, 2 lateral bodies and a biconcave-shaped nucleoid which seems to consist of a number of folded or coiled tubular structures not unlike the S-shaped structure or triad of the pseudo-cow pox nucleoid. The virus particles stained with uranyl acetate and shadowed with platinum appear to have a 'knobbly' surface and resemble a mulberry. Beneath this the interior of the particle shows a detail of intertwining, short, criss-cross strands or threads which is quite distinct from the spiral coils seen in parapoxviruses.

Growth cycle

The developmental cycle studied by electron microscopy of fowl pox infected chorioallantoic membranes shows that the virus becomes adsorbed and phagocytosed by invagination of the membrane of the ectodermal cells within 2 hours post infection. After an incubation period of 48 hours, immature viral particles appear within discrete intracytoplasmic areas or zones of reticulo-granular material. The viral particles are surrounded by a double membrane and contain eccentrically situated dense nucleoids. After 72 hours, 'myelin' structures composed of numerous layers of tightly-woven concentric membranes appear and are probably lipid in nature. At 96 hours, inclusion bodies are recognisable inside which are seen mature viral particles composed of a central biconcave nucleoid covered by a thick layer of viroplasm. Surrounding this is a wide clear zone which is limited by an outer dense layer of lipid material, possibly derived from the inclusion body itelf. This suggestion is supported by recent evidence that isolated mature fowl pox virus contains approximately 30 per cent of extractable lipid. After separation from the inclusion bodies, the particles apparently migrate to the cell membrane where, at about the 120th–140th hour, they bud from the cell surface and thereby obtain a thick additional outer membrane. Occasionally, mature viral particles appear within the nuclei and whilst it is conceivable that nuclear penetration by virus is an integral part of the infective process, its exact meaning is not yet known.

Physicochemical characters

The fowl pox virus is highly resistant to adverse environmental factors and, in epithelial masses, is said to withstand dessication and sunlight for several weeks. It is inactivated by heating at 60°C for 8 minutes or 50°C for 30 minutes. It is readily destroyed by 1–2 per cent caustic potash or caustic soda but only after being freed from the matrix of inclusion material in the cytoplasm of infected tissue cells. It withstands 1 per cent phenol and 1 in 1000 formalin for periods of up to 9 days and is readily preserved by drying or freeze-drying for periods of several years. It is also preserved by 50 per cent glycerol. Fowl pox virus is sensitive to chloroform but reports of its activity in the presence of ether are variable since some strains seem to be moderately sensitive although the majority are resistant.

Haemagglutination

Many workers have failed to demonstrate haemagglutination by fowl pox virus, but it is now generally agreed that haemagglutinins are produced and that the presence of the virus in cell cultures of chick embryo fibroblasts can be detected in the absence of visible cytopathic effects by haemadsorption.

Antigenic properties

Although avian strains have the general characters of poxviruses and share the nucleo-protein (NP) antigen, they are not related immunologically to vaccinia virus or other viruses of the group. Nevertheless, all avian poxviruses show varying degrees of cross-protection among themselves and some workers consider that, irrespective of the natural avian host, they should all be regarded as variants of a single virus. Fowl and pigeon pox viruses, and to a somewhat lesser extent canary pox virus, are fairly closely related serologically as shown by neutralization tests in fertile eggs and diffusion tests in agar gel.

Cultivation

Avian pox viruses grow well on the chorioallantoic membrane of hens' and ducks' eggs producing large, raised, whitish pocks within 3 days, that later develop dark necrotic centres. (Plate 42.3a, facing p. 480). In cell cultures, most avian pox strains grow well but do not produce cellular changes in chicken or duck fibroblasts. On whole chick embryo cell cultures, however, a marked cytopathic effect is produced and large intracytoplasmic inclusions (Bollinger bodies) can be seen in the infected cells.

Pathogenicity

All ages of birds are susceptible but the disease is mostly seen in stock from 5–12 months of age. Following an incubation period of 4–8 days, the clinical condition runs a course of 3 or 4 weeks. The mortality rate varies widely but is highest in the diphtheritic form of the disease particularly when the lesions are affected with secondary bacterial infections. After entering the skin, multiplication of the virus results in the proliferation of epithelial cells giving rise to a typical pox-like eruption, scabbing or nodule formation on the skin, especially of the comb, wattles, commissures of the mouth, feet and, sometimes, the vent. (Plate 52.3b, facing p. 692). Involvement of the eyes may lead to conjunctivitis and temporary blindness, and caseous material may accumulate in the infra-orbital sinuses. The process is almost entirely limited to the epithelial layers and the dermis is only slightly involved. The same process occurs in the diphtheritic type where small caseous white nodules appear at the side of the tongue, on the roof of the mouth and around the epiglottis. These may coalesce to form an extensive yellow to white necrotic membrane which may result finally in death from suffocation by occlusion of the larynx. When the lesions involve the larynx and trachea, the affected birds show severe respiratory symptoms. The exudates from these birds contain large amounts of virus and may serve as a source of infection for susceptible contacts. Usually, the course of the disease is chronic with signs of anorexia, loss of weight and fall in egg production, and the infection may persist for long periods on an affected farm due to its relatively slow spread.

Histologically, affected epithelial cells show characteristic ballooning or hydropic degeneration, and also the formation of single acidophilic intracytoplasmic inclusion bodies (Bollinger bodies) that are frequently larger than the nucleus of the cell. Aggregates of mature virus particles (Borrel bodies) are frequently found embedded in the acidophilic matrix of the Bollinger body. Proliferation of the epithelial layer is characteristic of fowl pox infection, but subcutaneous involvement is rare. (Plates 52.3c, d, facing p. 692).

The experimental disease is very similar to that occurring naturally and birds of practically all species can be infected by a variety of routes.

Ecology

The disease is disseminated in healthy flocks by direct contact with actively infected birds, by indirect contact with exudates and contaminated utensils or through mechanical transfer by biting insects. Mosquitoes are known to harbour the virus for as long as 210 days. The virus does not penetrate the intact skin of the host and it is assumed that infection mostly occurs through minor abrasions in the mouth region by rough feed or through injuries to the comb, wattles or skin as a result of fighting, pecking and scratching. Virus may also enter by way of the feather follicles. Apart from blood-sucking flies, poultry ticks and lice may play a part in transmitting the infection. The virus is usually conveyed from affected birds either in desquamated epithelium from lesions, or in exudates from the mouth or nares expelled during sneezing and coughing. The importance of wild birds in the transmission of fowl pox to domestic fowls is not known. The virus is very stable and can remain viable in dried scabs and exudates for many months or even years.

Diagnosis

The slow spread of the infection and the appearance of typical proliferative pox lesions on the head and skin in natural cases of the cutaneous form of the disease are usually sufficient to justify a diagnosis of fowl pox. The diphtheritic form, however, is more difficult to diagnose as it may be confused with a number of other conditions including avitaminosis-A and respiratory infections. Histologically, the presence of large intracytoplasmic inclusions (Bollinger bodies) in ballooned epithelial cells is helpful, and the virus can be regularly isolated and identified in fertile hens' eggs and in some tissue culture systems. Virus neutralization tests can be performed in eggs and tissue cultures and even on the skin or wattles of susceptible birds. Specific antibodies are revealed by agar gel diffusion, complement-fixation and neutralization tests.

Control

Recovered birds develop a lifelong active immunity and various types of vaccines have been used successfully to control the disease. The 2 vaccines most commonly employed are live fowl pox vaccines which produce a solid long-lasting immunity following a severe systemic reaction, and live pigeon pox vaccines which are safer to use but may only produce an immunity of about 6 months' duration. Both types may be used in turkeys but only pigeon pox vaccine should be given to pigeons. Pigeon pox vaccine prepared on the skin of the breast of pigeons is applied to poultry by light scarification of the feather follicles of the thigh; whereas fowl pox vaccine, usually prepared by growing the virus in embryonated chicken eggs, is applied either by the feather follicle method or by pricking the skin of the wing-web with a sharp needle dipped in the vaccine. In successfully vaccinated birds, small pock-like lesions develop at the site within 6–10 days and antibodies are formed after 14–21 days. Vaccinated birds must be protected from exposure to field infection during this period. In some countries, these vaccines have largely been replaced with a strain of pigeon pox virus which has unusually high immunizing properties but does not produce a severe reaction and has little tendency to spread. In endemic areas, birds on badly affected farms are vaccinated during the first few weeks of life and revaccinated 8–12 weeks later.

Recent work in Italy suggests that young chickens may be safely vaccinated with the TE-A strain of fowl pox which was found, after 30 passages in the allantoic cavity, to be of reduced virulence for day-old chicks by intramuscular inoculation, and gives rise to a solid immunity. Cell culture vaccines are also being developed and a strain of turkey pox has been successfully adapted to growth on pig kidney cell cultures with some degree of attenuation for birds after about 40 passages. Fowl pox and pigeon pox viruses grown in embryonic duck and chick fibroblasts produce local reactions in chickens inoculated by wing-web application. However, the lesions disappear within 2 weeks, and the chickens thus vaccinated, resist challenge between 2 and 4 weeks later.

LEPORIPOXVIRUS

Myxomatosis

Synonyms

La myxomatose (Fr.): die Myxomatose der Kaninchen (Ger.):

Definition

Myxomatosis is an infectious disease of rabbits named from the mucinous nature of the exudate from the cut surface of the 'tumours' or swellings which develop in the skin of infected animals.

Hosts affected

The native wild rabbit of Uruguay and Brazil (*Sylvilagus brasiliensis*) is the natural host for myxomatosis, and infection in this species is manifested by a single benign localised skin 'tumour' in which the causative virus (myxoma) is present. The wild and domestic European rabbit (*Oryctolagus cuniculus*) is much more susceptible and affected animals suffer a severe generalised infection characterized by oedema of the head and ano-genital region, blepharoconjunctivitis and widespread tumour-like swellings over the body. In these species myxomatosis is almost uniformly fatal. In parts of North America, the jack-rabbit or hare (*Lepus californicus*) and some species of cottontail rabbits e.g. *Sylvilagus floridanus* and *S. floridanus mallanus*, are almost wholly resistant. In Europe, the brown hare (*L. europaeus*) and the mountain hare (*L. timidus*) have an innate resistance to the infection although several cases of naturally occurring myxomatosis in hares have been reported from time to time mainly in France, the U.K., Poland and Australia. Man and other animal species are not affected.

History and distribution

Myxomatosis first occurred as a new and fatal disease among laboratory rabbits in Uruguay in

1898, and in 1930 it was recognised in commercially raised rabbits in California. In 1950 the causative virus was deliberately introduced into Australia in an attempt to reduce the population of wild European rabbits which were regarded as a serious pest to agriculture, and 2 years later similar action was taken in France by a private landowner. Widespread and severe infection caused considerable reduction in the rabbit populations but later the disease became endemic and less severe. As a result, myxomatosis spread over all parts of Australia and to many countries in Europe, including the U.K., wherever rabbits occurred in large numbers. Myxomatosis is now an enzootic disease of native *Sylvilagus* rabbits in South America and California and of *Oryctolagus* (European) rabbits in Australia, Europe and parts of South America.

Properties of the virus

The causative agent of myxomatosis is a pox virus (*P. myxomatis*) which is morphologically very similar to vaccinia. The virus particle is brick-shaped and measures about 280 x 230 nm. Negative staining techniques show that the surface of the virus has a beaded appearance and consists of a mass of threads or tubules, each of which is slightly wider than the surface tubules of other pox viruses. The central core almost certainly contains DNA since myxoma virus multiplication in cultured cells is inhibited by 5-bromodeoxyuridine (BUDR). The virus is sensitive to a pH of less than 4.6 and is very susceptible to heat, being inactivated more rapidly at 55°C than are most other poxviruses. It survives for many months in skins of affected animals at ordinary temperatures, is stable in 50 per cent glycerol or when frozen and dried. Myxoma virus is unusual in that it is ether-sensitive and sodium desoxycholate resistant whereas, with most other viruses, sensitivity to ether and bile salts are parallel. Haemagglutination has not been reported. Myxoma virus is a member of the family *Poxviridae* and, together with rabbit fibroma virus, squirrel fibroma virus and hare fibroma virus, constitutes the genus *Leporipoxvirus*.

Antigenicity

Like all other pox viruses, myxoma virus contains several antigens. In gel diffusion tests between myxoma antiserum and myxoma infected rabbit tissue, 3–5 precipitin lines are formed and cross-reactions are obtained between the soluble antigens of myxoma virus and the viruses of rabbit, hare and squirrel fibromas. Rabbits recovered from a fibroma virus infection are susceptible to challenge with myxoma virus but the disease is less severe and death does not ensue. No fewer than 8 myxoma antigens have been identified by immuno-electrophoresis. Substantial differences have also been found between the soluble antigens of myxoma virus of Californian and Brazilian strains, and each has antigens peculiar to it, the rest being common.

Cultivation

Myxoma virus grows and produces cellular changes in a variety of cell cultures including squirrel, rat, hamster, guinea-pig, chicken and human tissues, although the animals themselves are not susceptible. In rabbit kidney epithelial cells and in rabbit heart fibroblasts, strikingly different cytopathic effects are obtained. In the former, acidophilic intracytoplasmic inclusions are formed and there is vacuolation of the nucleus, whereas the latter show large stellate cells with basophilic granules in the nucleus and very little 'inclusion material' in the cytoplasm. (Plates 52.4 b, c, facing p. 693, and plate 52.5a, facing p. 708). In plaque assay experiments, myxoma virus produces microscopic plaques of damaged cells in rabbit kidney monolayers which reach a diameter of up to 3 mm. after 6 days and do not stain with neutral red. This is in sharp contrast to the plaques produced by fibroma viruses which are up to 1.5 mm. in diameter only, and are composed of clumps of cells which take up and retain neutral red as do the healthy cells of the monolayer. In nearly all cases, over 90 per cent of the virus remains cell-associated throughout the growth cycle. After serial passage of the Californian myxoma virus (MSD strain) in cultured rabbit kidney cells, the virus is sufficiently attenuated to be used for immunization. Myxoma virus can be serially passaged on the chorioallantoic membrane and dilute suspensions of virus produce discrete pocks of 0.5 to 1 mm. in diameter after 3 days of incubation without adaptation. (Plates 52.6a, b, facing p. 709). Fibroma virus also grows well on the chorioallantoic membrane but produces very minute lesions which are too small to be counted. Pocksize can be used to characterise certain strains of myxoma virus. Although pock-counting can be used for virus titration, eggs are 2–3 times less sensitive than rabbits' skin. The virus, and that of fibroma, can also be serially passaged in newborn mice inoculated intracerebrally without producing symptoms but weaned mice are insusceptible.

Pathogenicity

In Uruguay and Brazil myxomatosis persists in native wild rabbits (*Sylvilagus brasiliensis*) in a harmless form and mosquitoes are responsible for spreading the infection. Following mosquito bite, the only sign of infection in the rabbit is a localised swelling which appears at the site of inoculation about a week later. Although the tumour-like swelling may persist for at least 3 months there is no generalization and the disease is not fatal. In other parts of the world, feral and domestic (*Oryctolagus*) rabbits are generally highly susceptible to the disease. Following insect bite, the virus multiplies initially at the inoculation site. Thereafter, it spreads via the lymph nodes and blood to the internal organs where it replicates, probably in the cells lining the small arterioles. The subsequent viraemia enables the virus to reach the skin where further multiplication gives rise to generalised tumour-like swellings. In most natural outbreaks subcutaneous gelatinous swellings usually appear by the third or fourth day and by the end of a week they have increased in size and spread all over the body. On first contact with the new host, virulent strains will kill almost all infected rabbits within about 12 days of infection. The first characteristic symptom is that of blepharo-conjunctivitis which rapidly becomes more marked and is accompanied by a milky discharge from the inflamed eyes which leads to sealing of the eyelids with inspissated pus. Other early signs include swelling of the nose, muzzle and ano-genital region. Generalised swelling of the head gives the animal a characteristic leonine appearance. (Plate 52.5c, facing p. 708). In severe acute outbreaks, the rabbits appear listless, the temperature frequently reaches 42.0°C and many of the animals die within 48 hours of showing symptoms. With less virulent strains, or in rabbits which have become genetically resistant, the signs are much less severe, less rapidly progressive and many infected animals may linger on for several weeks before death ensues, but some may recover. In these cases fibrotic nodules may be found on the nose, ears and feet. The subcutaneous swellings consist of undifferentiated mesenchymal cells and exude a sero-mucinous exudate when they are cut. Histologically, the lesions are characterised by the presence of numerous 'myxoma' cells. These are large stellate cells derived from the mesenchymal tissues, some of which contain acidophilic cytoplasmic inclusions. (Plate 52.5b, facing p. 708). In rabbits that survive, serum neutralizing and complement-fixing antibodies are produced from about the 10th. day onwards and the animals themselves are immune.

Reactivation

The phenomenon of non-genetic reactivation is a general property of the poxvirus group, but does not occur with other groups of viruses. Thus, when a mixture of heat- or ether-inactivated myxoma virus and active rabbit or squirrel fibroma virus is inoculated into rabbits, reactivation of the myxoma virus occurs and most of the experimentally infected animals develop clinical myxomatosis.

Ecology

Myxomatosis spreads with difficulty via the respiratory tract and by contact, but rabbit to rabbit spread is usually possible only across distances of a few inches. Such infection is probably due to mechanical transmission of the virus by the rabbit louse or the rabbit flea. In Britain and France the rabbit flea, *Spilopsyllus cuniculi*, is the principal vector. In South America and Australia, as in most parts of the world, mosquitoes (*Aëdes* and *Anopheles*) constitute the most important vehicle of infection, but the virus does not multiply in those vectors although infection can take place as long as 7 months after the infective feed.

Diagnosis

The nature and distribution of the subcutaneous swellings and the very high mortality in rabbits exposed to the virulent virus for the first time are so characteristic of the disease that laboratory confirmation is seldom necessary. Diagnosis is much more difficult, however, when the disease is less severe due to attenuation of the virus or to an increase in genetic resistance in the rabbit population. In those atypical cases, the virus can be isolated on the chorioallantoic membrane of fertile eggs and identified by neutralization and cross-immunity tests. Histological examination of lesions for the presence of 'myxoma cells' and intracytoplasmic inclusions is also of value.

Control

Prophylactic vaccination of domestic rabbits can be carried out by inoculation of Shope's fibroma virus. Although this produces a lesion and should not be used in young rabbits of under 3 weeks of age, an active immunity is produced and usually protects the rabbit against fatal myxomatosis. Domestic rabbits should also be protected against attack by mosquitoes and other biting insects. In some countries a live vaccine prepared from an attenuated strain of myxoma virus is available commercially.

Fibromatosis of rabbits

In 1932, Shope described a benign subcutaneous fibrous tumour of cotton-tail rabbits which was transmissible to both wild and domestic rabbits by the inoculation of cell-free filtrates. The causative virus belongs to the pox group of viruses and is regarded at present as a member of the genus *Leporipoxvirus*. Rabbit fibroma virus is immunologically related to myxoma virus and to the fibroma viruses of hares in Europe and grey squirrels in North America. The relationship to myxoma virus is extremely close and only minor differences are revealed in cross-complement-fixation or precipitation tests. Vaccination of rabbits with Shope's fibroma virus will confer considerable protection against myxomatosis. Some strains of fibroma virus can be cultivated on the chorioallantoic membrane of fertile hens' eggs but, unlike myxoma virus, do not produce focal lesions. Most strains grow and produce a cytopathic effect on cell cultures derived from rabbit, guinea-pig, rat and man.

In natural infections in cotton-tail (*Sylvilagus*) and European rabbits (*Oryctolagus*), firm spherical loosely attached tumours occur in the same animal. The lesions normally remain localised and are usually found on the foot. Histological examination shows that the swellings are composed of numerous spindle-shaped connective tissue cells. Experimental infection in cotton-tail rabbits leads to an immediate inflammatory reaction followed by fibroblastic proliferation. The growth of the tumour continues over a long period of time and the virus persists for 10–12 weeks or more. In domestic rabbits, however, growth is rapid and regression of the tumour may begin 10–14 days after infection and quickly disappears. Although the virus has been propagated successfully by intracerebral inoculation of 1-day-old mice, other laboratory animals including chickens, rats and guinea-pigs are not susceptible.

The method of transmission is not yet known but the virus does not pass from animal to animal by contact, nor is it passed from mother to young through the placenta or milk. The disease is produced in experimental rabbits only by inoculation and it is suggested that natural transmission may occur by *Aëdes* and *Culex* mosquitoes, or other biting insects, as in myxomatosis.

CAPRIPOXVIRUS

Sheep Pox

Synonyms
Variola ovina: Clavelée (Fr.): Schafpocken (Ger.).

Definition
Sheep pox is a highly contagious febrile and often fatal illness characterised by epithelial hyperplasia and micro-vesicle formation in the epidermis which is particularly noticeable on the more exposed parts of the body. It is the most severe pox disease of domestic animals.

Hosts affected
Sheep are the only natural hosts but the susceptibility of different breeds is extremely variable. Merinos are probably the most susceptible. Coarse-woolled sheep are less susceptible and the disease is very mild or even inapparent in the so-called resistant Algerian breed.

History and distribution
Sheep pox is known to have existed in Asia since the second century A.D. and was first mentioned in England as long ago as 1275. The disease is enzootic in many parts of the world being particularly prevalent in the Near and Middle East (apart from Cyprus), Asia and areas of Northern Africa through to Ethiopia, Kenya, Somalia and the Sudan. Sheep pox does not occur in the continents of America and Australasia and it has been eradicated from Great Britain (in 1862), Scandinavia, the Netherlands, Germany and many other countries in Europe. Small foci of infection may still persist in parts of France, Russia, Greece, Portugal and Spain. In 1973, sheep pox was known to exist in 29 countries and was suspected in 16 others.

Properties of the virus
Mature elementary bodies, which are visible in smears stained by Paschen's method, are smaller and more elongated than other pox viruses and measure approximately 200 x 115 nm. The virus survives dessication for long periods and is said to remain active in particles of dry scabs for 3 months, in unused sheep pens for 6 months and in grazed pastures for 2 months. It is inactivated in 15 minutes by 2 per cent phenol and by formalin. A relatively low resistance to heating at 55°C for 30 minutes is a characteristic of the virus. Unlike most other poxviruses, sheep pox is rapidly inactivated by exposure to 20 per cent ethyl ether or to chloroform. The nucleic acid core contains DNA. Little is known about the haemagglutinin activity of sheep pox virus but Russian workers have recorded low haemagglutination titres with fowl red blood cells.

Antigenicity
Specific complement-fixation is reported and it has long been known that antigen from the subcutaneous tissues of experimentally infected sheep will fix complement in the presence of antibody in the sera of convalescent or vaccinated sheep. Neutralization of sheep pox virus by specific antiserum was studied by Borrel in 1903 who developed a method for immunisation (sero-clavelization) using incompletely neutralized virus. Surprisingly little information is available regarding the antigenic structure of this, one of the most important and destructive of all the animal pox viruses, and a good deal of confusion exists about the possible antigenic relationships with other pox viruses. Agar gel diffusion and cross complement-fixation tests indicate that sheep and goat pox viruses in India share a common antigen, while the latter test also shows that some cross reaction may occur between orf, sheep pox and goat pox viruses. However, this latter observation is not acceptable to other workers and more

recent studies employing indirect flourescent antibody staining failed to reveal cross-fluorescence between orf virus and the viruses of sheep pox, goat pox, camel pox, cowpox and vaccinia. Tissue culture studies show cross neutralization between goat pox, sheep pox and lumpy skin disease viruses in East Africa, and also some crossing with vaccinia and cowpox. Gel diffusion tests using convalescent serum show 2 lines of precipitation with homologous goat pox antigen and only one line with the heterologous sheep pox antigen. Using hyperimmune goat pox rabbit serum, no fewer than 6 lines of precipitation are distinguishable with the homologous goat pox antigen compared with only 3 lines with sheep pox antigen. It has also been suggested that strains of sheep and goat pox viruses exist that are completely host specific and cannot be transmitted to chick embryos, unweaned mice, rabbits, guinea-pigs or hamsters.

The many variable and conflicting reports regarding antigenic relationships between sheep pox, goat pox and other animal poxviruses may be due to differences in the geographical location, the breeds of sheep and goats affected, and the stage of adaptation reached in natural as well as in closely related hosts, but further work in this field is urgently required.

Cultivation
Several unsuccessful attempts have been made to propagate the virus in rabbits and other laboratory animals and only very limited successes have been achieved in attempts to adapt the virus to fertile hens' eggs. A Chinese strain of sheep pox virus passaged in chicken embryos became attenuated after 90 passages and was of low virulence for the chicken embryos. It did not agglutinate fowl red blood cells and was harmless for sheep but induced a strong immunity when injected intradermally or subcutaneously. Sheep pox virus replicates in sheep and goat kidney cell cultures and produces specific cytopathic changes within 4–6 days but the infection tends to be self-limiting and rarely involves more than half of the monolayer. On the other hand, an extensive cytopathic effect can often be obtained in tissues from very young animals. Monolayers of sheep testis fibroblasts produce high titred virus with a cytopathic effect that becomes visible within 24 hours and generalised 3 days later. By the fourth day of incubation most of the cells contain eosinophilic cytoplasmic inclusions that become larger, more basophilic and acquire a well-marked 'halo'. Within the inclusions small elongated elementary bodies may be visible. Basophilic inclusion material and other abnormalities can be found in the nuclei of infected cells from about the 3rd day onwards. Similar nuclear changes have been described in cells infected with other pox viruses including myxoma, lumpy skin disease and swine pox. Calf testis cells are equally susceptible to 'culture-virus' as those derived from sheep despite the fact that sheep pox virus does not initiate local or generalised lesions in calves. The 'culture virus' can, however, be transmitted to goats but serial passage of the virus in this species does not attenuate the virus for sheep. The Chinese and Russian (Stavropol) strains of sheep pox give identical changes in cultures of sheep embryo lung cells, a cytopathic effect developing after 7 to 10 days, or within 4 days after several passages. Although intra-cytoplasmic inclusions are present in infected cells the most characteristic changes are related to destruction of the cell nuclei, a phenomenon which has also been observed with some African isolates. The Kazakhstan strain of sheep pox has been successfully adapted to cell cultures derived from skin and muscle of mouse embryos giving an unusual diffuse-type of cytopathic effect but with titres up to 10^5 TCID$_{50}$/ml. This strain has been adapted to KEM-La cells after only 5 to 7 passages, losing its virulence for sheep in the process but retaining its full immunological properties.

Pathogenicity
The first sign of infection following an incubation period of about 4–8 days is a rise in temperature, increase in respiration rate, swollen eyelids and a mucous discharge from the nose. On the second day of the clinical illness there is an intense inflammatory reaction in the dermis. Dermal oedema becomes marked, the skin proliferates until it is 12–15 cells thick and raised circular thickened plaques with congested borders develop on the skin. In many respects the cutaneous reaction is similar to that produced by other poxviruses and passes through the various stages of papules, micro-vesicles, pustular pocks and scabs. The eruptions may be widely distributed over the body but are most prevalent on the cheeks, lips, ears and wool-free skin. (Plate 52.5d, facing p. 708). Viraemia frequently follows the development of the primary pock and may give rise to generalisation resulting often in tracheitis and caseous nodules in the lungs. At this stage the virus can be isolated from almost any tissue. When the clinical reaction starts to regress, the temperature falls and during resolution of the pocks there is often severe itching, shedding of wool and exfoliation of the epidermis. The course of the uncomplicated form of the disease is about 3 to 4 weeks. In addition, post-mortem examination may reveal haemorrhagic inflammation and ulcers of the mucous membranes of the respiratory and intestinal tracts as well as swelling of the lymph nodes, petechiation of the serous membranes and numerous small spherical nodules in the lungs, kidneys and occasionally in

some other tissues. A gelatinous oedema of the subcutaneous and intramuscular tissues is not uncommon. Histological examination of tissues taken during the period of resolution reveals dramatic changes in the dermal vessels. These include severe vasculitis, with necrosis of the vessels and the formation of thrombi. Elsewhere, the mesodermal cells contain numerous stellate histiocyte-like cells with vacuolated nuclei, enlarged nucleoli and cytoplasm swollen by large vacuoles, the so-called 'cellules claveleuses'. In a number of cells single, round or oval inclusions can be seen in a juxta-nuclear position, and are considered to be the sites of viral replication. The mortality rate varies from 5 to 50 per cent, and occasionally as high as 80 per cent, depending on the breed susceptibility and the type of strain of virus involved. Sheep inoculated intradermally in the tail-fold with sheep-adapted sheep pox virus develop a viraemia in 3 to 4 days, reaching its maximum on the 5th day and disappearing by the 9th day. On the 8th day there are considerable quantities of the virus in the oedematous subcutaneous tissues (c. 8×10^6) and precrural lymph nodes, moderate amounts in the spleen, liver and kidneys (c. 5×10^2) and some in the lungs (c. 1×10^1). Some strains of sheep pox virus may produce local lesions in artificially infected goats and cattle.

Ecology
In naturally occurring cases, transmission probably occurs from contact with infected animals or with objects contaminated with the virus. Infected sheep are particularly liable to spread the virus after the pustules have developed. Air-borne infections are probably the most important, especially with the sheep specific strains, and there are reports of air-borne transmission taking place over distances of 20–25 yards. The virus survives well under natural conditions and unused sheep pens are said to harbour the virus for 6 months or longer. The less species-specific strains and some of the milder types of infection do not spread readily by contact, and there is evidence that biting insects may play a part in the mechanical transmission of the disease.

Diagnosis
The clinical diagnosis of sheep pox is based on the history, course, and symptoms of the disease, together with the post-mortem findings. Confirmation is obtained in a laboratory by examination of suitably stained smears and tissue sections for the presence of elementary bodies and 'cellules claveleuses'. Gel diffusion slide tests using hyperimmune anti-sheep pox rabbit serum are of value for the rapid diagnosis of sheep pox in skin nodules and scabs. Isolation and identification of the virus can be carried out in various tissue culture systems depending on the strains of virus likely to be involved in the outbreak. The cytopathic effect on tissue monolayers can be neutralized by means of specific antisera, although complete neutralization of the virus does not occur. Neutralization tests in cell cultures may also be used to detect rising antibody titres in paired serum samples. Cross-protection tests can also be carried out if pox-susceptible and immune sheep are available.

Control
Animals which recover from natural infections of sheep pox develop a solid, sometimes life-long active immunity. Vaccination by scarification (ovination) or intradermal injection of glycerine-preserved lymph obtained from artificially induced cases, is commonly employed to control infection in an endemic area. To prevent outbreaks of clinical sheep pox attributable to the use of virulent lymph, a mixture of the virus and immune serum will produce a satisfactory level of immunity without formation of lesions. In Russia an avianized strain ('K') grown on the chorioallantoic membrane of embryonated hens' eggs is used to prepare a dried vaccine. The use of this vaccine in 1 ml. amounts into the caudal fold of the tail produces no side effects and is said to confer 100 per cent protection after 2 months and, in most cases, for as long as 5 months. Freeze-dried vaccines prepared from the Russian and Chinese avianized strains can be stored satisfactorily for at least 13 months. Inactivated virus is less efficient and only protects for a few months even when adjuvants are incorporated in the vaccine. In some countries promising results are obtained when virus is first adsorbed on to aluminium hydroxide and then formolised, whereas in other regions β-propiolactone inactivated oil adjuvant vaccines are used. Cell culture vaccines are also being developed in which large quantities of virus are propagated for 30–40 passages in calf kidney, lamb kidney or lamb testis cells and adsorbed on to aluminium hydroxide. First reports indicate that they confer a solid immunity on susceptible sheep which persists for about a year or longer.

Lambs born of immune ewes may acquire passive protection through ingestion of antibodies in the colostrum, and immune serum may be used to confer a passive immunity. The protection thus conferred is immediate but short-lived.

Goat Pox

Synonyms
Variole des chèvres (Fr.): Ziegenpocken (Ger.): Variola caprina.

Definition

Goat pox is a well recognised epizootic disease that closely resembles sheep pox and is characterised by fever, a mucopurulent nasal discharge and the development of a generalised cutaneous eruption.

Hosts affected

Natural infections occur mostly in goats but it is generally believed that some strains may produce the clinical disease in sheep. Man may not be entirely immune as an eruption of small vesicles on the hands and arms is sometimes observed in those who handle goats, but confirmation is still awaited that this condition is due to the virus of goat pox.

History and distribution

Goat pox has probably existed since early times but its presence as a distinct disease entity was first recorded in Norway in 1879. Since then the disease has been recognised in Africa, parts of Europe, many near Eastern Countries, India and the Far East. Suggestions that the disease might occasionally occur in South America and Australasia have not been confirmed.

Properties of the virus

Very little is known about the properties of the virus but most workers are agreed that it is very similar to that of sheep pox. It resists freezing and thawing and remains viable for many months in the dried state. The virus is believed to be ether-sensitive. Agar gel diffusion and cross complement-fixation tests indicate that goat and sheep pox viruses share a common antigen and that some cross reaction occurs between orf, sheep pox and goat pox, but not vaccinia. Detection of precipitinogens in skin nodules and vesicles by means of homologous and heterologous pox sera has been reported. Hyperimmune sera prepared in rabbits and tested in cell culture show cross neutralization between lumpy skin disease virus and some strains of goat pox and sheep pox.

Cultivation

Goat pox grows readily in cell cultures of lamb kidney, kid kidney and kid testis, producing cyto-pathic changes and inclusions similar to those described for sheep pox. There is usually complete degeneration of the infected monolayers within 5 days. It has been reported that growth occurs on the chorioallantoic membrane of fertile hens' eggs after a short period of adaptation and that the virus becomes attenuated for goats after 4–8 passes.

Pathogenicity

Natural cases of goat pox are commonest in younger animals or females in milk, and the mortality rate ranges from 0–50 per cent, although on rare occasions it may be even higher. The clinical picture is similar to that of sheep pox. Following an incubation period of some 5–14 days, small papules appear on the hairless regions of the body around the eyes, nose and mouth, on the udder, teats or scrotum and on the inner aspects of the thighs. Later, lesions develop which are of different sizes, sometimes confluent and umbilicated, and after forming crusts they heal uneventfully within 3–4 weeks, leaving well-defined radiating cicatrices. Some affected goats show fever, and nasal and lachrymal discharges that become mucopurulent. Recovered animals develop a solid, life-long immunity.

With some strains of goat pox virus, experimentally induced infection of sheep can be achieved and there are unconfirmed reports of successful transmissions to cattle, monkeys and rabbits.

Ecology

The saliva may contain large quantities of virus and it is claimed that transmission can occur by contact with infected animals or with objects contaminated with the virus. Spread is usually rapid among the members of the herd and commonly affects all the animals. Frequently, however, the disease remains confined to the infected herd and there is little tendency to further extension. Many observers believe that mechanical transmission by biting insects is an important factor in the spread of this disease, but little information is available about the hazards of airborne transmission.

Diagnosis

Diagnosis is invariably based on the course and symptoms of the disease. In the laboratory, gel diffusion tests have proved helpful in detecting specific precipitinogens in affected tissues, and tissue cultures can be used to isolate the virus. Antibody titres in paired serum samples are generally low and may be of little diagnostic value.

Control

In the Near East live vaccines are being developed from goat and chicken embryo adapted strains of goat pox virus. Attempts are also being made to attenuate strains of goat pox virus on lamb and kid testis cultures and preliminary field trials have given promising results.

Lumpy Skin Disease

Synonyms

Knopvelsiekte: Exanthema nodularis bovis: Dermatose nodulaire (Fr.): Knotenansschlag des Rindes (Ger.): Pseudo-urticaria.

Definition

Lumpy skin disease is an acute, febrile infectious disease of cattle characterised by the sudden appearance of an eruption of skin nodules of varying size and extent which usually undergo necrosis.

Hosts affected

The disease is known to affect only cattle and it does not spread to other species of animals. All ages and breeds are susceptible but Channel Island cattle and other thin-skinned breeds are most severely affected.

History and distribution

This was an unknown disease until it first appeared in Northern Rhodesia in 1929 and was called 'pseudo-urticaria'. In 1944 the same condition was reported in the Transvaal and, by 1945 and 1946, it had become widespread in the Union of South Africa. By the late 1950s the disease had appeared in a number of other territories including Kenya, Uganda, Tanzania, Zaire and Madagascar. More recently, lumpy skin disease has been spreading Westwards and outbreaks have been reported in the Sudan (1971), Tchad (1973), Niger (1974) and, possibly, Northern Nigeria (1974).

Properties of the virus

Three different groups of cytopathic agents have been associated with lumpy skin disease of cattle one of which, the Group III or 'Neethling' strain is now known to be the causative virus of this condition. The Group I 'Orphan' strains and the Group II, 'Allerton' type viruses are discussed in the chapter on Herpesviruses. The Neethling virus is related to African sheep pox which is now thought to resemble closely goat pox virus.

Negatively-stained preparations show that the particles of lumpy skin disease virus are morphologically similar to those of vaccinia. The virion measures approximately 350 nm in length by 300 nm in width, and its outer-coat consists of a complex interwoven network of strands presenting an irregular surface structure.

The virus is readily inactivated by treatment with ether or chloroform, suggesting that lipid is incorporated in the outer layers of the virion. It is remarkably stable between pH 6.6 and 8.6 and is thermostable for 5 days at 37°C. The virus withstands repeated freezing at −25°C and thawing at room temperature without significant drop of titre, and it will survive in glycerol-saline or in tissue culture fluid kept at 4°C for 4–6 months. It is also known to persist in skin lesions of affected cattle for at least 33 days even though the necrotic material has become completely dry.

Antigenic properties

There is only one immunological type of virus responsible for true lumpy skin disease and all strains of virus show complete reciprocal cross-neutralization with the 'Neethling' prototype strain.

Cultivation

Neethling virus multiplies on the chorioallantoic membrane of embryonated hens' eggs causing the production of macroscopic 'pocks', but it is not lethal to the chick embryo. After 20 serial passages in fertile eggs the virus becomes attenuated for cattle. The highest yield of virus is obtained by inoculating 5-day-old embryonated eggs and harvesting the membranes after 6 days' further incubation at 33.5°C. No 'pocks' are formed under these conditions but the average infectivity for cell cultures is approximately $10^{4.5}$ TCID$_{50}$.

Group III viruses, of which Neethling is the prototype strain, can be readily propagated in a wide variety of cell cultures including lamb and calf kidney, testes, adrenal and thyroid cells and chick embryo fibroblasts. Continuous cell lines such as bovine kidney and baby hamster kidney (BHK-21) cells will also support the growth of the virus. Progress of the degenerative changes is slow and the cytopathic effect does not become evident before the 10th day of incubation, but after several serial passages in susceptible cultures the cellular abnormalities appear after only 3–4 days but may take a further 3–5 days to reach completion. However, the reaction can be speeded up by increasing the concentration of lactalbumin hydrolysate in the growth medium to 2 per cent, and cytopathic effects become evident with primary field isolates after only 3 days of incubation. Infected cells initially appear as discrete foci of rounded, highly refractile cells and stained monolayer cultures show intracytoplasmic inclusions. These are large rounded or oval moderately acidophilic masses often surrounded by a halo and situated close to one pole of the nucleus. Some of the inclusions are frankly basophilic but become more acidophilic as they increase in size. Many of the cells show finely granular intracytoplasmic acidophilic matrices with basophilic inner bodies, often in the shape of a broken arc or continuous hoop towards the periphery of the cell. Some inclusions are spherical but others have irregular outlines and show small protuberances at their margins. Cells may contain one to several intracytoplasmic inclusions of varying size and the affected cells become rounded and shrunken. There is no evidence of syncytial formation. Immunofluorescence studies show that the cytoplasm is the site of viral replication and that the inclusion material contains viral antigen. In infected cell cultures the virus is mostly cell-bound but can be released into the supernatant fluid by disruption of the cells by sonication.

Rabbits inoculated intradermally develop local erythematous lesions at the site of inoculation followed, perhaps, by generalization within 4 days.

Pathogenicity

Cattle are the natural hosts of the virus and all breeds and both sexes are equally susceptible. Sheep and goats may be susceptible and the first outbreak of lumpy skin disease in cattle in Kenya was believed to have been associated with a disease in sheep. Spontaneous outbreaks have not been described in game animals although several species are susceptible to experimental infection.

The natural incubation period is unknown but is probably about 7–14 days, and cases can be expected within 2–4 weeks following the introduction of healthy cattle into an infected herd. The first sign of the disease is a rise in body temperature which varies from 38–41°C followed in 4–14 days by a generalised eruption of firm, circumscribed, raised and painful nodules involving the skin and underlying muscle. In most cases there is marked enlargement of the superficial lymph nodes which are freely palpable and cause visible swellings of the skin. The nodules are circular and discrete and vary greatly in size but are usually about 2–3 cm. in diameter, and may number from 1 or 2 to more than 100. They may occur on any part of the body but are generally most numerous on the head and neck, brisket, thighs and back. In very severe cases lesions may extend all over the body from muzzle to tail. Granulomatous lesions may also be found in the tongue, dental pad and inner surface of the cheeks in severely affected calves. The nodules usually undergo complete necrosis but indurated skin lesions may persist for many years. They begin to separate from the surrounding tissue after about 7–14 days and become hard and dry to form 'sitfasts' which may take 2–3 months or longer before complete recovery. Affected animals are often unwilling to move and there is frequently oedema of the brisket, limbs and udder, a drop in milk yield and abortion of pregnant cows. In some animals breathing is laboured and there may be inappetence, depression, excessive salivation and a nasal discharge which may be mucopurulent. Although the morbidity rate varies between 5 and 45 per cent in certain areas of Africa, the mortality rate rarely exceeds 1 per cent. Nevertheless, the economic loss is considerable especially in the hide trade where affected skins may be so pitted and holed that the majority are quite unsaleable.

At necropsy there is general lymphadenitis and the affected glands are oedematous and 4 or 5 times the normal size. Raised plaques are commonly found in the buccal cavity and sometimes in the wall of the rumen. Microscopical examination shows the presence of acidophilic intracytoplasmic inclusions in the epithelial cells of affected tissues.

Following intradermal or subcutaneous inoculation of virus into susceptible experimental cattle a local, firm, painful swelling develops at the site of inoculation after an incubation period of 4–7 days. The regional lymph nodes are enlarged but the infection is usually benign. Generalization is rare but may occur 2–3 weeks after inoculation with the formation some weeks later of typical dry necrotic sequestrae. In artificially infected cattle, the virus may be recovered from the skin nodules, underlying musculature, saliva, blood and spleen.

A mild transient infection has been described in sheep and goats following inoculation of infective cattle skin suspensions as the source of virus.

Immunity

Cattle that recover from a natural infection develop neutralizing antibodies in their sera which persist for a number of years. Following immunization with modified live virus vaccine, circulating antibodies appear about the 10th day, reach a high titre by the 30th day and persist for more than 3 years. Calves derive a passive immunity via the colostrum which persists for up to 6 months. A report that experimentally infected cattle which fail to develop local reactions are often resistant to challenge despite the absence of neutralizing antibodies in their sera awaits confirmation, and no explanation has been given to account for this phenomenon.

Ecology

The method of natural infection and transmission is not known but the disease can be transmitted experimentally to cattle by the inoculation of blood taken at the height of the fever and of material obtained from fresh nodules. The virus has also been demonstrated in the saliva of clinically affected cattle but infection by direct contact has not yet been proved. Because many of the original outbreaks in South Africa occurred during the wet summer months, and were particularly prevalent in low-lying and moist areas, many workers are of the opinion that the infection may be transmitted mechanically by a variety of biting arthropods particularly mosquitoes. This theory is supported by the failure of quarantine methods to confine the infection, and the fact that the disease often appears to jump many miles from one area to another and spreads along water courses and valleys. However, outbreaks are known to occur also during winter when the insect population is at its lowest. Recovered animals harbour the virus for 3 weeks at least but the existence of symptomless carriers has not been proven.

Diagnosis

A presumptive diagnosis of lumpy skin disease is usually based on the erratic method of spread of the infection from farm to farm and the appearance of the distinctive nodules on the skin, together with lesions in the mouth, oedema of the limbs and marked swelling of the superficial lymph nodes. The disease is more readily diagnosed where there is necrosis of the nodules giving rise to the characteristic tightly adherent 'sitfasts'. Confirmatory diagnosis is obtained by microscopical examination of stained sections of excised skin lesions for the presence of intracytoplasmic inclusions, by the isolation and identification of the causative pox-like virus on cell culture monolayers and the demonstration of a rise of neutralizing antibody titre in the sera of suspect animals.

Differential diagnosis

The disease may be confused with several other conditions including Allerton-type infection, cowpox, pseudo-cowpox, papular stomatitis, globidiosis, demodicosis, mycotic dermatitis, urticaria, mange, ringworm and photosensitization.

Control

Recovered cattle are believed to be immune for several months at least and, in East Africa, virulent strains of sheep pox virus, propagated in tissue culture, have proved successful as vaccines for controlling lumpy skin disease in infected areas. It is claimed that these live virus vaccines are safe for cattle and even sheep in close contact. Strains of Neethling virus attenuated by egg-passage are also being used as vaccines and are said to produce a good immunity. It has also been reported that certain African strains of 'sheep pox', which are believed to be more closely related to goat pox, give better protection against lumpy skin disease than true sheep pox virus.

UNCLASSIFIED POXVIRUSES

All members of the family *Poxviridae* are related immunologically by a common internal antigen which is extractable from the virion by 1 N sodium hydroxide. They can be divided into a number of genera (Table 38.1, pp. 414–5) on the basis of their more specific antigens, morphology and natural hosts. But some, such as those responsible for horse pox, swine pox, camel pox, molluscum contagiosum, Yaba monkey pox and Tana poxvirus infection, have not been investigated sufficiently to permit accurate classification and are placed temporarily in the unclassified group of poxviruses.

Horse Pox

Synonyms

Contagious pustular stomatitis: Variola equina. Grease, grease-heels and sore-heels are also regarded as synonyms but some workers consider them as separate entities due to a different virus.

Definition

A benign but highly contagious viral disease of horses that is characterized by typical pox-like eruptions on the pasterns (grease) or on the buccal mucous membrane (contagious pustular stomatitis). It should not be confused with the condition known as grease or seborrhoea which is a chronic dermatitis of the fetlock and pastern region and bears no relationship to horse pox.

Hosts affected

Only horses are the true natural hosts but hand lesions on animal attendants have been reported.

History and distribution

The first critical appraisal of horse pox was made by Jenner who regarded it as a vesico-pustular contagious eruption of the pasterns, and so convinced was he of its identity with cowpox that he vaccinated a number of children against smallpox with material from affected horses. The buccal form of horse pox (contagious pustular stomatitis or contagious pustular dermatitis of horses) was not described until much later, and chiefly occurs as a stall infection of young horses. With the rapid world-wide decline in the number of horses in recent years, horse pox in either of its clinical forms is now very rare and in 1964 only a few sporadic outbreaks were recorded from Mexico, Denmark, France, Norway, Hungary, Spain and Jordan. The disease has not been reported in the U.S.A.

Aetiology

The 2 clinical forms of the disease may be caused either by different strains of the same virus, which is closely related to cowpox, or by 2 different but related viruses one of which causes Jenner's grease-heel and is probably true cowpox virus. Unfortunately, the specific agents have not yet been adequately characterized and numerous reports of cross-immunity with vaccinia, cowpox and other poxviruses await confirmation. There is general agreement, however, that the causal agent of horse pox is closely related to cowpox virus since both diseases are reciprocally transmissible and give rise to reciprocal immunity.

Pathogenicity

Although natural infections occur in horses the

existence of a primary horse pox virus is doubtful, and it is probable that the disease first arose from human patients affected with cowpox or from recently vaccinated animal attendants.

Grease or greasy-heel is characterized by tenderness and pain of the affected pasterns and fetlocks. The skin becomes red and oedematous as the lesions progress rapidly through the typical papule, vesicle and pustule stages, becoming transformed into brownish adherent crusts after rupturing. In the buccal form there is usually a mild transient fever and the animal has difficulty in masticating its food and may salivate profusely. Papules appear on the mucous membranes of the lips and gums, which are hot and painful, and quickly develop into vesicles containing clear serous fluid. These may become confluent and rupture leaving small erosions on the mucous membranes, or become larger and develop into pustules which eventually leave deep crateriform ulcers. Extension of the lesions may occasionally give rise to catarrhal symptoms and to an eruption of papules, pustules and ulcers on other parts of the body such as the nares, chest, upper limbs, perineum and, sometimes, the whole body. In such exceptional circumstances the course of the disease may run for 4–6 weeks, instead of the more usual 10–24 days, and a few horses may die.

The virus produces a typical skin eruption in experimentally infected horses, cattle, dogs, pigs and poultry, after a short incubation period of 2–3 days, and recovered animals are solidly immune to challenge with active calf lymph.

Ecology
Horse pox virus survives for very long periods on harness and other equipment, and spreads quickly in large studs of susceptible horses. In the buccal form, the primary mode of natural transmission is probably via contaminated food and water-troughs, but droplet infection may also occur. Greasy-heel can be acquired through contact with animal attendants suffering from cowpox or who have recently been vaccinated against smallpox; and it may also be transmitted indirectly by contact with contaminated equipment, harness and kicking posts.

Diagnosis
The diagnosis of horse pox is usually based on the history and clinical findings. The disease usually runs a mild course and the assistance of the laboratory is rarely sought, and confirmation of the disease is seldom achieved.

Control
Recovered horses possess a solid, long-lasting immunity to artificial infection and vaccinia has been used successfully to produce protection. However, owing to the benign nature of the disease little attention is being given to the preparation and use of vaccines to control the infection. Most spontaneous outbreaks of horse pox can be controlled by rigorous quarantine measures and the thorough cleansing and disinfection of buildings and equipment.

Camel Pox

Synonyms
Variole du chemau: Kamelpocken: Photo-Shootur.

Definition
A mild, occasionally severe, contagious disease of camels which is characterised by pox-like eruptions on the head and other parts of the body having few hairs.

Hosts Affected
Natural cases of the disease occur only in camels and dromedaries, but there are many unconfirmed reports that camel drivers may develop lesions on their hands and arms from contact with affected animals. In East Africa it is believed that people drinking milk from affected camels may develop ulcers on the lips and in the mouth.

History and distribution
The disease probably existed but remained unrecognised for many centuries before being first described about the middle of the 19th century. It is known to occur in the Middle East, North and East Africa, Pakistan and in the far eastern states of Asiatic Russia, and may be endemic in all countries having large camel populations.

Properties of the virus
Little information is available about the properties of camel pox virus and, as in most other animal pox diseases, it is not known whether the infection is due to a species-specific strain of virus or whether other pox viruses can initiate infection after becoming adapted to a secondary host. The clinical disease is typical of a pox virus infection and the causative agent is highly resistant to the natural environment. Most strains are sensitive to pH 3–5 and pH 8.5–10, and are ether sensitive but chloroform resistant.

Cultivation
East African strains of camel pox replicate and produce cytopathic effects in a variety of cell culture systems including baby hamster kidney (BHK-21), Vero, lamb testis, lamb kidney and calf kidney cells. Small, roughly circular plaques measuring 0.4–0.8 mm in diameter are formed after 5 days' incubation

and many of the infected cells contain acidophilic intracytoplasmic inclusions. Infected monolayers haemadsorb chicken red blood cells and their supernatant fluids contain low titres of haemagglutinins. Raised, greyish-white pocks are formed on the chorioallantoic membrane of embryonated hens' eggs when incubated at 37°C, but not at 39°C. Rabbits and sheep do not react to scarification or intradermal inoculation with the Iranian, Russian or East African viruses. On the other hand, it has been reported that an Egyptian strain (Fayoum-71) produces erythematous lesions in rabbits 3–4 days after intradermal inoculation and that the virus can be isolated and serially transferred through rabbits without difficulty. No reaction ensues, however, following scarification of the cornea with this virus.

Antigenicity

Little is known about the antigenic properties of camel pox virus, but there appears to be a close relationship with cowpox, vaccinia and variola viruses, and it has been recorded that Arab tribes protect their children from smallpox by vaccinating them with camel pox virus.

Indirect immunofluorescence studies reveal cross-fluorescence between camel pox, vaccinia and cowpox viruses but not with sheep pox, goat pox or lumpy skin disease viruses. Nor do cross-reactions occur with fowl pox or with orf viruses. Moreover, it has been shown repeatedly that sheep pox hyperimmune serum does not protect camels against camel pox. There is general agreement that the Iranian, Russian and East African strains are antigenically closely related, if not identical, and although there are minor antigenic differences between camel pox and variola, most strains so far studied have many of the characteristics of the orthopox group of viruses. In contrast to this, a recent report from Egypt suggests that camels inoculated with vaccinia virus are not protected against subsequent infection with the Fayoum-71 camel pox virus and that this has been confirmed by cross-immunity tests in rabbits.

Pathogenicity

Natural infections occur in camels after an incubation period of about 6–15 days in adults and 4–7 days in younger stock. In Turkmenia, as in some other regions, camel pox seems to flare-up every 3rd to 5th year, usually between the months of July and September. In other territories, however, there is no apparent seasonal incidence although it is recognised that the prevalence of the infection is greatest during the rainy season. The majority of outbreaks are in a mild form but a more 'malignant' type can occur which is associated with abortions and deaths of young camels. In small herds nearly all camels become infected within a period of 2–4 months and most make an uneventful recovery after 1–2 weeks.

Early in the disease there is mild fever, and pustules begin to appear on the skin of the lips, nose, eyelids and mucous membranes of the mouth and nares. The skin lesions take about 8–15 days to develop fully, and lesions may also appear later on the skin of other parts of the body which are relatively hairless. The vesicles soon become pustular and brown crusts form over the lesions and drop off a few weeks later leaving round scars underneath. In some cases there is swelling of the lips, general facial oedema and, occasionally, keratitis and corneal opacity. Camels that recover from the natural disease are immune for 20–25 years, whilst the young born of recovered females are said to resist infection for about 3 years.

Diagnosis

The diagnosis is based on the course and symptoms of the infection, and confirmation by laboratory methods is rarely if ever attempted.

Control

Suitable vaccines are not yet available for the control of camel pox. In some rural areas camel owners attempt to control the disease by scarifying the lips of young camels with infected material prior to the next rainy season.

Swine Pox

Synonyms

Pig pox: Variola suilla.

Definition

Swine pox is a benign infection of young pigs characterised by transient fever and a generalised eruption of pocks of about 1 cm. in diameter.

Hosts affected

The natural disease occurs in pigs of any age or breed, but very young actively growing animals and especially suckling pigs are most commonly affected.

History and distribution

Swine pox was first described in Europe in 1842 and is now thought to occur in almost all pig-raising countries of the world. It is prevalent in the U.S.A., particularly in the Midwest where 1–5 per cent of all herds may be affected. Its importance in the U.K. may well be underestimated.

Properties of the virus

It seems fairly certain that 2 different viruses are responsible for pox-diseases in swine. One is probably vaccinia caused by the virus of that name whilst the other is true swine pox, a distinct entity caused by the virus known as swine pox. Morphologically, swine pox virus is similar to but slightly larger than vaccinia and other pox viruses, measuring about 320×280 nm. Although agar gel diffusion tests reveal a minor component common to vaccinia and swine pox, it is generally agreed that the virus of swine pox is antigenically distinct from vaccinia and other animal poxes. Moreover, pigs infected with vaccinia are fully susceptible to swine pox virus and *vice versa*. Swine pox virus is relatively heat-stable and is said to survive for 10–12 days even at 37°C. Unlike vaccinia virus, the swine pox virus has a very restricted host range and cannot be propagated on embryonated hens' eggs. However, after a few blind passages on tissue cultures, swine pox virus can be induced to grow on monolayer cultures of pig kidney and testis as well as on embryonic lung and brain, giving rise within about 5 days to very small plaques on agar-overlay cultures. The cytopathic effect consists of nuclear vacuolation, the formation of acidophilic intracytoplasmic inclusions, cytoplasmic stranding and cell death. The virus may also produce large intracytoplasmic crystalline bodies (800 nm in diameter) which are not seen with other poxviruses. Unlike vaccinia, swine pox virus does not grow on cell systems derived from cattle and sheep tissues.

Pathogenicity

The incubation period in natural cases is probably about 5–7 days and rarely as long as 12 days. The infection is usually very mild and in the early stages is marked by a transient low-grade fever. Small areas of erythema, about 4–5 mm in diameter, appear on the skin of the lower abdomen and inner aspects of the limbs, increasing rapidly in size as they pass through the various stages of papules, vesicles and pustules until, finally, scabs with depressed centres are formed within 8–11 days after the appearance of the papules. All lesions do not necessarily arise at the same time and secondary pocks may develop after the first ones are fully formed. The resultant crusts soon fall off and, in uncomplicated cases, healing with minimal scar formation is usually complete 2–4 weeks later. In some outbreaks there are papules and crusts, but no vesicles, on the back and sides of affected animals. The morbidity rate is generally high in young stock but the mortality rate in uncomplicated cases rarely exceeds 3 per cent. In histological sections, hyperplasia of the epidermis is seen and the cytoplasm of affected cells contains both basophilic and acidophilic inclusions with, on occasion, characteristic vacuolation of the nuclei. These vacuoles in the nuclei of the stratum spinosum cells may be of diagnostic value since they have not been described in swine pox caused by vaccinia virus, which is the only other known cause of pox in pigs. The basophilic intracytoplasmic inclusions in swine pox can be separated into 2 types. The first, resembling the type B poxvirus inclusion, occurs more frequently and varies in size and shape, but is strongly basophilic with a somewhat granular appearance. The second, resembling the type A poxvirus inclusion, is less frequently present, is oval or spherical in shape, moderately basophilic and of an homogeneous appearance. Inclusion material in the cytoplasm of the swollen superficial cells is believed to contain masses of mature virus particles. Unlike vaccinia, the virus of swine pox is highly species-specific and will not multiply in cattle, sheep, goats or laboratory animals such as guinea-pigs or mice. Rabbits injected intradermally may develop papular lesions but the virus cannot be passed more than 2–3 times in series. Cross neutralization tests in pigs and rabbits fail to show any serological relationship between swine pox and vaccinia.

Ecology

Whereas vaccinia infection of swine may be passed by direct or indirect contact, the swine pox virus is only rarely transmitted by pig to pig contact but sows nursing their first litter may become infected by their young. Biting insects are thought to play a part in the spread of the infection to adjacent premises, and there is a good deal of evidence to show that local spread within a sty and extension of the lesions on the body of an affected pig is largely due to mechanical transmission of the virus by the biting parts of the pig louse (*Haematopinus suis*). The virus of swine pox is said to survive or be maintained in lice for about a year even in the absence of pigs. The disease can also occur in pigs which are not infested with lice and it has been suggested that other insects may act as mechanical carriers of the virus. Swine pox is found throughout the year but occurs most frequently in the warmer months, and many fresh outbreaks cease with the onset of winter.

Diagnosis

The disease is usually diagnosed on clinical grounds but differentiation of the causative virus from that of vaccinia infections in pigs is rarely attempted Unlike vaccinia, swine pox has a very restricted host range and does not grow in fertile hens' eggs but a cytopathic effect is produced in porcine cell cultures. Agar gel diffusion tests with concentrated swine pox antigens yield 2 lines of precipitation against sera of swine pox convalescent pigs, and a recent report suggests that the method is of value in the detection of precipitating antibodies against swine pox in serological surveys.

Control

Pigs recovered from swine pox probably develop a solid life-long immunity but the disease is usually mild and of low incidence, and vaccination is not considered necessary. The most effective control measure is good hygiene and the eradication of lice from infected pigs and piggeries.

Molluscum Contagiosum

Definition

A benign viral infection of man, characterized by the appearance of multiple, soft, rounded wart-like swellings restricted to the epithelium of the skin of the face, axilla, arms, legs, back, buttocks and genitalia.

Hosts affected and distribution

Molluscum contagiosum is exclusively a human disease which occurs throughout the world in both sporadic and epidemic forms. Individuals of any age may be affected but the disease is commonest in children and young adults. In 1966, an epidemic in Alaska affected 77 per cent of young boys exposed to the infection.

Properties of the virus

Although the benign tumour or wart-like appearance of the disease suggests that the causal agent might be an oncogenic virus, it has been definitely established that molluscum contagiosum virus is a poxvirus having most of the characteristics of that group. The virions are large (350 x 230 nm), oval or brick-shaped structures with an eccentric nucleoid surrounded by a single or double limiting membrane. The nucleoid is 50–100 nm in diameter and contains DNA. In negatively-stained preparations the mature viral particles may have a 'ball of wool' appearance similar to orf and other members of the poxvirus group. In thin-sections of infected cells the matrix of the large intracytoplasmic inclusions, so-called molluscum bodies, is divided into compartments by extremely fine septa, with clusters of poxvirus particles filling the cavities.

Antigenic properties

A heat-labile soluble antigen can be used for complement-fixation, but antibodies are rarely demonstrable in the sera of patients with molluscum contagiosum. There are no cross-reactions with other members of the poxvirus group.

Cultivation

The virus does not grow in embryonated hens' eggs but is cytopathic in tissue cultures of human and monkey cells. It has not yet been serially propagated *in vitro* even when organ cultures are used but developing virus particles have been seen in ultra-thin sections under the electron microscope. Virus in extracts from lesions interferes with the growth of certain other viruses in cultures of mouse embryo cells, and the effect is weakly neutralized by sera of patients.

Pathogenicity

The incubation period is probably about 14–50 days and the lesions, which are confined to the skin, develop as pimples which later increase to form small reddish waxy nodules with a diameter of 2 mm. They generally become pearly-white and persist for many months. The lesions are characterized by the presence of acidophilic intracytoplasmic structures in the basal layers of the epithelium, which gradually enlarge to 20–40 μm in diameter, crowding the nucleus to one side and eventually filling the cell. Affected cells lying just above the germinal layer of the epidermis show proliferation and hyperplasia.

Ecology

The infection is commonly spread by direct skin-to-skin contact, especially among young people in swimming baths and gymnasia. Transmission by fomites is also possible.

Diagnosis

Laboratory diagnosis is generally based on the histological appearance of sections of lesions taken at biopsy, or the demonstration of the elementary particles in Giemsa-stained smears made by expressing the exudate from a 'molluscum nodule' obtained by curettage from a lesion.

Control

There is no specific treatment nor are vaccines available, but the lesions usually regress spontaneously.

Yaba Virus

A virus causing subcutaneous tumours in monkeys was isolated, in 1958, from a naturally occurring disease of captive rhesus monkeys at Yaba in Nigeria. The infection spread rapidly to companion monkeys and also to a baboon. The spontaneous disease has not been observed in other parts of the world.

The causative agent has typical poxvirus morphology, does not produce an haemagglutinin and is inactivated after 1 hour at 56°C or pH 3 at room temperature. No immunological relationship has been found between Yaba virus and other members of the poxvirus group, with the possible exception

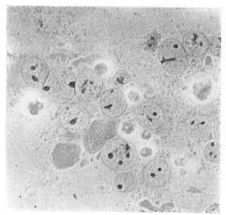

52.5a

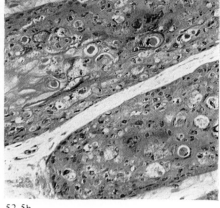

52.5b

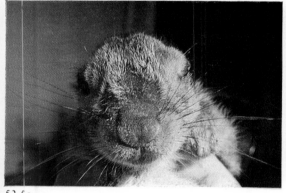

52.5c

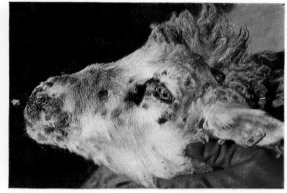

52.5d

52.5a Syncytium produced in a secondary culture of pig kidney cells 3 days after inoculation with myxoma virus. There are a number of large, irregularly-shaped acidophilic cytoplasmic inclusions, each surrounded by a clear halo. The cytoplasm also contains two large basophilic masses consisting of a closely woven mesh of fine fibrillary tubules. Haematoxylin eosin stain, ×420.

52.5c Naturally occurring myxomatosis in the rabbit. Generalized swelling of the head gives the animal a characteristic leonine appearance.

52.5b Section through the skin of a rabbit with myxomatosis. The epithelium shows varying degrees of ballooning and degeneration of affected cells, and the presence of numerous acidophilic intracytoplasmic inclusion bodies. Haematoxylin eosin stain, ×170.

52.5d Lesions of sheep pox, 19 days after experimental inoculation. Early papules have passed through various stages of vesicles, pustular pocks and scabs. Typical eruptions are present on the cheeks, lips and nostrils. (Courtesy of Dr W. B. Martin.)

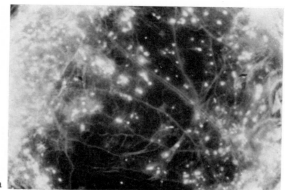

a

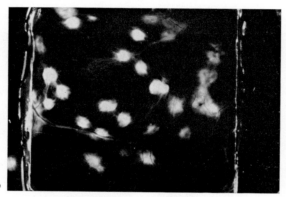

b

Chorioallantoic membrane of 12-day-old chick embryo 4 days after inoculation with a field strain of myxoma virus.

52.6a Excised membrane shows numerous tiny white pocks less than 1 mm in diameter.

52.6b The same strain occasionally produces large pocks with unstained necrotic centres. Membrane stained with methyl violet.

of Tanapoxvirus which causes localised skin lesions in children in Kenya and, possibly, a disease in captive monkeys.

Yaba virus can be cultivated on the chorioallantoic membrane of embryonated hens' eggs and in human or monkey kidney cell cultures. Infected monolayers show lytic and proliferative cytopathic effects and the cells contain acidophilic intracytoplasmic inclusions. Viral antigens can be readily identified in cell cultures by immunofluorescence staining. Subcutaneous or intramuscular inoculation of the virus into monkeys gives rise to benign histiocytomas after 1–3 weeks, while intravenous administration induces multiple histiocytomas in the lungs, heart and skeletal muscles. Cytoplasmic inclusion bodies can be found in the tumour cells. Unweaned mice, hamsters and other commonly used laboratory animals are not susceptible.

The naturally occurring disease is characterized by the appearance of tumour-like growths on the head and limbs of rhesus and cynomolgus monkeys. Although some of the growths may become very large and tend to break down and ulcerate, spontaneous regression usually begins after approximately 5 weeks and is complete in 6–12 weeks.

The method of spread is not known, but it is believed that the virus can be transmitted by blood-sucking arthropods as is myxoma virus in rabbits. There are no specific vaccines, and monkeys recovered from infection with monkey pox or vaccinia are not immune to challenge with Yaba tumour virus.

Further reading

ABDUSSALAM M. (1957) Contagious pustular dermatitis. II. Pathological histology. *Journal of Comparative Pathology*, **67**, 217.

ALEXANDER R.A., PLOWRIGHT W. and HAIG D.A. (1957) Cytopathic agents associated with lumpy-skin disease of cattle. *Bulletin of Epizootic Diseases of Africa*, **5**, 489.

ANDREWES C.H. AND HORSTMANN D.M. (1949) The susceptibility of viruses to ethyl ether. *Journal of General Microbiology*, **3**, 290.

ARITA I. AND HENDERSON D.A. (1968) Smallpox and monkeypox in non-human primates. *Bulletin of the World Health Organization*, **39**, 277.

BEDSON H.S. AND DUCKWORTH M.J. (1963) Rabbit pox: an experimental study of the pathways of infection in rabbits. *Journal of Pathology and Bacteriology*, **85**, 1.

BERGOIN M. AND DALES S. (1971) Comparative observations on poxviruses of invertebrates and vertebrates. In, Comparative Virology, eds. K. Maramorosch and E. Kurstak, p. 135. London: Academic Press Inc.

BRIODY B.A. (1966) The natural history of mousepox. In, Viruses of Laboratory Rodents. *National Cancer Institute Monographs*, **20**, p. 105.

CHO C.T. AND WENNER H.A. (1973) Monkeypox virus, *Bacteriological Reviews*, **37**, 1.

DAVIES F.G., MUNGAI J.N. AND SHAW T. (1975) Characteristics of a Kenyan camelpox virus. *Journal of Hygiene, Cambridge*, **75**, 381.

DEBOER G.F. (1975) Swinepox. Virus isolation, experimental infections and the differentiation from vaccinia virus infections. *Archives of Virology*, **49**, 141.

DOWNIE A.W. AND DUMBELL K.R. (1956) Poxviruses. *Annual Review of Microbiology*, **10**, 237.

FENNER F. (1948) The clinical features and pathogenesis of mousepox (infectious ectromelia of mice). *Journal of Pathology and Bacteriology*, **60**, 529.

FENNER F. (1959) Myxomatosis. *British Medical Bulletin*, **15**, 240.

FENNER F. (1965) Viruses of the myxoma-fibroma subgroup of the poxviruses. II. Comparison of soluble antigens by gel diffusion tests, and a general discussion of the subgroup. *Australian Journal of Experimental Biology and Medical Science*, **43**, 143.

FENNER F. AND BURNET F.M. (1957) A short description of the poxvirus group (vaccina and related viruses). *Virology*, **4**, 305.

FENNER F. AND RATCLIFFE F.N. (1965) Myxomatosis. London: Cambridge University Press.

FENNER F. AND WOODROOFE G.M. (1953) The pathogenesis of infectious myxomatosis. The mechanism of infection and the immunological response in the European rabbit (*Oryctolagus cuniculus*). *British Journal of Experimental Pathology*, **34**, 400.

JENNER E. (1798) An enquiry into causes and effects of the Variolae vaccinae, a disease discovered in some of the western counties of England, particularly Gloucestershire, and known by the name of Cowpox. Reprinted by Cassell and Co. Ltd., available in Pamphlet Volume 4232. Washington: Army Medical Library.

JOKLIK W.K. (1966) The poxviruses. *Bacteriological Reviews*, **30**, 33.

JOKLIK W.K. (1968) Poxviruses. *Annual Review of Microbiology*, **22**, 359.

KATO S., TAKAHASHI M., KAMEYAMA S. AND KAMAHORA J. (1959) A study on the morphological and cyto-immunological relationship between the inclusions of variola, cowpox, rabbitpox, vaccinia (variola origin) and vaccinia IHD and a consideration of the term "Guarnieri body". *Biken's Journal*, **2**, 353.

KLUG A. AND FINCH J.T. (1965) Structure of viruses of the papilloma-polyoma type. *Journal of Molecular Biology*, **13**, 961.

MURRAY M., MARTIN W.B. AND KOYLU A. (1973) Experimental sheep pox. A histological and ultrastructural study. *Research in Veterinary Science*, **15**, 201.

NAGINGTON J. (1968) The growth of paravaccinia viruses in tissue culture. *Veterinary Record*, **82**, 477.

NAGINGTON J. AND HORNE R.W. (1962) Morphological studies of orf and vaccinia virus. *Virology*, **16**, 248.

NAGINGTON J., LAUDER I.M. AND SMITH J.S. (1967) Bovine papular stomatitis, pseudo-cowpox and milker's nodules. *Veterinary Record*, **81**, 306.

PLOWRIGHT W. AND FERRIS R.D. (1958). The growth and cytopathogenicity of sheep-pox virus in tissue cultures. *British Journal of Experimental Pathology*, **39**, 424.

PLOWRIGHT W. AND FERRIS R.D. (1959) Papular stomatitis of cattle in Kenya and Nigeria. *Veterinary Record*, **71**, 718.

PLOWRIGHT W., MACLEOD W.G. AND FERRIS R.D. (1959) The pathogenesis of sheep pox in the skin of sheep. *Journal of Comparative Pathology and Therapeutics*, **69**, 400.

PLOWRIGHT W. AND WHITCOMB M.A. (1959) The growth in tissue cultures of a virus derived from lumpy-skin disease of cattle. *Journal of Pathology and Bacteriology*, **78**, 397.

PLOWRIGHT W., WHITCOMB M.A. AND FERRIS R.D. (1959) Studies with a strain of contagious pustular dermatitis virus in tissue culture. *Archiv für die gesamte Virusforschung*, **9**, 214.

PRYDIE J. AND COACKLEY W. (1959) Lumpy skin disease — Tissue culture studies. *Bulletin of Epizootic Disease of Africa*, **7**, 37.

ROMERO-MERCADO C.H., MCPHERSON E.A., LAING A.H., LAWSON J.B. AND SCOTT G.R. (1973) Virus particles and antigens in experimental orf scabs. *Archiv für die gesamte Virusforschung*, **40**, 152.

SAUER R.M., PRIER J.E., BUCHANAN R.S., CREAMER A.A. AND FEGLEY H.C. (1960) Studies on a pox disease of monkeys. 1. Pathology. *American Journal of Veterinary Research*, **21**, 377.

TANTAWI H.H. (1974) Comparative studies on camel pox, sheep pox and vaccinia viruses. *Acta Virologica*, **18**, 347.

WESTWOOD J.C.N., HARRIS W.J., ZWARTOUW H.T., TITMUSS D.H.J. AND APPLEYARD G. (1964) Studies on the structure of vaccinia virus. *Journal of General Microbiology*, **34**, 67.

WOODROOFE G.M. AND FENNER F. (1962) Serological relationships within the poxvirus group: an antigen common to all members of the group. *Virology*, **16**, 334.

CHAPTER 53

PARVOVIRUSES (Picodnaviruses)

CHAPTER 53

Parvoviruses

(Picodnaviruses)

The first of a rapidly increasing number of small DNA-containing viruses known as parvoviruses (Latin, *parvus* = small) or picodnaviruses (Greek, *pico* = very small) was Kilham's latent rat virus isolated in 1959 from tumours in rats. Since that time, the group has been extended to include a large number of similar viruses isolated from a wide variety of hosts. These include several parvo- or minute viruses of rats, mice, hamsters, chickens and dogs, the haemadsorbing enteric virus HADEN from cattle, feline panleucopenia virus, mink enteritis virus, porcine parvovirus and the adeno-associated or satellite viruses (AAV) from human and simian sources.

Properties of the virus
The diameter of parvovirus particles ranges between 18–24 nm but, because of their small size and closely-packed capsids, details of their ultra-structure have proved very difficult to determine. It is generally agreed, however, that they show cubic symmetry, and the surface of the capsid consists of 32 or, possibly, 42 knob-shaped capsomeres (2–4 nm in diameter) arranged either as an icosahedron or pentagonal dodecahedron. In some preparations hollow, ring-shaped subunit structures have been observed.

The nucleic acid of parvovirus is composed of linear, single-stranded DNA (mol. wt. between 1.5 and 2.2 $\times$ 10^6 daltons). Until recently, all members had been classified into two subgroups or subgenera according to the strandedness of the nucleic acid component and the ability to replicate with or without participation of a 'helper' virus. However, in 1975, members of the group were established as a family, *Parvoviridae*, with three genera *Parvovirus*, *Adeno-associated virus* and *Densovirus*, based on differences in the mode of replication. Members of the genus *Parvovirus* (e.g. Kilham's rat virus, minute virus of mice and feline panleucopenia virus) multiply without a 'helper' virus in susceptible cell cultures and the mature virus particles contain only plus (positive polarity) strands of DNA. In contrast, adeno-associated viruses (AAV) are defective and cannot multiply in the absence of a replicating 'helper' adenovirus. (See also Chapter 55, page 728). Mature AAV particles contain either plus or minus strands of DNA that are complementary and come together *in vitro* to form a double strand. Densoviruses occur naturally in arthropods (*Lepidoptera* and *Diptera*) and are capable of autonomous replication, but, as in AAV, the single strands of DNA are complementary and hybridize *in vitro* to form double strands. It should be noted that ⊘X174 and other very small bacteriophages with cyclic single-stranded DNA do not belong to the *Parvoviridae*, and have recently been assigned to a new group with the generic name *Bullavirus*.

All parvoviruses are non-enveloped, lack essential lipids and are ether- and chloroform-resistant. They are stable between pH 3 and 9, and are resistant to high temperatures (70°C for 60 minutes). They remain infective for long periods of time at low temperatures or in 50 per cent glycerol, and can remain viable in fomites for many years.

Haemagglutination
Some members of the parvovirus group e.g. AAV types 1, 2 & 3, do not haemagglutinate red blood cells but others show varied ability to agglutinate different species of erythrocytes. For example, the bovine HADEN strain agglutinates guinea-pig and human group O erythrocytes but not rat cells. Porcine parvoviruses agglutinate a wide range of erythrocytes whereas canine parvo-, feline panleucopenia and mink enteritis viruses agglutinate pig erythrocytes at 4°C. but not at 37°C. There is no spontaneous elution of the virus from red blood cells when exposed to temperatures of 37–40°C for 60 mins.

Antigenic properties
The antigenic properties of parvoviruses have not

been well characterized and although there appears to be no antigen common to the whole group, the feline panleucopenia and mink enteritis viruses are immunologically closely related as has been shown by serum neutralization tests. Four distinct immunological types of AAV have been identified as contaminants of human and simian adenoviruses, and AAV antibodies are frequently found in humans and monkeys.

Cultivation

Many species of parvoviruses have been propagated in different types of cell cultures and some produce marked cytopathic effects. Most multiply within the nucleus, often with the formation of large intranuclear inclusions, and all apparently need rapidly dividing cells for replication. Adeno-associated viruses [AAV] are defective and are completely dependent upon the multiplication of an unrelated adenovirus for their own replication and the production of infectious AAV. Thus, they will only multiply in cultures supporting the growth of an adeno 'helper' virus and can be readily transferred from a culture of one adenovirus-type to another. Cultures of adenoviruses can be freed from AAV by treatment with specific antisera.

Recent observations appear to indicate that parvoviruses have an affinity for tissue cell lines where they are often present as inapparent infections. Since it is now known that porcine parvoviruses occur in most farm pigs as a latent infection, it has been suggested that a possible source of the virus in contaminated cell lines is in trypsin (derived from pig pancreas) which is used in the process of trypsinization.

Pathogenicity

The prototype strain of parvovirus, Kilham's rat virus, was originally isolated from liver sarcomas of the rat associated with *Cysticercus fasciolaris*. The virus is probably latent in many rat colonies but is capable of inducing fatal disease when inoculated into unweaned hamsters. The canine parvovirus occurs in the faeces of normal dogs, and many of the rodent strains were isolated from animals in which transplantable tumours were growing. Parvoviruses have been associated with acute non-bacterial gastroenteritis in humans, enteritis in calves, acute hepatitis in goslings and with reproduction failures in pigs. One of the few naturally pathogenic parvoviruses is feline panleucopenia virus which produces an acute, sometimes fatal enteritis with leucopenia in cats. Parvoviruses exhibit tissue tropism and most strains have an affinity for rapidly multiplying tissues, especially the vascular epithelium, the external germinal layer of the cerebellum, the hepatic parenchyma, fetal tissues and tumours.

Feline Panleucopenia

Synonyms

Panleucopenia of cats: feline infectious enteritis: feline agranulocytosis: feline distemper: cat plague: cat fever: show fever. Mink enteritis.

Definition

An extremely contagious and generally fatal viral disease of cats characterized by high fever, anorexia, vomiting, depression and leucopenia.

Hosts affected

The disease occurs primarily in kittens but all ages of cats may be affected. Panleucopenia has been reported in leopards, tigers, lions and panthers, and there is evidence that other members of the family *Felidae* are equally susceptible. Natural outbreaks have been observed in racoons in the family *Procyonidae* but, of *Mustelidae*, only mink are naturally susceptible, although neonatal infections can be induced in ferrets. The condition known as mink enteritis is caused by strains of virus indistinguishable from those of feline panleucopenia.

History and distribution

Feline infectious enteritis or panleucopenia has been recognised as a specific disease entity of cats for many years. Although a viral aetiology was first suspected in 1928 when it was discovered that the disease could be transmitted by means of filtrates prepared from infected cat tissues, further progress was greatly hampered by the lack of a convenient laboratory host in which to propagate and study the virus. In 1964, however, a major advance was made towards an understanding of the aetiology of the condition when a virus was isolated from the spleen of a leopard which died from an infection resembling feline panleucopenia. Subsequently, strains of virus with similar properties were isolated in cell cultures from a number of domestic cats showing symptoms of panleucopenia, and these produced the typical disease when inoculated into susceptible kittens.

At the present time, feline panleucopenia has a world-wide distribution and is considered to be the most important infectious disease of cats in Europe and North America.

Properties of the virus

Virions are morphologically indistinguishable from other parvoviruses. They are very small (20–25 nm), are non-enveloped and have cubic symmetry. The nucleic acid component probably contains double-stranded DNA and, for this reason, the virus of panleucopenia is only provisionally included with the parvoviruses.

It is ether-, chloroform- and trypsin-resistant but is readily inactivated by 0.05 per cent phenol and 0.2 per cent formalin. It is resistant to heating for 30 minutes at 75°C, but not between 80° and 85°C, and is stable between pH 3–9. Although the virus may be inactivated when dried at room temperature, fomites and infected premises retain infectivity for up to one year.

Haemagglutination

Some strains, especially from mink, have a weak haemagglutinin for pig red blood cells at 4°C. The haemagglutinin is probably closely associated with the virus particle. Elution occurs at 22°C, and haemagglutination is inhibited by specific antisera.

Antigenic properties

All strains of feline panleucopenia virus are similar antigenically, and cross-protection tests show a very close immunological relationship between the viruses of feline panleucopenia and mink enteritis. More recent studies employing reciprocal serum neutralization tests with many isolates and their antisera indicate that these two viruses are very similar antigenically, if not identical; but there is no evidence that they are related to other parvoviruses.

Cultivation

The virus does not multiply in fertile hens' eggs and numerous attempts to adapt feline panleucopenia virus to growth in a wide range of laboratory animals, other than cats, have been unsuccessful.

The virus can be cultivated in feline kidney cell cultures producing a cytopathic effect which is not easily recognizable in unstained monolayers. In stained coverslip preparations, however, the first sign of infection (in 10–12 hours) is enlargement of the nucleolus surrounded by a clear halo. By about 24 hours, a small proportion of the cells contain intranuclear inclusions which develop through acidophilia to basophilia. (Plate 53.1a, facing p. 720). The appearance of the cellular changes is transient and there is complete recovery of the cell sheet after several cycles of virus growth. The virus shows an unusual tropism for actively dividing cells in the mitotic phase and, for best results, the virus is added to the kidney cell suspension before it is allowed to monolayer. The presence of *Mycoplasma* contaminants in cell cultures should be avoided since they readily inhibit the growth of panleucopenia virus. A wide range of primary and established cell cultures have been tested but only those derived from cat, tiger, mink and ferret show the characteristic cytopathic effect.

Pathogenicity

Of all the parvoviruses, only those of feline panleucopenia and mink enteritis appear to be naturally pathogenic for animals.

Feline panleucopenia is a highly contagious disease affecting principally young cats. The incubation period varies from 4–10 days and the mortality rate in animals showing clinical symptoms often exceeds 60–70 per cent and may approach 100 per cent in some outbreaks. The clinical signs vary widely, ranging from peracute to mild or inapparent. In the peracute form the cat is found dead leading the owner to suspect that it has been poisoned, whereas in acute infection the cat is *in extremis* and usually dies within 24 hours. The course of the disease is characterized by high fever (40°–41°C.), anorexia, marked depression and dehydration. Persistent vomiting of yellow frothy liquid occurs, the patient becomes dehydrated and the breath has a foetid odour. Although many animals have a desire for water they seem to be unable to drink and are frequently found lying near their drinking bowl. The animal shows abdominal pain when handled and diarrhoea may occur 2 or 3 days after the initial temperature rise. There is no evidence of respiratory illness. In less acute cases, death may occur suddenly on or about the 5th day of illness but cats surviving beyond the 6th day may recover after a prolonged period of convalescence.

The disease is transmissible to cats and mink by various routes of inoculation. Shortly before the temperature rises there is an initial leucocytosis followed by a decrease of both lymphocytes and polymorphs from the circulation. As the infection progresses, the leucopenia becomes pronounced and the white blood cells are difficult to find. The virus has a selective affinity for cells which are undergoing active mitosis and most of the damage occurs in tissues showing active development. Thus, the pathogenicity of the virus is reflected by its activity on the stem cells of the bone marrow, lymphopoietic tissue and intestinal mucosa which are the most actively dividing cells in the maturing cat, and by its selective action on the actively dividing cerebellar germinal cells of the neonate to cause feline ataxia. When infection occurs in the latter part of pregnancy, the virus may pass the placental barrier to cause cerebellar hypoplasia. Invasion of the lymphatic tissues and bone marrow usually results in lymphopenia and neutropenia, respectively. In experimentally infected cats, the virus can be isolated from the nasal passages, most of the viscera, the faeces and, irregularly, from the urine.

At necropsy there is evidence of dehydration and emaciation, except in peracute cases where gross abnormalities may be negligible. In less acute cases there is often localised congestion of the jejunum or ileum, enlargement of the spleen and hyperplasia, oedema and necrosis of the mesenteric lymph nodes. In many cases the red marrow of the long bones becomes fluid or semi-fluid in consistency and is often considered diagnostic of panleucopenia. Histologically, intranuclear inclusions which develop through acidophilia to basophilia are present in the intestinal epithelium, germinal layers of lymph nodes and in bone marrow cells early in the disease, but may not be found in cats surviving 3–4 days.

Animals that recover from panleucopenia show a slow but progressive rise in neutralizing antibodies as demonstrated by immunofluorescence and neutralization tests in cell cultures. Subclinical or inapparent infections are common and the fact that the clinical illness is seldom seen twice in the same animal suggests that a durable immunity results. Recovered cats are solidly immune and kittens usually derive protection from maternal antibodies in the colostrum. Passively-derived immunity lasts for 3–12 weeks, depending on the immune status of the dam.

Ecology
All secretions and excretions of affected animals contain virus and recovered cats may shed viable virus in their urine or faeces for about a year. In spontaneous outbreaks the infection spreads readily by direct contact particularly between kittens 3–4 months of age. The oral and respiratory passages are probably the natural portals of entry of the virus. The high resistance of the virus to physical and chemical agents suggests that the infection can be transmitted by indirect means and that contamination of infected premises may persist for long periods. Since virus is frequently present in the bloodstream of affected cats during the incubation and early clinical phases of the disease, the infection may also be transmitted by fleas and other biting insects.

Diagnosis
Provisional diagnosis is based largely on clinical and histological findings together with the presence of leucopenia in blood smears. In general, any cat showing fever, agranulocytosis, semi-fluid aplastic bone marrow and intranuclear inclusions in the intestinal epithelial cells suggests a diagnosis of panleucopenia. Confirmation can be obtained by immunofluorescence staining, by isolating the virus from spleen or other tissues in feline kidney cell cultures and by demonstrating a significant increase in antibody titres in paired sera from affected cats. Although the serum neutralization test is most commonly used for detection of antibodies to feline panleucopenia, it is often difficult to obtain reproducible endpoints because of the variability of the cytopathic effect in cell culture. For this reason a

haemagglutination-inhibition test has been devised which, although less sensitive than serum neutralization, is simpler to use and gives satisfactory results. Porcine red blood cells are employed and the test, using chilled reagents throughout, is read at 4 hours or after overnight incubation at 4°C.

Control
Formalinized vaccines prepared from the tissues of experimentally infected cats and combined with an adjuvant have been used successfully for a number of years in healthy cats over 6 weeks old. Alternatively, formalin inactivated cultures of feline infectious enteritis virus adsorbed onto aluminium phosphate and aluminium hydroxide may also be used. Two subcutaneous injections are given 14 days apart. Satisfactory immunity results approximately 7 days after the second dose and lasts for 8–12 months. Thereafter, repeated annual vaccination is recommended.

Adaptation of the virus to feline kidney cell cultures is quickly followed by attenuation, and live modified cell culture vaccines administered to fully susceptible cats confer an effective immunity within 7 days that gives lifelong protection. To overcome the inhibitory effects of maternally derived antibodies in kittens, two doses of live attenuated vaccine should be given at about 10 and 16 weeks of age, respectively. In these animals, annual revaccination gives maximum protection. Live virus vaccines must not be administered to pregnant cats nor to kittens less than 4 weeks old.

Porcine Parvoviruses

In 1967, small, spherical virus-like particles were observed by electron microscopy in preparations of swine fever virus. Subsequently, the contaminating particles were isolated and found to possess many of the properties of typical parvoviruses. In the same year, it was reported that a large number of isolations had been made of small haemagglutinating DNA viruses from pig-breeding establishments in the U.K. with histories of abortions, stillbirths and neonatal losses. The strains appeared to be serologically identical and one, 59e/63, was chosen as a prototype. In 1969, similar strains were isolated from cases of infertility in swine.

Properties of the virus
The virus particle is small (20–28 nm in diameter), non-enveloped, and shows cubic symmetry. It is ether and chloroform resistant and is stable at pH3–7 for 3 hours at 37°C. It can be stored at −20° to −70°C for 6 months or longer, with little loss of titre. Virus held at 70°C for 2 hours, 56°C for 48

hours and 37°C for 7 days retains its infectivity but is inactivated after 5 minutes at 80°C.

Inhibition of replication by IUDR together with positive Feulgen staining, indicates that the nucleic acid component contains DNA.

Porcine parvoviruses agglutinate chick, rat, guinea-pig, human 'O', rhesus and patas monkey red blood cells, but do not agglutinate other species of erythrocytes including quail, sheep and calf. Haemadsorption is weak or absent.

Cultivation

The virus does not multiply in embryonated hens' eggs or in unweaned mice inoculated intracerebrally or intraperitoneally.

It produces a cytopathic effect in pig kidney cell cultures, especially in monolayers of young actively dividing cells. The cellular changes are clearly visible in stained coverslip preparations and consist of cytoplasmic vacuolation, sometimes followed by necrosis of the cell sheet by the 7th or 8th day, and the development of intranuclear inclusions about 18 hours post-inoculation. The inclusion bodies stain as for DNA by Feulgen's method.

Pathogenicity

The repeated isolation of 59e/63 and other strains of parvoviruses from aborted fetuses and still-born piglets suggests that they may be the causative agents of embryonic and neonatal losses throughout the pig industry of the U.K. Isolations from semen and vaginal mucus seem to indicate that the virus may also be associated with infertility in pigs. Introduction of the virus into susceptible herds generally gives rise to viraemia in all stock. Clinical signs are absent but the majority of pigs develop high titres of haemagglutination-inhibiting antibodies.

Antibodies to parvoviruses are widespread in this country and have also been detected in the pig populations of Holland, Germany, Canada and the U.S.A.

Parvoviruses from other Animal Hosts

In 1970, a 'minute virus of canines' was isolated from the faeces of clinically healthy dogs. It has many of the properties of parvoviruses but grows only in a line of dog epithelial cells. Large intranuclear inclusions are formed which give green fluorescence when stained with acridine orange suggesting the presence of double-stranded DNA. Haemagglutination-inhibition tests show that strains of canine parvoviruses are antigenically distinct from minute virus of mouse, and other rodent parvoviruses. Although antibodies to minute virus of canines have been demonstrated in a large proportion of healthy dogs in breeding colonies the significance of the virus to canine disease is not yet known.

The HADEN or haemadsorbing enteric virus which was isolated from the urino-genital tract of cattle has been provisionally classified with the parvoviruses. Other bovine strains may be the same virus and all of them agglutinate guinea-pig and human 'O' erythrocytes but not rat red blood cells.

The presence of small, DNA-containing particles in preparations of avian adenoviruses derived from cases of quail bronchitis has been reported.

Further reading

BACHMANN P.A., HOGGAN M.D., MELNICK J.L., PEREIRA H.G. AND VAGO C. (1975) Parvoviridae. *Intervirology*, **5**, 83.

BINN L.N., LAZAR E.C., EDDY G.A. AND KAJIMA M. (1968). Minute virus of canines. Bacteriological Proceedings, 68th Annual Meeting, American Society for Microbiology, p. 161 (Abstract).

CARTWRIGHT S.F., LUCAS M. AND HUCK R.A. (1969) A small haemagglutinating porcine DNA virus. I. Isolation and properties. *Journal of Comparative Pathology and Therapeutics*, **79**, 371.

GORHAM J.R., HARTSOUGH G.R., SATO N. AND LUST S. (1966) Studies on cell culture adapted feline panleucopenia virus — virus neutralization and antigenic extinction. *Veterinary Medicine*, **61**, 35.

HOGGAN M.D. (1971) SMALL DNA viruses. In, Comparative Virology, eds. K. Maramorosch and E. Kurstak, p. 43. London: Academic Press Inc.

JOHNSON R.H. (1965) Feline panleucopaenia virus. II. Some features of the cytopathic effects in feline kidney monolayers. *Research in Veterinary Science*, **6**, 472.

JOHNSON R.H. (1969) Feline panleucopaenia. *Veterinary Record*, **85**, 338.

JOHNSON R.H. AND COLLINGS D.F. (1969) Experimental infection of piglets and pregnant gilts with a parvovirus. *Veterinary Record*, **85**, 446.

JOHNSON R.H., SIEGL G. AND GAUTSCHI M. (1974) Characteristics of feline panleucopaenia virus strains enabling definitive classification as Parvoviruses. *Archiv für die gesamte Virusforschung*, **46**, 315.

KILHAM L., MARGOLIS G. AND COLBY E.D. (1967) Congenital infections of cats and ferrets by feline panleukopenia virus manifested by cerebellar hypoplasia. *Laboratory Investigation*, **17**, 465.

MAYOR H.D. AND MELNICK J.L. (1966) Small deoxyribonucleic acid — containing viruses (picodnavirus group). *Nature*, **210**, 331.

O'REILLY K.J., PATERSON J.S. AND HARRISS S.T. (1969) The persistence in kittens of maternal antibody to feline infectious enteritis (Panleucopenia). *Veterinary Record*, **84**, 376.

TINSLEY T.W. AND LONGWORTH J.F. (1973) Parvoviruses. *Journal of General Virology*, **20**, (Supplement), 7.

CHAPTER 54

PAPOVAVIRUSES

CHAPTER 54

Papovaviruses

The term papova is derived from the first two letters of the names of viruses originally included in the group: *PA*pilloma, *PO*lyoma and *VA*cuolating agent. Although papovaviruses exist in many animal species and may or may not be capable of producing disease, the fact that they share certain fundamental biological properties led to their being classified in the same family. In 1974, a study group of the International Committee on the Taxonomy of Viruses (ICTV) divided the family *Papovaviridae* into two genera named *Papovavirus A* and *Papovavirus B*, with the virus species designated by numbers. The former contains viruses causing papillomas of man, monkeys, horses, cattle, sheep, goats, dogs, rabbits, and other species while the latter includes polyomavirus, K or pneumonitis virus of mice, rabbit kidney vacuolating virus and the SV40 or simian vacuolating virus. (Table 54.1).

Papovaviruses contain double-stranded DNA which is often circular or super-coiled. They have a guanine plus cytosine ratio of 41–48 per cent and the viral genome has a molecular weight of about $3–5 \times 10^6$. Electron microscopy reveals naked icosahedral capsids 45–55 nm in diameter, composed of 72 capsomeres (each 8 nm across) in a skew arrangement but hollow tubular or filamentous forms may also be present. (Plate 54.1a, facing p. 721). All members of the family are ether- and acid-stable, and most withstand heating for 30 minutes at 56°–65°C. They survive well in 50 per cent glycerol, when frozen or lyophilized. Some species haemagglutinate by reacting with neuraminidase-sensitive receptors. Papovaviruses are antigenically distinct from each other and cross reactions do not occur between members of the group. Assembly is mainly intranuclear and the majority of species cause latent or chronic infections, and are oncogenic in certain hosts. Members of the genus *Papovavirus-A* induce papillomas in the hosts of origin, while those of *Papovavirus-B* are oncogenic in hosts (chiefly immunodeficient newborn hamsters) different from the species of origin. Transformation of cells by papovaviruses have been achieved both *in vitro* and *in vivo*, and the viral DNA integrates into the cellular chromosomes of the transformed cells.

TABLE 54.1   A classification of the papovaviruses

Family:	Papovaviridae			
Genus:	Papovavirus-A		Papovavirus-B	
Species:	Type 1	Human papilloma (wart) virus	*Type 1	Polyoma virus
	*Type 2	Shope rabbit papilloma virus	Type 2	Simian vacuolating virus (SV40)
	Type 3	Bovine papilloma virus	Type 3	K-papovavirus (pneumonitis virus of mice)
	Type 4	Canine papilloma virus	Type 4	Rabbit kidney vacuolating virus (RKV)
	Type 5	Hamster papilloma virus	Type 5	BK virus from human urine after renal transplantation
			Type 6	JC virus from progressive multifocal leucoencephalopathy in man

* = Type species

717

The characteristics of papova- and other potentially oncogenic DNA viruses are summarised in Table 54.2.

Cellular transformation

Two types of virus-cell interactions can occur following infection of cell cultures with papovaviruses. Either there is a productive or lytic cycle resulting in synthesis of progeny virus followed by death of the infected cells or the infection is abortive whereby little or no infectious virus is released and the infected cell survives although it is permanently altered or 'transformed'. Transformed cells are readily recognised by their altered morphology, loss of contact inhibition and their ability to cause tumours when artificially inoculated into susceptible hosts. Characteristically, transformed cells produce 2 new types of viral antigens distinct from the structural proteins of the virion and these have been named 'T' (for tumour) and transplantation antigens, respectively. Fluorescent antibody staining has shown that 'T' antigens occur mainly in the nucleus whereas transplantation antigens mostly occur in the plasma membrane of transformed cells. The continued synthesis of these 'new' proteins is due to permanent retention of viral genetic material within the transformed cell which is, nevertheless, incapable of releasing mature infectious virus. However, recent investigations have shown that infectious virus can be released by the technique of co-cultivation whereby the transformed cells are fused artificially with 'permissive' cells by means of inactivated Sendai virus. Alternatively, production of infectious virus can also be induced following exposure to ultra-violet irradiation. Thus, the virus-cell relationship in transformed cells in which the viral DNA is integrated in the cellular DNA closely resembles the lysogenic bacteriophage systems.

PAPOVAVIRUS-A

Virions of *Papovavirus-A* are larger (55nm) than those belonging to *Papovavirus-B*, and their nucleic acid component has a molecular weight of 5×10^6 daltons. The virus species induce papillomas in the host of origin but rarely cause cell transformation or cytopathic effects in cell culture.

Bovine papillomatosis

The contagious nature of bovine papillomatosis has been known for many years and its viral aetiology was confirmed in 1929.

All ages of cattle are affected by warts but the incidence is higher among calves and yearlings than adults. The lesions appear more frequently when the animals are housed than when on pasture, and in dairy cattle they are mostly found on the teats and udder. In beef cattle, warts (sometimes in immense numbers) occur on the skin around the eyes, mouth and ears and on the neck and shoulders, but rarely on the limbs. The lesions vary from small firm nodules to large cauliflower-like growths. Occasionally warts are found in the prepuce of bulls, the vulva and vagina of heifers, the urinary bladder of calves and the oesophagus or omasum of older cattle but whether all of these are caused by papilloma viruses is not known.

Properties of the virus

In ultra-thin sections, the virus particles are morphologically similar to those of papillomaviruses and are found in the nuclei of the cells of the stratum granulosum and corneum of the skin. In negatively-stained preparations, the virions appear as mulberry-like particles composed of 72 capsomeres clearly distinct one from the other. The diameter of the virions is between 47–53 nm and each capsomere is approximately 7.5 nm long by 5–6 nm wide, with a longitudinal central cavity. The nucleic acid component consists of circular, double-stranded DNA, with a right-hand twist. All strains are antigenically similar and antibodies can be detected in sera of affected cattle by means of gel diffusion tests.

Cultivation

Growth on the chorioallantoic membrane of fertile hens' eggs has not been reported and it would appear

TABLE 54.2. Some properties of potentially oncogenic DNA viruses.

Characteristic	Papovavirus Type A	Type B	Adenovirus	Herpesvirus	Poxvirus
Multiplication	Nuclear	Nuclear	Nuclear	Nuclear	Cytoplasmic
Symmetry	Icosahedral	Icosahedral	Icosahedral	Icosahedral	Complex
Outer membrane	Naked	Naked	Naked	Enveloped	Enveloped
Ether-sensitivity	Resistant	Resistant	Resistant	Sensitive	Variable
Acid-sensitivity	Resistant	Resistant	Resistant	Sensitive	Sensitive
Capsomeres	72	72	252	162	—
Size (nm)	55	45	70–90	100–150	170–250 x 300–325
Genome mol. wt. $\times 10^6$	5	3	20–25	54–92	160
G + C ratio (%)	41–47	41–49	48–57	57–74	35–40

that the virus does not induce lytic cytopathic effects in cell culture. On the other hand, non-productive infections with cellular transformation have been observed within 6–8 weeks on embryonic cells of hamsters, mice and cattle. Staining of the transformed cells does not reveal any inclusion bodies in the cytoplasm or nucleus. Although there is still no definite evidence for the successful replication of animal strains in cell culture, it is claimed that serial passage of bovine papilloma virus occurs on embryonic hamster cells.

Subcutaneous inoculation of the virus gives rise to connective tissue tumours in experimental horses while intracerebrally injected calves may develop meningeal fibromata. Unweaned hamsters and certain strains of mice (C₃H/eB) inoculated subcutaneously may develop tumours at the site of inoculation within about 100 days. The tumours are firm, multiple or single and measure about 8–15 mm in diameter. They generally persist for 4–6 months but do not show evidence of metastasis.

Transmission

The virus probably gains entry through abrasions in the skin by direct contact with infected animals or indirectly by means of contaminated halters and equipment or by syringe needles and tattooing machines.

Diagnosis

The disease can readily be confirmed by demonstrating the presence of viral particles in negatively-stained specimens of wart tissues.

Control

For many years, formalinized wart tissues have been used as autogenous vaccines either for prophylaxis or cure, and satisfactory results have been claimed by some workers. The dosage for cattle is 10 ml. given subcutaneously and repeated after 10–14 days. Warts on the teats and udder respond poorly to vaccine therapy and the use of bovine autogenous vaccines in cases of canine papillomatosis is of questionable value. It is very difficult to assess the efficacy of wart vaccines since the lesions usually clear-up spontaneously.

Equine papillomatosis

Warts may occasionally be seen on the skin around the lips and muzzle of young horses between 1 and 3 years of age. They may be few in number or numerous, and generally appear as small, elevated, horny lesions between 2–10 mm. in diameter. The condition has a protracted course and lesions of equine papillomatosis may persist for up to 18 months. The agent is readily transmissible to horses, but not to other animals. Microscopical examination shows intranuclear inclusion bodies and virus particles arranged at random or in crystalline arrays.

Similar viruses have been observed in benign connective-tissue tumours ('sarcoids') of horses which are probably caused by the same virus as bovine papillomatosis. The sarcoids occur locally on the skin but are often multiple and can spread to secondary sites. All ages of horses may be affected and the lesions may persist for up to 8 months.

Canine oral papillomatosis

This type of wart usually begins on the lips and spreads to the buccal mucosa, tongue, palate and pharynx of young dogs. They rarely become malignant and tend to disappear spontaneously after a few weeks. The infection can be transferred to other young dogs by scarification of the inside of the mouth. The incubation period is probably 4–8 weeks and the development of lesions is usually confined to the oral mucosa and neighbouring skin. The condition of dermal papillomatosis in dogs may be caused by a different virus.

Formalinized wart suspensions given intramuscularly may have prophylactic but no curative value.

Rabbit papilloma

In 1933, a filterable agent was isolated on a number of occasions from the horny papillomatosis growths in wild cottontail rabbits but not from papillomas induced by this agent in domestic rabbits: nor could the agent produce tumours in mice, rats, guinea-pigs, dogs, pigs or goats. Experimentally inoculated domestic rabbits bearing tumours in which the infectious agent could not be detected were capable, nevertheless, of developing antibodies in their sera and were resistant to reinfection.

Naturally occurring rabbit (Shope) papillomatosis is restricted to wild cotton-tail rabbits (*Sylvilagus floridanus*) in the Midwestern states of the U.S.A. The lesions are mostly present on the skin of the head, neck, shoulder, abdomen and inner aspects of the thighs. They are never found on the mucous membranes of the mouth. Lesions often regress spontaneously, and if the rabbit has several separate papillomas they may regress simultaneously, suggesting an immunological reaction. In warts of wild cotton-tail rabbits, the nuclei of the keratinized layer contain viral capsid antigen recognizable by immunofluorescence, and mature virus particles detectable by electron microscopy and infectivity.

Domestic rabbits (*Oryctolagus*) may be infected experimentally by rubbing infected material on to the scarified skin, but the infection cannot readily be passaged serially. Although the virus tends to die out in domestic rabbits, large fleshy benign tumours are produced which usually regress spontaneously or, sometimes, become malignant and metastasize. In contrast to the naturally occurring infection, the virus in experimentally induced papillomatosis in domestic rabbits appears to be masked or defective; thus cells from the tumour may contain infectious DNA and novel enzymes (e.g. arginase) but not infectious virus,

The virions of rabbit papilloma contain circular double-stranded DNA of the left-handed skew form. The capsids mostly show icosahedral symmetry but filamentous forms also occur. The virus is more resistant to X-radiation than are most viruses and can be stored for up to 20 years in 50 per cent glycerol. It does not haemagglutinate red blood cells. Rabbit papilloma virus has not yet been propagated in fertile eggs or tissue cultures. Only one antigenic type of virus has been recognized, having no relation to papilloma viruses in other animals.

Natural transmission probably occurs by direct contact. Although arthropod vectors can transmit the infection experimentally there is no evidence that they do so under field conditions.

Oral papillomatosis of rabbits

A second type of wart, oral papilloma, occurs naturally in domestic rabbits only. The lesions are small (5 mm. across), greyish-white, benign nodules located on the gums and undersurface of the tongue, but never on the skin as in Shope papilloma. Despite their persistence for one or more months, they show no tendency to become malignant. The virus does not spread quickly by contact, even in crowded animal houses, but infection can be readily transmitted to other domestic rabbits and to several species of wild rabbits by inoculation into the oral mucosa.

The virus is morphologically similar to other papillomaviruses and is present in crystalline arrays in infected nuclei. It is heat stable and survives in 50 per cent glycerol for several years. Recovered rabbits develop an immunity which lasts for a number of months, but there is no cross-immunity with the Shope papilloma.

Infectious warts of man

In 1894, human wart virus was transmitted experimentally from host to host by inoculation, and the ability of cell-free filtrates from wart material to induce the disease was confirmed in 1970. The virus was first seen under the electron microscope in 1949 and its intranuclear development was discovered in 1953.

Various clinical types of warts are described. The most common form is *verruca vulgaris* which occurs most frequently on the fingers, hands and wrists particularly of children, where it persists for months or years. Other types that can be recognised are juvenile (flat warts), plantar, digitate, filiform, laryngeal and genital warts.

Human warts can be spread by auto-inoculation through scratching, or by direct and indirect contact.

Histologically, the lesions are characterized by proliferation of the prickle cells in the upper layers of the dermis. Thin sections of warts show intranuclear inclusion bodies, cytoplasmic masses and virus particles in crystalline arrays.

The virus probably does not grow in fertile hens' eggs, but proliferative changes have been described in cell cultures of human embryonic skin and muscle. In 1976, the human wart virus was found to replicate and produce a cytopathic effect in a line of human epitheliod (BE) cells provided the cells were inoculated in the logarithmic phase of growth, incubated at pH 6.5 to allow the virus to adsorb on to the cells and then stressed by raising the pH rapidly to 8.0. Antibodies to wart virus can be detected by agar gel precipitation tests but the fact that they are of the 19S (IgM) type suggests that the antigenic stimulus is low. Regression of warts may not depend on humoral antibodies and it is well known that the lesions may disappear at one site while new warts appear elsewhere.

PAPOVAVIRUS-B

Virions are smaller (45 nm) than those belonging to Papovavirus-A, and their nucleic acid has a molecular weight of 3×10^6 daltons. The virus species are oncogenic in immunodeficient newborn hamsters and other hosts different from the species of viral origin. The viral DNA integrates into the cellular chromosomes of transformed cells.

Polyoma virus

Properties of the virus

In general, the polyoma virus is spherical in shape but electron micrographs of negatively-stained preparations frequently show a number of hollow, tubular to filamentous forms. There is no outer envelope and the virus resists treatment with ether, chloroform or other lipid solvents. The outer protein shell or capsid consists of 72 capsomeres, shows icosahedral symmetry and is slightly smaller in diameter (35–45 nm) than papillomaviruses (45–55 nm). Ultra-thin sections of infected tissues stained with uranyl acetate reveal an electron-dense central core, about 25 nm in diameter, and its nucleic acid component consists of circular, double-stranded DNA which represents about 12 per cent of the virus mass. The molecular weight of polyoma DNA is 3×10^6 compared with $5–6 \times 10^6$ daltons for papillomaviruses. Group B papovaviruses are very resistant to inactivation by formalin and one of them, SV40

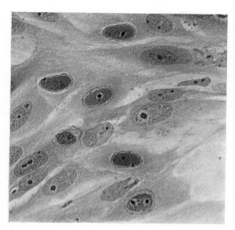

53.1a   The parvovirus of feline panleucopenia can be
isolated and propagated on kitten kidney monolayer
cells. In stained coverslip cultures the cytopathic effect is
characterized by the formation of intranuclear inclusion
bodies in a proportion of the cells. The inclusions appear
singly and develop through eosinophilia to basophilia.
Notice the wavy outline of the nuclear membrane and the
clear halo surrounding the swollen nucleoli in affected
cells. Haematoxylin eosin stain, × 420.

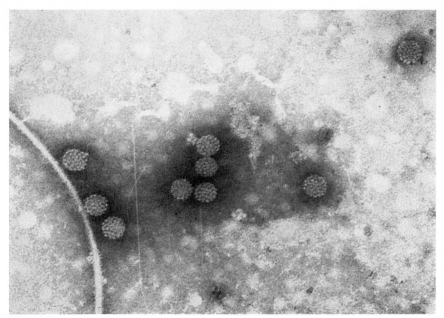

54.1a

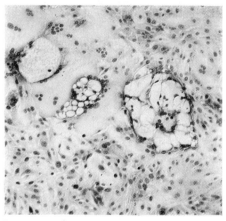

54.1b

54.1a Electron micrograph of a papovavirus; direct smear of bovine wart. The arrangement of the surface capsomeres of the virion is clearly defined by negative staining with phosphotungstic acid. The capsid is an icosahedron of skew form, ×100 000. (Courtesy of Dr J. B. McFerran.)

54.1b Monolayer of kidney cells prepared from a seemingly healthy monkey in which a latent monkey virus—the Simian Virus 40 (SV40) or vacuolating agent—is growing. Freed from the influence of immune mechanisms in the monkey's body, the contaminating virus produces numerous cytoplasmic vacuoles which give parts of the monolayer a characteristic 'foamy' appearance. Giemsa stain, ×44.

virus, is known to have survived in some early batches of formalin-inactivated poliovirus vaccines. However, most strains of papovavirus can be readily inactivated at 50°C in the presence of molar solutions of dibasic salts such as magnesium chloride, and the method has been used to eliminate contaminant particles of SV40 from stocks of poliovaccines (*vide infra*) since the infectivity of poliovirus is stabilised under these conditions.

Haemagglutination
Polyoma virus, unlike most other papovaviruses, agglutinates erythrocytes at 4°C over a pH range of 5.4–8.4. Many species of red blood cells may be used but guinea-pig cells are probably the most reliable. Non-enzymatic elution occurs at 37°C.

Antigenic properties
Only minor antigenic differences between strains have been described.

Pathogenicity and cultivation
Polyoma virus is endemic in wild mice living in dense colonies and in some stocks of inbred laboratory mice. Under natural conditions the virus causes no demonstrable disease but affected mice remain silent or latent carriers of the infection. Virus is shed in the milk, urine and faeces, and survives for long periods outside the body. Thus, the great majority of mice within the colony are affected and baby mice acquire the infection within a few hours of their birth. Transmission is probably by the intranasal route.

Polyoma virus grows in primary and secondary cultures of mouse, rat and hamster cells. It multiplies in permissive cells (e.g. mouse embryo and mouse kidney) giving rise to cell death, plaque formation and the release of infectious progeny virus. In non-permissive cells (e.g. secondary hamster and rat embryo cells) it produces an abortive infection usually without cell death but sometimes resulting in cellular transformation. B-type papovaviruses have a narrow host range and high yields of virus are obtained only in tissues from the appropriate species. Thus, for efficient virus growth, mouse embryo or baby hamster kidney cells are used for polyoma, monkey kidney cells for SV40 and rabbit kidney for the rabbit kidney vacuolating agent.

Infected cell cultures inoculated into newborn mice, rats or hamsters produce an astonishing variety of histologically diverse tumours (hence the term 'poly-oma'), after a latent period of several months. Although more than 20 types of tumour have been described, parotid tumours are the most frequent in mice and sarcomas in hamsters. Because a wide range of tumours can be induced by virus that has been cloned from a single cell culture plaque, their diversity probably depends on the nature of the target cell infected. It is emphasised that polyomavirus rarely, if ever, induces malignant tumours in natural infections because, presumably, the concentration of virus in the secretions and excretions of naturally infected mice is insufficient to induce tumour formation, and because older animals are already immunologically competent when infected.

SV40
Simian vacuolating virus 40, or SV40, was isolated in 1960 from uninoculated rhesus monkey kidney cell cultures in which the virus apparently grew without causing a cytopathic effect. Freed from the influence of the immune mechanisms of the monkey's body, the virus grows uninhibited in secondary cultures of African green monkey kidney cells (e.g. Vero and BSC-1), producing foci of affected cells with vacuolation of the cytoplasm. (Plate 54.1b, facing p. 721). Many strains of SV40 cause cellular transformation when grown in non-permissive cells of many animals including hamsters, mice, rabbits, cattle, pigs and humans. Subsequently it was discovered that SV40 was capable of producing sarcomas when inoculated into unweaned hamsters and, since millions of people had been exposed to poliovirus vaccines prepared in monkey kidney cultures, a considerable amount of research was devoted to studying the properties of this unusual virus. As a result, it was soon established that the virus could be recovered from both live and inactivated polio vaccines and that after ingestion of live poliovaccine young children continued to excrete SV40 for as long as 5 weeks. It was also discovered that SV40 was capable of transforming both human and hamster cells growing *in vitro* and that transformed hamster cells, even when free of infectious virus, were oncogenic when introduced into young hamsters. Although SV40 infection does take place in human patients, as shown by the presence of specific antibodies in their sera, no evidence of tumour induction has been reported.

Rabbit kidney vacuolating virus
In 1964, a hitherto unrecognised papovavirus was shown to be present in Shope rabbit papillomas. This new isolate was named rabbit kidney vacuolating virus because of its ability to induce vacuolization in rabbit kidney cell cultures. Cells of other species are not susceptible.

Virions are morphologically indistinguishable from polyoma and SV40 viruses and tubular filaments are frequently found under the electron microscope. It is immunologically distinct from rabbit papillomavirus, and haemagglutinates guinea-pig red blood cells at 4° and 20°C. It is present as a latent infection in cotton-tail rabbits but is non-pathogenic and does not induce papillomas on the skin of rabbits of any species.

K virus

K or pneumonitis virus of mice was originally isolated from C3H mice known to carry Bittner's mammary gland virus. It is not known to have oncogenic properties but causes fatal pneumonia and, sometimes, liver lesions in young experimentally infected mice. Virus is present in high titres in all affected tissues and is shed in the urine and faeces for up to 4 weeks after inoculation. Intranuclear inclusions are found in the endothelium of lung arterioles.

The virus causes transformation in cultures of embryonic mouse lung and the transformed cells induce tumours in new-born mice.

Kidney tumour virus

The kidney tumour agent is a member of the neoplasm-associated fish viruses which includes fish or carp 'pox', papillomas of salmon, epitheliomas of brown bullhead trout and, possibly, lymphosarcomas of pike.

The kidney tumour virus was isolated in 1959 from a common aquarium species *Pristella riddlei* bearing multiple tumours of the body cavity and musculature which were transmissible to some other species of aquarium fish by feeding and injection of cell-free homogenates. The clinical signs in the naturally occurring disease were not described but the mortality rate in susceptible experimental fish reached 75 per cent. The guppy (*Lebistes reticulatis*) was particularly susceptible and most succumbed to infection after a short illness of 25–40 days. Very young fish were resistant but became susceptible as they grew older.

At necropsy, tumours were most commonly found in the kidneys but lesions also occurred in the heart, intestine, skin, musculature, swim bladder and testis. The liver, spleen, ovaries and brain were not affected. The tumours, which consisted of undifferentiated mesenchymal cells, were invasive but did not show any tendency to metastasise.

Little is known about the nature of the causative virus since all the experimental fish were accidentally destroyed and the virus has not been subsequently recovered. The available evidence suggests that it passes Seitz and membrane filters (of unspecified APD), is sensitive to drying and cannot be preserved in glycerol. Replication takes place in the cytoplasm but inclusions have not been described in any of the infected cells. Most workers in this field consider it to be a type of papovavirus. They also suggest that viral particles seen in electron micrographs of certain other fish neoplasms may prove to be members of the papovavirus group.

Further reading

ALMEIDA J.D., HOWATSON A.F. AND WILLIAMS M.G. (1962) Electron microscopic study of human warts, sites of virus production, and nature of the inclusion bodies. *Journal of Investigative Dermatology*, **38**, 337.

BOIRON M., LEVY J.P., THOMAS M., FRIEDMAN J.C. AND BERNARD J. (1964) Some properties of bovine papilloma virus. *Nature*, **201**, 423.

CRAWFORD L.V. AND CRAWFORD E.M. (1963) A comparative study of polyoma and papilloma viruses. *Virology*, **21**, 258.

EDDY B.E. (1969) Polyoma virus. *Virology Monographs*, **7**, 3.

FINCH J.T. (1974) The surface structure of polyoma virus. *Journal of General Virology*, **24**, 359.

FUJIMOTO Y. AND OLSON C. (1966) The fine structure of the bovine wart. *Pathologia veterinaria*, **3**, 659.

HUCK R.A. (1965) Bovine papillomatosis. Synonyms: warts, infectious verrucae. *Veterinary Bulletin*, **35**, 475.

McPHERSON I. (1967) Recent advances in the study of viral oncogenesis. *British Medical Bulletin*, **23**, 144.

MELNICK J.L. (1962) Papovavirus group. *Science*, **135**, 1128.

MELNIK J.L., ALLISON A.C., BUTEL J.S., ECKHART W., EDDY B.E., KIT S., LEVINE A.J., MILES J.A.R., PAGANO J.S., SACHS L. AND VONKA V. (1974) Papovaviridae, *Intervirology*, **3**, 106.

MELNICK J.L., KHERA K.S. AND RAPP F. (1964) Papova virus SV40: Failure to isolate infectious virus from transformed hamster cells synthesizing SV40 induced antigens. *Virology*, **23**, 430.

OLSON C. (1948) Equine sarcoid, a cutaneous neoplasm. *American Journal of Veterinary Research*, **9**, 333.

OLSON C., SIEGRE D. AND SKIDMORE L.V. (1960) Further observations on immunity to bovine cutaneous papillomatosis. *American Journal of Veterinary Research*, **21**, 233.

OLSON C., JR. AND COOK R.H. (1951) Cutaneous sarcoma-like lesions of the horse caused by the agent of bovine papilloma. *Proceedings of the Society for Experimental Biology and Medicine*, **77**, 281.

RAPP F. AND MELNICK J.L. (1966) Papovavirus SV40, Adenoviruses and their 'hybrids': transformation, complementation, and transcapsidation. *Progress in Medical Virology*, **8**, 349.

ROWE W.P. (1961) The epidemiology of mouse polyoma virus infection. *Bacteriological Reviews*, **25**, 18.

ROWSON K.E.K. AND MAHY B.W.J. (1967) Human papova (wart) virus. *Bacteriological Reviews* **31**, 110

STEWART S.E. AND EDDY B.E. (1960) The polyoma virus. *Advances in Virus Research*, **7**, 61.

SWEET B.H. AND HILLEMAN M.R. (1960) The vacuolating virus, SV40. *Proceedings of the Society for Experimental Biology and Medicine*, **105**, 420.

TAJIMA M. GORDON D.E. AND OLSON C. (1968) Electron microscopy of bovine papilloma and deer fibroma viruses. *American Journal of Veterinary Research*, **29**, 1185.

TAKEMOTO K.K., MATTERN C.F.T. AND MURAKAMI W.T. (1971) The papovavirus group. In, Comparative Virology, eds. K. Maramorosh and E. Kurstak, p. 81. London: Academic Press Inc.

VOGT M. AND DULBECCO R. (1962) Properties of cells transformed by polyoma virus. *Cold Spring Harbor Symposia on Quantitative Biology*, **27**, 367.

CHAPTER 55

ADENOVIRUSES

Adenoviruses

The term adenovirus was first used in 1953 to describe a number of viruses which were isolated from fragments of adenoids removed surgically from human patients and grown in 'clotted plasma' cultures. Characteristically, these viruses could not be isolated by the usual cell culture methods from swabs of the adenoids and tonsils or even by preliminary grinding of the tissues to release infectious virus. In most cases it was necessary to prolong the growth of the apparently healthy cell cultures for 4 or 5 weeks before the virus was released and cytopathic changes developed. The first report that an adenovirus could cause disease was made in 1954 when a strain, subsequently identified as type 4 adenovirus, was isolated from the throat washings of young army recruits during an epidemic of respiratory disease.

Distribution and hosts affected

The adenovirus group now consists of a large number of viruses that inhabit the ocular, upper respiratory and digestive systems of man, animals and birds. Most species are capable of living for prolonged periods in a latent or inapparent form in the absence of clinical symptoms, and some are responsible for causing disease. Many types of human adenovirus occur almost exclusively in the intestinal tract while others are frequently associated with such conditions as coryza, pharyngitis, acute respiratory tract infections or, sometimes, conjunctivitis and other eye infections.

Although adenoviruses have been isolated from various animal sources, they appear to be responsible for only a few clinical syndromes such as fox encephalitis, infectious canine hepatitis, infectious canine laryngotracheitis, conjunctivitis amongst captive monkeys, and pneumo-enteritis of calves. Comparatively little is known about the pathogenicity of equine, ovine or porcine adenoviruses. In rodents, an adenovirus has been described which proved fatal when inoculated into unweaned mice, but other strains isolated from the faeces of healthy mice are probably of little pathogenic importance. Healthy poultry and other species of birds harbour adenoviruses in their intestines but the great majority are non-pathogenic. A notable exception is the Quail bronchitis virus which causes a highly fatal respiratory disease in young quail. There is no known isolation of an adenovirus from cats.

The host range of adenoviruses is usually limited to the naturally susceptible animal species but, under experimental conditions, infections may be induced in laboratory animals with or without clinical symptoms.

Morphology

The mature virus particle is uniform in shape, and measures between 70 and 85 nm in diameter. The nucleic acid core consists of 3 species of arginine-rich polypeptides in association with a linear, double-stranded DNA molecule of molecular weight $20-25 \times 10^6$ daltons, and is enclosed in a protein shell or capsid, composed of 252 surface subunits or capsomeres, arranged in icosahedral symmetry. (Plates 55.1 a, c, facing p. 726). There is no envelope surrounding the nucleocapsid. The capsomeres measure about 7 nm in width and are generally described as spherical although recent evidence suggests that they may be prismatic with a tubular or otherwise hollow structure. Of the 252 capsomeres, 240 are designated as non-vertex capsomeres or 'hexons' and the remaining 12 as vertex capsomeres or 'penton bases'. The 'hexons' are distributed on the faces and along the edges of the 20 triangular facets of the icosahedron, and each adjoins 6 neighbouring capsomeres. The 'penton bases' are located at each vertex of the icosahedron and are bounded by 5 capsomeres. Extending outwards from the 'penton base' is a single projection or fibre, about 2 nm wide and 10–25 nm long, with a terminal knob; and the complex of base plus fibre is referred to as the 'penton'. The fibre contains a type-specific antigen (haemagglutinin) and is probably responsible for attachment of the virus to the host cell.

Physicochemical characters

Adenoviruses contain DNA, as shown by staining of the particles in infected cells by Feulgen's method or with acridine-orange. They are resistant to ether treatment and are acid stable. Most types are relatively stable at temperatures below 50°C and show no significant loss in titre at 37°C, after 7 days; they remain viable at room temperature after 14 days, and for over 2 months at 4°C. They are, however, sensitive to heat and most types are inactivated by a temperature of 56°C for 10–15 minutes, but some avian strains are more tolerant to heat.

Haemagglutination

Various species of red blood cells are agglutinated by human adenoviruses. Rat cells have been most successfully employed but strains which do not agglutinate rat erythrocytes are generally capable of agglutinating rhesus monkey red cells. The capacity of the individual serotypes to agglutinate rat and monkey red cells has enabled members of the group to be further subdivided into 4 sub-groups.

Certain animal adenoviruses are also capable of agglutinating red blood cells but few data are available concerning the presence of haemagglutinins in the majority of recent isolates. Present knowledge of the haemagglutinating activity of animal adenoviruses is summarised in Table 55.1.

Two incomplete and 3 complete soluble haemagglutinins have been demonstrated in human adenoviruses whereas in dog strains most of the haemagglutinin activity resides in the virion. Avian adenoviruses do not agglutinate fowl, human, guinea-pig, sheep or mouse erythrocytes but the majority of strains agglutinate rat red cells. Spontaneous elution of the haemagglutinin does not occur. Although many types of adenovirus show haemagglutinating activity, the presence of virus in cell cultures cannot be detected by the haemadsorption reaction.

Antigenic properties

Virus neutralization tests indicate that the number of adenovirus serotypes from all animal sources is of the order of 78, but there are also numerous sub-types including strains which are distinguishable only by haemagglutination-inhibition tests. At the present time there are more than 30 human types, 23 simian (7 ape and 16 monkey), at least 7 bovine, 4 porcine, 2 canine, 2 murine and 8 or 9 avian types.

All human and animal adenoviruses, except avian strains, share a group-specific soluble antigen which is readily detectable by complement-fixation, gel-diffusion and indirect haemagglutination tests; but they have different antigens in neutralization tests. Because of the common group-specific antigen, serological cross-reactions have been described between adenoviruses of human and animal origin.

The adenovirus capsid components (*vide supra*) are of some importance since it has recently been shown that the 'hexons', 'penton bases' and some 'penton fibres' carry antigenic specificities which are shared between the adenoviruses of human origin (Table 55.2). These antigenic components

TABLE 55.1. Haemagglutination by some animal adenoviruses.

Species of origin	Serotype	Agglutination of red blood cells			
		Rat	Mouse	Human	Guinea-pig
Bovine	1	+	−	−	−
	2	+	+	−	−
	3	−	+		
Porcine	1	+	+	+	+
	2	−	−	−	−
	3	−	−	−	−
Canine	ICH	−	−	+	+
	ICL	−	−	+	−
Murine	—	−	−	−	−

ICH = Infectious canine hepatitis
ICL = Infectious canine laryngotracheitis

TABLE 55.2. Antigenic specificities of capsid components of mammalian adenoviruses.

Designation	Location	Characterization
∝	Hexons, oriented inwards in the assembled capsid	Group specific
β	Penton base	Group specific
γ	Distal part of fibre	Type specific
δ	Proximal part of fibre	Sub-group specific
∈	Hexons, oriented outwards	Type specific

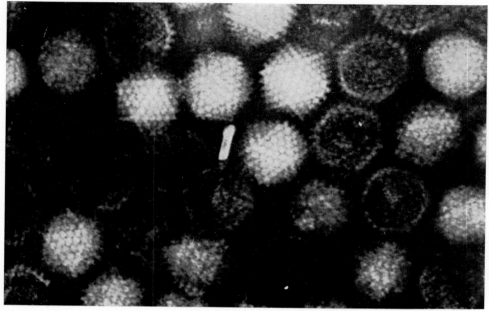

55.1a

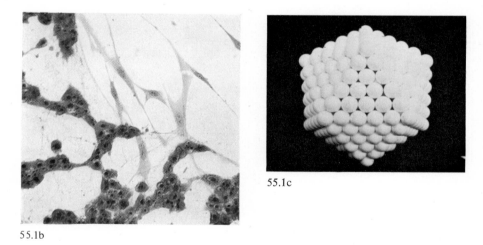

55.1b

55.1c

55.1a Electron micrograph of semi-purified particles of ovine adenovirus. The arrangement of the spherical capsomeres on the surface of the virion is identical to that of the model illustrated in 55.1c, × 220 000. (Courtesy of Mr J. M. Sharp.)

55.1b Monolayer of the MDBK line of bovine kidney cells 2 days after inoculation with a type 2 strain of bovine adenovirus. Infected cells round up and aggregate in clusters, and their nuclei contain single, deeply staining basophilic inclusions. Haematoxylin eosin stain, × 170.

55.1c Model of adenovirus particle made of 252 polystyrene spheres, representing the protein sub-units or capsomeres. The capsid shows icosahedral symmetry and the edge of each triangular facet consists of 6 capsomeres.

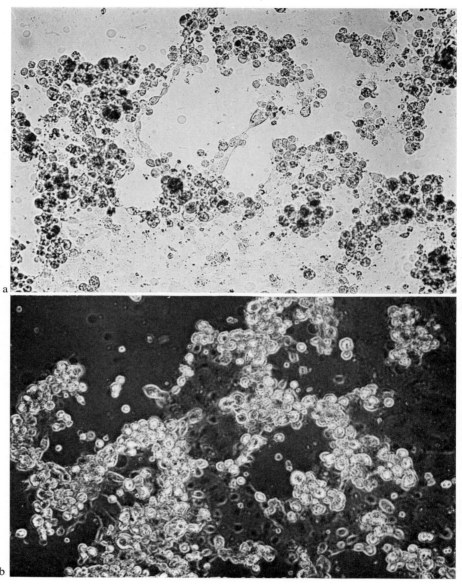

Unstained monolayer cultures of pig kidney cells seen 3 days after inoculation with the 25R strain of porcine adenovirus, ×160.

55.2a   The cytopathic changes include rounding and swelling of the infected cells.

55.2b   Under phase contrast microscopy, affected cells have the appearance of irregular clusters of rounded, highly refractile cells resembling bunches of grapes.

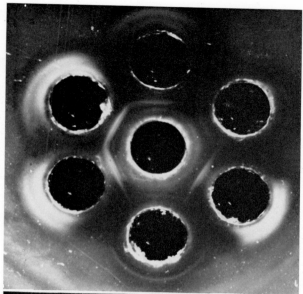

a

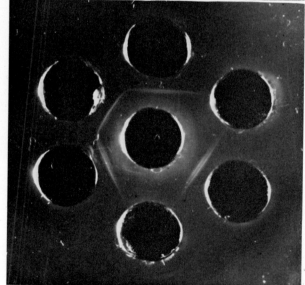

b

Diagnosis of Rubarth's disease (infectious canine hepatitis) by the agar-gel double diffusion test.

55.3a Suspected liver tissues are placed in the 4 lateral wells of an agar plate and the central well filled with a specific immune serum. Positive and negative control tissues are added to the top and bottom wells, respectively. The reaction was observed after holding the plate overnight at room temperature.

55.3b The same test after tissue proteins have been removed by treating the medium with trypsin at 37°C, until clear. Notice the distinct double lines of precipitation between the central well and the positive control well, and between the central well and 3 of the 4 lateral wells.

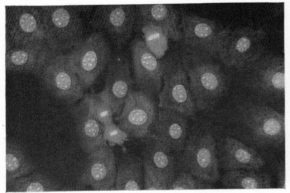

55.4a

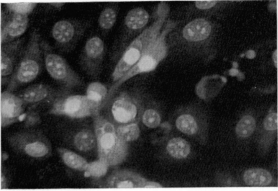

55.4b

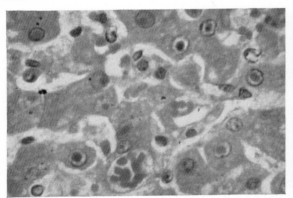

55.4c

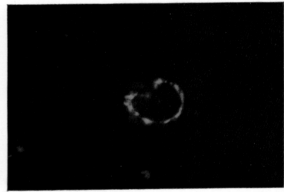

55.4d

55.4a   Healthy growing culture of the MDCK line of dog kidney cells, stained with acridine orange and viewed under the ultraviolet light microscope. Notice the brilliant yellow fluorescence of the mitotic figures in a few of the cells, × 280.

55.4c   Section of liver from a puppy dying from Rubarth's disease. Detail of an area of centrilobular necrosis showing dilation of the sinusoids and the presence of several large acidophilic intranuclear inclusion bodies. Notice the margination of the nuclear chromatin. Haematoxylin eosin stain, × 240.

55.4b   Three days after inoculation with Rubarth's disease virus, the accumulation of DNA in a number of affected cells causes increased nuclear fluorescence. Notice that the yellow-green masses do not fill the nuclei completely, × 350.

55.4d   Immunofluorescence photomicrograph of cultured puppy kidney cell inoculated with Rubarth's disease virus. Diffusion of viral antigen into the perinuclear zone is revealed by its combination with specific fluorescein-conjugated antibody which emits green fluorescence under ultraviolet light, × 650.

have not yet been detected, in the capsids of avian adenoviruses.

In general terms, the non-vertex capsomeres (hexons) contain the group-specific complement-fixing antigen while the vertex projections (fibres) largely represent the type-specific antigen. The pentons, which consist of the vertex capsomeres plus their attached fibres are associated with viral haemagglutination and, it is believed, with the toxic or cell-detaching component.

Cultivation

Adenoviruses are highly species-specific and few strains are capable of producing clinical illness in animals other than their natural host. Their limited host range is also reflected *in vitro* and most unadapted strains can only be propagated success-fully in cell cultures of the natural host or closely related species. In many cases, however, adaptation to 'foreign' cell types is accomplished by rapid serial passage of the unmodified virus.

Human strains grow best in continuous lines of human malignant cells, e.g. HeLa, KB and HEp-2, or in primary human amnion or primary human kidney cell cultures. They will grow in monkey kid-ney cell cultures only in the presence of papovavirus SV40. The cytopathic effect may be very characteris-tic with rounding and clumping of the affected cells into irregular clusters resembling "bunches of grapes". (Plates 55.2a, b, between pp. 726–7). In general, adenovirus replication is associated with a late cytopathic effect due to the inefficiency of viral adsorption and the incompleteness of virus release, and incubation periods of 7–10 days or longer (2–4 weeks) may be required to produce obvious changes in the cells and their nuclei. Nuclear changes include the formation of single, large basophilic inclusions in the form of honeycombs or rosettes, or acidophilic inclusions followed by nuclear enlargement and the formation of irregular basophilic inclusions from which threads of chroma-tin sometimes radiate to the periphery of the nucleus. (Plate 55.4b, facing p. 727). The intranuclear inclusion bodies represent aggregations of pro-teinaceous material and crystals of mature and immature virus particles. In electron micrographs of ultra-thin sections of infected cells the intranuclear masses of virus particles are themselves arranged in crystalline array. Most avian adenovirus-infected cells are characterized by the development of large, strongly basophilic intranuclear inclusion bodies.

Replication of adenoviruses in cell culture leads to the arrest of mitosis of affected cells with increased glycolysis and increased acid production. The colour change of the pH indicator in the medium occurs early in cell infection. This enables cultures of adenoviruses to be distinguished from those infected with most other viruses where there is destruction of the infected cells and the pH becomes more alkaline than in the controls.

It is emphasised that cultures infected with high multiplicities of adenovirus generally produce an early cytopathic effect which may be visible within a few hours of incubation. This is not due to viral replication but to a toxic protein present in the 'penton' which causes the cells to detach from the glass.

Despite their limited host-range, strains of human adenovirus have been adapted to growth in cultures of rabbit or swine kidney. In certain systems, human adenoviruses can be induced to replicate in non-permissive cells with the assistance of a 'helper' virus and, in one such experiment, a type 7 strain propagated together with SV40 virus on monkey kidney cells, was shown to have incorporated part of the SV40 genome, thereby acquiring the capacity to produce SV40 tumours in hamsters.

Pathogenicity

Human adenovirus infections are transmitted directly from man to man and cause catarrhal inflammation of the mucous membranes of the eye and respiratory tract, sometimes with enlargment of the regional lymph nodes. They may also affect the intestinal tract, giving rise to symptoms of nausea, vomiting and diarrhoea. Many human adenovirus infections may be inapparent and at least 4 serotypes commonly become latent in the tonsils and adenoids; and there is good evidence that the virus tends to persist in host tissues, often for prolonged periods, following clinical recovery.

There are surprisingly few reports on the role of adenoviruses as causative agents of specific animal diseases, the most notable examples being infectious canine hepatitis (Rubarth's disease), infectious canine laryngotracheitis, fox encephalitis and, perhaps, quail bronchitis. Nevertheless, numerous strains have been isolated from a wide range of animal species including apes, monkeys, horses, cows, sheep, pigs, dogs, foxes, an opposum, chickens and geese; and precipitating antibodies to the adenovirus group have been identified in sera from horses, cattle, sheep, goats, deer and pigs. Thus, it is probable that all mammalian species will eventually be found to be susceptible to natural adenovirus infections although they may not develop clinical signs of illness.

Oncogenic activity

Many adenovirus serotypes are capable of inducing the development of malignant tumours when inoculated into newborn hamsters but animals more than 7 days old are almost completely resistant. The oncogenicity of adenoviruses is generally expressed by their ability to transform rodent cells *in vivo* and *in vitro*, but not all types produce neoplastic transformation *in vivo*, although they may do so in rat cell culture.

Human adenovirus types 12, 18 and 31 cause undifferentiated sarcomas within 1–4 months, usually at the site of inoculation. Type 7 induces tumours in less than 25 per cent of animals after a long latent period of at least 160 days, but the tumours are usually malignant lymphomas or lymphosarcomas. Sarcomas are also produced by types, 3, 8, 14 and 21 but the latent period is even longer than that for type 7.

There are also a number of oncogenic animal adenoviruses. These include bovine type 3 (which induces undifferentiated sarcomas), infectious canine hepatitis, some avian CELO strains (which cause fibrosarcomas) and at least 5 simian serotypes, which give rise to lymphomas in unweaned rodents.

Infectious virus particles cannot be recovered from tumours but their relationship to the tumour is confirmed by the presence of type-specific, virus-induced, cellular proteins called tumour or "T" antigens; and by the development of type-specific antibody to the tumour antigen in the sera of tumour-bearing animals.

It is of interest that the oncogenic activity of adenoviruses corresponds closely to the base composition of extracted nucleic acids. Thus, the highly oncogenic serotypes have a low (48–49 per cent) guanine plus cytosine ($G+C$) content in their DNA, the mildly oncogenic types have an intermediate $G+C$ (50–51 per cent) content, while the non-oncogenic types have the highest $G+C$ (55–60 per cent) proportion of all human adenoviruses.

In spite of their comparatively narrow host specificity, certain adenovirus serotypes are capable of initiating well-marked cytolytic infections in a variety of cells derived from different species of origin and, in doing so, may cause transformation of these 'non-permissive' cells. Whether or not animal adenoviruses can cause human infections and give rise to neoplastic formation is difficult to evaluate, but there are a number of reports which indicate that antibodies capable of neutralizing infectious canine hepatitis virus and some bovine adenoviruses are present in human sera.

Diagnosis

The complement-fixation test is the most useful single procedure for the serological diagnosis of adenovirus infections. The test is based on the fact that a complement-fixing antigen prepared from one type of adenovirus, e.g. in cell culture, will serve to detect the group-reactive antibody stimulated by infection with one of the other types. In general, there is a significant increase in titre (fourfold or greater) of complement-fixing antibodies in paired specimens of acute and convalescent sera, provided they are collected at least 10 days apart. The specific type of adenovirus involved can be distinguished by neutralization and haemagglutination-inhibition tests. In adenovirus infections of animals, specific precipitinogens can often be demonstrated in agar gel by diffusing infected tissue fragments against a known immune serum. (Plates 55.3a, b, between pp. 726-7).

Most mammalian adenoviruses can be isolated on primary, secondary or continuous cell cultures of the appropriate host species. The time required for the cytopathic effect to become evident varies considerably and depends mainly on the type of virus and its concentration in the inoculum. The cultures should be examined daily but, if they remain healthy for 10 days, the cells should be removed from the glass and passed in fresh cultures. Isolates are identified as belonging to the adenovirus group by their capacity to fix complement with a known positive antiserum, and the type is determined by neutralization and haemagglutination-inhibition tests using type-specific antisera prepared in animals.

Direct and indirect fluorescent antibody staining methods are also useful for detecting intranuclear and perinuclear viral antigens in infected cells. (Plate 55.4d, facing p. 727). Intranuclear inclusions can also be seen in smears, tissue sections and cell cultures stained with haematoxylin and eosin, Giemsa's stain or acridine-orange. (Plates 42.2a, facing p. 474a; 55.4c, facing p. 727; 55.1b, facing p. 726 and 42.11d, facing p. 488).

Adeno-associated parvoviruses

Virus growth cycles are not always productive and many animal viruses, including adenoviruses, reproduce imperfectly in one kind of host-cell although they do so adequately in another. Hence, infection may be said to be 'defective' when the virus initiates a replicative process which does not result in the formation of new infectious virus. Certain of these defective infections in which some or even all the viral components are synthesised but not assembled properly, and in which failure to produce infectious progeny virus is absolute, are termed 'abortive infections'. In some circumstances, a defective virus may be able to persist indefinitely as 'provirus' inside host cells and may succeed in replicating normally if the defective component is provided in the same cell by a related, non-defective virus (genetic recombination). On the other hand, some defective viruses can utilise the help of unrelated viruses and, in fact, may be found always in association with such 'helper viruses'.

It is now known that many laboratory stock

cultures of adenoviruses are contaminated with very small virus particles called adeno-associated viruses (AAV). They are about 20nm in diameter, show icosahedral symmetry with 32 surface capsomeres surrounding a central core of single-stranded DNA, and are so similar in morphology to small adenoviruses that they have to be distinguished from fragmented particles of the adenovirus capsid. The nucleic acid component of AAV is unusual in that the viral genome in each individual virion consists of either a 'plus' or 'minus' single strand of DNA. Following extraction, the complementary strands of opposite polarity from different virus particles band together *in vitro* to form double-stranded DNA helical molecules having twice the molecular weight of the individual strands. At least four serotypes of AAV have been described by neutralization, complement-fixation and precipitation tests but, although they were originally considered to be derived from adenoviruses, it is now known that they are antigenically distinct from their 'helper' viruses, and they have been classified as subgroup B parvoviruses (Chapter 53). None of the adeno-associated viruses is associated with pathogenicity although antibodies to AAV occur in human sera and the virus can be isolated from the faeces of children who are simultaneously excreting an adenovirus. Adeno-associated viruses appear to be defective since they cannot multiply in cell culture unless a typical adenovirus is also multiplying in the same cells. Moreover, normal human adenoviruses are themselves defective in monkey kidney cells but not, of course, in human cells, since they will only multiply if the non-permissive monkey cells are co-infected with the unrelated papovavirus SV40, or with a simian adenovirus, either of which can function as a 'helper' virus. Although it is generally agreed that the amount of genetic information contained within the AAV genome is too limited to code for all the necessary viral proteins, the part played by the unrelated 'helper' adenovirus is not fully understood. Recent data suggest that the replication of adenovirus is itself inhibited when it acts as a 'helper' to the defective AAV. Moreover, it is also known that AAV is capable of reducing adenovirus oncogenicity in experimentally infected hamsters, and it has been suggested that defective AAV's may play a role in the pathogenesis of 'slow virus' infections.

Adenovirus hybrids

During passage of human adenovirus in non-permissive monkey kidney cell cultures, the DNA constituents of the SV40 papovavirus and some adenoviruses may form hybrid molecules which become enclosed within capsids formed by the adenovirus proteins. These hybrid particles, con-sisting of the SV40 genome (genetic material) inside an adenovirus capsid, are capable of potentiating human adenovirus replication. In this case, however, the effect is reciprocal since the hybrid molecule is itself defective and is unable to replicate in cell cultures unless an adenovirus is present. These hybrid populations consist of two types of particles. The first consists of a complete adenovirus genome surrounded by an adenovirus capsid while the second type contains a defective SV40 genome linked to defective adenovirus DNA enclosed within an adenovirus capsid. The latter type of particle has been named PARA (particle aiding the replication of adenovirus) because it aids the replication of adenovirus in *monkey* kidney cell cultures. When hybrid populations are inoculated into *human* kidney cell cultures, only the adenovirus particles replicate and PARA do not. Hence, the progeny virions are free of the SV40 genome and behave once more as non-hybridized adenovirions.

Recent work has shown that the adenovirus capsid of the PARA-adenovirus hybrid can be exchanged for the specific protein coat of other adenovirus serotypes by a process called transcapsidation. This transfer of the oncogenic SV40 genome into the protein coat of non-oncogenic adenoviruses has resulted in the acquisition of oncogenic properties by these viruses. It is also possible that the phenomenon of transcapsidation might enable the host range of a virus to be extended should it acquire a novel capsid from a second unrelated virus.

Bovine adenoviruses

Compared with human infections, comparatively little is known about the role of adenoviruses in diseases of cattle. However, there is evidence from serological and histological surveys that adenoviruses are commonly associated with respiratory disorders of calves and adult cattle, and a number of strains have been isolated from calves with pneumonitis, polyarthritis or enteritis. In the U.K., precipitating antibodies are present in about 25 per cent of bovine sera and in one survey of more than 100 outbreaks of respiratory disease in cattle, no less than 29 per cent were associated with adenoviruses.

In 1959, the first 2 bovine strains of adenoviruses, representing serotypes 1 and 2, were isolated in the U.S.A. from the faeces of apparently healthy calves. Neutralizing antibodies to both strains were widely distributed among cattle but neither serotype produced clinical illness when inoculated intravenously into calves. In 1956, a third serotype of bovine adenovirus, designated WBRI, was isolated in the U.K. from the conjunctiva of an apparently healthy cow. This isolate produced typical adenovirus cytopathic changes in bovine kidney cell cultures and induced mild respiratory infections and enteritis when inoculated intravenously or intratracheally into colostrum-deprived calves. Other strains of adenovirus have been found in the lungs, intestinal tracts and nasal discharges of calves, many of which were affected with diarrhoea. By 1974, no fewer than 8 serotypes of bovine adenoviruses had been defined and a 9th type has been proposed recently. The duration of immunity in cattle to the various serotypes of adenovirus is not known.

Probably all bovine adenoviruses agglutinate rat erythrocytes and some types are capable of agglutinating mouse or monkey red blood cells.

Bovine strains possess the group-specific complement-fixing antigen which is common to all mammalian adenoviruses and are distinguished from each other and from human serotypes by virus neutralization and, in some cases, by haemagglutination-inhibition. Gel diffusion tests show that human and canine adenoviruses have only a one-way crossing whereas bovine types cross two ways with each of those viruses.

Primary, secondary and continuous cell cultures of bovine kidney or bovine testis are capable of supporting the growth of bovine adenoviruses and the cytopathic changes, which may be delayed, are typical of adenoviruses with rounding of the affected cells and the development of large basophilic or acidophilic intranuclear inclusions. (Plate 55.1b, facing p. 726). None of the serotypes produces infection in embryonated hens' eggs or in laboratory animals including chickens, mice, guinea-pigs or rabbits, but the WBR I (type 3) strain may induce tumours in newborn hamsters.

Ovine and equine adenoviruses

Little information is available about adenoviruses from sheep and horses. In 1969, however, 8 isolates were obtained from sheep faeces in Northern Ireland and were classified into 3 antigenic types. In Australia, adenoviruses of unknown type have been isolated from sheep while in Scotland a fourth serotype of adenovirus has been isolated from housed lambs affected with respiratory disease. A more recent report suggests that a fifth serotype has been obtained from the faeces of healthy lambs in Germany.

Several adenoviruses have been isolated from apparently healthy foals, pneumonic foals and from adult horses with mild respiratory symptoms. In Australia and the U.S.A., a uniformly fatal syndrome has been described in certain Arabian foals which begins at about 25 days of age and runs a course of about 23 days (range 13 to 42 days). The infection gives rise to a progressive, intractable, bronchopneumonia in foals which have a combined T and B cell immuno-deficiency that is inherited as a simple recessive autosomal gene. Serological evidence of equine adenovirus infection has been demonstrated in horse sera in several countries including the U.K., but the relationship of the virus to clinical disease has not yet been established.

Porcine adenoviruses

The possibility that adenoviruses might cause natural infections in pigs was suggested by the fact that the virus of infectious canine hepatitis and some human adenoviruses grew readily in pig kidney cell cultures and produced characteristic intranuclear inclusions. Moreover, four human serotypes (1, 2, 5 and 6) inoculated intratracheally into colostrum-deprived, 'pathogen-free' piglets produced both gross and microscopical lesions of broncho-pneumonia. Inoculation of adult pigs sometimes resulted in latent infections with virus persisting in the tissues for several months.

The first porcine adenovirus was isolated in 1964 from a rectal swab of a 12-day-old piglet with diarrhoea, and was designated Compton strain 25R. Complement-fixation tests showed that the virus possessed the adenovirus group antigen and produced intranuclear changes in cell culture consistent with those of human serotypes 3, 4 and 7. Since then, a number of porcine adenoviruses have been isolated in monolayer cell cultures of kidney tissue obtained from healthy pigs, from the rectal swabs of both healthy and scouring piglets and from the brain of a piglet showing signs of encephalitis. It is also of interest that several porcine adenoviruses have been isolated as "contaminants" in pig kidney cell cultures infected with swine fever virus. This observation might account for earlier, unconfirmed reports of the existence of so-called "cytopathic strains" of swine fever virus.

At the present time, the number of established porcine serotypes is 4, and all possess the common adenovirus group antigen as judged by complement-fixation and gel diffusion tests. Although the 4 serotypes, designated 1, 2, 3 and 4, were identified by cross-neutralization tests using rabbit antisera, none of them is neutralized by antisera against human adenovirus types 1–33.

Studies of the incidence of adenoviruses in the rectal swabs of pigs in conventional and "minimal disease" herds suggest that the virus is more prevalent during the post-weaning period than in unweaned piglets or adults; and that infection with adenoviruses is not related to the presence of diarrhoea. Antibodies to all 4 serotypes have been demonstrated in the sera of many healthy pigs but none of the serotypes produces illness or gross lesions when inoculated intranasally into colostrum-deprived piglets.

Strains of serotype 1 are capable of agglutinating

the red blood cells of rats, mice, guinea-pigs, rhesus monkeys and human group O, but pig, ox, sheep, rabbit and fowl cells are not affected.

Growth of porcine adenoviruses occurs in embryonic and young pig kidney cell cultures, and is enhanced by serial passage. Most strains will also grow, or can be adapted to grow, in cultures prepared from pig lung and testis as well as embryonic bovine kidney. The cytopathic effect is typical of adenoviruses with acidophilic intranuclear inclusions containing basophilic central granular masses similar to those produced by human types 3, 4 and 7.

Electron micrographs of thin sections of infected cells show mature and immature virus particles lying within the nuclei. Most of the viruses are circular in outline but occasional hexagons are seen. Three main types of internal viral morphology have been described; first, those with a dense centre surrounded by an inner clear halo and an outer dense envelope; second, those with a very dense wide centre surrounded by an envelope; and third, those with a mottled circumscribed centre. The number of virus particles per section of infected nucleus varies from several to, more rarely, a massive packing of virions in regular crystalline arrays.

Canine adenoviruses

There is general agreement that canine adenoviruses are the causative agents of infectious canine hepatitis (Rubarth's disease), infectious canine laryngotracheitis (kennel cough) and fox encephalitis. The viruses causing infectious canine hepatitis and fox encephalitis are probably identical, but the strain associated with infectious canine laryngotracheitis can be distinguished from those other canine adenoviruses by haemagglutination-inhibition and, to a limited extent, by virus neutralization. Nevertheless, the general characters of all canine adenoviruses are very similar, but the most important disease is infectious canine hepatitis.

Infectious canine hepatitis

Synonyms
Rubarth's disease: Hepatitis contagiosa canis: fox encephalitis.

Definition
A febrile disease which affects mainly foxes and young dogs, and is associated with centrilobular necrosis of the liver.

Hosts affected
Dogs and foxes are the natural hosts but guinea-pigs, coyotes, racoons and wolves are susceptible to experimental infection; grey foxes and ferrets are said to be resistant.

History and distribution
The disease is widespread in the U.K. and on the continents of Europe and North America. It was originally described in 1928 as an enzootic fox encephalitis. In 1947, Rubarth was the first to recognise infectious canine hepatitis as a clinical entity in dogs and, in 1949, the immunological identity of the causative viruses of Rubarth's disease and fox encephalitis was confirmed by independent workers. The presence of the common adenovirus group-specific complement-fixing antigen in infectious canine hepatitis virus and its typical adenovirus morphology were established in 1959 and 1961, respectively.

Properties of the virus
The virus of infectious canine hepatitis has the typical icosahedral capsid of an adenovirus, with a particle diameter of about 55–80 nm. The DNA nature of its nucleic acid component was confirmed by suppressing virus synthesis in dog kidney cell cultures with FUDR (5-fluorodeoxyuridine) and by staining infected cell monolayers with acridine-orange which gives the characteristic yellow-green colour to the intranuclear inclusions. (Plate 42.11d, facing p. 488). Electron micrographs of thin sections of infected cells show clusters of virus particles arranged in characteristic crystalline arrays within the nuclei.

The virus resists inactivation by heat and acid and, since it contains no lipid, its infectivity is not affected by treatment with lipid solvents including ether and bile salts. It survives in cell culture fluid for 10–16 weeks at room temperature, for 6–9 months at 4°C and for several years in 50 per cent glycerol at 4°C. It also withstands 0.5 per cent phenol for several days but is inactivated by 0.2 per cent formalin within 24 hours. Infectious canine hepatitis virus may retain its infectivity for 10–14 days in solid fomites and, because it is generally more resistant than distemper virus, kennels remain infected for longer periods.

Haemagglutination
Canine adenoviruses contain a haemagglutinin for human group O red cells. Infectious canine hepatitis, but not infectious canine laryngotracheitis virus, is also capable of agglutinating guinea-pig erythrocytes. None of the canine types agglutinates erythrocytes of dogs, mice, sheep or other species tested.

Interference
Interferons are not produced by cells infected with canine adenoviruses and these viruses are not affected by the action of interferon. For this reason, there is no interference between the viruses of infectious canine hepatitis and canine distemper in

live attenuated bivalent vaccines and both will replicate satisfactorily in the inoculated animal. Indeed, fluorescent antibody staining shows that the viruses can multiply in the nucleus and cytoplasm, respectively, of the same infected cell.

Antigenic properties

Infectious canine hepatitis virus, like all other animal adenoviruses, shares the soluble complement-fixing antigens of human strains. Hence, they probably all share at least one of the major antigenic components on the 'hexon' polypeptide, and another on that of the 'penton base'.

Precipitating antigens are often present in the organs of infected dogs and are readily identified by agar gel diffusion tests. (Plates 55.3a, b, between pp. 726–7). One of the two soluble antigens produced by infectious canine hepatitis virus, as demonstrated on agar gel, is specific for canine hepatitis whereas the other is shared with human adenovirus types 5 and 7. Infectious canine hepatitis virus appears to have only one immunological type but differences in virulence may occur among strains.

It is emphasised that the virus of infectious canine hepatitis is unrelated to the agent of human infectious hepatitis.

Cultivation

The virus is readily propagated in kidney and testis cell cultures of dogs, other canidae and also in cultures of pig, ferret, racoon and guinea-pig cells. Growth in rabbit, hamster, calf, mouse, monkey or human cells has not been recorded. Virus replication in cell cultures is associated with rounding and swelling of infected cells, sometimes to twice their original volume, and the formation of intranuclear inclusions. The initially small, acidophilic inclusions enlarge, frequently turn basophilic, and are connected to the nuclear periphery by strands of chromatin Many infected nuclei are seen to contain aggregates of virus particles arranged in crystalline arrays when examined under the electron microscope.

Pathogenicity

Classical Rubarth's disease is most frequent in young dogs but has been reported in almost all age groups. Recently weaned puppies are particularly susceptible and show the highest mortality rates, whereas relatively few adult dogs become sufficiently ill to show definite clinical symptoms. The usual incubation period after natural exposure is 2–5 days but periods of 10–14 days may occur, depending upon the virulence of the strain. In the most severe form, an apparently healthy dog suddenly collapses with acute abdominal pain, vomiting and diarrhoea, and dies within 12–14 hours. The presence of blood in the vomit and faeces generally indicates impending

death. In less acute and recovering cases there is high fever accompanied by leucopenia, enlargement of the tonsils and submaxillary lymph nodes and, sometimes, oedema of the cornea giving rise to transient corneal opacity ('blue eye'). A number of dogs may show intermittent vomiting and diarrhoea. In older dogs the disease is mild and symptoms may be few or absent.

In foxes, the disease is usually characterized by acute encephalitis with convulsions followed within 24 hours by paralysis, coma and death.

At necropsy, the predominant features are subcutaneous oedema and the presence of an haemorrhagic exudate in the peritoneal cavity and intestinal tract. The liver is enlarged, generally pale in colour and often shows a distinct mottled or lobular pattern. The spleen is also enlarged and haemorrhagic, and the wall of the gall bladder is oedematous and several times its normal thickness.

Histological examination of the liver shows a massive centrilobular necrosis and numerous local dilatations of the sinusoids with an accompanying atrophy of the liver cells. The endothelial cells are often swollen and many of them, like the liver cells, contain large acidophilic or basophilic intranuclear inclusions. (Plate 55.4c, facing p. 727). Basophilic inclusion bodies are also present in the lymph nodes and kidneys. Fluorescent antibody staining reveals viral antigens in the nuclei or perinuclear area of serosal, hepatic, Kupffer and vascular endothelial cells of the liver, as well as in the endothelial nuclei of renal vessels.

Dogs, foxes, wolves, racoons and some other species may be experimentally infected by any route, but the intra-ocular route is particularly sensitive. The ferret, which readily succumbs to canine distemper infection, is not susceptible to Rubarth's virus. There are conflicting reports of the susceptibility of mice and rabbits to the virus of infectious canine hepatitis but hamsters are probably susceptible. Guinea-pigs inoculated intraperitoneally may show fever and some may develop fibrinous peritonitis over the serosal surfaces of liver, spleen, kidney and urinary bladder.

Ecology

Infectious canine hepatitis is highly contagious and the virus is discharged in secretions from the respiratory tract as well as in the urine and faeces during clinical illness. In recovered animals the virus may continue to be produced in certain tissues, as is the case in many adenovirus infections, and some dogs are known to shed virus in the urine for at least 200 days after the acute phase of the illness.

The disease is probably transmitted by direct contact with infected animals or indirectly from contaminated buildings, clothing, syringes, etc.

Indirect airborne spread is unlikely because susceptible dogs kept in separate but adjacent pens do not become infected.

Diagnosis

The clinical signs, post-mortem picture and the presence of intranuclear inclusions in smears or tissue sections, usually permit a diagnosis of infectious canine hepatitis. (Plate 42.2a, facing p. 474a.).

In the early stages of disease, the virus can be isolated in primary or secondary cultures of dog kidney cells from blood, tonsils and, sometimes, the conjunctival sac. The isolate may be identified as an adenovirus by complement-fixation. Alternatively, viral antigens may be demonstrable in the blood by the complement-fixation test, using specific antisera produced in experimentally infected animals. Among survivors, a diagnosis can be obtained by demonstrating precipitating antibodies in the sera or by showing a four-fold or greater rise in neutralizing or complement-fixing antibodies in acute and convalescent paired sera taken at 14-day intervals. The antigen used may be in the form of purified cell culture virus or an extract of infected liver tissue.

Haemagglutination-inhibition tests using albino rat or human group O red cells can also be used for the detection of serum antibodies, and the titres are believed to correlate more closely with neutralizing than with complement-fixing titres.

At necropsy, agar gel diffusion tests are especially useful for the rapid detection of specific precipitinogens in infected tissue fragments. Virus can be readily isolated from the affected tissues by inoculation of cell cultures and its identity confirmed by complement-fixation or virus neutralization.

Fluorescent antibody staining can be employed for detecting antigens in smears, tissue sections or infected cell monolayers, and for demonstrating antibodies in unknown dog sera by a blocking method using a known positive liver section.

Immunity

Complement-fixing and precipitating antibodies appear in the blood of infected dogs in about 14–21 days and reach their maximum titres within 10–12 weeks. Thereafter, the titres gradually decline until they are often barely detectable by the 12th month. The immunity resulting from an active infection with Rubarth's virus is solid and long-lasting, hence the absence of complement-fixing antibodies is not a reliable indication of susceptibility. Dogs without complement-fixing antibodies may still be immune to challenge with virulent virus and it is perhaps significant that these animals mostly show measurable amounts of neutralizing antibodies in their sera. Although this suggests that serum neutraliza-tion is a more reliable measure of immunity to canine hepatitis than complement-fixation, it is possible that the immunity is related not only to the development of neutralizing antibodies but also to persistence of the virus in the tissues of recovered animals for very long periods. This form of latent or inapparent infection could give rise to a state of premunition.

Passive immunity is transferred to puppies via the colostrum of recovered or vaccinated bitches, and the protective antibodies have a 'half-life' of about 8 days.

Control

Canine immunglobulins can confer temporary passive immunity lasting for about 3 weeks, and may prove useful in dogs which have recently been exposed or are likely to be exposed to the infection. Simultaneous inoculation with immune serum and virulent virus produces a solid immunity but will not eliminate the carrier status of the animal.

Formolized and attenuated virus vaccines have been used successfully in many countries to induce an active immunity against canine hepatitis. The inactivated vaccines were originally prepared from infected dog tissues but in recent years they have mostly been produced from infected dog kidney cell cultures. The vaccine virus was 'modified' by several serial passages in dog kidney cultures but a more stable strain was obtained after further passages in cultures of pig kidney cells. Live virus attenuated in pig culture or inactivated virus from dog kidney cell culture, may be used as a monovalent vaccine or in combination with live permanently attenuated distemper virus as a bivalent vaccine. Multiple vaccines are also available commercially in which both of the dog viruses have been combined with inactivated *Leptospira icterohaemorrhagiae* and *Leptospira canicola*.

Infectious canine laryngotracheitis

In 1962 Ditchfield and his colleagues in Canada reported on the association of a canine adenovirus with an outbreak of laryngotracheitis or kennel cough. Affected dogs showed symptoms of subacute to chronic repiratory distress and the disease was characterised by laryngitis, tracheitis, bronchitis and tonsillitis.

The causative virus, Toronto A26/61, produced typical adenovirus cytopathic effects in dog kidney cell culture, including rounding of the affected cells and intranuclear inclusions. Human group O red cells were agglutinated by the virus but fowl and guinea-pig erythrocytes were not.

Complement-fixing cross-reactions occurred with infectious canine hepatitis and human adenoviruses, but the Toronto strain could be distinguished from canine hepatitis virus by haemagglutination-inhibition and, to some extent, by virus neutralization.

Simian adenoviruses

Interest in simian adenoviruses arose when it was discovered that many kidney cultures from clinically healthy rhesus and cynomolgus monkeys used for producing inactivated poliovirus vaccines were latently infected with a cytopathic agent. Many of the isolates were identified as adenoviruses and several distinct serotypes were designated SV (for simian virus) followed by numerals in sequence for each virus. Many additional simian adenoviruses have now been isolated, some from monkey faeces, tonsils and other tissues, including one from the faeces of a chimpanzee.

All simian viruses of the adenovirus group share the soluble complement-fixing antigen with human adenoviruses, but are distinct by neutralization tests. Twenty of the early isolates have been reclassified by Pereira and his colleagues, and the total number of distinct antigenic types has been reduced to 12 and designated M1–M12. Many strains recovered subsequently from monkeys and chimpanzees are related to one or other of the M types but several have not yet been fully characterized. Like most adenoviruses, simian strains agglutinate a variety of red blood cells at 37°C. or 4°C. and, on this basis, 4 simian sub-groups have been established.

Simian adenoviruses grow better in monkey kidney cell cultures than in human cells, with rounding of the cells, the formation of grape-like clusters and the presence of small acidophilic inclusions throughout the nucleus.

Simian adenoviruses are not related to any known clinical illness in free-living monkeys or chimpanzees but a few strains can cause disease when inoculated into susceptible monkeys. One strain, M6 (SV17) may produce rhinitis and conjunctivitis in captive patas monkeys and three strains, M2 (SV23), M4 (SV15) and M6 (SV17) have been associated with acute respiratory illness, including deaths, in captive rhesus monkeys.

Although simian adenoviruses do not usually produce illness in experimentally infected rats, mice, rabbits or chickens, 6 of 18 serotypes are capable of inducing tumour formation in unweaned hamsters. One of these may also produce tumours in baby mice and another is believed to be oncogenic in unweaned rats.

Avian adenoviruses

Several adenoviruses have been isolated from the tissues, faeces and secretions of healthy chickens as well as from birds showing symptoms of respiratory disease and diarrhoea. Studies on their classification, antigenic relationships, biological characters and cytopathology clearly indicate that they belong to the adenovirus group, although none of them possesses the soluble group-specific complement-fixing antigen which is shared by all mammalian adenoviruses.

Members of the avian adenovirus group are generally considered under 3 headings: (a) Quail bronchitis virus (QBV), (b) CELO virus (chick-embryo-lethal-orphan) and (c) GAL (Gallus adeno-like) virus. At least 8 serologically distinct avian adenoviruses have been established by virus neutralization tests among which GAL and CELO strains are mostly represented. All chicken strains share a common antigen which is revealed by gel diffusion and, to a lesser extent, by complement-fixation tests.

Adenoviruses have been isolated in Hungary from goose embryos that failed to hatch and from the droppings of adult geese, but the strains are serologically distinct from other avian adenoviruses.

Quail bronchitis virus

Quail bronchitis virus was identified as the causative agent of a highly fatal respiratory disease of quail in Virginia, in 1950, and in Texas, in 1958. The clinical illness was characterized by coughing and sneezing, and a sudden fall in egg production. At necropsy, affected birds showed thickened crops, opacity of the cornea and yellow mucus plugs in the trachea. Inoculation of the virus into embryonated chicken eggs produced death with dwarfing and curling of the embryos similar to the picture induced by avian infectious bronchitis virus. The amniotic sacs were thickened and small, necrotic foci were found in the livers of dead embryos. Inoculation of tracheal exudates, ocular fluids and other tissues into chicken kidney cell cultures produced typical adenovirus cytopathic changes with rounding of the cells and basophilic nuclear inclusions.

Birds recovered from the clinical disease develop neutralizing antibodies in their sera and will resist a second exposure to the virus if the antibody titres are sufficiently high. Studies of the serological relationships among avian adenoviruses showed that 2 antigenically identical strains of quail bronchitis virus could not be distinguished from 3 CELO chicken isolates when examined by reciprocal serum-neutralization tests although they differed from them in pathogenicity.

CELO virus

The name CELO (chicken-embryo-lethal-orphan) was originally used to describe an agent that was recovered from a number of "dead-in-shell" chicken embryos. Since then, a large number of adenoviruses have been isolated from spontaneously degenerating 'normal' chicken embryo cell cultures and from a variety of tissues, faeces and eggs of apparently healthy chickens, and many are serologically indistinguishable from the original CELO isolates.

CELO virus infections appear to be widely distributed and naturally acquired antibodies to CELO virus are frequently present in the sera of domestic poultry. There are also numerous reports of virus isolations from flocks in the U.S.A., Germany and Japan.

CELO virus grows well in fertile hens' eggs following allantoic or yolk sac inoculation, and generally produce death and dwarfing of the embryos within 7–14 days. At least one strain of CELO virus is said to be capable of inducing tumour formation when inoculated into unweaned hamsters. Despite this, there is very little evidence that CELO viruses can cause natural disease in birds.

GAL virus

Strains of avian (GAL) adenoviruses do not appear to be associated with clinical illness in poultry. The first isolate was obtained from chicken liver cell cultures inoculated with filtrates of avian lymphomas and was assumed, wrongly, to be the causative agent of the disease. The virus failed to induce visceral lymphomatosis when inoculated into highly susceptible chickens but, because of its close similarity to human adenoviruses, it was designated Gallus adeno-like, or GAL virus.

The isolation of GAL virus has been reported from the U.S.A. France and the U.K., and the high incidence of neutralizing antibodies in chicken sera suggests that sub-clinical infections are common in those countries. GAL virus grows in fertile eggs and adapted strains readily kill the developing embryos, irrespective of the route of inoculation. It produces a marked adenovirus type of cytopathic effect in chicken kidney cell cultures and the nuclei of infected cells contain large, clearly defined, strongly basophilic inclusions surrounded by a clear halo.

Further reading

CABASSO V.J. (1962) Infectious canine hepatitis virus. *Annals of the New York Academy of Sciences*, **101**, 498.

CLARKE M.C., SHARP H.B.A. AND DERBYSHIRE J.B. (1967) Some characteristics of three porcine adenoviruses. *Archiv für die gesamte Virusforschung*, **21**, 91.

COFFIN D.L., COONS A.H. AND CABASSO V.J.A. (1953) A histological study of infectious canine

hepatitis by means of fluorescent antibody. *Journal of Experimental Medicine*, **98**, 13.

CORIA M.F., McCLURKIN A.W., CUTLIP R.C. AND RITCHIE A.E. (1975) Isolation and characterization of bovine adenovirus type 5 associated with 'weak calf syndrome'. *Archives of Virology*, **47**, 309.

Darbyshire J.H. (1968) Bovine adenoviruses. *Journal of the American Veterinary Medical Association*, **152**, 786.

DARBYSHIRE J.H., DAWSON P.S., LAMONT P.H., OSTLER D.C. AND PEREIRA H.G. (1965) A new adenovirus serotype of bovine origin. *Journal of Comparative Pathology and Therapeutics*, **75**, 237.

GINSBERG H.S. (1962) Identification and classification of adenoviruses. *Virology*, **18**, 312.

HAIG D.A., CLARKE M.C. AND PEREIRA M.S. (1964) Isolation of an adenovirus from a pig. *Journal of Comparative Pathology and Therapeutics*, **74**, 81.

HOGGAN M.D. (1970) Adenovirus associated viruses. *Progress in Medical Virology*, **12**, 211.

NORRBY E. (1971) Adenoviruses. In, Comparative Virology. eds. K. Maramorosch and E. Kurstak, p. 105. London: *Academic Press Inc.*

PHILIPSON L., PETTERSSON U. AND LINDBERG U. (1975) Molecular biology of adenoviruses. *Virology Monographs*, **14**, 1.

PRYDIE J., BATTY I. AND WALKER P.D. (1966) Lack of interference in tissue culture between the viruses of canine distemper and infectious canine hepatitis as demonstrated by immunofluorescence. *Veterinary Record*, **79**, 354.

ROWE W.P. AND HARTLEY J.W. (1962) A general review of the adenoviruses. *Annals of the New York Academy of Sciences*, **101**, 466.

ROWE W.P., HUEBNER R.J., GILMORE L.F., PARROT R.H. AND WARD T.G. (1953). Isolation of a pathogenic agent from human adenoids undergoing spontaneous degeneration in tissue culture. *Proceedings of the Society for Experimental Biology and Medicine*, **84**, 570

RUBARTH S. (1947) An acute virus disease with liver lesions in dogs (*hepatitis contagiosa canis*). A pathologic-anatomical and etiological investigation. *Acta pathologica et microbiologica Scandinavica*, Supplement 69.

SOHIER R., CHARDONNET Y. AND PRUNIERAS M. (1965) Adenoviruses. Status of current knowledge. *Progress in Medical Virology*, **7**, 263.

VALENTINE R.C. AND PEREIRA H.G. (1965) Antigens and structure of the adenovirus. *Journal of Molecular Biology*, **13**, 13.

CHAPTER 56

HERPESVIRUSES

Herpesviruses

The herpesvirus group (Gr. herpein = to creep), originally consisted of the three species, *Herpes simplex* of man, B-virus of monkeys and pseudorabies or Aujeszky's disease virus of animals. In recent years the group has been greatly extended by the addition of viruses from a wide variety of vertebrate hosts and at least 40 species have now been included in the family.
(Table 56.1).

Properties of the virus

All herpesviruses consist of a central core of double-stranded DNA surrounded by a protein capsid which in turn is usually enclosed in a loose outer envelope derived from one of the host cell membranes. The surface of the nucleocapsid is in the form of 162 short projecting capsomeres arranged in the form of an icosahedron. Each capsomere, or protein sub-unit, measures 12.5×9.5 nm in

TABLE 56.1. Some herpesviruses and their primary hosts.

Mammalia—Primates	
Herpes simplex	Man.
B-virus	Old World Monkey.
M-virus (Marmoset virus)	New World Monkey.
Cytomegaloviruses	Man, chimpanzees and monkey.
Varicella—zoster	Man.
Burkitt's lymphoma	Man.
Mammalia—Non Primates	
Pseudorabies	Pig.
Infectious bovine rhinotracheitis	Ox.
Malignant catarrhal fever	Sheep, wildebeest
"Allerton" virus infection	Ox.
Bovine ulcerative mammillitis	Ox.
Equine rhinopneumonitis	Horse.
Feline viral rhinotracheitis	Cat.
Canine herpesvirus infection	Dog.
Virus III	Rabbit.
Cytomegaloviruses	Pig, sheep, guinea-pig, mouse, rat, mole and hamster.
Inclusion-body rhinitis	Pig.
Jaagsiekte	Sheep.
Aves	
Infectious laryngotracheitis	Poultry.
Herpesvirus infection of pigeons	Pigeon.
Duck plague	Duck.
Pacheco parrot disease	Parrot.
Cormorant disease	Cormorant.
Marek's disease	Poultry.
Amphibia	
(?) Renal carcinoma (Lucké's virus)	Leopard frog.

diameter and resembles a short hexagonal or pentagonal tube with a hollow centre. Particles may be found with or without envelopes and nucleoids. The enveloped virion is about 180 nm in diameter whereas the 'naked' less infectious form is 110 nm in diameter. The surrounding envelope contains essential lipids and viral activity is, therefore, markedly reduced by exposure to 20 per cent ether. The envelope contains both host cell and viral components, and is important for adsorption to susceptible host cells. (Plate 37.3 facing p. 430).

The molecular weight of the nucleic acid component of herpesviruses varies from $3-9 \times 10^7$ daltons. The guanine+cytosine (GC) content also varies from values as low as 45 per cent for avian infectious laryngotracheitis virus to as high as 74 per cent for Aujeszky's disease virus.

The herpesvirus is relatively unstable at room temperature and also is fairly heat-labile, being inactivated in 30 minutes at 50°C. Virus can be preserved in the frozen state at −50°C or at 4°C, but storage of many strains at −20°C reduces infectivity more than ten-fold in 2 weeks. However, infected tissue homogenates suspended in glycerol, or after being ground up in skimmed milk, can be stored at −20°C without appreciable loss of titre.

Haemagglutination
Most herpesviruses do not agglutinate red blood cells when examined by the usual methods but some are adsorbed on to sheep erythrocytes treated with tannic acid which can then be agglutinated by specific antisera. The reaction is best carried out at 25°C and at pH 6.4.

Antigenic properties
On the basis of serum neutralization, cross-protection, complement-fixation and gel diffusion tests, a number of serological relationships have been established between herpes simplex virus and B-virus. Pseudorabies is related to these two viruses by a common precipitating antigen only. There is also evidence of crossing between herpes simplex and canine herpesvirus, between infectious bovine rhinotracheitis and equine rhinopneumonitis viruses and even minor ones between varicella/zoster and herpes simplex. Recent unconfirmed reports suggest that the herpesviruses associated with Lucké adenocarcinoma, Burkitt lymphoma and Marek's disease of poultry are also serologically related.

Cultivation
All herpesviruses can be grown in cell cultures derived from one or more of a wide range of animal sources and, with the exception of varicella and avian infectious laryngotracheitis, most of the viruses multiply well in monolayer cultures of rabbit kidney cells. Some herpesviruses can also be propagated in embryonated hens' eggs and a few produce surface pocks on the chorioallantoic membranes. All strains produce intranuclear inclusions of Cowdry's type A both *in vivo* and *in vitro*. With most members of the group, active virus is readily found in the fluid phase of the infected cultures, whereas a few species such as cytomegalovirus, varicella, Marek's virus and the EB (Epstein Barr) virus are more firmly associated with the infected cell and are probably transmitted from one cell to another by direct cell-to-cell contact or during the process of cell division. The experimental host range of selected herpesviruses is shown in Table 56.2.

Viral multiplication
Replication of herpesviruses occurs in the cell nucleus. Following assembly of their component parts the progeny virus particles approach the inner nuclear membrane which becomes thicker and

TABLE 56.2.   Experimental host range of selected herpesviruses.

Virus	Range of Susceptible Cell Cultures	Eggs	Rabbits	Mice
Herpes simplex	Broad	+	+	+
Herpes B (and M)	Broad	+	+	+
Pseudorabies	Broad	+	+	+
Avian infectious laryngotracheitis	Limited	+	−	−
Equine rhinopneumonitis	Broad	−	+	−
Infectious bovine rhinotracheitis	Broad	−	−	−
Feline viral rhinotracheitis	Limited	−	−	−
Canine herpesvirus	Limited	−	−	−
Bovine mammillitis virus	Limited	−	−	−
Malignant catarrhal fever	Limited	−	−	−
Cytomegalovirus	Limited	−	−	−
Marek's virus	Limited	−	−	−
EB virus	Limited	−	−	−

progressively envelops the virion. The membrane eventually pinches off, leaving the nuclear membrane intact and the enveloped particle free in the perinuclear cisterna. Alternatively, some particles may acquire envelopes by budding into nuclear vacuoles which are probably formed by indentations of the nuclear membrane and are continuous with the perinuclear cisterna. The newly-formed enveloped nucleocapsid is transported through the cytoplasm to the extracellular environment, either within vesicles formed by the endoplasmic reticulum or, more probably, travels along canaliculi in the endoplasmic reticulum where it is protected from cellular enzymes until it reaches the surface of the cell and is released through the plasma membrane. The biochemical events responsible for herpesvirus replication are similar to those of many other DNA-containing viruses, e.g. adenoviruses.

During the multiplication cycle of herpesvirus, a basophilic mass appears within the nucleus which corresponds to the accumulation of newly synthesized viral DNA. Assembly of incomplete virus particles begins within the matrix of this inclusion and as assembly and release of the infectious virions proceeds, accompanied by diffusion of soluble antigens into the cytoplasm, the original basophilic mass is converted into an acidophilic intranuclear inclusion. Since this structure does not contain visible virus particles or detectable specific viral antigens, it probably represents the residual scar of an area of nuclear damage.

Pathogenicity

An important characteristic of many herpesvirus infections is the ability of the virus to persist in a quiescent state for very long periods. When the initial infection recedes, virus is not completely eradicated from the host and a chronic or latent type of infection is produced at the major site of the primary disease despite the presence of high levels of circulating antibody. Frequently, the infection is reactivated in patients subjected to some form of stress such as heat, cold, ultra-violet light, hypersensitive reactions, hormonal or emotional disturbances, and the clinical disease reappears. In many instances, however, neutralizing antibodies are present and, since the virus cannot disseminate, the lesions remain localized. Despite this, some infectious virus particles may spread to adjacent susceptible cells by direct transfer or via intercellular cytoplasmic bridges similar to those seen in many infected cell culture systems. An additional feature of some herpesvirus infections is the fact that transmission of a latent viral infection in the natural host to another susceptible species frequently results in a severe and often fatal illness, e.g. herpes B-virus of monkeys in man, and pseudorabies virus of adult pigs in cattle. Many members of the herpes group grow in the nervous tissues of their hosts and travel along nerves to reach the central nervous system from a peripheral site.

Diagnosis

Most herpesvirus infections can be readily confirmed by laboratory procedures. Specific antigens can be detected in cells from the lesions by immunofluorescence or gel diffusion techniques, and in many primary infections significant increases in neutralizing or complement-fixing antibody titres can be demonstrated in sera obtained early in the illness and again 14–21 days after onset. The causative virus can often be isolated in cell cultures, laboratory animals or embryonated hens' eggs, and identified serologically. The presence of intranuclear inclusions and syncytial formation is characteristic of many herpesvirus infections, both *in vitro* and *in vivo*.

Herpes simplex and varicella-zoster viruses

Herpesviruses are responsible for two of the most common diseases of man, viz. "fever blisters" (herpes simplex) and chickenpox (varicella). Primary infection with herpes simplex occurs mostly in young children but the virus often becomes latent and recurrent attacks of "fever blisters' or "cold sores" are frequently induced by conditions of stress. Similarly, herpesvirus varicellae or varicella-zoster (V–Z) virus which causes the papular rash of chickenpox in children, frequently lies dormant in the body for many years until it is reactivated by various stimuli to cause herpes zoster (shingles) in adults. Zoster is a painful local condition with skin lesions resembling those of varicella. Not only has typical varicella been contracted from patients with zoster, and zoster material produced varicella in children, but comparison of the viruses isolated in cell culture has conclusively proved that the two diseases are caused by the same agent, the varicella-zoster virus.

Properties of the virus

Herpes simplex virus is the type species of the group and its principal characteristics closely resemble those of varicella-zoster virus.

Antigenic properties and immunity

Patients susceptible to recurrent attacks of "fever blisters" possess reasonably high titres of neutralizing and complement-fixing antibodies, whereas those not susceptible to attack and those who have not experienced infection show no antibodies in their sera. This unusual feature is underlined by the fact that multiple recurrence of the disease in susceptible humans does not usually affect the serum titres although these are significantly increased following a primary infection. In chickenpox (varicella) and shingles (zoster), convalescent zoster sera usually have higher antibody titres than post-varicella sera, probably because a secondary antigenic stimulus is concerned.

Although there is no antigen common to the herpes group of viruses, serological cross-reactions occur between a few members, e.g. herpes simplex, B-virus and pseudorabies; or infectious bovine rhinotracheitis and equine rhinopneumonitis. The human herpesviruses are antigenically distinct except for types 1 (oral herpes) and 2 (genital herpes) which show some cross-reactivity. These are distinguished by the use of sera with high homotypic titres and by certain growth properties in different cell species. Antibodies to type 2 herpesvirus do not develop in the general population until the age of adolescence and increased sexual activity.

Cultivation
Herpes simplex grows well on the chorioallantoic membrane of embryonated hens' eggs producing small, white surface pocks of about 1–2 mm. in diameter. Varicella-zoster virus has not been cultivated in fertile eggs.

Growth of herpes simplex occurs readily in many types of tissue cultures including rabbit, chicken embryo and human cells. The formation of intranuclear inclusion bodies and multinucleated syncytia is usually followed by marked cell destruction. Human kidney, human amnion and rabbit kidney cultures are the cells of choice and the optimum temperature for growth is probably 35°C. Varicella-zoster virus grows in cell cultures of human-embryo skin and muscle, prepuce, thyroid, and HeLa cells as well as various monkey tissues. Supernatant fluids from many of these infected cultures contain a complement-fixing antigen but are free of infective virus and it is presumed that the infection passes to contiguous cells rather than through the medium in the fluid phase of the culture. On the other hand, fluids harvested from infected human thyroid cells generally yield infectious virus. Cytopathic effects, including intranuclear inclusions, appear in 2–7 days, and are generally focal in character but gradually involve the whole monolayer.

Pathogenicity
Herpes simplex virus gives rise to different forms of disease and these are classified either as primary or recurrent infections. Many of the primary infections are inapparent but the most common clinical response is a mild vesicular eruption of the skin or mucous membranes. Primary infections occur mainly in young children (2–4 years) and the commonest sites for "fever blisters" are the muco-cutaneous junctions such as around the lips or nostrils. Other forms of the disease include kerato-conjunctivitis associated with corneal opacity, Kaposi's varicelliform eruption in which there is widespread superinfection of eczematous skin, herpes genitalis and cervicitis (both of which are transmitted venereally), fatal meningoencephalitis and a generalised neonatal infection which is usually due to the genital type 2 strain of herpes simplex virus and is often fatal. The most common manifestation of recurrent herpes are the "cold sores" which appear as a crop of vesicles around the anterior nares or lips, and progress to pustules with crust formation. Between attacks the virus remains latent in the tissues of the host, probably in the sensory cells of the trigeminal nerve ganglion.

Varicella (chickenpox) also affects mainly children, causing a papular rash which becomes vesicular and then scabby. On the other hand, zoster (shingles) is a sporadic, painful and localized condition of adults (rarely in children) which is characterized by an inflammatory reaction of the posterior nerve roots and ganglia, accompanied by crops of vesicles over the skin supplied by the affected sensory nerves. The disease is due to reactivation of virus latent in thoracic or cranial nerve ganglia many years after an attack of chickenpox in childhood. Zoster, unlike varicella, is not acquired by contact with cases of varicella or zoster, although it may give rise to varicella in susceptible contacts.

Diagnosis
Herpes simplex infections can be readily diagnosed by the isolation of the virus in tissue cultures of BHK-21, HeLa or other cells, and observing the monolayers for cytopathic effects. The virus is identified by neutralization tests using standard antisera. Isolation of varicella-zoster virus is rarely attempted but cases of chickenpox and shingles can be confirmed by complement-fixation tests. Other serological tests which may be employed are immunofluorescence and a precipitation test in agar gel.

B-virus of monkeys

Synonym
Herpesvirus simiae. Cercopithecid herpesvirus 1.

Definition
A natural herpes-like infection of normal Asiatic monkeys, especially rhesus and cynomolgus species, which causes an acute ascending highly fatal myelitis of man.

Properties of the virus
The mature virus particle measures about 110 nm in diameter and is very similar in its morphological,

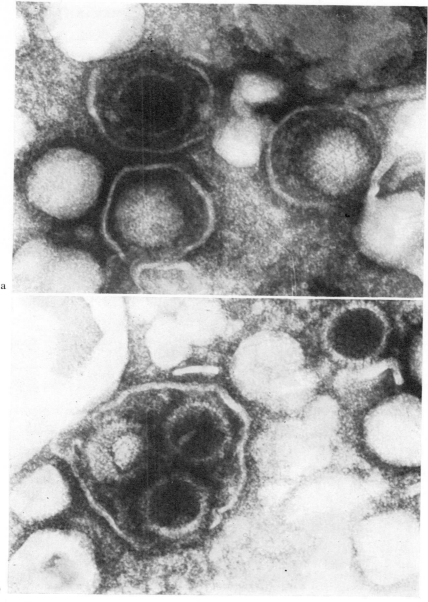

Electron micrographs of partially purified pseudorabies (herpesvirus) particles, negatively stained with phospho-tungstic acid. (Courtesy of Dr Sakkubai Ramachandran.)

56.1a Three enveloped virus particles in different stages of development. One of the capsids (right) reveals icosahedral symmetry and the edge of each triangular facet consists of five hollow prismatic capsomeres, × 160 000.

56.1b Three penetrated virus particles are enclosed by a single envelope. A fourth non-enveloped particle (top right) clearly shows the hollow longitudinal capsomeres on the surface of the virion, × 140 000.

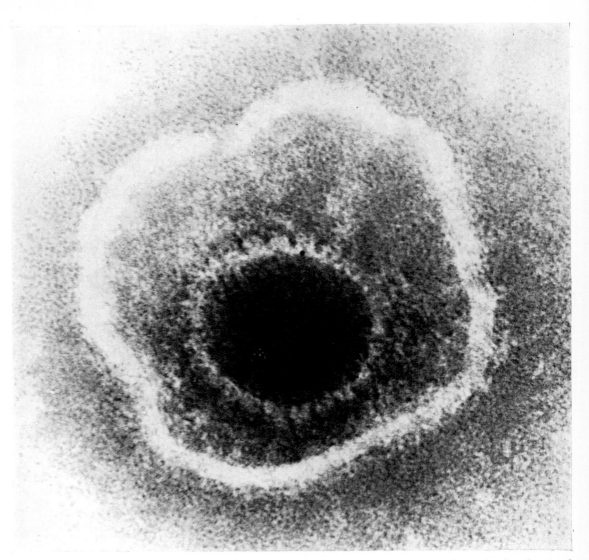

56.2 Electron micrograph of a single particle of the McFerran strain of Aujeszky's disease virus. The phosphotungstic acid stain has penetrated inside the core, giving the virion an empty appearance. The capsid is composed of a regular radial arrangement of hollow capsomeres and is surrounded by a thick-walled outer membrane or envelope, × 520 000.

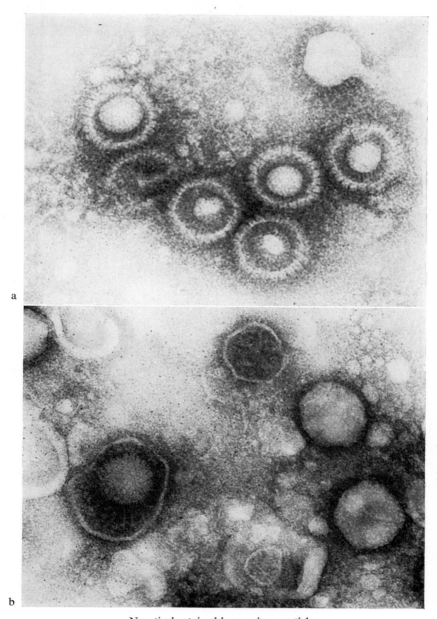

a

b

Negatively stained herpesvirus particles.

56.3a Non-enveloped virions, each showing a distinct halo between the outer shell of the capsid and the electron-dense core. Notice the hollow zone running longitudinally through the radially arranged capsomeres and the hexagonal shape of some of the capsids, × 180 000.

56.3b Penetrated and unpenetrated particles. The envelopes surrounding two of the virions have been disrupted during penetration of the specimen. The icosahedral symmetry and the arrangement of the surface capsomeres are clearly defined in the particle (lower, left), × 140 000.

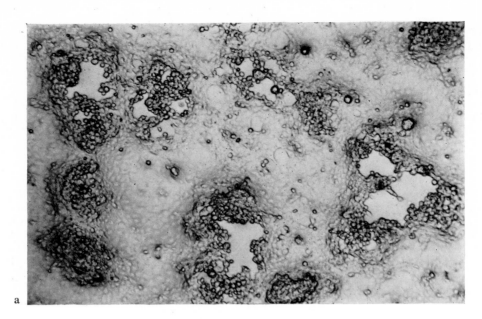

a

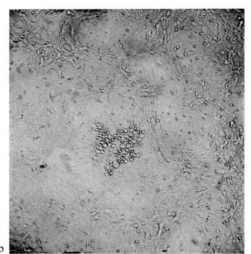

b

56.4a Unstained Petri dish culture of the PK15 line of pig kidney cells 24 hours after inoculation with Aujeszky's disease virus. The early cytopathic effect of the virus is characterized by foci of rounded refractile cells and disruption of the monolayer, × 80.

56.4b Unstained primary culture of chick kidney cells showing a small focus of rounded degenerating cells induced by Marek's disease virus. (Courtesy of Mr G. N. Woode.)

biochemical and biological characters to herpes simplex virus. It is labile at room temperature but may be preserved at —70°C, or in 50 per cent glycerol at 4°C, or in the lyophilized state. It can be inactivated by formaldehyde within 48 hours and is ether- and chloroform-sensitive.

Antigenic properties
Most members of the herpes group are antigenically distinct but some serological relationships exist (*vide supra*). For example, a variety of serological tests has established a group relationship between B-virus and herpes simplex, between B-virus and pseudorabies, but not between herpes simplex and pseudorabies viruses. It is emphasised, however, that sera from animals immunized against B-virus neutralize herpes simplex, whereas immune herpes simplex sera do not neutralize B-virus; indeed, a fatal human case of B-virus infection has been described in a patient known to have antibodies to herpes simplex. Thus, B-virus has a broader antigenicity than herpes simplex virus.

Cultivation
The virus grows well in embryonated hens' eggs and produces small opaque pocks on the surface of the chorioallantoic membrane. It can also be propagated in cultures of rabbit, monkey or human cells and has frequently been isolated from cell cultures derived from apparently normal rhesus monkey kidneys. The virus is transmissible to monkeys, rabbits, unweaned mice and day-old chicks. Growth of virus in these cell systems is characterized by the formation of intranuclear inclusions and multinucleated 'giant-cells'.

Pathogenicity
Naturally infected monkeys may show vesicular herpes-like lesions that develop into ulcers on the dorsal surface of the tongue and on the mucoepithelial borders of the lips. There is little change in the animal's body temperature and the ulcers tend to heal spontaneously within 10–14 days. Herpetic lesions are found most commonly in monkeys that are crowded together, and recently imported animals constitute the greatest danger to attendants dealing with monkeys. Clinical infection in human subjects may develop 10–20 days after exposure to the virus. Fortunately, human cases are rare but the incidence is increasing as the number of people handling monkeys and preparing monkey tissue culture vaccines increases. Of 15 cases known to have occurred in man, only 2 survived and both showed severe residual damage to the central nervous system. One of the fatal cases was a veterinary surgeon with a wound on a finger that became contaminated with saliva when examining a monkey.

In every case but one, human infection with B-virus has been associated with the handling of monkeys. The one exception occurred in a laboratory worker who became infected after handling glassware used for tissue cultures of monkey kidneys.

About 3 days after a bite from an infected monkey there is usually local inflammation at the site of the wound followed by the formation of papules and vesicles, and then necrosis of the area. About 7 days later the virus at the site of the skin lesion reaches the central nervous system by way of the peripheral nerves, giving rise to ascending myelitis, acute encephalitis or encephalomyelitis, and death. Besides the destructive lesions in the brain and cord, which show intranuclear inclusions, there is also focal necrosis of the lymph nodes, adrenals, spleen and liver. In most fatal cases, virus can be recovered from the brain, spinal cord and spleen. Suspensions of infected tissues inoculated intradermally into rabbits give rise to necrotic skin lesions, which may not appear for 10–12 days, followed by severe pruritus when the central nervous system becomes involved, leading to encephalitis and death.

Ecology
The virus spreads by direct contact between monkeys, especially in monkeys crowded together in captivity. B-virus sets up a latent infection much as herpes simplex does in man. About 10 per cent of newly caught rhesus monkeys have B-virus antibodies in their sera and the incidence rises to over 60 per cent when they are confined together in captivity. Virus has been recovered from the saliva, brain and spinal cord of clinically healthy, persistently infected monkeys and is frequently present in primary monkey kidney cell cultures. Both of these are possible sources of infection for human subjects.

Diagnosis
B-virus can be readily isolated from the brain, spinal cord and spleen of fatal human cases or from the saliva, brain and other tissues of latently infected monkeys by the inoculation of rabbit kidney cell cultures, embryonated hens' eggs, or experimental animals such as rabbits, young mice or day-old chicks. The virus is irregularly fatal for guinea-pigs. Because the infection is invariably fatal in man, serological tests for the detection of neutralizing and complement-fixing antibodies are of little practical value.

Control
There is no specific treatment for B-virus infection in human patients and vaccination of man with formolized vaccines has been attempted without success. Human gamma globulin, if known to contain B-virus antibodies, should be given in large

doses immediately after the patient is bitten and the wound should also be infiltrated with antiserum.

Workers wishing to examine the mouths of recently imported monkeys for ulcers must wear protective clothing such as gowns, heavy gloves, face masks and eye shields and, whenever possible, the monkeys should be anaesthetised or heavily sedated before being handled. Primates should only be attended by responsible and adequately trained animal-house personnel and laboratory workers should be warned about the dangers of handling and breaking glassware containing monkey tissue cultures.

Marmoset virus

A virus has been isolated from throat swabs and necropsy material of South American marmoset monkeys (*Tamarindus nigricollis*) which has all the properties of a herpesvirus. It is usually known as marmoset or M-virus but is sometimes called Herpes-T (Tamarindus), Herpesvirus platyrhinae or Callitrichid herpesvirus 1.

The virus grows well in marmoset, rabbit and human tissue cultures but poorly in rhesus monkey kidney cells, and produces pocks on the surface of the chorioallantoic membrane of developing chicken embryos. Typical Cowdry type A intranuclear inclusions are produced. Most strains are highly virulent for marmosets and are pathogenic for rabbits and mice infected intracerebrally and for unweaned mice and hamsters inoculated intraperitoneally. Although some cross-protection between marmoset and herpes simplex has been described, other workers failed to show an antigenic relationship between marmoset virus and either herpes simplex virus or B-virus.

Marmoset virus has been isolated from owl monkeys and squirrel monkeys, and it is possible that squirrel monkeys are the natural hosts for the virus since they develop latent infections and sometimes show labial and oral lesions similar to those of B-virus infections.

In the diagnostic laboratory the three primate herpesviruses can be distinguished by their different cell susceptibilities. Thus, rhesus monkey kidney cultures are highly susceptible only to B-virus; green monkey cultures to B-virus and M (marmoset) virus; and rabbit cultures to B-virus, M-virus and herpes simplex virus.

Aujeszky's disease

Synonyms
Pseudorabies, Mad itch, Infectious bulbar paralysis, Herpesvirus suis. Pig herpesvirus 1.

Hosts affected
Aujeszky's disease occurs naturally in a wide range of animals including swine, cattle, sheep, dogs, mink, ferrets, foxes, cats and rats: in all but adult swine it is characterized by marked localized pruritus and an invariably fatal termination. Reports of the natural disease in horses are not supported by virological data. The causative agent is a member of the herpes group of viruses which closely resembles herpes simplex of man and B-virus of monkeys. The most common primary hosts are swine, and adult pigs are probably the main reservoir of the virus. Typical Aujeszky's disease has not been described in man, but there are a number of reports of mild illness, including pruritus, following accidental infection of laboratory workers. Fortunately, none of these cases was described as serious.

History and distribution
The disease was first described by Aujeszky in Hungary in 1902 and its viral aetiology was confirmed in 1910. There is evidence, nevertheless, that the infection had existed for several decades before this in parts of Western and Central Europe. The paucity of reliable accounts of the disease in the earlier literature is probably due to the quiescent and insidious nature of the disease in adult pigs which rendered diagnosis difficult, together with the furious manifestations of the illness in cattle and sheep which were probably mistaken for rabies. On the other hand, there seems little doubt that Aujeszky's disease existed in the USA in the 19th century, because the early American farm literature contains a number of detailed accounts of a highly fatal pruritic condition described as "mad-itch" in dairy cattle. The description of this infection, which was contracted by dogs feeding on infected beef, bears a striking similarity to the later accounts of Aujeszky's disease. At the present time, Aujeszky's disease is enzootic in many European countries, particularly in areas where there has been intensification of pig-rearing in recent years: and outbreaks continue to occur in Bulgaria, Czechoslovakia, Denmark, France, Hungary, Italy, the Netherlands, Poland, Portugal, Rumania and Yugoslavia. The disease is not so important in the United Kingdom as it is in Europe but sporadic outbreaks are encountered in Northern Ireland. Although Aujeszky's disease is still prevalent in the Mid Western United States and in parts of South America it does not have a world-wide distribution and, apart from occasional reports of the disease in China, Algeria, Tunisia and Angola, it is almost entirely confined to Europe and the Americas.

Morphology
In negatively-stained preparations the virions of Aujeszky's disease measure about 110–150 nm in diameter, but particles up to 230 nm may be

observed depending upon the techniques that are employed in preparing the specimens. In thin-sections of infected cells, the viral particles sometimes appear round but more frequently oval and contain an electron-dense core surrounded by a double membrane. The dense central body or nucleoid, contains the viral nucleic acid which consists of double-stranded DNA with a molecular weight of $68-70 \times 10^6$ daltons.

The ultrastructure of Aujeszky's disease virus is indistinguishable morphologically from that of herpes simplex, B-virus or other herpesviruses. The capsid, which probably corresponds to the inner membrane seen in thin-section, is composed of 150 hexagonal and 12 pentagonal hollow elongated subunits or capsomeres, about 12 nm in length and 9 nm in width, with a central hole of approximately 4 nm in diameter. The capsomeres are regularly arranged on the surface of the icosahedral capsid in such a way that each edge of the 20 triangular facets consists of 5 equally spaced hollow prismatic capsomeres. (Plates 56.1a, b, facing p. 740, and 56.3a, b, between pp. 740–1). Many of the capsids are enclosed by envelopes of varying shape and size with an average diameter of about 180 nm. In some preparations tiny radially arranged projections (8–10 nm in length) are seen on the surface of the envelope but the function of these structures is not entirely clear. (Plate 56.2, between pp. 740–1). Although there is a strong correlation between the presence of envelopes and infectivity, naked virions can also be infectious.

Physicochemical characters
The virus is frequently stable between pH5 and 9. It retains its infectivity in glycerol saline or skimmed milk at refrigeration temperatures but is best preserved at $-70°C$ when stored in saline, buffered with Tris at pH 7.5, containing 1 per cent serum albumin. Although Aujeszky's disease virus is more thermostable than herpes simplex virus it should not be held at temperatures between 4°C and $-30°C$, otherwise infectivity is reduced more than tenfold in 2 weeks. It is inactivated in an exponential manner by X-ray or ultra-violet light irradiation and is extremely susceptible to lipid solvents such as ethyl ether, sodium desoxycholate and chloroform. Trypsin and certain other enzymes inactivate the virus without destroying the viral capsid: the effect being due either to total destruction of the envelope or to removal of specific sites essential for attachment to cells. Aujeszky's disease virus can withstand 3 per cent phenol but not 5 per cent, and may persist in swine fever vaccines. It is inactivated almost immediately by 0.5–1 per cent NaOH, but is said to survive on hay for a month or longer.

Haemagglutination
In spite of repeated attempts, there is no evidence that Aujeszky's disease virus can agglutinate avian or mammalian species of red blood cells.

Antigenic properties
All strains of Aujeszky's disease virus are antigenically similar but unrelated to most other members of the herpesvirus group. However, a small but definite antigenic relationship exists between Aujeszky's disease virus and B-virus since monkeys with antibodies to B-virus may be resistant to Aujeszky's virus and a common antigen is evident in gel diffusion tests. Antisera to Aujeszky's virus are usually prepared in adult swine since the virus is lethal to most other species and inactivated virus does not readily immunize. Adult hens, on the other hand, are generally highly resistant to the virus and are suitable for the production of immune sera.

Cultivation
Aujeszky's virus is a typical herpesvirus and grows readily on the chorioallantoic membrane of embryonated hens' eggs forming moderately large, raised, white 'pocks' after 3–4 days of incubation. (Plate 42.3c, facing p. 480). Many strains of the virus are lethal to the embryo and haemorrhagic destruction of the nervous system frequently gives rise to protrusion of the cranium of the embryo. The virus can also be passaged serially via the yolk sac giving rise to increased virulence for the embryo. All strains of Aujeszky's virus will multiply in a wide variety of cells cultivated *in vitro*, but the different types of cells vary in their sensitivity to the virus. Rabbit kidney cells are particularly susceptible and are more sensitive to the virus than fertile eggs and laboratory animals. Infection with virulent virus usually causes a rapid and marked cytopathic effect which is characterized by cellular degeneration and, eventually, death of the susceptible cells. In general, the cytopathic effects are of 2 types: 1) early cytoplasmic granulation followed by rounding or ballooning of the infected cells, which tend to form discrete foci of heaped-up refractile cells, and 2) fusion of the contiguous membranes of infected cells, giving rise to scattered ill-defined foci of syncytia (polykaryons). (Plates 56.4a facing p. 741 and 56.5a, facing p. 748). The process of cell-fusion proceeds rapidly and numerous large syncytial masses are formed consisting of multinucleated cells many of which contain basophilic or acidophilic intranuclear inclusions of Cowdry type A. (Plate 56.5c, facing p. 748). Monolayer cultures of cells on which agar has been laid after adsorption of the virus will form plaques of necrotic and dead cells after about 4–6 days of incubation, and these will appear as colourless areas against a red background if a vital dye such

as neutral red is added to the agar. The kind of cytopathic effect (rounding or syncytial formation) and the size and shape of the plaques formed under agar varies according to the strain of virus and the type of cell. However, variants of both types of virus can be separated from each other either by centrifugation in density gradients of caesium chloride or by 'cloning' methods.

Pathogenicity

Spontaneous outbreaks of Aujeszky's disease have been confirmed in a wide range of domestic, captive and free-living mammals in several genera of the orders *Lagomorpha, Rodentia, Carnivora* and *Artiodactyla*, but of these, the most commonly affected are pigs, cattle, sheep, dogs, cats and rats. In most natural hosts the virus generally produces a highly fatal infection, but in swine the occurrence of clinical symptoms is inversely related to the age of the affected animal. Thus, adolescent and adult pigs usually undergo only a subclinical or mild febrile illness.

In its fully developed state, Aujeszky's disease in ruminants, carnivores and laboratory rodents is usually of an explosive nature. There is, invariably, profound central nervous involvement that is characterized by restlessness, staggering gait, convulsions and paralysis leading to exhaustion, prostration and coma. Hyperaesthesia of the skin is a pathognomonic symptom of the disease in most susceptible species, but may be entirely absent in adult swine.

Cattle and sheep are among the most susceptible of the domestic animals to Aujeszky's disease virus. Affected animals lick some part of the body, rub violently against solid objects and, as the disease progresses, bite frantically at the skin of the affected area, but at no stage is there any fever. The animal becomes progressively weaker and coma and death usually follow within 18–48 hours after the first signs of the disease. Although the virus produces a mild or inapparent infection in adult swine, younger pigs usually develop a highly fatal illness which is characterized by pyrexia, paralysis, coma and death within 24 hours. Infected sows may abort and most produce stillbirths or mummified fetuses at full term.

Following artificial infection by any route, the virus travels centripetally along the peripheral nerves to the central nervous system, giving rise eventually to the characteristic nervous symptoms. Virus can be readily isolated from the brain of almost all species of affected animals but is rarely found in the cerebro-spinal fluid, blood or viscera. In pigs, on the other hand, virus is frequently present in the nasal and oral secretions for 10–14 days following infection and spreads by contact to other animals.

Many species of laboratory animals are susceptible to Aujeszky's disease and peripheral inoculation generally gives rise to intense pruritus, terminating in death. Following subcutaneous or intramuscular injection, the virus multiplies at the site of inoculation, invades the local nerve and reaches the central nervous system along the peripheral nerves. Depending on the route of inoculation and the age and species of animal, virus may be found in the brain, head lymph nodes, spinal cord and, occasionally, lungs and certain other organs. Rodents are readily infected by the oral and respiratory routes and, since their carcases invariably contain virus, these animals may constitute an important source of infection for pigs. Chicks are also highly susceptible to experimental infection by different routes during the first 24 hours after hatching, but intramuscular inoculation fails to induce mortality in birds over 48 hours of age.

Pathological lesions

There are no gross changes of a specific nature. Microscopically, the principal lesions in all animals are those of a diffuse, lymphohistiocytic, nonsuppurative, meningo-encephalitis and ganglioneuritis characterized by a moderate to pronounced neuronal and glial necrosis, diffuse or focal gliosis and marked perivascular cuffing. Although the distribution of the lesions is often dependent on the site of pruritus and duration of the illness, the cerebrum is invariably severely affected; the cellular exudation being especially prominent in the corpus medullare around the lateral ventricles. The lesions diminish in intensity caudally and intranuclear inclusions of Cowdry type A are usually prominent. In ruminants and carnivores the disease is also characterised by involvement of the lumbo-sacral segments of the cord and the related dorsal root ganglia on the affected side.

Ecology

The method of transmission of Aujeszky's disease virus in naturally occurring infections is not fully understood, but the disease is highly contagious in swine since adult pigs with inapparent infection frequently shed virus in their nasal and oral secretions. In many outbreaks of Aujeszky's disease in Europe there is often a close association with rodents which are naturally susceptible to the infection. Many workers believe that pigs contract the disease from eating carcases of infected rats or mice, and that cattle may become infected directly by rat bite. In dogs, the disease usually occurs on farms where there has been close contact with pigs and rats or where they have fed on infected beef. Although the virus can be readily transferred by bites or through abraded areas of skin, there is increasing evidence that the respiratory route plays an important part in the spread of infection especially in pigs, rats and mice. It is emphasised that Aujeszky's disease is not contagious among cattle, sheep and other domestic animals, except swine, and that outbreaks of disease in these animals is invariably of a sporadic nature.

Diagnosis
In the U.K., the disease in cattle and sheep is so characteristic and striking that laboratory confirmation is usually not required, but in some countries it may be necessary to eliminate the possibility of rabies. Clinical diagnosis is, however, more difficult in adolescent and adult swine especially since the overt disease is not common in these animals and is suspected only when the infection spreads to cattle. Classically, the diagnosis of Aujeszky's disease has been made by the subcutaneous inoculation of rabbits with material removed from the brain or spinal cord of the affected animal. If positive, the rabbit will begin scratching and biting furiously at the site of inoculation within 48–72 hours and will die in 3–5 days. Although young mice, day-old chicks and embryonated hens' eggs are also highly susceptible, it is now known that the virus can be readily isolated in a wide range of cell cultures and produce a rapid and characteristic cytopathic effect which is neutralized by specific antiserum. Evidence of infection may be determined by testing the animal's serum for the presence of neutralizing and complement-fixing antibodies.

Control
There are no satisfactory therapeutic or prophylactic measures for Aujeszky's disease, and cattle and most other mammalian species invariably die. In endemic areas, the practice of running pigs with other animals should be avoided. and breeding sows should not be kept with fattening pigs. Pigs and offal should not be introduced from infected areas and rodent-free quarters must be ensured.

Swine recovered from Aujeszky's disease develop neutralizing antibodies which may be transferred to their new-born piglets by way of the colostrum. Maternally derived antibodies protect piglets for about the first 2 months of life and probably reduce the degree of infection to the subclinical form.

Although workers in Eastern Europe have successfully attenuated Aujeszky's disease virus by successive passages in chick- or calf-tissue cultures, difficulty has been experienced in producing a wholly avirulent and immunogenic strain that can be used in cattle and sheep with safety. On the other hand, promising results have been obtained with a strain of virus grown in chick embryos and inactivated by ultraviolet light irradiation, but this vaccine has not yet been critically evaluated in cattle. Therapeutic treatment with immune serum is generally unsuccessful.

Infectious bovine rhinotracheitis

Synonyms
Viral bovine rhinotracheitis: necrotic rhinitis: red nose. The causative virus (Bovid herpesvirus 1) also gives rise to infectious pustular vulvovaginitis and bovine coital exanthema.

Definition
Infectious bovine rhinotracheitis (IBR) is an acute contagious viral disease of cattle characterized by fever, dyspnoea, rhinitis, sinusitis and other inflammatory changes in the upper respiratory tract. The virus may also invade the placenta and fetus causing abortion or stillbirth subsequent to the respiratory infection.

History and distribution
IBR has been recognised as a distinct clinical entity since 1950 when it was first observed in dairy cattle in Colorado, and later in California where the virus was first isolated. It spread rapidly to other regions of the USA and Canada and, in recent years, has been recorded in almost all parts of the world with the exception of South America.

Hosts affected
Cattle are the natural host for the virus, but wild deer show a high incidence of neutralizing antibody in their sera. Man is not susceptible.

Properties of the virus
Electron microscopy shows that IBR virions are morphologically indistinguishable from those of other members of the herpesvirus group and in thin sections they appear in the cytoplasm of infected cells as spherical structures, measuring about 130–180 nm in diameter, composed of a double limiting membrane and an electron-dense central core. The exact composition of the core or nucleoid is not known but recent evidence indicates that it contains double-stranded DNA and some other material in addition. The base composition of its DNA is similar to that of Aujeszky's disease virus but its molecular weight of 84×10^6 daltons is greater than that of Aujeszky's virus (68 to 70×10^6 daltons). IBR is relatively thermolabile with a half-life at 37°C of approximately 10 hours; and the inactivation curve appears to be exponential. Its infectivity is destroyed by ether, acetone or alcohol and by irradiation with ultraviolet light. The virus is labile at pH 4.5–5 but is very stable at pH 6–9, and remains viable at optimum pH for at least 9 months when stored at −60°C.

Antigenic properties

Neutralization tests in cell culture show that the virus is antigenically homogeneous, only minor differences existing between strains. It is antigenically distinct from most other herpesviruses but is probably related to the virus of equine rhinopneumonitis. Although there is no reciprocal neutralization between these two viruses, they appear to be related by common antigens that cross-react in complement-fixation and gel diffusion precipitation tests.

Cultivation

IBR grows well in cell cultures of calf kidney, testis, lung and skin, producing a well-marked cytopathic effect within 1–2 days. Characteristically, intranuclear inclusions appear in affected areas of the monolayer cultures. In bovine embryonic cells, rounding and shrinking of cells are visible in unstained preparations 24–48 hours after infection, and plaques are readily produced in agar-overlay cultures. Growth also occurs in monolayers of pig, sheep, goat, horse and monkey kidney cells, in rabbit spleen, human amnion and HeLa cells, but generally only after adaptation. There is no growth in fertile hens' eggs.

Pathogenicity

The natural infection varies in severity from an inapparent or mild febrile reaction to an acute illness involving the whole of the upper part of the respiratory tract including the sinuses, pharynx, larynx and trachea. In severe cases, the entire respiratory tract may be involved with swelling and inflammation of the mucous membranes. These changes, together with the accumulation of muco-purulent exudates frequently cause dyspnoea and coughing leading to bronchitis and, in some cases, to bronchial pneumonia. Badly affected cattle usually show severe depression, emaciation and bloodstained diarrhoea. In the natural disease, the incubation period of 2–6 days is followed by a rise in body temperature as high as 41°–42°C. The morbidity rate varies from 30–90 per cent but the mortality is much lower and seldom exceeds 3 per cent of affected cattle, but higher losses may occur in calves. The course of the illness, which may be sudden in onset, varies from 7–14 days but very mild cases may pass unrecognized. By the third day, virus is present in the nasal and ocular discharges and this, undoubtedly, represents the principal means by which the disease is spread. Many recovered animals become carriers and shed the virus for variable periods.

The virus may also cause meningoencephalitis in 2 to 3-month-old calves, and abortion in pregnant cattle may be a direct result of virus infection and localization in the placental membranes. The virus of IBR is also capable of causing a disease of the genital tract known as infectious pustular vulvovaginitis (IPV), and there is evidence from retrospective serological surveys that the genital manifestation of infection has been present in cattle in the USA at least since 1941. Genital disease of bulls has also been reported and the infection may be transmitted by venereal contact. In female cattle, IPV is characterized by inflammation, necrosis and pustular formation on the mucosa of the vulva and vagina, but vesicle formation does not occur.

The IBR virus appears to be highly host-specific although young goats can be infected experimentally and develop fever. In artificially infected calves, the virus is confined mainly to the upper respiratory tract but some develop lesions of bronchopneumonia. Other workers have reported a febrile reaction accompanied by anorexia, lachrymation, nasal discharge and coughing following administration of virus by the intra-tracheal route. In some animals inoculation of mixed cultures of IBR virus and *Pasteurella haemolytica* results in a more severe reaction, sometimes with pneumonia, and it has been suggested that the virus may be an important exciting factor in "shipping fever".

At necropsy, the main pathological lesions in the natural disease are those of acute inflammation and necrosis of affected mucous membranes. In very severe cases, the tracheal mucosa is diphtheritic and there may be bronchopneumonia in some fatal cases. The pharyngeal and pulmonary lymph nodes may be extensively swollen and haemorrhagic, and petechial haemorrhages may be found in the nasal cavity and paranasal sinuses. Gross lesions of a specific nature are not evident in aborted fetuses although some may show severe damage to the spleen and liver.

Histologically, typical Cowdry type A intranuclear inclusions are present in some epithelial cells but they are not usually discernible in animals which die after a short illness.

It should be noted that the virus of IBR has many clinical features in common with other members of the herpesvirus group. As with equine rhinopneumonitis (type 1) virus, it gives rise to a respiratory illness which tends to be more severe in younger animals. It sometimes causes conjunctivitis and genital infections as do the viruses causing 'cold sores' of man, and infectious laryngotracheitis of chickens. Liver damage in aborted fetuses is similar to that of human cytomegalovirus infections and its ability to invade the central nervous system resembles that of herpes simplex, pseudorabies and B-viruses.

Ecology

Virus is present in the nasal and ocular secretions

and in the placental tissues of cattle which abort. Transmission is by contact, particularly in conditions where there is much overcrowding. Since spontaneous outbreaks of IBR frequently occur one to several weeks after the introduction of animals into a herd, it is suggested that cattle recovered from the disease may act as carriers and shed the virus in the nasal secretions for several weeks after an attack. In IPV, the virus has been isolated from the vagina of a cow on two occasions about a year apart. The virus has also been isolated from bull semen and may be spread by coitus.

Diagnosis

In endemic areas, a presumptive diagnosis of IBR or IPV can usually be made from the characteristic lesions and clinical symptoms. A confirmatory diagnosis can be obtained by isolation and identification of the causal virus in cell cultures, demonstration of neutralizing antibodies in the sera of affected animals and the occurrence of intranuclear inclusions in necropsy material. An indirect haemagglutination test using tanned sheep erythrocytes is now frequently employed and is of considerable diagnostic value.

Control

A number of modified live-virus vaccines are available commercially for the control of IBR and IPV, and their extensive use in enzootic areas has greatly reduced the incidence of the disease. Immunity to IBR develops within 10–14 days after vaccination and may last for several years, but annual revaccination is recommended for the control of IPV. Most vaccines are prepared from strains of virus which have been attenuated by serial passage in bovine or porcine cell cultures.

The equine rhinopneumonitis – mare abortion complex

Synonyms

Equine herpesvirus (Equid herpesvirus 1) infection: mare abortion: equine virus abortion: epizootic abortion of mares: equine 'influenza'.

Definition

A benign but highly contagious viral infection characterized by an acute febrile respiratory catarrh which is most severe in young horses, and by abortion in mares usually during the latter half of the gestation period.

Hosts affected

Only equines are naturally affected.

History and distribution

Although equine virus abortion, or mare abortion, was recognised as a virus infection before its relationship to respiratory disease was established, it is now known that equid herpesviruses can cause two distinct syndromes: acute respiratory catarrh in young horses and fully susceptible adults, and abortion in pregnant mares. Whilst both terms accurately reflect the principal clinical features of the disease, equine rhinopneumonitis seems preferable since another virus, that of equine arteritis, can also cause abortion in mares. In 1936, a form of epizootic abortion of mares caused by a filterable agent was recognized in the USA and, as early as 1942, it was demonstrated that the causal virus could be supported in cell cultures. In 1954, it was reported that some outbreaks of respiratory disease in young horses were caused by this same virus and the name equine rhinopneumonitis virus was introduced in 1959. Since then, the disease has been observed in parts of Canada, Japan, South Africa and Europe, including the UK.

Properties of the virus

Equid herpesviruses are morphologically indistinguishable from other members of the group. In ultra-thin sections, spherical viral particles with a featureless electron-dense central core are seen in the nuclei of affected hepatic cells, whereas in infected cell cultures the nucleoid is frequently shaped like a star or cross. The viral nucleic acid consists of double-stranded DNA which has a relatively high proportion of guanine and cytosine and a molecular weight of about 92×10^6 daltons.

Although equid herpesviruses retain their infectivity for over a year at $-18°C$., they are delicate structures that do not survive for long outside their hosts and are readily inactivated by lipid solvents, by 0.35 per cent formalin and by heating at 56°C. for 10 minutes.

Haemagglutination

In contrast to most other herpesviruses, tissues of horses or hamsters infected with rhinopneumonitis virus agglutinate horse red blood cells between 4° and 37°C. The haemagglutinin is labile at 56°C. Guinea-pig erythrocytes are also agglutinated, preferably after treatment with formalin. The reaction is inhibited by sera of horses hyperimmunized against infected hamster tissues but not by sera from convalescent horses.

Antigenic properties

Three antigenically distinct species of herpesviruses are recoverable from horses. The first, EHV 1 or equine rhinopneumonitis virus (ERP), is primarily a respiratory pathogen and is probably the major cause of acute respiratory disease in young horses, but may also be isolated from the genital tract or from aborted fetuses. Although they are antigenically similar, strains of EHV 1 recovered from fetal material are said to be more infective, grow better in cell culture and are released to a greater extent than is virus isolated from horses with respiratory infections. The second, EHV 2 or equine cytomegalovirus (ECM), includes two antigenically distinct slow-growing strains which are widespread among horses especially during the early months of life and are probably non-pathogenic. They are mostly found in leucocytes, kidneys or spleen of young foals but may also occur in respiratory and genital mucous membranes. The third, EHV 3 or equine coital exanthema virus (ECE) causes genital infections but is also frequently associated with mild or inapparent infections of the respiratory tract. Strains of ECE virus are antigenically homogeneous. Complement-fixing and neutralizing antibodies are present in the sera of infected horses. Titres of the former begin to decrease after 30 days and have usually disappeared in 3–6 months, while the latter persist at moderate to high titres for a year or more. An interesting feature of equine rhinopneumonitis is that occasional mares showing a high titre of specific neutralizing antibody may become reinfected and then abort.

Cultivation

Freshly isolated equine herpesviruses cannot be propagated in embryonated hens' eggs, but several strains of EHV 1 obtained from the respiratory tract and tissues of aborted horse fetuses have been adapted to growth on the chorioallantoic membrane, yolk sac and amnion by alternate serial passages between hamster kidney cells and fertile hens' eggs. Intranuclear inclusions are formed in the cells of the ectoderm and mesoderm. EHV 1 also grows well and produces high titres of cell-free progeny virus in human amnion and HeLa cells, as well as on horse, sheep, pig, cattle, cat and chick embryonic tissues. The cytopathic effects in roller tube cultures of horse and rabbit kidney cells are characterised by rounding and ballooning of the infected cells. Multinucleated syncytia develop later and several small acidophilic inclusions, each surrounded by a clear halo, tend to precede the more deeply staining and centrally placed type A intranuclear body. Growth of EHV 3 on cell culture is similar to that of EHV 1 and the presence of nuclear inclusions is accompanied by rounding up, detachment and lysis of the affected cells. Both types of virus grow rapidly and EHV 3 strains regularly produce large multinucleate syncytia. The slowly growing equine cytomegalovirus (EHV 2) differs from the other two viruses in that it produces delayed cellular changes and remains closely cell-associated. Its cytopathic effect is particularly striking in that foci of up to 100 cells may contain intranuclear inclusions without evidence of cell disruption. In unstained preparations these apparently normal infected cells ultimately degenerate, round up and detach from the glass. Plaque formation occurs on several species of host cells and the differences in the growth rates of the 3 types of EHV are related to the different diameter of the plaques which each produces. After 6 days of incubation under a methyl cellulose overlay the sizes of the foci are approximately 4, 2 and 10 nm for EHV 1, 2 and 3, respectively.

Unweaned hamsters are readily infected with EHV 1 by intraperitoneal inoculation and develop a fatal hepatitis within 18–21 hours. High titres of virus are present in sera and liver extracts from the affected animals. The virus has also been adapted to cause a fatal infection in adult hamsters and unweaned mice. It may also give rise to catarrhal inflammation of the upper respiratory tract of guinea-pigs and induce abortion in pregnant females. In contrast to EHV 1, most other types of equine herpesviruses are less virulent and do not produce fatal infections in rabbits or unweaned mice following intracerebral inoculation.

Both complement-fixing and neutralizing antibodies develop in experimentally infected animals. The complement-fixing antibodies usually appear first and develop to maximum titres more quickly than neutralizing antibodies, but the neutralizing titres persist longer. These observations suggest the possibility of 2 distinct antigenic components in the virion.

Pathogenicity

The incubation period in experimental animals is usually from 18 to 30 days but in natural infections it may vary from 9 days to as long as 60 days. Most outbreaks of equine rhinopneumonitis occur suddenly and disappear quickly at the end of the foaling season. The stud is seldom affected 2 years in succession but the infection may return 3–4 years later, sometimes affecting the same mare a second time. When young horses are affected there is fever and acute rhinopneumonitis characterized by serous rhinitis, conjunctivitis, congested nasal mucosa, cough, pyrexia (39°–41.5°C) and inappetance. The cough and watery nasal discharge may persist for several weeks. In older horses the disease is usually mild or inapparent but pregnant mares may abort. The period between the respiratory infection and abortion varies from 1–4 months but mostly occurs during the 8th to 11th months of pregnancy. Lesions are not present in aborting mares and further breeding performance is not affected but there is extensive viral invasion of the fetus with multiple, white or yellow-coloured foci of degeneration in the liver just beneath the capsule. In some instances the aborted fetuses show icterus, subcutaneous oedema, petechiation of the heart

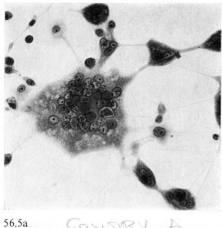

56.5a   COWDRY   A

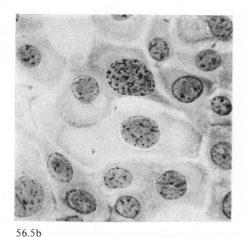

56.5b

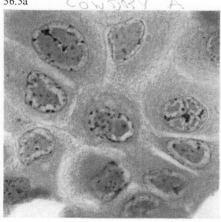

56.5c

56.5d

56.5a   Detail of a syncytium in monolayer culture of ox kidney cells inoculated 4 days previously with a herpes-virus. The aggregated nuclei contain large acidophilic inclusion bodies. Giemsa stain, × 170.

56.5c   Detail of a pig kidney cell culture infected with Aujeszky's disease virus showing various morphological forms of Cowdry type-A intranuclear inclusions. The presence of four small inclusions in one of the nuclei (right, centre) probably represents four portions of a single multilobulated type-A inclusion. Haematoxylin eosin stain, × 645.

56.5b   Nuclear changes induced in pig kidney cells by Aujeszky's disease virus. Changes in the distribution of the nuclear chromatin give recently infected nuclei a speckled appearance. Notice also the presence of a large single intranuclear inclusion in some of the cells. Giemsa stain, × 420.

56.5d   Monolayer of pig kidney cells growing on the base of a two-inch Petri dish, 48 hours after inoculation with Aujeszky's disease virus. Small plaques with a regular outline are clearly visible when the agar overlay is removed and the monolayer is stained with neutral red.

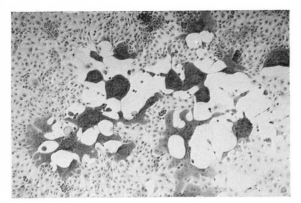

56.6a

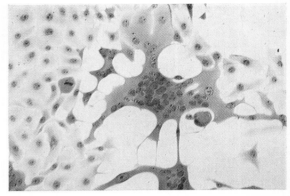

56.6b

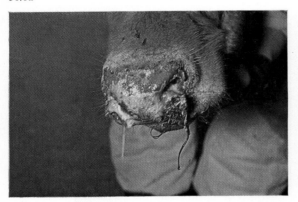

56.6c

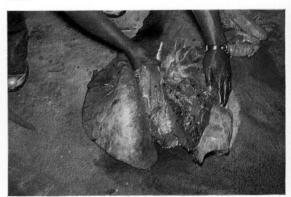

56.6d

56.6a Cytopathic effects of bovine mammillitis virus on the MDBK line of ox kidney cells; three days after inoculation. The syncytia are characterized by extensive deeply staining cytoplasmic masses devoid of cell membranes. Haematoxylin eosin stain, × 44.

56.6c Muzzle of a cow affected with malignant catarrhal fever, showing erosions of the muzzle epithelium and characteristic long strings of yellow tenacious material from the anterior nares. (Courtesy of Dr H. Reid.)

56.6b Most nuclei in syncytia induced by bovine mammillitis virus contain basophilic or acidophilic Cowdry type-A inclusions. There is also margination of the nuclear chromatin. Haematoxylin eosin stain, × 106.

56.6d In the 'head and eye' form of bovine malignant catarrh the lungs are congested and oedematous, and plugs of mucus may be found in the larger bronchi. Lesions pathognomonic of the disease are seldom present.

muscle and serous membranes, and excessive pleural fluid. In many respects the lesions are similar to those of neonatal cytomegalovirus inclusion disease in children. If foals are carried to term they may be born alive but are weak and die shortly afterwards.

The gross lesions in horses affected with the respiratory form of the disease include oedema of the lungs and bronchopneumonia especially of the apical lobes. Purulent exudates may be present in the bronchi and trachea, and in some cases there is conjunctivitis, oedema of the limbs and acute haemorrhagic gastroenteritis. Meningoencephalitis has been recorded rarely. Histologically, Cowdry type A intranuclear inclusions are most likely to be found in fetal liver, spleen, lungs, adrenal and thymus.

The role of the slowly growing equine herpesvirus (EMC or EHV 2) in producing disease has not been established but there is evidence that the ubiquitous nature of the virus is due to the fact that infected horses become life-long carriers and persistent shedders of the virus. In contrast to this, equine-coital exanthema virus (ECE or EHV 3) causes an acute but relatively mild genital infection which is characterized by the formation of pustular lesions on the prepuce, penis, vagina and perineal region. In uncomplicated cases healing is usually complete by the 14th day and there is no evidence that recovered animals act as carriers of the virus.

Ecology
Virus inoculated intravenously into susceptible mares gives rise to a febrile illness associated with conjunctivitis, nasal catarrh and coughing, and horses placed in contact with aborting mares develop bronchopneumonia. The introduction of an infected horse into a herd may cause abortion in about 60 per cent of in-foal mares. Under natural conditions, virus may be maintained in the upper respiratory tract of carrier animals but virus disseminated during spontaneous outbreaks in the nasal discharges of young affected horses is the principal source of infection. Other sources of infection include aborted fetuses, placental membranes and uterine discharges. Although the infection frequently spreads from mare to mare by the respiratory route, transmission by carrier stallions has been alleged but is not generally accepted. It is possible, nevertheless, that the virus may give rise to a chronic latent-type of infection as in human herpes simplex infections and be spread by venereal contact as in infectious bovine rhinotracheitis to which it is related serologically.

Diagnosis
Presumptive diagnosis is usually based on the clinical symptoms and the history of abortions in a number of pregnant mares. Histopathological studies are of value for the detection of intranuclear inclusions in the lungs, liver, spleen, thymus, myocardium, kidney, and small intestines of aborted fetuses.

Positive diagnosis may be obtained by isolating the causative virus, especially from aborted fetuses and the upper respiratory tract of older animals. Various primary cell culture systems can be used but horse kidney cells produce a well-marked cytopathic effect and are usually preferred. Bovine kidney cells are not useful, however, for primary isolations. Neutralizing and complement-fixing antibodies can be readily demonstrated in paired sera from recovered animals but tests on sera of aborting mares cannot be used for diagnosis of the disease.

Control
Vaccines prepared from equine fetal tissues have been abandoned because they contribute to haemolytic disease of newborn foals, and inactivated vaccines prepared from hamsters have been discarded because of the resulting poor protection.

In recent years, live hamster and mouse adapted virus vaccines have been used with safety. Young horses are given 3 intranasal inoculations as sucklings, weanlings and yearlings, respectively; and are revaccinated annually thereafter. Alternatively, in the Northern Hemisphere, vaccination by intramuscular injection can be carried out during July and October in all horses in a breeding establishment regardless of age, sex or breeding status. The procedure is useful for controlling fetal death and abortion but has little effect on the respiratory form of the disease.

Administration of the vaccine causes an elevated temperature lasting for several days and may occasionally induce abortion (about 0.5 per cent). It is recommended, therefore, that such a vaccination programme be used only in enzootic areas or on farms with known infection during the previous foaling season.

Malignant catarrhal fever

Synonyms
Malignant catarrh: bovine malignant catarrh: Snotsiekte.

Definition
An acute and generalised highly fatal infectious disease of cattle, characterized by fever, a catarrhal mucopurulent inflammation of the respiratory and alimentary epithelia, extensive lymphoid hyperplasia, keratoconjunctivitis, encephalitis and rapid loss of condition.

Hosts affected

The disease occurs naturally in cattle and buffalo, but sheep and wildebeest may act as symptomless carriers of the infection.

History and distribution

Malignant catarrhal fever has been recognised as a specific disease of cattle for more than a century. It occurs throughout Europe, in parts of North and South America, Asia and Australasia and is fairly widespread in South and East Africa. It is usually sporadic in occurrence and does not generally spread to any extent through a herd. In many countries the disease is very rare but in parts of Africa severe and widespread losses may occur especially where cattle are allowed to live in close association with black wildebeest (*Connochaetes gnu*). All ages and breeds of cattle may be affected.

Properties of the virus

The causal agent is a member of the herpesvirus group. (Bovid herpesvirus 3). The virus particle is very fragile and does not readily withstand alternate freezing and thawing. Although it may be stored for a few days in citrated blood at 5°C it will not survive for more than a week at —60°C or after lyophilization. In common with other herpesviruses, it is ether- and chloroform-sensitive. Blood from an infected animal contains the virus in fairly high concentration but soon loses its virulence and is rapidly destroyed by putrefaction or by exposure to 30°C for 5 days. The virus may remain viable in 50 per cent glycerol-saline for about one week.

Antigenic properties

Recovered cattle develop a solid immunity which may persist for 2 or 3 years. A report that there are different immunological strains of virus and that cattle which survive infection with one type of virus subsequently withstand challenge with a homologous but not a heterologous strain awaits confirmation. Although it is generally believed that the South African form of the disease (Snotsiekte) is identical with that of European malignant catarrh, recent work in East Africa suggests that more than one strain of virus, if not more than one disease, might be involved.

Cultivation

In Africa, the virus of malignant catarrhal fever has been isolated from blood leucocytes and splenic tissues of apparently healthy blue wildebeest (*Gorgon taurinus taurinus*). It is apparently non-pathogenic for the natural host but gives rise to the typical clinical disease when inoculated into cattle. The virus produces a marked cytopathic effect with syncytia and Cowdry type A intranuclear inclusions when cultivated on bovine thyroid, bovine adrenal or calf kidney cell cultures, but there is little evidence of extracellular virus in the supernatant fluids during early passages. In this respect the virus may be likened to the sub-group of herpesviruses which includes the varicella-zoster agents and also, perhaps, the cytomegaloviruses. Additional similarities between malignant catarrhal fever virus and cytomegaloviruses lie in the fact that Feulgen-positive granules have been described in the cytoplasm of infected cells and the intranuclear inclusions formed by both viruses show an increasing basophilia as they mature. Once growth has been initiated, cultivation is also possible in cell cultures of sheep thyroid, rabbit kidney and wildebeest kidney. Transmission experiments in young susceptible calves have shown that cultures up to the 19th passage are still infectious and that infectious extracellular virus is produced by modified strains adapted to growth in thyroid cells.

The virus cannot be cultivated in embryonated hens' eggs. Rabbits may be artifically infected but attempts to infect other laboratory animals such as guinea-pigs and mice have not proved successful.

Pathogenicity

Malignant catarrhal fever occurs sporadically at all times of the year. In most areas the morbidity of the disease is low but the mortality rate is generally high, reaching 60–90 per cent. Under natural conditions, the incubation period varies from 4–20 weeks or longer, but most often is between 28 and 60 days. In experimentally infected calves the incubation period is usually 10–30 days. Several clinical syndromes have been described, these being the peracute, alimentary, head and eye, benign and chronic forms. The 'head and eye' form may be considered as the most typical and is the one usually seen in Africa. In Europe, the benign and alimentary forms are commonest. The first signs of infection are high fever, which may persist throughout the course of the disease, accompanied by slight ocular and nasal discharges. Within 24–72 hours there is inflammation of the oral and nasal mucous membranes followed by congestion, necrosis and erosion of the oral mucosae. In the course of a few days, the discharges from the anterior nares become thick and purulent and in typical cases form long strings of yellow tenacious material reaching to the ground. (Plate 56.6c, facing p. 749). As they dry, the discharges tend to accumulate in the nasal chambers causing obstruction of the air passages and severe respiratory distress. Necrosis and erosions resembling those of rinderpest become widespread in the oral cavity and there is excessive salivation and a fetid odour from the mouth. Nearly all cases of malignant catarrhal fever, particularly those in

Africa, are characterized by marked swelling of the joints, hyperplasia of the lymph nodes and a progressive, severe depression, but diarrhoea is not a feature of the 'head and eye' form. Nervous signs may develop and the animal becomes excited and aggressive. In many cases there is photophobia and marked corneal opacity leading to complete blindness. Cystitis is also frequently present. Death may occur within 24 hours but in some instances the disease may last a fortnight or more.

The infection can be transmitted to susceptible cattle by the inoculation of large amounts of blood or lymph node tissue from reacting animals, provided the material has not been stored for more than a few days. The disease can also be induced with cell suspensions from infected monolayer cultures or, as has been reported more recently, with suspensions of extra-cellular virus obtained by serial passage in calf kidney or thyroid cells.

At necropsy, the lymph nodes are enlarged, congested and oedematous, and the cut surface presents a granular, cherry-pink appearance. The brain, myocardium and other tissues may show petechiae and there is generally severe congestion, haemorrhages and diphtheresis in the larynx and trachea. The lungs are congested and oedematous and, occasionally, there is a terminal bronchopneumonia. (Plate 56.6d, facing p. 749). In some cases there is abomasitis and enteritis, while in others small grayish foci representing accumulations of lymphoid cells may be observed in the liver and kidneys.

Ecology

In most countries, outbreaks of malignant catarrhal fever are rare, except in areas where cattle are kept in contact with sheep which may have symptomless infections. In East Africa, the Masai have long believed that Snotsiekte occurs when cattle are allowed to graze on veld contaminated by the after-births of wildebeest or where a wildebeest calf has lain and shed its coat: and it is significant that most outbreaks occur during the period February to June following the wildebeest calving season. The actual method of virus transmission to cattle is not known but laboratory investigations suggest that adult wildebeest may act as healthy carriers of the virus and that their fetuses may acquire the infection *in utero*. It has also been shown that viraemia is present in about 40 per cent of wildebeest calves 1–3 months old, and that during this period of symptomless infection they are capable of transmitting the virus to other wildebeest and to cattle. It is also possible that outbreaks of malignant catarrh in other parts of the world are spread during the viraemic phase of the infection in carrier sheep.

In the naturally occurring disease, the virus of malignant catarrhal fever is intimately associated with the intact cell and remains active outside the body only for a short time. It has not been detected in the secretions and excretions of sick animals and contact transmission among cattle seems not to occur.

Diagnosis

In Africa, a provisional diagnosis of malignant catarrhal fever can readily be made if animals that have been in contact with wildebeest show the characteristic symptoms of the 'head and eye' form of the disease. A confirmatory diagnosis can be obtained from the histopathological findings and by the isolation and identification of the causal virus. Blood leucocytes or lymph node suspensions from affected animals produce marked cellular changes in calf thyroid tissue cultures after 6–9 days of incubation. The cytopathic effects, which include syncytia and intranuclear inclusions, are neutralized by specific antisera.

Strains of European origin may be isolated by inoculating freshly obtained whole blood or lymph node material into rabbits by the intracerebral route. Infected rabbits show nervous symptoms and generally die within 28 days.

As regards differential diagnosis, the diseases most likely to be confused with malignant catarrhal fever are East Coast fever, mucosal disease, rinderpest, bovine rhinotracheitis, foot-and-mouth disease, bluetongue, papular stomatitis, and pasteurellosis.

Control

Although the virus is neutralized by sera of recovered cattle, the degree of immunity that follows a natural attack of malignant catarrhal fever is often so poor that attempts to produce a means of artificial immunization are unlikely to succeed. Moreover, the incidence of the disease is generally low and the use of vaccines is unlikely to be an economic proposition. Contact with wildebeest should be prevented, and the separation of sheep from cattle may result in the complete disappearance of the disease.

Allerton virus infection

Three distinct groups of cytopathic viruses have been associated with the condition known as Lumpy skin disease of cattle in South Africa. (See page 701). The first (Group I) produces rapid degenerative changes in monolayer cell cultures with the formation of large acidophilic intranuclear inclusions but fails to elicit the clinical disease in experimental cattle, and is generally regarded as one of the 'orphan viruses' that are widespread among cattle in Africa. The second (Group II) or 'Allerton' virus also gives rise to a rapid cytopathic effect in cell cultures with syncytia and intranuclear inclusions, and causes a marked clinical reaction in susceptible cattle. Although this naturally occurring skin infection resembles Lumpy skin disease it has not the same economic importance. The third (Group III) or 'Neethling' virus is characterized by the formation of large intracytoplasmic inclusion bodies and is the true causal agent of classical Lumpy skin disease. This virus is classified as a member of the poxvirus group. (See Chapter 52).

Hosts affected
Cattle are the only natural hosts of Allerton virus infection.

History and distribution
The disease occurs in several areas of South and East Africa and the causative virus was first isolated and identified in 1957. A similar if not identical virus causes bovine ulcerative mammillitis in Britain and parts of North America.

Properties of the virus
Allerton virus is a member of the herpesvirus group (Bovid herpesvirus 2). Virions are present in the nucleus, and those in the cytoplasm have a double-layered limiting membrane. The diameter of the intact virus particle is about 130–150 nm and its ultrastructure is identical to that of other herpes-viruses. The nucleoid contains double-stranded DNA with a guanine+cytosine (GC) content of approximately 65 per cent.

Antigenic properties
Allerton virus is antigenically indistinguishable from that of bovine mammillitis, and neutralizing antibodies are present in the sera of recovered cattle.

Cultivation
The virus does not grow in developing chicken embryos but can be readily propagated in a number of cell culture systems. Three separate strains of Group II viruses were isolated in South Africa and named Allerton, Elsias' River and Pentrick Grange. All are characterized by the very rapid development in primary calf kidney cultures and by the formation of large multinucleated syncytia. The cytopathic changes may appear as early as 8 hours after inoculation or as late as 8 days. Most of the nuclei contain Cowdry type A inclusions. Similar cytopathic effects are obtained on primary cultures of lamb testis and on cell lines of bovine kidney and baby hamster kidney. In some cultures the infection is so progressive that complete destruction of the monolayer takes place within 18–24 hours.

Pathogenicity
Naturally occurring Allerton virus infection may be confused with true Lumpy skin disease caused by the Neethling strain of poxvirus. In both diseases the lesions are of similar size and extent but those caused by Allerton virus tend to involve only the superficial layers of the dermis, and heal without complications. The scabs can be readily removed leaving intact hairless skin or areas of bleeding granulation tissue. There is no evidence of 'sit-fast' formation which is characteristic of Neethling-type infections. In experimental cattle, Allerton virus causes a mild febrile reaction followed by the development of skin nodules on all parts of the animal's body but especially on the face, neck, back and perineum. There is frequently a generalised lymphadenitis.

Allerton virus causes transient lesions when inoculated intradermally into rabbits. In unweaned mice, hamsters and rats it may produce skin rashes, stunting and deaths.

Ecology
The mode of natural infection and transmission is not known but virus is excreted in the urine and faeces, and there is evidence that the infection can be transmitted mechanically by biting insects.

Diagnosis
Although Allerton virus infection may be confused with Lumpy skin disease, the two conditions can readily be differentiated histopathologically and by the isolation and identification of the causative viruses. Allerton virus grows rapidly in cell cultures and induces an early cytopathic effect with syncytia and intranuclear inclusions, whereas Lumpy skin disease virus grows more slowly and produces intracytoplasmic inclusions. Moreover Neethling virus, unlike Allerton virus, grows readily on embryonated hens' eggs and produces surface 'pocks' on the chorioallantoic membrane. The neutralizing antibodies present in the sera of recovered animals are also distinctive.

Control
The disease is not of major economic importance and vaccination has not been attempted to any great extent. Formalinized vaccines give poor protection and attenuated live virus vaccines have not been developed.

Bovine ulcerative mammillitis

Synonyms
Bovine mammillitis: Herpesvirus mammillitis: Bovine herpes mammillitis.

Definition

Bovine mammillitis is the name given to an ulcerative infection of the teats and udder of dairy cows caused by a member of the herpes group of viruses. (Bovid herpesvirus 2).

History and distribution

Milking cows on several farms in the west of Scotland were affected with a severe ulcerative condition of the teats during the autumn of 1963 and the causative agent, named bovine mammillitis virus (BMV), was isolated in cell cultures. The disease has since been reported from other parts of the U.K. The virus is very similar, if not identical, to the Group II viruses (prototype Allerton) associated with bovine Lumpy skin disease, and which are known to produce extensive erosions on the teats of cows in Ruanda-Urundi and other parts of Central and South Africa.

Properties of the virus

The mature virus particle is morphologically identical to herpesviruses. Its nucleocapsid is approximately 80 nm across, whereas the mature enveloped particle measures up to 250 nm in diameter and is sensitive to ether and chloroform. The virion contains a core of DNA with a GC base composition of 64 per cent and a molecular weight of 34×10^6 daltons, compared with a GC content of 65 per cent and molecular weight of 32×10^6 daltons for Allerton virus. Thus, within the precision of the methods used, the nucleic acid content of the two viruses is identical. The virus can be held at $-50°C$ for up to a month without significant loss in titre, but storage at $5°C$ is not recommended.

Antigenic properties

Neutralizing antibodies are present in the sera of recovered animals. Serologically, bovine mammillitis virus differs from infectious bovine rhinotracheitis, bovine malignant catarrh and other herpesviruses but it cannot be distinguished in neutralization and agar precipitation tests from Allerton virus. In double-diffusion tests in agar, concentrates of bovine mammillitis virus and Allerton virus form two bands of precipitate with homologous or heterologous antisera. Complete fusion of the respective bands confirms the similarity of the antigen-antibody systems involved. There is also evidence of a serological relationship between bovine mammillitis virus and herpes simplex viruses 1 and 2 of man.

Cultivation

Mammillitis virus can be readily cultivated in a variety of cell cultures including bovine lymph node, calf kidney, bovine conjunctiva, calf thyroid, lamb testis, pig kidney, kitten kidney, feline lung and baby hamster kidney cells. The cellular changes consist of large cell masses of bizarre shape, often with long cytoplasmic processes, and are rapidly progressive until there is total cell destruction of the monolayer within 2–6 days. (Plates 56.7a, b, facing p. 764). In stained monolayer cultures, large syncytia are seen containing 30–40 nuclei or, sometimes, several hundred in one 'giant cell'. (Plates 42.11a, facing p. 488 and 56.6a, b, facing p. 749). Many of the nuclei contain single, basophilic or acidophilic inclusions of Cowdry type A which stain bright yellow with acridine orange. (Plates 42.8b, c, d, between pp. 480–1). Maximum yield of virus occurs after maximal CPE is observed. The characteristic cytopathic effects may not be obtained, however, on established cell cultures of HeLa, pig or rabbit kidney cells. The virus cannot be grown on embryonated hens' eggs, but in unweaned mice, rats and hamsters it may produce rashes, stunting and death.

Pathogenicity

The incubation period of naturally occurring mammillitis infection is approximately 5–10 days and many lactating cows in a milking herd develop lesions within a fortnight of the first case being-observed. Affected animals show little or no systemic illness unless acute mastitis occurs as a complication of the disease. Acute cases of sudden onset are characterized by a painful swelling of the entire teat, often with blue discolouration, which precedes sloughing of the skin. In less severe cases there are localised painless swollen plaques which develop within the thickness of the teat-wall, and the overlying skin quickly assumes a blue-black discolouration. At other times, raised circular plaques appear with shallow ulcers on the surface of the lesion. Some of the ulcerated areas may remain moist through much of the illness but others become dry and form thick brown or black scabs from 3 mm. to several centimetres in diameter, and sometimes encircle the teats. Occasionally, large vesicles occur in the initial stages of infection, especially at the teat-udder junction, and rupture of the lesions may lead to sloughing and gangrene. In cows calved less than 3 weeks, lesions may appear at the base of the teat and spread to the udder until the whole escutcheon becomes affected. The disease, which is self-limiting, only occurs in autumn or early winter. The course of the illness varies in individual animals from about 10 days in mild cases to 12 weeks or longer in more severely affected animals.

The condition can also be reproduced experimentally by injecting the virus into the teats of heifers and cows, the lesions persisting for at least 5 weeks. Young calves inoculated intradermally with infected cell culture fluids develop plaques at the sites of inoculation within 2–4 days. These increase in size and become hard and painful, but the reaction gradually recedes after the fifth day without evidence of spread or a febrile reaction. Calves inoculated intravenously develop numerous firm nodules on the skin of the neck after 5–8 days and, later, on the skin of the face and tail. Within a few days the scabs can be removed, leaving an apparently normal skin surface. In this respect the reaction is similar to that described with Allerton virus.

Rabbits inoculated intradermally show circumscribed pox-like lesions within 5 days and scarification of rabbits or guinea-pigs may produce an erythematous rash which later becomes covered with a scab of dried serous exudate.

Lesions have been observed on the hands and forearms of cattlemen working in contact with affected cows but virus isolations have not been reported so far, nor has the disease been produced in human volunteers.

Ecology
The exact method of transmission is not known but the infection is probably spread within a herd by milking machines or milkers' hands since non-lactating cows do not develop lesions in affected herds. A report that the virus can be transmitted mechanically by biting insects has not been confirmed by other workers.

Diagnosis
Laboratory confirmation is usually necessary to distinguish ulcerative mammillitis from other viral conditions affecting the bovine teat and udder. The causative virus can be readily isolated in a variety of cell cultures if vesicular fluids are available in a fresh state. Attempts to isolate the virus from scabs and ulcer swabs are less frequently successful. Direct electron-microscopical examination of negatively-stained material from suitable lesions is proving increasingly helpful in the differential diagnosis of teat conditions of cattle.

Control
Cattle inoculated with unattenuated cell culture virus show neutralizing antibodies in their sera as early as 7 days post-infection. Neutralizing antibodies are also present in sera of cattle recovered from a natural attack of the disease, and these may persist for 8 months or longer. Attempts to control the disease by means of live modified cell culture vaccines or formalinized virus vaccines coupled with aluminium hydroxide gel adjuvants have been largely unsuccessful. However, more recent findings suggest that concentrated aluminium hydroxide vaccines prepared from non-inactivated cell culture virus containing saponin or Freund's adjuvant are

harmless for cattle, and heifers react to immunization by developing specific antibody with the highest titres between the 20–30th days after inoculation. Heifers vaccinated in this manner resist infection when challenged on the 45th day after immunization.

Canine herpesvirus infection

Synonyms
Herpesvirus infection of puppies: Canine tracheo-bronchitis.

Definition
An acute and fatal generalised viral infection of neonatal and infant puppies.

Hosts affected
The disease occurs only in puppies under 3 weeks of age, but a virus causing tracheo-bronchitis in older dogs is probably the same.

History and distribution
This recently recognised infection of puppies was first reported in 1965 in the U.S.A., and has subsequently been confirmed in the U.K. and other countries in Europe. The virus of canine tracheo-bronchitis was first described in 1968.

Properties of the virus
The causative virus (Canine herpesvirus 1.). is morphologically similar to other herpesviruses. Naked capsids and hollow 'immature' morphological sub-units measure 90–100 nm in diameter but enveloped forms are generally about 115–175 nm across. The nucleoids in some of the virions show cross and star forms similar to those of equine rhinopneumonitis virus. (Plate 56.8 facing p. 765). The virus particles are ether-sensitive and acid labile. Infectivity is reduced by 50 per cent after 5 hours at 37°C and is lost below pH 4.5 after 30 minutes. Haemagglutinin activity has not been reported.

Antigenic properties
Virus is not neutralized by immune sera prepared against equine rhinopneumonitis, pseudorabies or feline viral rhinotracheitis, but a plaque-reduction test reveals a low degree of crossing with herpes simplex. Complete cross-neutralization occurs with immune sera prepared against strains of American and British canine herpes viruses.

Cultivation
Primary isolates in dog kidney cultures cause a cytopathic effect within 2–3 days which is characterized by the formation of discrete tightly packed foci of rounded, highly refractile cells scattered throughout the monolayer. Small discrete plaques of necrotic

cells (1.5 to 2.0 mm. in diameter) are produced in monolayer cultures under agar. In stained coverslip preparations, margination of the chromatin is common and many cells at the edges of the foci contain faintly acidophilic intranuclear inclusions. Only limited viral replication takes place in human lung cultures and in monkey, calf, pig, rabbit and baby hamster kidney cells. Pocks are not formed on the chorioallantoic membrane of embryonated hens' eggs, nor are lesions produced in baby mice and hamsters following intraperitoneal inoculation.

Pathogenicity

The disease in puppies is characterized by anorexia, laboured breathing and abdominal pain. Puppies less than 4 weeks old usually die within 24 hours after the onset of the illness and show small, disseminated focal areas of necrosis (2–3 mm. in diameter) and haemorrhages throughout the livers, kidneys and lungs. In most cases there is serous or serohaemorrhagic fluid in the large body cavities, with pulmonary congestion and oedema. Sometimes, there is acute lymphadenitis, splenomegaly, tonsillitis and non-suppurative meningoencephalomyelitis. Histological sections reveal necrotic lesions in most organs and intranuclear inclusions that are either pale purplish in colour surrounded by smaller intensely basophilic thickenings of the nuclear membrane, or single basophilic inclusions in swollen nuclei without marked thickening of the nuclear membrane. Faintly acidophilic inclusions are less commonly seen. Experimentally, the virus causes vaginitis in bitches, and puppies that are infected *in utero* die 1–3 weeks after birth.

Ecology

Little is known about the epidemiology of this disease or of the means of dissemination and excretion of the virus. Transmission by droplet infection has been observed between older dogs. The virus has been recovered from pups obtained by Caesarian section and the canine tracheo-bronchitis virus has been isolated from apparently normal dogs, which could be carriers.

Diagnosis

In cases of 'fading puppy disease' a canine herpes-virus infection may be tentatively diagnosed on the basis of the post-mortem findings and the presence of the characteristic basophilic bodies at the nuclear membrane of the degenerating cells. The virus is readily isolated in dog kidney cell cultures from affected livers and kidneys and can be identified by specific neutralization tests.

Control

The degree of immunity is not known and vaccines against canine herpesvirus infections are not available at present.

Feline viral rhinotracheitis

Definition

Feline viral rhinotracheitis (FVR) is an acute viral disease affecting the upper respiratory tract of the domestic cat, and is caused by a member of the herpesvirus group. (Feline herpesvirus 1.). The disease is difficult to differentiate on clinical grounds from feline rhinoconjunctivitis (Calicivirus), feline panleucopoenia (Parvovirus) and feline pneumonitis (Chlamydia), although they are caused by distinct and unrelated agents.

Hosts affected

Cats are the only natural hosts of feline viral rhinotracheitis.

History and distribution

The disease was recognised in 1957 as a new viral respiratory infection of kittens in the U.S.A. Since then, the virus has been isolated from affected cats in Canada, the U.K., Holland, Switzerland, Germany and Hungary.

Properties of the virus

The causal agent of FVR has been identified as a member of the herpesvirus group and is morphologically identical to other herpesviruses. It is very labile and is able to survive for only a few days outside the host. It is also sensitive to acid, ether and chloroform, and is readily inactivated by formalin. The virus survives storage at —60°C for 3 months; is most stable at pH6 and is inactivated at 56°C in 4–5 minutes.

Antigenic properties

All strains so far examined appear to be serologically identical to the original prototype strain. Neutralizing antibodies are present in sera of recovered cats but the immunity seems to be of short duration.

Cultivation

The virus grows readily in cell cultures of cat kidney, lung and testis producing patchy foci of rounded cells, strands of cytoplasm and small syncytia in 2–6 days. Degeneration of the cells spreads fairly quickly and there is complete disruption of the monolayer within 36–48 hours of the first appearance of the cytopathic effect. Most strains do not grow well in tissues other than those of the natural host and cytopathic effects are not obtained in cultures of bovine, human and monkey cells. Stained coverslip preparations of susceptible cell cultures show the presence of numerous intranuclear inclusions in the areas of syncytial formation.

The virus is non-pathogenic for laboratory animals and chickens, and growth is not obtained in developing hens' eggs.

Pathogenicity

In natural cases of the disease the morbidity is high and the incubation period is usually short, about 2–5 days. The mortality rate is high in kittens but low in older cats. Deaths are often associated with secondary bacterial invasion. Affected animals show pyrexia and severe upper respiratory infection with sneezing, coughing, excessive salivation and acute dyspnoea. These are usually accompanied by conjunctival oedema, lachrymation and serous nasal discharges which later become muco-purulent. The clinical picture is similar to that of feline pneumonitis, feline rhinoconjunctivitis and feline pan-leucopoenia. At necropsy, inflammatory changes are seen in the mucosa of the upper respiratory tract ranging from a mild congestion to areas of focal necrosis. There may also be purulent conjunctivitis, catarrhal bronchitis and ulceration of the tongue. The carcases are frequently dehydrated and debilitated. Intranuclear inclusions are present in the respiratory epithelium. Similar changes occur in experimentally infected kittens and intranuclear inclusions can be readily demonstrated in the epithelial cells of the nictitating membrane, trachea and turbinates.

Ecology

Recent reports suggest that the majority of recovered cats become carriers of the virus and a few may be capable of transmitting the infection to susceptible contact animals. However, the clinical response in those contact cats is very variable and may range from frank disease to a mild, subclinical, afebrile type of illness depending on the age, breed, immune status and, probably, other unknown factors relating to the contact animals. The naturally occurring illness is highly contagious to younger animals due, presumably, to droplet infection by inhalation, but attempts to transmit the disease experimentally are often unsuccessful.

Diagnosis

Because FVR resembles a number of other upper respiratory infections of cats, an accurate diagnosis can only be obtained by isolation and identification of the virus in susceptible cell culture. Ocular, nasal and orthopharyngeal swabs taken for virus isolations must be kept moist or placed in a suitable transport medium and used as soon as possible because viable virus rarely survives on swabs held longer than 18 hours at room temperature. Intranuclear inclusions are present in histological sections and there is generally a rise in neutralizing antibody titre following infection.

Control

Commercially prepared anti-viral vaccines or anti-sera are not yet available for the control of feline viral rhinotracheitis.

Infectious laryngotracheitis of poultry

Definition

Infectious laryngotracheitis (ILT) is a highly contagious respiratory disease of poultry characterized by moist rales, sneezing, coughing and marked dyspnoea. Lesions and exudates are constantly found in the pharynx, trachea and larynx, but less frequently in other parts of the respiratory system.

Hosts affected

All breeds and ages of fowls are susceptible. Pheasants may also be affected and occasional infection of ducks, pigeons and turkeys is reported.

History and distribution

Infectious laryngotracheitis was first described in the U.S.A. in 1923, in Canada in 1925 and in Holland in 1929. Since then, it has been reported from many other countries throughout the world. It has been known to exist in the U.K. since 1935.

Properties of the virus

The virus is classified as a member of the herpesvirus group (Phasianid herpesvirus 1.) and its physical, chemical and biological properties are similar to those of herpes simplex. The virion contains double-stranded DNA with a relatively low guanine+cytosine (GC) content of 45–50 per cent. It is ether-sensitive.

Virus in saline suspension is readily destroyed by exposure to moderate temperature (55°–75°C) and does not survive longer than 90 minutes at room temperature. In glycerol-saline, it may remain viable for 7–14 days at 37°C, 14–21 days at 22°C and 100–200 days at 4°C. Virus in tracheal exudates is inactivated by exposure to direct sunlight within 6–8 hours but survives for up to 110 days in the dark at room temperature. It also survives in the carcases of dead chickens until decomposition begins but is readily destroyed by 3.0 per cent cresol or a 1 per cent solution of sodium hydroxide.

Haemagglutination

A report that ILT virus haemagglutinates fowl red blood cells has not been confirmed by other workers.

Antigenic properties

The virus appears to be antigenically homogeneous and is readily neutralized by specific antisera. Nevertheless, some strains though fully antigenic are poorly neutralized by antisera. A similar phenomenon has been observed with certain strains of influenza virus.

Cultivation

The virus can be readily propagated on the chorioallantoic membrane of 10-day-old chicken embryos producing isolated 'pocks' with an opaque raised edge and a depressed grey central area of necrosis. Well developed surface foci attain a diameter of 4–5 mm. but smaller ones are often seen and, with some strains, the foci are without the central necrotic area. (Plate 42.3b, facing p. 480). Histologically, the foci consist of a zone of cellular proliferation surrounding an area of central necrosis. After 36–48 hours of incubation, Cowdry type A intranuclear inclusions appear in the infected ectodermal cells. The virus of ILT cannot be grown satisfactorily in the yolk sac of developing hens' eggs but amniotic inoculation causes lesions in the trachea and bronchi of the infected chick embryo. The virus can also be grown on the chorioallantoic cavity of turkey eggs but, unlike fowl pox virus, it does not grow on the chorioallantoic membrane of guinea fowl or pigeon eggs.

In 1932, ILT virus was grown successfully in suspended cell cultures of the Maitland type and, in 1957, it was observed to produce a cytopathic effect in chick embryo cell cultures. More recently, growth has been obtained on chick embryo respiratory epithelium, chick embryo lung, and chick embryo kidney. In general, the cytopathic effects of ILT virus are confined to epithelial cell cultures although growth occurs without cellular changes on chicken fibroblasts and HeLa cells. In chicken kidney cell cultures most strains of ILT virus produce a marked cytopathic effect within 3–5 days which is characterized by the appearance of large syncytia or 'giant cells' (Plate 56.9, facing p. 772) many of which contain typical Cowdry type A intranuclear inclusions.

Infectious laryngotracheitis has a narrow host specificity, and chickens and pheasants are the only species that are susceptible to natural or experimental infections. The disease can be reproduced by intranasal, intraocular and intratracheal inoculation of infected material, but irregular results are obtained by the intravenous or intraperitoneal routes.

Pathogenicity

The disease is usually sudden in onset and early symptoms suggest a cold or mild coryza: but these are rapidly followed by respiratory distress of varying degree. The virus attacks the tracheal mucosa causing inflammation, proliferation and necrosis. This frequently causes haemorrhagic tracheitis which results in spasms of gasping, coughing or sneezing, and the bird frequently shakes its head vigorously in an attempt to dislodge blood-stained or caseous exudates obstructing the trachea or larynx. In the acute form of the disease, the fowl extends its neck and takes a prolonged inspiration through a wide open beak. This is often accompanied by a gurgling or wheezing sound, and paroxysms of coughing are sometimes accompanied by haemorrhage or dislodgement of blood clots. In outbreaks associated with a virulent strain of virus, the incubation period lasts for 2–6 days and the course of the disease varies from 1–2 weeks, but some birds may cough for about a month. The morbidity varies, but most birds in a flock may become affected with a mortality rate ranging from 10–60 per cent. A milder form of the disease, due to a less virulent strain of virus, runs a more protracted course and is characterized by coughing, sneezing, lachrymation and conjunctival oedema. A considerable number of recovered birds become carriers and may serve as a source of infection. The main pathological changes include haemorrhagic inflammation and oedema of the larynx, trachea and bronchi, the presence of a diphtheritic membrane in the trachea or a caseous exudate in the air passages and air sacs. The lungs occasionally appear normal except for small areas of congestion, but other organs are not involved. Histological examination shows a desquamative necrotizing tracheitis with typical Cowdry type A intranuclear inclusions in many of the affected epithelial cells early in the disease.

Ecology

Fowls and pheasants of all ages and breeds are naturally susceptible and virulent strains of virus produce severe illness with rapid spread of the infection. In most spontaneous outbreaks, the virus and lesions are mainly confined to the respiratory tract, and transmission is invariably by droplet infection. In many instances the actual means by which infection gains entrance to a flock is unknown but it is unlikely that contaminated footwear, clothing, utensils or equipment play an important role in transmission. The virus of ILT is not present in the yolk sac of chick embryos, and day-old chicks from infected parents are unlikely to be a source of infection to susceptible stock. There is no evidence that insect vectors are infected or are capable of mechanical transmission of the virus. Most affected birds recover completely from the disease but a large number continue to harbour the virus and may remain infective for more than 2 years. Small well-isolated farms seldom suffer from ILT but the concentration of large numbers of chickens in confined areas predisposes to the spread of infection. Once the disease has been introduced on to a farm, usually by newly purchased stock, the infection is carried over from year to year by symptomless but persistently infected recovered birds which may continue to excrete virus for very long periods.

Diagnosis

The acute form of the disease is readily recognised by its sudden onset, the characteristic symptoms of rales accompanied by blood, mucous and caseous exudates in the trachea, its rapid spread and high mortality. Other forms of the clinical disease, however, are not sufficiently characteristic to be pathognomonic and may resemble other respiratory infections of the fowl. In these cases, a confirmatory diagnosis can only be made in the laboratory.

The most common method of diagnosis is by inoculating a suspension of suspected material into 10 to 12-day-old embryonated hens' eggs and examining the chorioallantoic membranes for the presence of typical surface 'pocks' after 5 days of incubation. The presence of ILT virus is confirmed by demonstrating intranuclear inclusion bodies in the lesions and by serum neutralization tests. Inclusion bodies can also be detected in smears prepared from the epithelium of the trachea or conjunctiva and stained by Giemsa's method. For best results, the material should be obtained from fresh carcases of birds which had shown symptoms for only 2 or 3 days. Agar gel diffusion and immuno-fluorescence methods are also useful for detecting ILT antigens in affected tissues and for differentiating sera of fowls which have been infected with ILT, fowl pox, Newcastle disease or other respiratory viruses. Additional laboratory methods include the isolation of the virus in susceptible cell cultures or by infraorbital sinus inoculation or cloacal scarification of suceptible and immune chickens. Specific neutralizing antibodies can be demonstrated in the sera of birds that are, or have been, infected.

Control

Eradication of ILT is achieved by complete depopulation and disinfection of infected premises, followed by restocking with healthy birds not less than one month afterwards. In enzootic areas it may be possible to control the disease or to shorten the course of an epidemic by the use of living virus vaccines. Virulent strains may be introduced into the bursa of Fabricius by applying the vaccine-virus to the vent mucosa. In a satisfactory 'take' there is an inflammatory reaction of the cloaca which usually runs its course in about 5–7 days and produces a solid immunity by the 9th day. Birds which do not react must be revaccinated immediately lest they develop the natural disease from their vaccinated pen-mates. These early 'virulent' virus vaccines consisted of infected tracheal exudates and are seldom used at the present time owing to the risk of spreading avian leukosis, Newcastle disease or other infections. It is best to use strains of lower virulence which have been modified by serial passage in eggs. These can be applied by the brush method to the vent mucosa or introduced into the conjunctival sac. Although broiler flocks must be protected as early as possible, vaccination against ILT should be delayed, if possible, until the birds are at least 4 weeks old.

Attenuated virus vaccines have also been prepared in duck embryo tissue cultures and are administered either by aerosol or by conjunctival inoculation.

Herpesvirus infection of pigeons

Synonym

Inclusion disease of pigeons.

Definition

An infectious viral disease of pigeons giving rise to conjunctivitis, dyspnoea, diarrhoea, dehydration and emaciation, with lesions of the liver and other internal organs.

Hosts affected

So far as is known, only pigeons are susceptible.

History and distribution

The disease was first described in the U.S.A. in 1943 during an investigation of an unusual outbreak of ornithosis in pigeons. The presence of the disease was confirmed in England in 1947 in stock founded on birds imported from America. In Denmark, the disease accounted for 3 per cent of all pigeon diseases during the 15-year period following 1950.

Properties of the virus

The causative agent is a herpesvirus (Pigeon herpesvirus 1.) which is morphologically similar to that of ILT virus but differs from it antigenically. Inhibition by IUDR confirms that the viral nucleic acid is DNA. The virus is ether-sensitive and shows a relatively high degree of thermal resistance. It is destroyed by exposure to a pH of 4 and can be stored for several months at —20°C. No haemagglutinin has been described.

Cultivation

The pigeon virus produces a cytopathic effect in cultures of chicken embryo kidney and liver, but does not multiply in HeLa cells or in primary cultures of dog kidney. The cytopathic effect is characterized by the appearance of foci of round refractile cells and, in some cell cultures, a number of large syncytia with multi-nucleate 'giant cells' may be seen. Unlike ILT virus, which is non-pathogenic for fibroblasts, the pigeon virus grows well in tissue cultures of fibroblasts from whole chicken embryos and can also multiply in chicken hepatic epithelial cells. Growth occurs on the chorioallantoic membrane of embryonated hens' eggs with the formation of small cream-white pocks and the embryos may die about the fifth day. The pocks are about 1 mm. in diameter and sections of infected membranes show that intranuclear inclusions appear within the ectodermal cells on the second day of incubation. The inclusions may be basophilic or acidophilic. Foci of necrosis may be present in chick embryonic livers by the fourth day. In contrast to ILT virus, the pigeon herpesvirus may infect the mesoderm of the chorioallantoic membrane.

Pathogenicity

The disease occurs most commonly in younger birds of 1–6 months old, and seldom in older pigeons. Most cases probably occur between 5–6 weeks of age and show symptoms of rhinitis, conjunctivitis, dyspnoea, diphtheroid foci in the pharynx and larynx and generalized weakness. The most constant postmortem finding is focal hepatic necrosis and, in some cases, renal necrosis. Intranuclear inclusions are usually to be found in the parenchymal cells adjacent to the necrotic foci.

Ecology

The infection is probably spread by the respiratory route and is commonest in pigeon lofts and conditions of overcrowding. Domestic pigeons can be affected experimentally but the virus cannot be transmitted to chickens or any other species.

Diagnosis

Laboratory assistance is required to confirm the presence of the infection and to enable the disease to be distinguished from that of pigeon-pox. The presence of Cowdry type A inclusions in smears and sections prepared from the mouth and trachea will eliminate pox-virus infections. On the other hand, ILT and pigeon herpesvirus infections can be differentiated from each other by the fact that there is no cross-neutralization of the viruses in eggs or cell cultures using specific antisera. Moreover, the pigeon virus differs from ILT virus in the character of the lesions produced in the chorioallantoic membrane and in tissue cultures.

Control

There are no suitable vaccines at present for the control of herpesvirus infections of pigeons and control can best be achieved by drastic culling of affected birds, good management and the maintenance of a closed flock.

Other avian herpesvirus infections

Other avian herpesviruses associated with disease include Pacheco's disease of parrots and a disease of owls. The former, which was isolated from South American parrots, may be related to the virus of ILT although the presence of necrotic foci in the liver and spleen of diseased birds suggests that it is closer to the herpesvirus of pigeons. Symptoms in affected parrots consist of debility, diarrhoea, coma and death. Type A intranuclear inclusions may be seen in some affected tissues. The virus is pathogenic for budgerigars and chicks, and produces pocks on the chorioallantoic membrane of embryonated hens' eggs.

A highly fatal disease of owls associated with a herpesvirus causes necrosis of the liver and spleen with large acidophilic intranuclear inclusions in the hepatic cells. The infection is not transmissible to other birds.

A herpesvirus has been isolated on the chorioallantoic membrane of fertile hens' eggs inoculated with blood from a little pied cormorant. Pocks were produced on the egg membrane but chicks, pigeons, parrots and laboratory rodents could not be infected.

Duck plague

Synonyms

Duck virus enteritis: eendenpest (Dutch): peste du canarde (Fr.): entenpest (Ger.).

Definition

An acute, contagious viral infection of ducks, geese and swans characterized by ocular and nasal discharges, diarrhoea, extensive vascular damage with tissue haemorrhages, and high mortality.

Hosts affected

The disease occurs naturally in domestic ducks but wild *Anserinae* (ducks, geese and swans) may occasionally become infected. The disease has not been reported in the domestic chicken, wild waterfowl or other species of birds. Man and animals are not affected.

History and distribution

The first account of a hitherto unrecognised acute haemorrhagic disease of domestic ducks was reported in the Netherlands in 1923. Since then, isolated outbreaks have occurred in Holland in 1930, 1942, 1952 and 1959 and, more recently, in India since 1963 and the U.S.A. since 1967. Serological evidence suggests that the infection may be present in wild mallard in Britain.

Properties of the virus

The causative agent is a herpes-type virus (Anatid herpesvirus 1.) which is similar to other herpesviruses in its structural, chemical and physical properties. It is ether and chloroform sensitive. Exposure for 18 hours at 37°C to trypsin, chymotrypsin and pancreatic lipase markedly reduces or inactivates the virus, but papain, lysozyme, cellulase, DNase and RNase have no effect. Heating at 56°C for 10 minutes inactivates the virus and storage at room temperature results in loss of infectivity within 30 days. The virus is stable at pH 7–9 but its titre is reduced at lower or higher pH levels.

Haemagglutination
Strains of duck plague virus do not agglutinate duck, chicken, sheep or horse red blood cells.

Antigenic properties
All strains are antigenically identical but are distinct from those of duck hepatitis (picornavirus), fowl plague (orthomyxovirus) and Newcastle disease (paramyxovirus).

Cultivation
Duck plague virus can be readily propagated on the chorioallantoic membrane of 9 to 12-day-old embryonated duck eggs. The infected embryos die with extensive haemorrhages after 4 days of incubation. The virus can be adapted to growth in chicken embryos and chicken fibroblasts but the adapted virus is non-pathogenic for ducks. Growth also occurs in duck embryo cell cultures and produces a cytopathic effect with microplaques of necrotic cells. Electron microscopy of ultrathin sections of infected cultures shows that immature virus particles appear within the nucleus 12 hours post-infection and that larger, enveloped forms are found in the cytoplasm a few hours later.

Pathogenicity
In Holland, outbreaks of the disease are usually confined to 1 or 2 farms or to small groups of neighbouring farms. In most of the early outbreaks the causal organism was extremely virulent and the disease invariably resulted in mortality rates approaching 100 per cent, but, in recent years, losses from duck plague have been appreciably lower.

Ducklings of all ages up to maturity are susceptible. The incubation period is between 3–7 days and death usually occurs within 1–5 days of the onset of clinical symptoms. Duck plague is an acute disease of a viraemic character which runs a very rapid course and is characterized by nasal and ocular discharges and diarrhoea. At necropsy, multiple petechiae occur in almost all parts of the carcase and, in many cases, there is diphtheritic inflammation of the oesophagus and cloaca. Large haemorrhages are also seen in the ovaries and some other organs, and blood lies freely in many of the body cavities.

Ducklings are susceptible to experimental infection by various routes including oral, intranasal, intravenous, intraperitoneal, intramuscular and cloacal administration but the virus, which is present in most tissues, has not been recovered from eggs laid by older infected birds. The domestic chicken is resistant to natural and experimental infection and although the virus cannot be isolated in embryonated hens' eggs, day-old chicks can be infected intramuscularly.

Transmission
The naturally occurring disease does not spread on a large scale and most outbreaks usually appear between January and July in areas where ducks have free access to water. The available evidence suggests that the infection is transmitted by direct contact between infected and susceptible birds or indirectly by contaminated water and food.

Diagnosis
A tentative diagnosis of duck plague can readily be made from the extensive vascular damage, large haemorrhages and multiple petechiae seen in many organs and tissues at necropsy. The isolation of a virus which fails to grow in embryonated hens' eggs, but which multiplies readily in fertile duck eggs and duck embryo cell cultures, and which produces the characteristic disease in experimentally infected ducklings is highly suggestive of duck plague. The identity of the virus isolate can be confirmed by neutralization tests with known duck plague antisera.

Control
Virus adapted to growth in embryonated hens' eggs forms a safe and effective live attenuated vaccine for the control of duck plague. Vaccinated ducklings develop a resistance to infection as early as the first day following vaccination due, it is believed, to the early formation of interferon. The vaccine is administered subcutaneously in 0.5 ml doses to ducklings over 2 weeks of age. Although the vaccine-virus does not spread to susceptible contact birds, persistent field infections have occasionally been observed in vaccinated ducks and, for this reason, the use of these live attenuated vaccines is not permitted in some countries. There are, unfortunately, no satisfactory inactivated duck plague virus vaccines available.

Marek's disease

Synonyms
Fowl paralysis: range paralysis: polyneuritis: neurolymphomatosis gallinarum.

Definition
A transmissible virus-induced disorder of chickens

characterized by mononuclear infiltration of peripheral nerves and, to a lesser degree, the iris, gonads, muscle, skin and various internal organs.

Hosts affected

The disease mainly affects domestic poultry and is commonest in young birds between 2 and 4 months of age. Natural infection has also been demonstrated in quail but it is not known if this species is an important reservoir for the virus. Lesions resembling those of Marek's disease have been described in other members of the order *Galliformes*, including pheasants, partridges, ducks, swans, geese, pigeons, canaries and budgerigars, but the causative agent of these lesions has not been determined. Virulent Marek's disease virus has occasionally been isolated from turkeys but the susceptibility of this species to naturally occurring infection is not known since many turkey flocks are infected with a non-pathogenic herpesvirus (HVT) which is closely related antigenically to that of Marek's disease.

History and distribution

Although there is evidence that the disease might have been present in the U.S.A. as early as 1878, the first detailed account of a 'polyneuritis' in poultry was published in Hungary by Marek in 1907. By 1914, the condition was prevalent in the U.S.A., and a few years later outbreaks were confirmed in Holland (1921), Germany (1927) and the U.K. (1929).

Early reports suggested that the lesions in typical cases of 'polyneuritis' were restricted to the peripheral nerves and central nervous system, but later workers showed that lymphoid tumours occurred occasionally in tissues and organs outside the nervous system. On account of this, they considered that the terms 'polyneuritis', or 'fowl paralysis' as it was sometimes called, were unsatisfactory and proposed instead the designation 'neurolymphomatosis gallinarum'. To add to the confusion, cases of neurolymphomatosis were sometimes present at the same time and in the same flock as another common lymphoid tumour disease of the chicken called lymphoid leukosis. Since the pathology of neurolymphomatosis is similar in many ways to that of lymphoid leukosis the two conditions were considered to be aetiologically related and were grouped together under the term 'avian leucosis complex'. Unfortunately, this encouraged the view that the two diseases were different manifestations of the same condition and the visceral lesions in both diseases were classified together as 'visceral lymphomatosis'. Further confusion arose from the fact that a small but experienced group of avian pathologists still believed that the leukosis complex

consisted of at least two distinct and unrelated diseases. In 1960–61, however, the World Veterinary Poultry Association accepted a plea to discard the term 'lymphomatosis' and to name the condition originally described by Marek in 1907 as Marek's disease. This decision to accept a major division between avian leucosis and Marek's disease was vindicated by the discoveries in 1967 and subsequently, that the causative agent of Marek's disease is a DNA virus of the herpes type and is, therefore, distinct from the RNA group of viruses (oncornaviruses) causing avian leukosis.

Marek's disease occurs in all poultry-producing countries throughout the world and is the source of considerable economic loss to the poultry industry. The incidence of the disease has increased markedly in recent years especially in areas where chickens are reared intensively. In the last decade a new and highly infectious form of the disease has appeared which differs from classical Marek's disease by the much higher incidence of malignant tumours involving the gonads and other tissues. Younger birds tend to be affected more frequently and the virulent nature of the virus usually results in severe losses.

Properties of the virus

On the basis of its morphological characters, nucleic acid type and cell-associated activity, the causative agent of Marek's disease has been identified as a herpesvirus. (Phasianid herpesvirus 2.). Electron microscopy of ultra-thin sections of infected cell cultures reveals hexagonal, non-enveloped viral particles about 85–100 nm in diameter, but larger enveloped virions 150–170 nm in size have occasionally been seen. The particles may or may not contain a dense electron-opaque nucleoid and are mostly located within the nucleus. The virus cannot readily be demonstrated in uncultured material but negative contrast preparations of lysed feather follicle epithelium usually reveals the presence of large, structureless particles measuring between 275–400 nm in diameter. In negatively-stained preparations of cultured cells typical herpes-type virions can be detected, showing icosahedral symmetry and 162 hollow wedge-shaped capsomeres. A fringe of fine projections is seen occasionally on the surface of the envelope.

Inhibition of infectivity by 5-iododeoxyuridine or 5-bromodeoxyuridine indicates that the virus contains DNA. Viral activity of blood cells or tumour tissues is reduced by freeze-thawing, sonication and lyophilization. Standard stocks of infected cells may be preserved by slow cooling (1°C per minute) to —60°C in growth medium containing 10 per cent calf serum and 7.5 per cent dimethyl sulphoxide (DMSO), and stored thereafter in liquid nitrogen. Infectivity is destroyed at pH 5.5 or below and at pH 8.4 or above; and within 18 hours at 37°C, 30 minutes at 56°C and 10 minutes at 60°C. Cell-free virus is stable at —70°C but loses its infectivity at —20°C.

Haemagglutination

A report, in 1970, that plasma from infected chicks may agglutinate sheep erythrocytes has not been confirmed by other workers. but indirect haemagglutination with tanned sheep red blood cells has been reported.

Antigenic properties

Chicken kidney cell cultures infected with Marek's disease virus produce a precipitating antigen which can be demonstrated by double-diffusion in agar with sera from affected birds. The sera are prepared in experimentally infected one-day-old chicks and the antibodies usually appear 4 weeks after inoculation. All field strains of Marek's disease virus so far tested have been antigenically identical but they appear to be unrelated to other avian herpesviruses except for the herpesvirus of turkeys (HVT). However, Marek's disease virus cross-reacts serologically with herpes simplex, Aujeszky's disease virus and bovine rhinotracheitis virus and with the Epstein-Barr (EB) virus from Burkitt's lymphoma.

Three antigens named A, B and C, have been detected in Marek's disease virus by means of agar gel diffusion and their identity confirmed by immunofluorescence tests. During serial passage, the virus tends to lose antigen A which is normally found in the supernatant fluids of infected cell cultures; but antigens B and C, which are present within the cells, are not affected. The turkey herpesvirus contains two A antigens as well as other antigens in common with Marek's disease virus. Antigens in both the nucleus and cytoplasm of cells infected with the turkey virus stain with homologous antiserum, whereas only the nuclear antigen stains with antiserum against Marek's disease virus. Cross-neutralization occurs between the two viruses but a 2-way cross has not been observed. Because of this, the non-pathogenic turkey herpesvirus is being used as a vaccine for the control of Marek's disease in chickens. In contrast to the oncornaviruses of lymphoid leukosis, all isolates of Marek's disease virus are RIF-negative and do not possess or induce the formation of COFAL antigen.

Cultivation

Early attempts to demonstrate the transmissibility of Marek's disease in experimentally infected birds frequently produced negative or inconclusive results. This was largely due to the lack of susceptible lines of chickens and to the low virulence of the great majority of strains causing clinical Marek's disease.

In recent years the increased availability of genetically susceptible birds together with the appearance of highly virulent strains of virus from 'acute leukosis' has enabled several groups of workers to confirm the transmissible nature of the disease. However, cell-free plasma is less effective as an inoculum than whole blood and some lines of fowls are more susceptible than others. It is stressed that the more chronic form of the disease is difficult to transmit experimentally although most workers are agreed that 'acute' and 'classical' Marek's disease have a common aetiology. Of the many strains examined some, including HPRS-B14 and HPRS-17, produce classical Marek's disease whereas others such as the JM strain and the HPRS-16, -18, -19, -20 strains produce the acute form. Additional evidence of strain variability is shown by the American strains GR and RPL-39 which are basically viscerotropic, whereas the JM strain tends to be neurotropic and produces fewer lymphoid tumours.

The virus can be readily propagated in newly hatched chicks producing lesions which can be detected histologically in the ganglia, nerves and certain viscera 2–4 weeks post-inoculation, or by gross examination after 3–6 weeks. In experimentally infected chicks, fluorescent-antibody staining shows that many tissues contain the virus, and specific viral antigen can be detected in apparently healthy kidney tubule epithelium or in the epithelium of the feather follicles.

Most strains grow well in the yolk sac of genetically susceptible chick embryos and some produce discrete pocks on the surface of the chorioallantoic membrane.

A major step towards an understanding of the aetiology of Marek's disease was the report, in 1967, of the isolation of a cytopathic agent in primary cultures of chick kidney cells inoculated with tumour or blood cells from birds with Marek's disease. The cytopathic effect was characterized by the development of discrete focal lesions consisting of clusters of rounded, highly refractile, degenerating cells about 7 days after inoculation. During the next 7 days the clusters of refractile cells enlarged and the cells became detached from the glass giving rise to microscopic plaques. Stained monolayer preparations contained typical Cowdry type A intranuclear inclusions and electron-microscopy revealed the presence of virions which were morphologically identical to herpesviruses. Further studies showed that the virus was strongly cell-associated and the characteristic cytopathic effect could only be passaged to healthy cell cultures by the transfer of intact infected cells. Cultures showing the cytopathic effect induced Marek's disease when inoculated into young susceptible chicks. Serial passage of the virus in chick embryo kidney cell cultures may induce attenuation of the virus and it has been suggested that the decrease in pathogenicity is accompanied by a loss of oncogenicity.

Also in 1967, a second group of workers obtained a cytopathic effect on duck embryo fibroblasts inoculated with blood collected from chickens infected with Marek's disease virus. The cellular changes occurred within 11–25 days, after a series of prolonged subcultures, and were characterized by focal lesions of rounded or shrunken spindle cells. Affected cells contained herpes-like particles and produced Marek's disease when inoculated into young chicks. Chicken embryo fibroblasts and other tissues derived from a variety of avian species have been found to be susceptible to the virus but established mammalian cell lines are probably resistant.

Spread of virus in infected monolayers is largely cell-to-cell but there is evidence that at least some infectious cell-free virus is present in the extracellular environment.

In a more recent study, herpes-type virus particles were observed in the nucleus of transformed lymphocytes from cases of acute and classical Marek's disease, after 3–5 days' culture *in vitro*. The viruses were found to be similar in morphology, antigenicity and nuclear staining activity to those isolated in cultures of chicken kidney cells. Electron-microscopy of thin-sections of cultured lymphocytes showed that the majority of the hexagonal herpes-type particles were immature, having a single envelope surrounding a nucleoid of variable density and measuring 74–94 nm in diameter. Budding of virus through the nuclear membrane and intracytoplasmic particles were not observed. Infected cells occasionally showed nuclei containing long double-walled tubules, about 74 nm in width, having a less dense central core which was sometimes exposed as a thread about 22 nm thick. These tubular structures were invariably associated with single-enveloped virus particles and where they were cut across, were similar in structure to the latter. It has also been reported that primary monolayer cultures prepared from kidney tissue of clinically normal chickens in a flock endemically infected with classical Marek's disease produced a spontaneous cytopathic effect after 3–8 weeks of incubation; but in secondary monolayers of this culture, typical cytopathic effects with extensive necrosis developed at 10 days. (Plate 56.4b, facing p. 741). Many of the infected cells showed Cowdry type A intranuclear inclusions which fluoresced brightly, as for DNA, when stained with acridine orange. They also contained viral antigens when examined by indirect immunofluorescence with either acute or classical Marek's disease antisera.

Other workers have observed that some chicken kidney and duck embryo fibroblast cultures infected with Marek's disease virus may not produce a marked cytopathic effect and that the affected cells become persistently infected with the virus.

Pathogenicity

Marek's disease is essentially a transmissible viral infection of young birds. In its original form the disease most commonly affected pullets and cockerels on the verge of sexual maturity but in recent years a more acute form has appeared in chickens only a few weeks old. Recovery from overt disease is unusual and mortality in an affected flock may range from a few per cent to over 60 per cent on rare occasions.

Marek's disease is a lympho-proliferative condition which affects the peripheral nerves and, sometimes, the visceral organs and other tissues. Symptoms of the disease are due to the lesions in the nervous system and range from slight paresis to spastic and, rarely, flaccid paralysis. Three forms of the disease have been described: 1) the *neural form* ('fowl paralysis') is characterized by infiltration of the peripheral nerves by lymphoid cells, causing progressive paralysis usually of a wing or leg. (Plate 56.11a, between pp. 772-3). In advanced cases of the disease the leg or wing is trailed on the ground, the perch reflex is impaired and paralysed birds often lie with one leg extended forward and the other directed backwards. In many cases, there is torticollis and, where the vagus nerve is affected, there may be respiratory distress or distension of the crop according to the site of the lesions: 2) the *visceral form* (including 'acute leukosis') in which lymphomas develop in the liver, spleen, gonads and other tissues: and 3) the *ocular form* ('pearly-eye') caused by lymphocytic infiltration of the iris. In these cases the normally bright coloured iris has a grey or pearly appearance and the pupil is contracted or distorted.

In younger birds, the acute form of the disease is generally characterized by severe depression, ataxia, diarrhoea, emaciation and high mortality.

The first observable lesion is a proliferation of lymphoid tissue in the nerves and visceral organs. These generally consist of small and medium-sized lymphocytes, 'blast' cells and an aberrant cell described as a 'Marek's disease' cell. The so-called Marek's disease cells are pyroninophilic degenerating blast-type cells with a vacuolated nucleus and cytoplasm, and are often present in proliferative lesions. The lesions are progressive and, in the neural form of the disease, one or more of the peripheral nerves show enlargement with the brachial, sciatic, coeliac and vagus nerves being most frequently involved. The affected nerves are often swollen, rounded and oedematous, and lose the characteristic, white, flat, cross-striations of the healthy nerve. In most cases the lesions are unilateral and even slight changes can often be distinguished by comparing opposite nerves. (Plate 56.10, between pp. 772–3). In addition to the inflammatory-like lesions of the nerves, affected chickens may also show visceral lesions which become gross lymphomatous tumours. These occur most frequently in the ovary but sometimes in the testes, liver, spleen, lungs, kidneys, heart, proventriculus and other tissues.

In Marek's disease, the proliferative lesions in the bursa of Fabricius usually appear as a diffuse thickening, in marked contrast to the discrete, nodular type of tumour formation characteristic of lymphoid leukosis caused by oncornaviruses (*Retraviridae*). In the acute form of Marek's disease there is a high incidence of the proliferative lymphomatous type of lesion but involvement of the peripheral nerves is less common. Small lymphomas are also common in the subcutis, especially in the feather follicles (skin leukosis). In the acute and classical forms of Marek's disease there are often lesions of a non-suppurative encephalomyelitis.

The incubation period in naturally occurring cases of Marek's disease is probably 3–4 weeks and most serious outbreaks generally occur when the chickens are between 8–16 weeks of age.

Day-old chicks infected experimentally excrete virus from the second to third week post-inoculation. At necropsy, microscopic lesions develop as early as the second week but gross lesions and clinical symptoms do not usually appear until the 4th week or later.

Ecology

In the naturally occurring disease, the infectious agent is present in the oral, nasal and tracheal secretions, the faeces and feather-follicle epithelium. Virus is rarely found in the plasma of infected chickens but is invariably present in the leukocytes of the blood, probably in either the macrophages or lymphocytes. These may be responsible for the spread of infection from one tissue to another. The available evidence shows that the first few days of life represent the period when the birds are most at risk and that the disease may be transmitted both by direct and indirect contact. Airborne transmission is probably responsible for the rapid spread between susceptible young birds, especially on farms where chickens are reared intensively. Moreover, since dust and litter from poultry houses remain infectious for 6 weeks or longer it appears that the virus is able to lead an independent extracellular existence. This observation has been largely confirmed by recent studies of the distribution of Marek's disease virus in affected tissues. Immuno-fluorescence tests have shown that specific viral antigen is frequently present in the feather follicles

as early as 5 days after infection and can also be detected in the medullary cells of the bursa of Fabricius. Small foci of fluorescent cells are less commonly seen in the kidney and various other epithelial organs including the proventriculus, testis and thyroid. Not only is the feather follicle the tissue most often positive in immunofluorescence tests, but Cowdry type A intranuclear inclusions and herpes-type virions can readily be demonstrated by light and electron microscopy, respectively. There is clear evidence that Marek's disease virus replicates in feather-follicle epithelium and can be detected in this tissue within 2–6 weeks after infection. Several workers have succeeded in isolating infectious cell-free virus from affected follicle epithelial cells and produced the disease in chickens. In view of these observations it is now generally agreed that shed follicle cells and feather dust are the most important means of spread of Marek's disease virus. Although the ovary is frequently affected, and the virus can survive in artificially infected chick embryos, most workers believe that egg transmission, if it occurs, is a rare event and is of little importance in the natural transmission of the disease.

Coccidiosis and Marek's disease are often present in the same bird and the presence of Marek's disease is believed to render birds more susceptible to infection with coccidia: but there is no evidence that Marek's disease virus is carried in the oocysts.

Diagnosis

A provisional diagnosis of Marek's disease is usually based on the symptoms produced by the lesions in the nervous system. These include unilateral or bilateral paralysis of the legs or wings, loss of the perch-reflex, curling of the toes, torticollis, dilatation of the crop, diffuse grey opacity of the iris and irregular outline of the pupil. In younger birds, the acute form of the disease is characterized by rapid spread, severe depression, emaciation and death. At necropsy, Marek's disease may be distinguished from lymphoid leukosis if the birds showing lymphoid tumours are under 18 weeks of age; in older birds there is no involvement of the bursa of Fabricius. Most cases of Marek's disease show diffuse or nodular oedematous swellings of the vagus and sciatic nerves and of the brachial, coeliac and lumbar plexuses. The nature of the cellular infiltrations in affected tissues can be readily identified histologically, and is of considerable diagnostic value.

In recent years, a number of virological procedures have been adapted successfully for confirming the diagnosis of Marek's disease. The most sensitive method available for isolating the causal virus is the intraperitoneal inoculation of day-old genetically susceptible chicks either with blood from suspected birds or with tumour-tissue suspensions. The birds

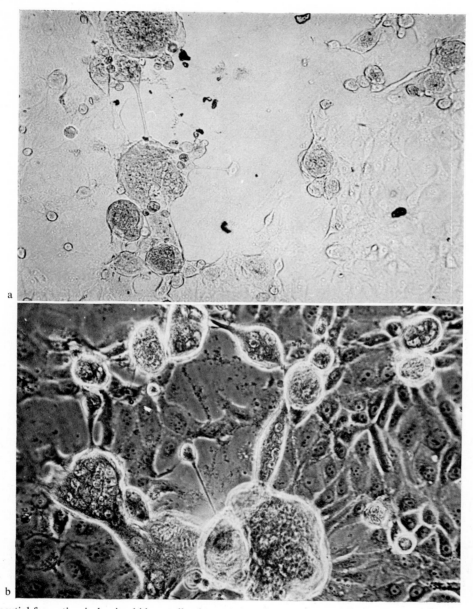

a

b

Syncytial formation in bovine kidney cell cultures 3 days after inoculation with bovine mammillitis virus.

56.7a Unstained preparation showing rounding of cells and fusion of the cytoplasm to form polykaryons, × 160.

56.7b Unstained monolayer viewed under phase contrast, showing several large refractile multinucleate polykaryons against the darker background of unaffected cells, × 240.

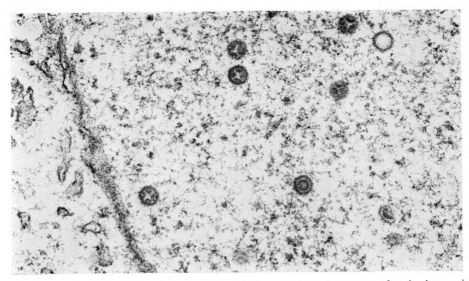

56.8 Electron micrograph of ultra-thin section of canine cerebellar astrocyte. Aggregates of canine herpesvirus particles are seen within the nucleus (right) of an infected cell. Notice the appearance of the nucleoid of the virions during different stages of development of the capsid; some show cross or star forms. (Courtesy of Dr H. C. Cornwell.)

are examined after 2–10 weeks for evidence of infection (e.g. gross and microscopical lesions), detection of specific antibodies in sera or specific viral antigens in tissue cells and isolation of the virus from avian tissues in chicken kidney cell cultures.

Primary monolayer cultures of chicken kidney cells or duck embryo fibroblasts are also useful for isolation of the virus from blood or tumour cells from field cases of the disease. Inoculated monolayers are incubated for 24–48 hours at 37°C., washed and refed with maintenance medium and reincubated for 2–3 weeks without sub-cultivation. Micro-plaques of necrotic cells and Cowdry type A inclusions develop within 5–14 days. A more sensitive method for detecting the causative virus is by direct cultivation of kidney cells from the suspect bird. Although the cytopathic effects are less marked and the plaques of round, refractile polykaryocytes tend to disappear after further incubation, intranuclear inclusions can be seen in many of the infected cells. Identification of virus isolated can be confirmed by chick inoculation or fluorescent antibody staining. For immunofluorescence studies, antisera against fractionated whole blood from infected chickens is produced in rabbits.

Serological evidence of infection can also be obtained by agar gel diffusion, indirect immunofluorescence or by an indirect haemagglutination test using tanned red blood cells treated with herpesvirus antigen.

Acridine orange staining of avian tumour cells may be useful for differentiating lymphoid leukosis cells, which stain orange, from cells affected with Marek's disease which do not take up the stain to the same degree.

Control

In 1965, it was reported that continuous passage of Marek's disease virus in cell cultures gave rise to an attenuated strain of virus which had lost its oncogenic potential for chickens. Birds vaccinated with this live attenuated strain were less susceptible than uninoculated birds to challenge or contact

infection with virulent virus, but the nature of the resistance has not yet been determined. These recent observations led to the development of the first commercially available vaccine against Marek's disease; and is, incidentally, the first vaccine to be developed against specific tumour-inducing viruses. Marek's disease is now being successfully controlled by vaccination with living non-pathogenic viruses. These include attenuated non-pathogenic Marek's disease virus, naturally occurring non-pathogenic Marek's disease virus and the herpesvirus of turkeys. It is interesting to note that these living virus vaccines do not prevent super-infection with pathogenic strains of virus, but they do protect against overt disease.

Jaagsiekte

Synonyms
Pulmonary adenomatosis: chronic progressive pneumonia: 'Jagziekte' (trail disease or driving sickness): epizootic adenomatosis.

Definition
A very slowly progressive chronic lung infection of sheep, characterized by gradually increasing dyspnoea, emaciation and eventually death.

History and distribution
The occurrence of a characteristic proliferation of epithelium in the lungs of sheep suffering from pneumonia was described in England and Germany towards the end of the 19th century. In 1904, a description was published of a chronic, catarrhal pneumonia of sheep in South Africa, which was known as 'Jagziekte' or 'drive sickness'. Since that time, progressive pulmonary conditions of sheep in which adenomatosis lesions are a prominent feature have been described in many areas of the world. In Europe, the disease is known to occur in the U.K., Germany, France, the Netherlands, Italy, Yugoslavia, Bulgaria, Israel, Greece, Turkey, and in parts of the U.S.S.R. The disease has also been described

TABLE 56.3. Differential diagnosis of avian lymphoid leukosis and Marek's disease.

	Lymphoid leukosis	Marek's disease
Age affected	16 weeks, or older	5–20 weeks, or older
Neural signs and lesions	No	Yes
Tumour formation:		
Bursa of Fabricius	Nodular	Diffuse or absent
Viscera	Yes	Yes
Skin and muscle	No	Yes
Eye	No	Yes
Cell type	Lymphoblasts	Small and medium-sized lymphocytes, blast cells, occasional lymphoblasts and pyroninophilic 'Marek's disease cells'
Virus	RNA, leukovirus	DNA, herpesvirus

in Peru, particularly among sheep grazing at high altitudes, and isolated outbreaks have been reported from India where goats are also believed to have been affected. In 1933, epizootic adenomatosis or jaag-siekte was introduced into Iceland by means of a diseased ram imported from Europe. The infection spread very rapidly over much of the island but was eradicated completely by the end of 1952.

Aetiology

Many attempts have been made to identify the causative agent of jaagsiekte and the most prevalent view among those who have worked with the disease is that it is caused by a virus.

A major step towards an understanding of the cause of jaagsiekte were the reports, published in 1969, of the presence of intranuclear inclusions in cultured macrophages from lungs of sheep suffering from pulmonary adenomatosis, and of the trans-mission of these effects in cultures of alveolar macrophages. Electron microscopic observations indicate that the cytopathic agent has many charac-teristics in common with the herpes group of viruses, and has been named Bovid herpesvirus 4. In negative-contrast preparations both complete and incomplete hexagonal capsids are present, measuring between 95–115 nm in diameter, with characteristic hollow elongated peripheral capsomeres. Occasional particles enclosed in envelopes are also seen. Ultra-thin sections of infected macrophage cultures show virus particles in the nuclei and, less frequently, in the cytoplasm also. The majority of particles are diffusely distributed within the nuclei and consist of a nucleoid surrounded by a single membrane. The particles vary in size from 80–100 nm and the diameter of the nucleoid is between 50 and 65 nm. Occasionally, particles with a double limiting mem-brane and a diameter of between 117–130 nm are found between the lamellae of the nucleus or in the vesicles near the nuclear membrane. In some preparations filamentous para-crystalline structures are closely associated with clusters of small intranu-clear virus particles of 30 nm in diameter.

Infectivity of the herpes-like particle is abolished by a temperature of 56°C for 60 minutes or by exposure to chloroform. It is also partially acid-labile. The agent cannot be propagated in em-bryonated hens' eggs and does not produce con-junctivitis in rabbits by corneal scarification, or deaths in day-old mice injected intracerebrally.

Although Scottish workers stress that the aetio-logical significance of their isolate in relation to that of pulmonary adenomatosis is at present unknown, they draw attention to the fact that herpes-type viruses have been reported as occurring in association with three other conditions which are of special interest in this context, viz. lymphoblast

cultures from Burkitt's lymphoma of man, tissue sections of Lucké's renal adenocarcinoma of the leopard frog and Marék's disease of chickens.

In 1971, Central European workers isolated a herpes-like virus from spontaneous cases of jaag-siekte which produced a cytopathic effect in cultures of fetal human fibroblasts and fetal sheep lung. They also reported that lesions of jaagsiekte were produced in lungs of lambs inoculated intratracheally 10–22 months previously with virus grown in cell cultures. On the other hand, American workers have described intracytoplasmic structures resembling A-type particles and extracellular elements resembling C-type particles of unknown aetiological significance in jaagsiekte. The importance of this last observation is underlined by the fact that reverse transcriptase and 60–70 S RNA have also been demonstrated in jaagsiekte tissue.

Pathogenicity

The signs of disease seldom occur in sheep under 2–3 years of age and are most common in animals 4 years old, or more. The incubation period is very variable but is probably longer than 6–9 months. The clinical illness, which usually lasts 2–8 months, is seen as a febrile, chronic, progressive respiratory condition, characterized by increasing dyspnoea particularly when the animal is under stress, cough-ing, abundant nasal discharge, inappetance, emacia-tion and death.

Although the average mortality rate in most endemic areas is low (about 1–3 per cent), affected animals seldom survive after the disease has reached the stage where clinical signs are obvious. Recovery from 'lunger disease', and similar forms of 'sheep pulmonary adenomatosis' (SPA) has not been reported.

The disease has been transmitted to susceptible sheep by the intranasal and intratracheal inoculation of extracts or filtrates from lesions of diseased lungs. Similar lung lesions had developed in these inoculated animals by the time they were slaughtered about a year later. Attempts to transmit the infection to laboratory animals have been unsuccessful.

At necropsy, the lesions of jaagsiekte consist of small grey or fawn-coloured multifocal nodules which are mostly confined to the apical and cardiac lobes and the lower parts of the diaphragmatic lobes of the lungs. In advanced cases, the lesions may be of different ages, although confluent, and there may be consolidated areas in which secondary bacterial infections are involved. If the lesion is squeezed, a thin frothy fluid usually exudes from the cut surface. The peribronchiolar lymph nodes are usually hyperplastic and markedly enlarged, although a number of typical cases may not show lesions in any other tissue or organ apart from the lungs.

Histologically, the primary lesion of pulmonary adenomatosis is characterized by accumulations of large mononuclear cells, and by proliferation and hyperplasia of the cells lining the bronchioles and alveolar ducts. Papilliform epithelial projections may extend from the alveolar septa causing partial obliteration of the alveolar spaces. The disease is essentially a progressive, transmissible infection and the proliferative nature of the pulmonary lesions, together with metastases, is strong evidence that jaagsiekte is neoplastic.

Ecology

There is good epidemiological evidence that the disease is infectious and that the causative agent can be transmitted naturally by herding healthy and diseased sheep together. In the 1930's, the contagious nature of jaagsiekte was dramatically illustrated in Iceland following the importation of an affected ram from Europe. The first clinical case occurred about one year later and in the next 2–3 years about 60 per cent of young breeding stock became affected and died. Thereafter, the mortality rate dropped to under 10 per cent and, when all sheep in affected areas were slaughtered 12–14 years after the disease was introduced, typical lesions were found in only 2–3 per cent of animals. Thus, the course of the disease in a previously 'clean' population had changed completely in a few years until it resembled the pattern of the disease in other parts of the world where the condition has been endemic for very long periods.

Diagnosis

The clinical symptoms of jaagsiekte are very similar to those of other chronic lung conditions of sheep and accurate diagnosis is only possible by careful histopathological examination of affected lungs.

The propagation of virus in cell cultures is, as yet, too uncertain to be useful in diagnosis and there are no serological tests for the detection of specific antibodies.

Control

No method of active immunization is yet available. The recommended method of control is the elimination of infected sheep as soon as they are recognised, and to seek replacement stock from another source. Epizootic adenomatosis was completely eradicated from Iceland by a slaughter policy.

Cytomegaloviruses

A group of viruses having a particular affinity for the salivary glands and kidneys are probably among the most common parasites of man and animals. They rarely cause disease but tend to persist for very long periods as latent or chronic infections. Unfortunately, on the rare occasions when recognizable disease occurs, the outcome is frequently serious (e.g. neonatal and postnatal cytomegalic inclusion disease of children and inclusion-body rhinitis in baby pigs), and the affected tissues show characteristic enlarged cells, hence the prefix 'cytomegalo'.

Properties of the virus

Morphologically, cytomegaloviruses are indistinguishable from other herpesviruses. Their nucleic acid component is DNA with a molecular weight of about 4×10^7 daltons and a guanine plus cytosine content of 58 per cent. The viruses are fairly sensitive to freezing and thawing and to prolonged storage at —70°C but are said to be stable at —90°C in the presence of 35 per cent sorbitol. They are ether-sensitive and lose their infectivity when heated at 56°C for 30 minutes or when held below pH5.0. They do not haemagglutinate fowl or other species of red blood cells. Complement-fixation tests suggest that human strains of cytomegaloviruses are serologically similar, although 2 and possibly 3 distinct antigenic types have been identified by neutralization tests. There is also evidence that a number of antigenically distinct species-specific cytomegaloviruses can infect domestic animals.

Cultivation

Human and animal cytomegaloviruses are highly species-specific and attempts to infect heterologous hosts are generally unsuccessful. In tissue culture, most cytomegaloviruses grow better in fibroblasts than in epithelial cells, although the latter are chiefly involved *in vivo*, and usually produce focal lesions but only after prolonged incubation. Replication takes place in the nucleus and the outer of the two coats of the virus is derived from the inner nuclear membrane. The growth cycle is slow and progeny virus, which is closely cell-associated, is often not demonstrable in the fluid phase of the cultures.

Stained monolayers contain large acidophilic or basophilic granular intranuclear inclusions up to 15 μm in diameter, surrounded by a clear halo together with small, round or crescent-shaped homogeneous basophilic intracytoplasmic structures (2–4 μm in diameter) lying next to the nucleus.

Pathogenicity

Human strains frequently give rise to inapparent infections of the salivary glands and it has been found that 80 per cent of healthy adults over 35 years of age have antibody to the virus. The most common human disease is a severe and generalised infection of neonates, usually acquired *in utero* from mothers with symptomless infections in which virus is excreted in the urine and saliva. The illness is often fatal in the first 6 months of life. Childhood infections acquired by the respiratory route may cause hepatitis, and adulthood infections may resemble glandular fever. A rare form of lesion is that of a localised granuloma. Reactivation of a latent cytomegalous infection commonly occurs in patients undergoing prolonged immunosuppressive therapy and causes a widely disseminated infection.

Cytomegaloviruses can infect a variety of animal species including monkeys, pigs, sheep, dogs, moles, guinea-pigs, opossums, hamsters and mice. In the natural host the infection is usually inapparent, e.g. salivary gland virus of guinea-pigs, and the characteristic inclusions in the salivary ducts are only discovered on histological examination. Some, however, cause clinical illness, e.g. abortions of rats and inclusion body rhinitis of pigs.

In South Africa, a number of herpes-like viruses have been isolated from the genital organs of cattle with either acute clinical vaginitis and epididymitis or a history of sterility and infertility. Further investigations have shown that these agents possess biological and physicochemical properties similar to those of cytomegaloviruses.

Ecology
Virus has been obtained from oral swabs and urine of 60 per cent of infants under 9 months old. About 10 per cent of normal children under five years of age with 'cytomegalic' cells in their salivary ducts excrete virus in their saliva or urine for many months or years. Older children and adults rarely secrete the virus even though primary subclinical infections continue to occur. Inclusions are rarely seen in the salivary glands of adults and their presence in other adult tissues is usually in association with other severe diseases.

In many species of laboratory animals, the virus is normally present in the saliva, salivary glands, kidneys and probably urine of the younger age-groups.

Diagnosis
Human cytomegaloviruses can be recovered from oral swabs, urine, kidneys, liver or other tissues by inoculating cultures of human embryonic fibroblasts. Small foci of swollen, rounded translucent cells usually appear within 1–2 weeks or longer and stained monolayers contain large intranuclear inclusions. Infected cell suspensions are required for serial passage of the virus to fresh cultures. Attempts to grow the virus on human epithelial cell cultures have failed.

Typical intranuclear 'owl's eye' inclusions may be demonstrated in cells of urinary sediment or in smears prepared from tissues at autopsy, and stained by Giemsa's method. (Plate 56.11b, between pp. 772–3).

Most animal strains of cytomegalovirus can be grown in fibroblast cell cultures derived from the homologous host. The cytopathic effects tend to appear sooner (9–12 days) than with human strains, higher virus titres are obtained and infective virus is often present in the fluid phase of the cultures.

African green monkey cytomegalovirus is unusual in that it grows in monkey kidney cells as well as in human embryonic fibroblasts while inclusion-body rhinitis virus of pigs grows better in pig epithelial than in pig fibroblastic cells.

In human cytomegalovirus infection, serum antibodies can be measured by neutralization tests in cell cultures and a complement-fixing antigen can be prepared from infected human embryonic fibroblasts. Antibodies in human sera can also be demonstrated by immunofluorescence.

Control
There is no specific treatment for cytomegalovirus infections and specific control measures are not yet available.

Inclusion-body rhinitis

Synonyms
Porcine cytomegalic inclusion disease: Einschlusskörpechen rhinitis biem Schwein (Ger.).

Definition
An infectious viral disease of swine characterized by degenerative and inflammatory changes in the nasal mucosa.

Hosts affected
Inclusion-body rhinitis is exclusively a disease of swine.

History and distribution
A disease called infectious atrophic rhinitis of swine has been recognized in Europe for a very long time, possibly since 1842 or earlier. In recent years it has appeared in the U.S.A., Canada and the U.K. The disease is characterized by atrophy of the turbinate bones and distortion of the nasal septum. Although *Bordetella bronchiseptica* and some other bacteria are capable of causing turbinate atrophy, the aetiology of atrophic rhinitis remains undetermined. In 1955, however, a viral inclusion-body rhinitis was reported in piglets in England and was recognized subsequently in many parts of Continental Europe, North America and Australasia. Although the symptoms and post-mortem findings of the 2 conditions are somewhat different, many workers are of the opinion that porcine inclusion-body rhinitis (PIBR) represents the early stages of atrophic rhinitis since the pathognomonic intranuclear in-

clusions found within the glandular epithelium of the mucosa in PIBR can only be detected for a very short time. This might explain the absence of inclusions in atrophic rhinitis which is generally a sub-acute or chronic condition.

Properties of the virus

The causative agent of inclusion-body rhinitis is generally considered to be a herpesvirus of the cytomegalo-type, called Porcine herpesvirus 2. However, like most cytomegalic diseases, porcine inclusion-body rhinitis and atrophic rhinitis are, perhaps, examples of 'opportunistic infections' in which the virus usually causes disease only when precipitating factors such as other concurrent infections (e.g. *Bordetella* or *Haemophilus*) are present which lower the normal resistance of the host.

Cell cultures prepared from the nasal mucosa, kidney, testes and salivary glands of experimentally infected piglets develop intranuclear inclusion bodies, and the 'inclusion agent' has been serially passaged in monolayer cultures of pig lung cells. 'Plasma-clot' cultures of nasal mucosa from experimentally infected piglets can induce the infection in young pigs by intranasal inoculation. Of the many primary and secondary porcine cell culture systems studied, pig lung macrophages are the most susceptible to infection with inclusion-body rhinitis virus. In monolayer cultures, the infected macrophages show a striking cytomegaly with the formation of DNA-positive intranuclear and intracytoplasmic inclusions.

Electron-microscopy of thin-sections of nasal mucosa from naturally infected piglets between 2 and 3 weeks of age, reveals numerous viral particles in the epithelial cells of tubuloalveolar glands. The nuclei of the infected cells are markedly swollen and contain large granular masses of chromatin-like material and various viral forms. The intranuclear virions mostly consist of non-enveloped capsids enclosing nucleoids of various electron densities, locations and shapes. Both enveloped and non-enveloped forms appear between the nuclear membranes. In the cytoplasm, which is often vacuolated, enveloped particles are frequently found within large membrane-bound sacs, whereas naked forms are usually lying free and are often arranged in crystalline arrays. The diameter of the different viral forms range between 45–65 nm, 90–100 nm and 120–150 nm for the nucleoids, non-enveloped virions and enveloped virions, respectively.

Examination of stained monolayer cultures by visible light suggests that the maturing intranuclear inclusion body probably develops from aggregates of small, acidophilic, homogeneous, oval or circular granules located within clear zones in the nucleoplasm. Nuclei each containing a single well-developed inclusion body may be elongated and curved or almost completely circular. In some nuclei reticulate masses of inclusion body material may be seen and it has been suggested that this may represent the final stage of the infective cycle in the cell. It is interesting to note that virus has been isolated from kidneys at a time when characteristic intranuclear inclusions are not present in the nasal mucosa, but not from the nasal mucosa when inclusions are no longer detectable histologically.

Little is known about the physicochemical properties of PIBR virus, but it appears to be ether sensitive and is inactivated at 56°C in 30 minutes. Nasal mucosa from affected piglets retains its infectivity for at least 5 months at —30°C and for 24 hours at 22°C. Virus in supernatant fluids from nasal mucosa cultures may be stored at —60°C for over 2 years.

Pathogenicity

Inclusion-body rhinitis affects particularly 2-week-old piglets but outbreaks often occur in young animals 2–5 weeks after weaning. Pigs over 4 months of age do not appear to develop the disease in a clinically recognizable form. The incubation period is about 7–10 days and the clinical illness is characterized by repeated sneezing and coughing followed by watering of the eyes, a serous nasal discharge and general depression. In very young piglets the nostrils may become blocked with mucopurulent discharges. They may be unable to nurse and frequently die. In a few cases there is nose-bleeding, and atrophy of the turbinates may result in distortion of the snout. The mortality rate is generally low, rarely exceeding 20 per cent, and most infected piglets recover normally within 3–4 weeks.

Pigs can be infected experimentally by intravenous inoculation or by direct infection of the nasal mucosa. Colostrum-deprived piglets are very susceptible and inclusion bodies can readily be produced, usually in 10–20 days, in the nasal mucosa of animals under 10 weeks of age. Pigs over 6 months old are difficult to infect and may be resistant. Small laboratory animals are not susceptible.

The main pathological findings in naturally or artificially infected animals are found in the upper respiratory tract. A variable amount of catarrhal or mucopurulent exudate is present on the nasal mucosa and numerous, small, pale-coloured foci of cellular aggregates can usually be seen in the depths of the mucosa. Similar foci may occur on the surface of the kidneys, but these are the only other organs showing macroscopical lesions.

Histologically, there are a number of large inclusion-bearing cells, up to 40 μm in diameter, in the affected gland cells. These enlarged cells are characteristic of the disease, and their swollen nuclei each bears a single large inclusion surrounded by a clear halo. The intranuclear or 'owl's eye' inclusions appear as granular, basophilic masses measuring about 8–10 μm across. (Plate 56.11c, between pp. 772–3). They are not, however, confined to the nasal mucosa and may occasionally be found in the tubule cells of affected kidneys, or in other organs. Thus, the infection may assume a more generalized form as sometimes occurs in cytomegalovirus infections of other animals. In atrophic rhinitis the characteristic inclusions tend to disappear after about a month and, consequently, the presence of the infection may be difficult to diagnose.

Transmission

Little is known about the natural methods of spread but piglets probably become infected from their dams in the first few weeks of life. Short-range droplet infection and contact with the udder of sows are possible methods of transmission.

Many recovered pigs become latently infected and are capable of shedding virus for a number of years despite the presence of antibodies in their sera. In contrast to cytomegalic disease in man, there is no clear proof, so far, that inclusion-body rhinitis can be contracted *in utero*.

Diagnosis

Symptoms of an infectious rhinitis in young piglets, especially 2–5 weeks after birth or at weaning, should lead to a tentative diagnosis of PIBR. The diagnosis can readily be confirmed by demonstrating clusters of enlarged cells bearing basophilic intranuclear 'owl's eye' inclusions in stained sections or scrapings of the nasal mucosa or, occasionally, of kidneys and other tissues. Characteristic intranuclear inclusions are also present in cell cultures prepared from the nasal mucosa, kidney, testes and salivary glands of affected animals. There are, as yet, no suitable diagnostic serological tests.

Control

Protection by vaccination has not been reported.

Burkitt's lymphoma

There can be no doubt that certain malignant neoplasms in animals are caused by viruses and a considerable amount of evidence for such an association has been accumulated over the past 60 years. On the other hand, no viral agent has been isolated consistently from any human cancer nor proved to be of aetiological significance. However, a highly malignant human tumour currently receiving much attention because of its possible viral aetiology is a malignancy of primitive undifferentiated lymphoreticular cells known as Burkitt's lymphoma.

Burkitt's tumour occurs mainly in tropical areas in Central Africa and, in Uganda, lymphomas of the jaw account for over half of all childhood cancers. Epidemiological evidence based on the unusually strict geographical distribution of this tumour suggests that it might be an arthropod-borne virus-induced neoplasm of the reticulo-endothelial system. Numerous investigations have resulted in the isolation of a variety of viruses associated with the disease, the majority being reoviruses, togaviruses and picornaviruses, but it is unlikely that any one of them is the primary causative agent of the tumour. In 1964, electron microscopy revealed that a high proportion of lymphoblast cell lines established from Burkitt lymphomas contained herpes-type particles, and this virus has been named 'EB' after its discoverers Epstein and Barr. The virus has not yet been cultivated in the conventional manner but its presence can be demonstrated in leucocyte cultures derived from patients with Burkitt lymphoma either by electron microscopy or by immunofluorescence using labelled sera from patients with the disease. The virion is morphologically indistinguishable from other herpesviruses and shows a high degree of cell-associated infectivity which can be transferred from intact infected cells to normal, uninfected human leucocytes. In some respects it most closely resembles the cytomegalovirus group.

The aetiological relationship of EB virus to Burkitt's lymphoma is not yet clear but the majority of workers in this field have shown that a herpes-type virus is associated constantly with the tumour. On the other hand, serological studies indicate that antibodies to EB virus are present in most 'normal' human sera, both in America as well as Africa, and in at least two human diseases other than lymphoma. A report that sera of patients convalescent from glandular fever (infectious mononucleosis) react specifically in the immunofluorescence test with cells of Burkitt's lymphoma, and that leucocytes from glandular fever patients bear the same chromosomal abberation as Burkitt's cells, suggests that EB virus is one cause of glandular fever. It has also been found that patients with carcinoma of the postnasal space invariably possess high titres of antibody to the Epstein-Barr virus. It is interesting to note that all three of these diseases in which EB virus can be epidemiologically implicated are of a lymphoproliferative nature.

Since EB infection is widespread and Burkitt's lymphoma is confined largely to tropical areas in Central Africa, it appears likely that the Epstein-Barr virus is not the only causal agent of the tumour. Several workers have suggested that an unknown mosquito-borne virus or endemic malaria parasites which stimulate the reticulo-endothelial system may play an important contributory role in the pathogenesis of the disease. EB virus, like other herpesviruses, can give rise to persistent latent infections of human tissues and it is possible that the virus in this state, either acting singly or together with other viruses, may induce an abnormal cellular response of the heavily parasitized reticuloendothelial system. As a result, EB virus, instead of persisting as a symptomless infection, becomes frankly oncogenic and induces cellular transformation in the lymphoid tissue and, consequently, tumour growth.

Fish 'pox'

Synonyms
Carp 'pox': epithelioma papillosum: hyperplastic epidermal disease.

Definition
A benign, localized, epidermal hyperplastic viral infection of fish.

Hosts affected
Principally a disease of European propagated fish. Carp are most frequently affected but smelt, pike and perch are also susceptible.

History and distribution
Fish 'pox' has been recognized in Europe for a very long time and an early description of the disease was published in 1563. It is a rare condition in North America.

Properties of the virus
Although the aetiology of fish 'pox' is not fully understood, electron microscopy has clearly shown the presence of viral particles, about 100 nm in diameter, in epidermal-lesion tissue of carp. The mature virions have a ring-shaped nucleoid, 50 nm across, surrounded by an outer membrane about 7 nm thick. Viral particles, 140–150 nm in diameter, with a double-layered limiting membrane are generally to be found scattered throughout the cytoplasm. Stained sections of affected tissues show numerous intranuclear inclusion bodies of Cowdry type A.

In most respects the fish 'pox' virus is morphologically indistinguishable from herpesviruses.

Pathogenicity
The disease is characterized by chronic localized cutaneous proliferations especially on the skin, fins and eyes, but other parts of the body may also be affected. The lesions consist of firm milky-white or grey papillary-like growths. There is little or no inflammatory response and the lesions are difficult to distinguish from true neoplasms although there

is no metastasis. Carp with extensive lesions may also show osteomalacia.

Cultivation
It is stressed that the causative virus has not yet been isolated from cases of fish 'pox' and there is no clear evidence that the condition is infectious. Nevertheless, independent workers have recently claimed successful transmission of infection by applying lesion homogenates to the pharynx and gills of healthy fish. It has also been reported that inoculated fish-cell cultures show multinucleated giant-cells, cytoplasmic inclusions and vacuolation of infected cells.

Ecology
Parasites are invariably associated with fish 'pox' and several workers consider that a vector might be involved in transmission of the infection.

Control
There is no known treatment and control is best achieved by strict attention to hygiene, including disinfection and removal of affected fish.

Further reading

BELL T.M. (1967) Viruses associated with Burkitt's tumor. *Progress in Medical Virology*, **9**, 1.

BOOTH J.C., GOODWIN R.F.W. AND WHITTLESTONE P. (1967) Inclusionbody rhinitis of pigs: attempts to grow the causal agent in tissue culture. *Research in Veterinary Science*, **8**, 338.

CARMICHAEL L.E., STRANDBERG J.D. AND BARNES F.D. (1965) Identification of a cytopathogenic agent infectious for puppies as a canine herpesvirus. *Proceedings of the Society for Experimental Biology and Medicine*, **120**, 644.

CARMICHAEL L.E., SQUIRE R.A. AND KROOK L. (1965) Clinical and pathologic features of a fatal viral disease of newborn pups. *American Journal of Veterinary Research*, **26**, 803.

CHURCHILL A.E. (1968) Herpes-type virus isolated in cell cultures from tumours of chickens with Marek's disease. I. Studies in cell cultures. *Journal of the National Cancer Institute*, **41**, 939.

CHURCHILL A.E. AND BIGGS P.M. (1967) Agent of Marek's disease in tissue culture. *Nature*, **215**, 528.

CORNWELL H.J.C. AND WRIGHT N.G. (1969) Neonatal canine herpesvirus infection: a review of present knowledge. *Veterinary Record*, **84**, 2.

CORNWELL H.J.C., WRIGHT N.G., CAMPBELL R.S.F., ROBERTS R.J. AND REID A. (1966). Neonatal disease in dogs associated with a herpes-like virus. *Veterinary Record*, **79**, 661.

CRANDELL R.A. (1967) The herpesvirus group. *American Journal of Veterinary Research*, **28**, 577.

CRANDELL R.A., REHKEMPER J.A., NIEMAN W.H., GANAWAY J.R. AND MAURER F.D. (1961) Experimental feline rhinotracheitis. *Journal of the American Veterinary Medical Association*, **138**, 191.

DITCHFIELD J. AND GRINYER I. (1965) Feline rhinotracheitis virus: a feline herpesvirus. *Virology*, **26**, 504.

DOLL E.R. AND BRYANS J.T. (1963) Epizootiology of equine viral rhinopneumonitis. *Journal of the American Veterinary Medical Association*, **142**, 31.

DONE J.T. (1958) An 'inclusion-body' rhinitis of pigs (Preliminary report). *Veterinary Record*, **70**, 525.

DOW C. AND MCFERRAN J.B. (1962) The pathology of Aujeszky's disease in the pig. *Journal of Comparative Pathology and Therapeutics*, **72**, 337.

DOW C. AND MCFERRAN J.B. (1962) The neuropathology of Aujeszky's disease in the pig. *Research in Veterinary Science*, **3**, 436.

DOW C. AND MCFERRAN J.B. (1966) Experimental studies on Aujeszky's disease in cattle. *Journal of Comparative Pathology and Therapeutics*, **76**, 379.

DUNCAN J.R., RAMSEY F.K. AND SWITZER W.P. (1965) Electron microscopy of cytomegalic inclusion disease of swine (inclusion body rhinitis). *American Journal of Veterinary Research*, **26**, 939.

EDINGTON N., SMITH I.M., PLOWRIGHT W. AND WATT R.G. (1976) Relationship of porcine cytomegalovirus and *B. bronchiseptica* to atrophic rhinitis in gnotobiotic piglets. *Veterinary Record*, **98**, 42.

EPSTEIN M.A. ACHONG B.G. AND POPE J.H. (1967) Virus in cultured lymphoblasts from a New Guinea Burkitt lymphoma. *British Medical Journal*, **2**, 290.

FRASER G. AND RAMACHANDRAN S.P. (1969) Studies on the virus of Aujeszky's disease. I. Pathogenicity for rats and mice. *Journal of Comparative Pathology and Therapeutics*, **79**, 435.

GALLOWAY I.A. (1938) Aujeszky's disease. *Veterinary Record*, **50**, 745.

GRATZEB J.B., CHENNEKATU P.P. AND RAMSEY F.K. (1966) Isolation and characterization of a strain of infectious bovine rhinotracheitis virus associated with enteritis in cattle: isolation, serologic characterization, and induction of the experimental disease. *American Journal of Veterinary Research*, **27**, 1567.

HANSHAW J.B. (1968) Cytomegaloviruses. *Virology Monographs*, **3**, 1.

HANSON R.P. (1954) The history of pseudorabies in the United States. *Journal of the American Veterinary Medical Association*, **124**, 259.

HARTLEY E.G. (1966) 'B' virus disease in monkey and man. *British Veterinary Journal*, **122**, 46.

HENLE G., HENLE W. AND DIEHL V. (1968) Relation of Burkitt's tumour-associated herpes-type virus to infectious mononucleosis. *Proceedings of the National Academy of Sciences of the United States of America*, **59**, 94.

HESS W.R. AND DARDIRI A.H. (1968) Some properties of the virus of duck plague. *Archiv für die gesamte Virusforschung*, **24**, 148.

JEFFCOTT L.B. AND ROSSDALE P.D. (1976) Practical aspects of equine virus abortion in the United Kingdom. *Veterinary Record*, **98**, 153.

JOHNSON R.H. AND THOMAS R.G. (1966) Feline viral rhinotracheitis in Britain. *Veterinary Record*, **79**, 188.

KAPLAN A.S. (1969) Herpes simplex and pseudorabies viruses. *Virology Monographs*, **5**, 1.

KAPLAN A.S. AND BEN-PORAT T. (1964) Mode of replication of pseudorabies virus DNA. *Virology*, **23**, 90.

MACKAY J.M.K. (1969) Tissue culture studies of sheep pulmonary adenomatosis (Jaagsiekte). I. Direct cultures of affected lungs. *Journal of Comparative Pathology and Therapeutics*, **79**, 141.

MACKAY J.M.K. (1969) Tissue culture studies of sheep pulmonary adenomatosis (Jaagsiekte). II. Transmission of cytopathic effects to normal cultures. *Journal of Comparative Pathology and Therapeutics*, **79**, 147.

MARTIN W.B., MARTIN B., HAY D. AND LAUDER I.M. (1966) Bovine ulcerative mammillitis caused by a herpesvirus. *Veterinary Record*, **78**, 494.

MCCRACKEN R.M., MCFERRAN J.B. AND DOW C. (1973) The neural spread of pseudorabies virus in calves. *Journal of General Virology*, **20**, 17.

MCFERRAN J.B. AND DOW C. (1964) Virus studies on experimental Aujeszky's disease (pseudorabies virus) in experimentally infected swine. *American Journal of Veterinary Research*, **26**, 631.

NAZERIAN K., SOLOMAN J.J., WITTER R.L. AND BURMESTER B.R. (1968) Studies on the etiology of Marek's disease. II. Finding of a herpesvirus in cell culture. *Proceedings of the Society for Experimental Biology and Medicine*, **127**, 177.

PAYNE L.N. AND BIGGS P.M. (1967) Studies on Marek's disease. II. Pathogenesis. *Journal of the National Cancer Institute*, **39**, 281.

PERK J., MICHALIDES R., SPIEGLEMAN S. AND SCHLOM J. (1974) Biochemical and morphologic evidence for the presence of an RNA tumour virus in pulmonary carcinoma of sheep (Jaagsiekte). *Journal of the National Cancer Institute*, **53**, 131.

PLOWRIGHT W. (1963) The role of game animals in the epizootiology of rinderpest and malignant catarrhal fever in East Africa. *Bulletin of Epizootic Diseases of Africa*, **11**, 149.

PLOWRIGHT W. (1965) Malignant catarrhal fever in East Africa. II. Observations on Wildebeest calves at the laboratory and contact transmission of the infection to cattle. *Research in Veterinary Science*, **6**, 69.

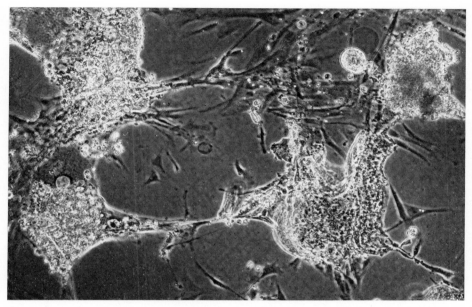

56.9 Monolayer of primary chick kidney cells 48 hours after inoculation with the virus of avian infectious laryngo-tracheitis. Phase contrast microscopy shows the presence of large, highly refractile, multinucleate syncytia, × 240.

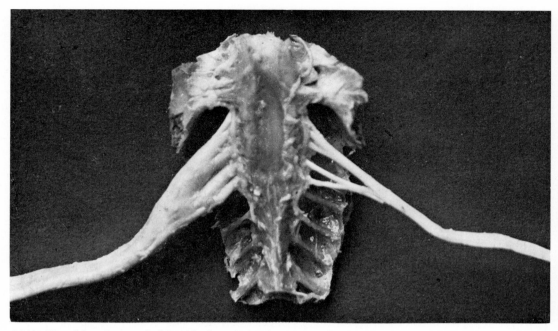

56.10 Neural lymphomatosis (Marek's disease) showing gross unilateral swelling of the right sciatic nerve plexus.

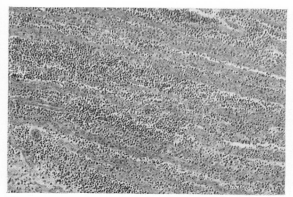

56.11a

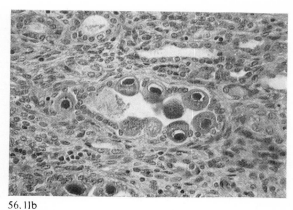

56.11b

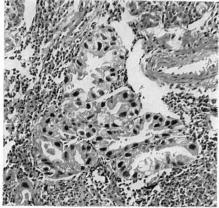

56.11c

56.11a Section through the sciatic nerve of a chicken dying from Marek's disease, showing massive lymphoid infiltration. Haematoxylin eosin stain, × 90.

56.11b Section of kidney from a fatal case of cyto-megalic disease in a child. The nuclei of enlarged epithelial cells contain basophilic inclusions. Shrinkage of the inclusion gives the cell its characteristic 'owl's eye' appearance. Haematoxylin eosin stain, × 240.

56.11c Section through the nasal turbinate of a piglet suffering from inclusion body rhinitis. Large basophilic (cytomegalic) inclusions almost completely fill affected cells in the subepithelial glands. Associated secondary bacterial infection causes epithelial desquamation and interstitial polymorph infiltration. Haematoxylin eosin stain, × 133.

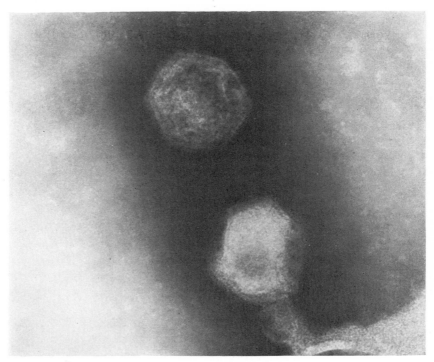

57.1 Negatively stained preparation of Tipula iridescent virus. The virions consist of an electron-dense centrally placed nucleoid surrounded by a clearly defined hexagonal outer shell, × 200 000. (Courtesy Dr C. R. Madeley.)

PLOWRIGHT W. (1968) Malignant catarrhal fever. *Journal of the American Veterinary Medical Association*, **152**, 795.

PLOWRIGHT W. (1967) Malignant catarrhal fever in East Africa. III Neutralizing antibody in free-living wildebeest *Research in Veterinary Science*, **8**, 129.

PLOWRIGHT W., MACADAM R.F. AND ARMSTRONG J.A. (1965) Growth and characterization of the virus of bovine malignant catarrhal fever in East Africa. *Journal of General Microbiology*, **39**, 253.

PLOWRIGHT W., PERRY C.T. AND GREIG A. (1974) Sexual transmission of African Swine Fever virus in the tick (*Ornithodoros moubata porcinus*. Walton). *Research in Veterinary Science*, **17**, 106.

PLUMMER G. (1967) Comparative virology of the herpes group. *Progress in Medical Virology*, **9**, 302.

PLUMMER G. AND WATERSON A.P. (1963) Equine herpesviruses. *Virology*, **19**, 412.

POVEY C. (1976) Viral diseases of cats: current concepts. *Veterinary Record*, **98**, 293.

POVEY R.C. AND JOHNSON R.H. (1967) Further observations on feline viral rhinotracheitis. *Veterinary Record*, **81**, 686.

PRYDIE J., HARRISON M.J. AND GRAHAM J. (1966) Isolation of a canine herpesvirus. *Veterinary Record*, **79**, 660.

PURCHASE H.G. AND BIGGS P.M. (1967) Characterization of five isolates of Marek's disease. *Research in Veterinary Science*, **8**, 440.

RAMACHANDRAN S. AND FRASER G. (1971) Studies on the virus of Aujeszky's disease. 11. Pathogenicity for chicks. *Journal of Comparative Pathology and Therapeutics*, **81**, 55.

REID H.W. AND ROWE L. (1973) The attenuation of a Herpes virus (Malignant Catarrhal Fever virus) isolated from hartebeest (*Alcelaphus cokei*. Gunther). *Research in Veterinary Science*, **15**, 144.

ROIZMAN B. AND SPEAR P.G. (1971) Herpesviruses: current information on the composition and structure. In, Comparative Virology, ed. K. Maramorosch and E. Kurstak, p. 510. London: Academic Press.

ROSS L.J.N., BASARAB O., WALKER D.J. AND WHITBY B. (1975) Serological relationship between a pathogenic strain of Marek's disease virus, its attenuated derivative and herpes virus of turkeys. *Journal of General Virology*, **28**, 37.

RWEYEMAMU M.M. AND JOHNSON R.H. (1967) Bovine herpes mammillitis virus. I. In-vitro behaviour of the virus. *British Veterinary Journal*, **123**, 482.

SCHWARTZ W.L. AND MARTIN W.D. (1966) Canine herpesvirus infection of puppies. *Veterinary Medicine*, **61**, 1171.

SINGH K.V. (1962) A plaque assay of pseudorabies virus monolayers of porcine kidney cells. *Cornell Veterinarian*, **52**, 237.

SICCARDI F.J. AND BURMESTER B.R. (1970) The differential diagnosis of lymphoid leukosis and Marek's disease. Technical Bulletin 1412, p. 1. Agricultural Research Service. U.S. Department of Agriculture.

STORZ J. (1968) Comments on malignant catarrhal fever. *Journal of the American Veterinary Medical Association*, **152**, 804.

STUDDERT M.J. (1974) Comparative aspects of equine herpesviruses. *Cornell Veterinarian*, **64**, 94.

VALICEK L., SMID B., PLEVA V. AND MENSIK J. (1970) Porcine cytomegalic inclusion disease virus. Electron microscopic study of the nasal mucosa. *Archiv für die gesamte Virusforschung*, **32**, 19.

WATRACH A.M. AND BAHNEMANN H. (1966) The structure of bovine rhinotracheitis virus. *Archiv für die gesamte Virusforschung*, **18**, 1.

WATT R.G., PLOWRIGHT W., SABO A. AND EDINGTON N. (1973) A sensitive cell culture system for the virus of porcine inclusion body rhinitis (Cytomegalic Inclusion Disease). *Research in Veterinary Science*, **14**, 119.

CHAPTER 57

IRIDOVIRUSES

Iridoviruses

In 1965, the name 'Iridovirus' was suggested to designate a number of large DNA viruses with cubic symmetry of the compound type. Members of this newly introduced genus, sometimes termed 'icosahedral cytoplasmic deoxyriboviruses' (ICDVs), include *Tipula* iridescent virus of the cranefly ("daddy longlegs") and, probably, *Aëdes* iridescent virus and other iridescent viruses of the mosquito. Viruses that have been provisionally grouped with the iridoviruses include amphibian icosahedral cytoplasmic deoxyriboviruses, African swine fever virus, cauliflower mosaic virus and lymphocystis virus of fish (*Stizostedion*); but many other members have been isolated from reptiles, insects, molluscs, protozoa, plants, fungi and algae.

All members of the group contain a single molecule of double-stranded DNA with a molecular weight of about 130×10^6 daltons and a guanine plus cytosine (G+C) base content of 29 to 32 per cent. Replication occurs in the cytoplasm and the accumulation of complex icosahedral viral particles in 'cytoplasmic factories' is readily demonstrated. The relatively large size (130–200 nm) of some of the iridoviruses is one of their most striking features and the largest, lymphocystis virus, may measure 240–300 nm in diameter. The surface shell of the capsid consists of between 812 and 1500 capsomeres, as compared with 252 for adenovirus or 162 for herpesvirus. Some possible members have a lipid-containing envelope and are sensitive to ether, but those affecting insects are apparently ether-resistant.

African swine fever

Synonyms
Wart-hog disease: East African swine fever.

Definition
A highly contagious often peracute viral disease of domestic swine characterized by high fever, marked cyanosis of the skin, pronounced haemorrhages of the lymph nodes and internal organs, with a mortality rate approaching 100 per cent. The clinical signs and lesions of African swine fever are strikingly similar to those of European swine fever (hog cholera) but the viruses responsible for these two diseases are quite distinct.

Hosts affected
African swine fever infection occurs naturally in domestic swine (*Sus scropa*), warthogs (*Phacochoerus aethiopicus*) and bushpigs (*Potamochoerus porcus*); and the virus has also been isolated from the third important species of pig indigenous to Africa, the giant forest hog (*Hylochoerus meinertz hageni*). Horses, cattle, sheep, goats, dogs, cats and poultry are not susceptible.

History and distribution
African swine fever is a relatively 'new' disease of swine which appeared in East Africa in the early years of this century following the importation of domestic pigs from Europe by the early settlers. It was quickly realised that this peracute type of 'swine fever' was occurring only in free-range pigs on farms where contact with other domestic pigs could definitely be excluded and, further, that bush pigs and wart-hogs were invariably present on land where fresh outbreaks occurred. In 1921, it was reported that pigs immune to classical swine fever were susceptible to this new disease and that hyperimmune swine fever serum would not protect pigs against challenge infection with the East African type of virus. It was also discovered that experimentally infected feral pigs developed sub-clinical or symptomless infections only. Earlier suggestions by the colonists in Kenya that wild pigs were associated with the spread of the disease were confirmed in 1932 when the causative virus of African swine fever was isolated from 3 out of 4 apparently healthy warthogs.

Since 1910, the disease spread rapidly to most African territories south of the Equator but caused little concern to the rest of the world until 1957 when it was observed for the first time in Europe, on a farm near Lisbon airport. Investigations showed that the epizootic which occurred in Portugal was due to pigs being fed food waste from planes arriving from Angola. The infection was quickly eradicated by a policy of slaughter but reappeared near Lisbon 2 years later, and spread to Spain in 1960. Since then, a number of isolated outbreaks have occurred in Southern France and Brittany and, in 1967, a case was confirmed in Italy on a farm near Rome.

Classification

Although African swine fever virus was first characterized in 1921, it has not been possible as yet to assign it to any recognised group of animal viruses. Suggestions that it might be a myxovirus, because it haemadsorbed swine erythrocytes, or that it was a type of herpesvirus, because it contained DNA and showed icosahedral symmetry, are no longer accepted and, in 1967, it was provisionally classified as a member of the iridescent virus group in the newly formed genus *Iridovirus*.

Morphology

Ultra-thin sections of infected cells show that African swine fever virus accumulates in the cytoplasm. The virus particle measures about 175–220 nm in diameter and consists of an electron-dense centrally placed nucleoid (70–90 nm across) surrounded by a clearly defined hexagonal outer shell. (Plate 57.1 facing p. 773). As the mature virion emerges from the host cell it seems to acquire an additional outer envelope which is probably derived by budding from the plasma membrane. In negative-contrast preparations the virions appear as large enveloped particles with cubic symmetry of the compound type. The edge-length of the icosahedron is about 85 nm and the outer shell of the capsid consists of a large number of irregular repeating sub-units in triangular arrangement. The number of capsomeres is probably 812 but possibly more.

Chemical composition

Evidence that the nucleic acid component contains DNA is provided by the fact that inclusions in infected cells stain as for DNA with Feulgen and acridine orange stains; growth is inhibited by treatment with IUDR, BUDR or FUDR and the effect is reversed by the addition of thymidine; viral activity is not affected by ribonuclease (RNase) but DNase digestion of the nucleoid is effective up to 1–4 hours on formalin—but not gluteraldehyde-fixed cells.

Physicochemical properties

African swine fever virus is less stable at high temperatures than swine fever (hog cholera) virus and is inactivated in 30 minutes at 55°C and in 10 minutes at 60°C. African swine fever virus is unusually stable in the presence of serum: the half-life of the virus at 37°C in a medium containing 25 per cent serum is 24 hours, but without added serum the half-life is reduced to 8 hours. The resistance of African swine fever virus at low temperatures is very marked and virus has been known to survive for years when dried at room temperature or frozen on skin or muscle. The virus is stable in pig blood held at 5°C for periods up to 18 months, and infected pig spleen retains its original infectivity for at least 2 years when stored at −70°C. It is unusually resistant to adverse environmental stresses and is able to survive in putrefying blood and excretions. It survives in chilled carcases for 15 weeks or longer, in processed hams for 5 months and in bone marrows for up to 6 months. It is stable over a wide pH range but is inactivated by 0.05 per cent β-propiolactone, acetylethyleneimine, or glycidaldehyde in 60 minutes at 37°C, by 1 per cent formaldehyde in 6 days, by 2 per cent sodium hydroxide in 24 hours and by lipid solvents such as ether and chloroform. The most practical method of disinfection is the application of 2 per cent NaOH in the proportion of 1 litre per square metre. The enveloped virion resists digestion by proteolytic enzymes but is readily inactivated by pancreatic lipase, while the outer hexagonal shell of the non-enveloped particle is removed by the action of pepsin but not trypsin.

Haemagglutination

Attempts to demonstrate specific haemagglutinins in the fluid phase of infected cell cultures or in tissue extracts from infected pigs have been unsuccessful. Despite the apparent absence of haemagglutinins, normal pig erythrocytes are readily adsorbed to the surface of infected leucocyte cultures due, it is believed, to the incorporation of a novel virus-specific antigen in the surface membrane of the infected leucocyte. The effect is inhibited by immune African swine fever serum and a haemadsorption-inhibition test is said to be strain specific.

Antigenic properties

African swine fever is quite distinct in cross-immunity tests from classical swine fever, but immunity, even to the homologous strain, appears to be transient. The complement-fixation test is group-reactive but specific antigens can be detected by means of gel diffusion and haemadsorption-inhibition tests. In agar gels, sera from pigs surviving infection with all known strains of African swine fever virus form six precipitin lines of identity, but the total number of lines depends upon the serum used and the source and concentration of the antigen.

The highest concentration of antigens is found in lymph nodes, spleen, liver and kidneys of pigs infected with virulent virus, but in pigs inoculated with attenuated strains no antigen is detectable in the viscera even though the avirulent virus stimulates antibody production. In Africa, at least eight different serotypes including the Uganda, Tengani and Hinde strains have been described by means of carefully controlled haemadsorption-inhibition tests and in Europe differences have been found between the 1957 and 1960 isolates from Portugal. It is emphasised, however, that these minor antigenic differences bear little relationship to the immunological status of different isolates.

Despite the fact that *in vitro* serological tests show considerable antigenic overlapping it has not been possible, so far, to demonstrate neutralizing antibodies in sera from pigs refractory to challenge infection. Nevertheless, more than one immunological type of virus must exist since it has frequently been shown that pigs refractory to one strain of virus may not withstand challenge inoculation with an heterologous strain. It is possible, however, that resistance to infection may not depend on the presence of detectable amounts of neutralizing antibodies and that the refractory state in African swine fever differs from that of classical immunity.

In Africa, a multiplicity of types exists but in European countries only the Portugal isolate of 1959 now appears to be dominant.

Cultivation

Growth occurs in the yolk sac of embryonated hens' eggs and some strains are capable of killing the embryos in 6 or 7 days provided the virus has been previously passaged through a series of alternating pig/rabbit passages.

Most strains can be readily propagated without previous adaptation in primary cultures of phagocytic mononuclear cells derived from the 'buffy-coat' or bone marrow of healthy pigs. Adapted virus can be propagated on cell cultures prepared from other pig tissues and on a variety of continuous cell-lines, with or without the production of a cytopathic effect. Adaptation of recently isolated strains may be enhanced by frequent changes of the growth medium and by repeated trypsinization of the infected cell monolayers. Virus adapted to growth in pig kidney cell-lines may be grown in chicken or bovine kidney cell cultures as well as in a variety of established lines such as BHK-21 and Vero cells with or without the production of nuclear and cytoplasmic inclusions. Serial passage of the virus in 'buffy' coat or bone marrow cultures at 5-day intervals for 60 or more transfers reduces the virulence of several virus strains for domestic swine.

Horses, cattle, sheep, dogs, cats, rats, mice, hamsters and poultry are resistant to the natural and experimental infection but virus adapted by a series of alternating passages in rabbits and pigs has been shown to induce haemorrhagic lesions in rabbits similar to those found in naturally infected pigs. Adapted virus has also been propagated in goats. Although rabbit and goat adapted strains after 100 passes may be less virulent for swine there is no evidence that they will immunize pigs against a virulent strain. Moreover, at least one lapinized strain is known to have reverted to full virulence following serial passage in pigs.

Pathogenicity

In most naturally occurring outbreaks, the onset of clinical symptoms may be sudden and the similarity to acute swine fever is striking. The incubation period varies from 5–15 days and the mortality rate may approach 100 per cent. In Angola, and more recently in Portugal and Spain, the strains of virus are less virulent and a relatively high percentage of pigs may survive. Surviving animals usually remain symptomless carriers for life. In peracute cases, death may be the first indication of the disease. In other acute infections, early symptoms include a rapid temperature rise to about 40.5°C or higher, and marked leukopenia. After 3–4 days of fever, affected animals stop eating, become weak, incoordinate and cyanotic. Some may show respiratory distress, coughing, vomiting and blood-stained diarrhoea, all of which resemble the signs of classical swine fever, but death usually occurs about 5–7 days after the onset of fever. In most African outbreaks, the few pigs that survive either develop a chronic form of the disease or become inapparent carriers, with a viraemia lasting for many months or even years, although the virus is not continually present in the secretions. The disease naturally affects warthogs (*Phacochoerus*) and bush pigs (*Potamochoerus*) which tolerate the infection without showing clinical signs of disease and also serve as carriers of the virus.

Following infection, mainly by ingestion or inhalation, the virus is adsorbed on to the red blood cells and undergoes haematogeneous dissemination. The virus has a marked affinity for the vasculo-endothelial cells and generalized viral damage to the walls of the small blood vessels usually gives rise to oedema, congestion, haemorrhage, infarction and thrombosis.

At necropsy, an almost unbelievable degree of haemorrhage may be seen .throughout the entire carcase, including the alimentary tract, and there is marked petechiation of the larynx, urinary bladder, renal cortex, heart, lungs and visceral surfaces of organs. The lymph nodes are enlarged and so severely haemorrhagic that they give the appearance of haematomas. Pleural, pericardial and peritoneal fluids are excessive and the spleen is up to 3 times its normal size. Perivascular haemorrhages and oedema may be widespread in the central nervous system in the early stages of the disease.

Under experimental conditions, the peracute form of African swine fever can be readily produced by instilling the virus into the nasal or oral cavities of domestic pigs. Following intranasal inoculation, the virus initially infects the lymphoid tissue of the pharyngeal mucosa whence it quickly spreads to the retropharyngeal lymph nodes, or it may invade the tonsillar crypts and mandibular lymph nodes. From these primary sites of infection the virus probably spreads via the lymph ducts and blood stream to almost all parts of the body. Generalized infection and the onset of fever usually occur by the 3rd or 4th day post-inoculation. African swine fever virus has a marked affinity for cellular elements of the reticulo-endothelial system. As the infection progresses, large concentrations of virus can be demonstrated in the bone-marrow, liver, spleen and lungs, and these tissues are considered to be the principal secondary sites of viral multiplication.

Ecology
In most endemic areas in Africa, spread of infection between apparently healthy carrier warthogs and domestic pigs follows indirect contact and is readily prevented by the erection of pig-proof fences. Serological and virus isolation studies indicate that most warthogs of approximately 6 months of age have precipitating antibodies in their sera and some may carry the virus in the blood, spleen, liver, lungs, kidneys, and especially the lymph nodes. Although warthogs do not usually excrete virus in their urine or faeces it has been suggested that the stresses of pregnancy and farrowing may activate the latent virus which then passes *in utero* to the fetus or overspills into the secretions and excretions.

Acutely-ill pigs are highly contagious and once the disease is established in a herd, the infection spreads rapidly by contact through muzzling or by ingestion of infected fomites. Chronically-ill animals and most apparently healthy survivors usually become carriers for life and shed the virus intermittently in their discharges. Since the virus is exceptionally hardy and persists in the tissues of carcases of carrier animals, the feeding of swill containing uncooked pork scraps constitutes the principal source of secondary epidemics and of virgin outbreaks in countries previously free of the disease.

It is surprisingly difficult, under experimental conditions, to establish contact transmission between infected warthogs and susceptible domestic pigs but the fact that the virus has been isolated from ticks found in piggeries where African swine fever had occurred suggested that arthropods may play an important role in the transmission of the natural infection. In some areas of East Africa, the argasid tick (*Ornithodoros moubata porcinus*) which is a frequent inhabitant of warthog burrows is not uncommonly infected with African swine fever virus, and there is evidence that viral replication and transovarial transmission can occur in these arthropods. In Spain, the virus has been isolated from *O. erraticus*. It seems likely, therefore, that argasid ticks play an important part in the maintenance of virus reservoirs and in the spread of the virus to pigs. Thus, African swine fever is the only icosahedral cytoplasmic DNA virus known to infect a mammal, and is the only DNA virus to qualify as an arthropodborne virus.

Immunity
The virus of African swine fever is unusual in that most strains are of high virulence but low immunogenicity. Although complement-fixing, precipitating, haemadsorption-inhibiting and other antibodies are usually produced within 7–21 days, it is extremely difficult to demonstrate significant levels of neutralizing antibodies in sera of pigs that have recovered from natural or experimental infections. Nor does incubation of immune sera with African swine fever virus prior to inoculation result in the inactivation of the virus. The protective antibody response, if produced, is of low potency and short duration whereas viraemia invariably persists for many months or even years. In this respect African swine fever resembles infectious equine anaemia and serum hepatitis in man, in that blood from symptomless viral carriers may induce the overt disease in the natural susceptible host. Despite the apparent lack of neutralizing or protective antibodies, pigs that survive the primary reaction usually withstand challenge with the homologous virus but never with heterologous strains, whether or not a viraemia is present. Thus, resistance to African swine fever does not appear to be associated with the presence of detectable amounts of serum antibodies nor with persisting infection and premunity. However, fully-attenuated strains administered prior to partially-attenuated strains may interfere with the ability of the latter to induce resistance and, for this reason, it has been suggested that resistance to reinfection might be associated with the formation of an interferon-like substance. More recently, it has been reported that a state of delayed hypersensitivity is produced in African swine fever and that the T and B immunocytes are apparently not impaired.

Diagnosis

African swine fever should always be suspected when a contagious, acute or peracute haemorrhagic syndrome, accompanied by high mortality, is encountered in domestic pigs that have been successfully vaccinated against classical swine fever. In other circumstances the clinical signs and post-mortem lesions are often presumptively diagnostic, particularly in enzootic areas where there has been possible contact with warthogs or bush pigs. On the other hand, provisional diagnosis may be extremely difficult in less acute or inapparent infections, and especially in outbreaks occurring in Europe where the current Portuguese strains have been modified as a result of natural serial passage in domestic pigs and following extensive use of attenuated vaccines. Because of this, the disease is becoming increasingly difficult to distinguish from classical swine fever. Accurate diagnosis requires laboratory confirmation by isolation and identification of the causative virus, by histopathological examination of the spleen and lymph nodes, and by demonstration of precipitins, complement-fixing and haemadsorption-inhibiting antibodies, if paired serum samples are available.

The oldest and still, perhaps, the most reliable diagnostic test for African swine fever is the inoculation of suspensions of spleen from a suspected case into groups of swine-fever-susceptible and swine-fever-immune pigs in conditions of strict isolation. Reactions will develop in both groups of animals if the suspected material contains African swine fever virus but only the susceptible pigs will react if the inoculum contains swine fever virus. These cross-immunity tests are accurate but laborious to perform, especially if swine-fever-immune pigs are not readily available. In these circumstances the test can be modified by injecting hyperimmune swine fever antiserum simultaneously with the suspected material into one group of susceptible pigs. Hyperimmune swine fever antiserum, even in massive doses, will not protect against African swine fever. Complement-fixation, immunofluorescence and gel diffusion tests can be used to demonstrate the presence of viral antigen in tissue suspensions of reacting animals provided a good African swine fever antiserum is available.

The detection of African swine fever antibodies in sera from clinically affected or carrier swine may be possible by complement-fixation and gel diffusion tests using concentrated antigen obtained from infected cell cultures rather than prepared directly from infected pig tissues. More recently, a reverse single radial immunodiffusion test has been developed for the detection of antibodies in swine infected with African swine fever virus. In this procedure, the suspect serum is added to wells cut in an agarose gel and impregnated with an appropriate concentration of African swine fever antigen. The plate is held overnight at room temperature. The efficacy of reverse radial immunodiffusion is much greater than that of the agar gel diffusion precipitin test and is particularly suitable for sera from acute cases but slightly poorer for sera from vaccinated animals and from pigs with chronic African swine fever.

The important discovery in 1960, that leucocyte cultures infected with African swine fever virus showed haemadsorption of healthy pig red blood cells provided a simple and reliable test for the rapid diagnosis of the disease. The method consists of bleeding a healthy pig, defibrinating the blood and removing the serum by centrifugation. The 'buffy-coat' (leucocyte) layer is then carefully harvested, together with a few erythrocytes, and suspended in the serum from which they were separated. Antibiotics are added and the leucocyte-serum mixture is dispensed in 2.0 ml. amounts in clean, sterile, culture-tubes, preferably the flat-sided Leighton type, tightly stoppered and incubated in the stationary position at 37°C for 24 hours. The procedure requires no special cell culture media and the healthy surviving leucocytes settle and become firmly attached to the glass. The leucocyte cultures are then inoculated with 0.2 ml. of a 20 per cent suspension of spleen from a suspect case of African swine fever, reincubated for 24–48 hours and examined for the presence of red blood cells adhering to the surface of those leucocytes infected with virus. Cytolysis usually follows within a few days. The specificity of the reaction can be confirmed by a haemadsorption-inhibition test.

All types of African swine fever virus isolated in Africa, and all strains recovered during the initial outbreaks in Europe, possess the property of haemadsorption. Unfortunately, however, recent isolates from Europe do so only after a number of passages in leucocyte cultures or when reinoculated into pigs. It is generally agreed that strains of classical swine fever virus do not induce haemadsorption of normal pig erythrocytes but recent reports from Germany suggest that under certain circumstances a few strains may possess this property. Despite these and certain other deficiencies, the haemadsorption test has proved to be of great practical value in the rapid diagnosis of African swine fever.

Histopathological examination of spleen, lymph nodes and brain may prove helpful, the most important distinguishing features being severe necrosis and karyorrhexis of lymphocytes in the lymphoid tissues, and a marked leucopenia.

Control

In endemic regions of Africa, there is a multiplicity

of types of virus and field vaccination is largely discouraged. In Europe, one type of virus appears to be dominant and, while the dangers of using live virus vaccines to control a disease in which persistent latently infected recovered animals is well recognised, attenuated strains have been widely used as vaccines in Spain and Portugal. Although vaccinated pigs may develop high-titre antibodies, they frequently fail to develop satisfactory resistance. Moreover, the extensive use of attenuated virus vaccines results in a marked increase in the number of healthy carriers and widespread dissemination of the virus.

Since a satisfactory vaccine is not yet available, the most effective means of controlling the disease is by preventing susceptible pigs gaining access to infected animals, carcases and food products including uncooked swill. The slaughter of all affected and in-contact pigs is usually effective provided the measures are carried out promptly and efficiently. In Africa, susceptible domestic swine must be prevented from coming into contact with wart-hogs and bush pig.

Lymphocystis disease of fish

Definition
A commonly occurring benign viral disease of fish characterized by tumour-like lesions of the skin and fins.

History and distribution
Hyperplastic and neoplastic diseases of fish have been recognised for many years and the oldest and perhaps best known fish virus is that of lymphocystis.

The presence of enormously enlarged connective tissue cells ('lymphocystis cells') in affected fish was described by several workers during the 19th century and it was generally believed that the causal agent was a form of protozoal parasite. In 1914, however, it was claimed that the disease was probably caused by an invisible, intracellular, filterable agent but this suggestion was not confirmed until 1966 when lymphocystis virus was first isolated and propagated in fish-cell fibroblasts.

The disease has a world-wide distribution but appears to be more prevalent in the Western Hemisphere. Natural outbreaks occur mainly during the summer months.

Hosts affected
Lymphocystis affects many species of fresh-water and marine fish, and is especially prevalent in walleyes and bluegills.

Morphology
The virus is hexagonal or pentagonal in outline, between 270 and 460 nm in diameter, and is morphologically similar to *Tipula* iridescent virus. The central nucleoid is about 150 nm across and is surrounded by a capsid about 12 nm thick. The number of surface sub-units has not been determined but electron microscopy shows an accessory membrane with several unusually long, delicate filaments associated with the apices of the virion.

Physicochemical properties
Infected cell cultures held at 23°C remain active for several months. The thermal stability of the virus is not known but it survives alternate freezing and thawing, is readily lyophilized but cannot be preserved in 50 per cent glycerol. It is ether-sensitive.

Haemagglutination
Lymphocystis virus does not haemagglutinate or haemadsorb red blood cells from fish, frogs, turtles, birds or mammals, including man.

Cultivation
Homogenates of lymphocystis lesions inoculated into fish-cell cultures produce cytopathic effects characterized by gross cellular proliferation and the formation of DNA-containing cytoplasmic inclusion bodies, some of which may measure up to 2,000 nm in diameter. The cellular changes develop slowly and are best seen after incubation at 23°–25°C.

Studies of the growth cycle of lymphocystis agent in young artificially infected bluegills indicate that the virus is temperature dependent and that adsorption and penetration occur at 25°C within 2–3 days of infection. By the 6th day, tiny particles staining Feulgen-positive as for DNA, are present in the cytoplasm of some of the affected cells and lesions develop on the skin or fins within 10 days of infection. Affected cells continue to enlarge until they are about 1 month old. Thereafter, they may be ruptured or burst spontaneously and the fish recovers, or a second wave of infection ensues.

Pathogenicity
Lymphocystis is a chronic but mild viral infection of fish in which multiple, raised, granular, wart-like masses occur on the skin or on the fins. The lesions are mostly grey to yellow in colour, sometimes with haemorrhagic foci, and tend to coalesce producing a mulberry-like appearance. The tumour-like masses, which consist of enlarged lymphocystic cells, usually persist for long periods but ultimately regress. Individual affected cells frequently attain a diameter of 2,000 μm, or even as large as 5,000 μm, and are clearly visible with the unaided eye.

Histologically, the mature lymphocystic cell shows an eccentrically positioned basophilic nucleus and numerous fragmented inclusions scattered through the cytoplasm, but especially towards the periphery of the cell. The cell is enclosed within a thick capsule which consists of acid mucopolysaccharide.

Although the condition is essentially of a dermatropic character, lesions have occasionally been described in the mouth, gut, ovary, spleen and cardiac musculature.

Ecology
Little is known about the exact mode of transmission of lymphocystis infection but the fact that natural outbreaks are often restricted in time and species suggests that arthropod vectors may play an important role in the spread of the disease. 'Contact' infection may occur due, perhaps, to rupture of the enlarged lymphocystis cells and the release of infectious virus into the water. This may represent the main method of spread, akin to aerosol transmission in mammalian infections.

Experimental infections can be produced by contact or implantation but attempts to spread the virus by feeding have so far been unsuccessful.

Diagnosis
The size and appearance of the grossly enlarged lymphocystis cells in the wart-like lesions of fish are so characteristic that the disease can be readily diagnosed histologically without the need for isolation of the slow-growing virus in susceptible fish or fish-cell cultures.

Control
In hatcheries, culling of all diseased adult stock prior to spawning helps to reduce the extent of infection.

Further reading
ALMEIDA J.D., WATERSON A.P. AND PLOWRIGHT W. (1967) The morphological characteristics of African swine fever virus and its resemblance to Tipula iridescent virus. *Archiv für die gesamte Virusforschung*, **20**, 392.

BREESE S.S. AND DE BOER C.J. (1966) Electron microscope observations of African swine fever virus in tissue culture cells. *Virology*, **28**, 420.

BREESE S.S. JUN. AND DE BOER C.J. (1967) Chemical structure of African swine fever virus investigated by electron microscopy. *Journal of General Virology*, **1**, 251.

COGGINS L. (1974) African swine fever virus. Pathogenesis. *Progress in Medical Virology*, **18**, 48.

COLGROVE G.S., HAELTERMAN E.O. AND COGGINS L. (1969) Pathogenesis of African swine fever in young pigs. *American Journal of Veterinary Research*, **30**, 1343.

DE BOER C.J. (1967) Antibody studies in animals infected with African swine fever virus (ASFV). *Federation Proceedings*, **26**, 7130.

DE BOER C.J. (1967) Studies to determine neutralizing antibody in sera from animals recovered from African swine fever and laboratory animals inoculated with African virus with adjuvants. *Archiv für die gesamte Virusforschung*, **20**, 164.

DEBOER C.J., PAN I.C. AND HESS W.R. (1972) Immunology of African swine fever. *Journal of the American Veterinary Medical Association*, **160**, 528.

DETRAY D.E. (1967) Persistence of viraemia and immunity in African swine fever. *American Journal of Veterinary Research*, **18**, 811.

DETRAY D.E. (1963) African swine fever. *Advances in Veterinary Science*, **8**, 299.

GREIG A. (1972) Pathogenesis of African swine fever in pigs naturally exposed to the disease. *Journal of Comparative Pathology*, **82**, 73.

KELLY D.C. AND ROBERTSON J.S. (1973) Icosahedral cytoplasmic deoxyriboviruses. *Journal of General Virology*, **20**, 17.

MALMQUIST W.A. AND HAY D. (1960) Haemadsorption and cytopathic effect produced by African swine fever virus in swine bone marrow and buffy coat cultures. *American Journal of Veterinary Research*, **21**, 104.

MAURER F.D., GRIESEMER R.A. AND JONES T.C. (1958) The pathology of African swine fever—a comparison with hog cholera. *American Journal of Veterinary Reseach*, **19**, 517.

PLOWRIGHT W., BROWN F. AND PARKER J. (1966) Evidence for the type of nucleic acid in African swine fever virus. *Archiv für die gesamte Virusforschung*, **19**, 289.

PLOWRIGHT W., PARKER J. AND STAPLE R.F. (1968) The growth of a virulent strain of African swine fever virus in domestic pigs. *Journal of Hygiene*, **66**, 117.

SCOTT G.R. (1972) Comments on African swine fever. *Journal of the American Veterinary Medical Association*, **160**, 532.

VIGARIO J.D., TERRINHA A.M. AND MOURA NUNES J.F. (1974) Antigenic relationships among strains of African swine fever virus. *Archiv für die gesamte Virusforschung*, **45**, 272.

CHAPTER 58

LATENT, CHRONIC AND SLOW
VIRUS INFECTIONS

Latent, chronic and slow virus infections

Viral latency

The majority of animal virus infections run an acute course and last for a relatively short period before culminating in death or clinical recovery. In the latter case, viral multiplication ceases and the virus rapidly disappears from the tissues due to the inhibitory effects of interferons or other antiviral substances, and to the development of active immunity.

In a few cases, however, animals that have made a complete clinical recovery from the disease continue to harbour the virus in their tissues and may shed the virus continuously or intermittently for many weeks or months and, as in infectious canine hepatitis or African swine fever, are capable of transmitting the infection to susceptible individuals. This type of infection is known by different names, but the term 'latent infection' is generally used.

Several types of latent infection have been described including inapparent persistent infections where animals may harbour the virus without giving visible evidence of its presence and where, because of its intracellular location and low level of multiplication, the virus is difficult to detect by the usual isolation and identification procedures. A good example of persistent viral infection is that which may follow an attack of varicella (chicken pox) in children. Here the virus may persist undetected in the nervous tissues for many years and its presence is only revealed when in adult life it gives rise to the characteristic clinical condition of herpes zoster or shingles.

There are many examples of latent or persistent viral infections in mice, hamsters, rats, guinea-pigs and other laboratory animals but the best known are probably mousepox (ectromelia) and lymphocytic choriomeningitis (LCM) of mice. The LCM virus is a good example of a natural inapparent infection which may spread horizontally by droplet infection or vertically, *in utero*. Susceptible baby mice exposed to LCM virus may develop the clinical disease and die or, if they become infected 2 days or more after birth, they may develop a durable resistance without showing clinical signs. On the other hand, if baby mice become infected *in utero*, or within 48 hours of birth, they may develop a chronic or symptomless 'persistent tolerant infection' which is characterised by a high level of viraemia throughout their life, absence of neutralizing antibody and the presence of the virus in their tissues. It is interesting to note that, in their later years, such mice may develop haemolytic anaemia and nephritis with lesions resembling those of an autoimmune disease.

Although the pathogenesis of LCM infection suggests that the virus persists because of failure by the host to produce specific neutralizing antibody, there are a number of other examples of persistent viral infection, e.g. visna in sheep, where the causative virus is readily demonstrable in the presence of specific antibody which neutralizes the growth of the virus in cell cultures but not in experimentally infected sheep.

In general terms, the effect of an animal virus on susceptible host cells takes one of 3 forms: 1) the replicative cycle is successfully completed and the virus destroys the cell (lytic action), 2) the cycle is completed and the virus induces cellular transformation without causing death of the cell (oncogenic action) or 3) the infection may not be accompanied by visible cell damage and the virus persists in a latent state within the cell, for very long periods (latency). There are numerous examples of this type of symbiotic relationship, both in cell culture and in the animal body; and while the virus may persist unsuspected in the tissues of latently infected animals, due to circumstances which are not well understood, it may be reactivated (e.g. by immunosuppressive drugs) to produce lesions of either the lytic or proliferative (oncogenic) type. In the case of leukoviruses and other RNA tumour producing viruses, the agent persists in the transformed cells and can usually be recovered from them, whereas in tumours induced by DNA viruses the genetic (hereditary) material of the virus is incorporated in the genome of the cell and the virus, as such, does not always persist within the altered cells.

Apart from their possible oncogenic role, there is increasing evidence that persistent infections with complete or defective virus particles may play an important part in many slow and chronic virus infections of man and animals.

Slow and chronic viral infections

The concept of 'slow virus infections' was first introduced by Sigurdsson, in 1954, in his account of a slowly evolving pulmonary disease of adult sheep in Iceland, called 'maedi'. Since then, the definition has been extended to include a number of virus diseases that are characterized by a very long incubation period and an insidious onset, followed by a slowly progressive and prolonged clinical illness which usually terminates in chronic disability or death. In a number of cases, the infection is limited to a single host species, e.g. kuru of man, and the characteristic lesions are confined to a single organ or tissue system. Unlike 'chronic infections' which generally run a protracted, irregular and often unpredictable course, 'slow virus infections' follow a set pattern which is just as regular as that of an acute infection except that following a long incubation period, the course of the illness is spread over a very long time and progresses continuously until death supervenes.

Other properties of slow viruses include, 1) their ability to multiply to high titre in the host for long periods of time without showing clinical symptoms, 2) they are often not recognised as foreign by the host, and an immune reaction occurs late or not at all, 3) they usually multiply on the cellular membrane or on the surface of cytoplasmic cisternae and 4) their pathological manifestations are unlike those normally associated with viral infections.

Studies of persistent myxovirus infections in cell cultures have clearly shown that defective virus particles, which also multiply by budding on the cell surfaces, frequently contain antigenic components specific for the animal species in which they are formed. Thus, it is tempting to suggest that this has occurred in vivo in scrapie, kuru and other slow virus diseases, and is responsible for some of the remarkable properties of these infections, including the prolonged incubation period, the lack of immune response and the mechanisms of spread of the agent.

The factors responsible for the onset of clinical disease in slow-virus infections are not clearly understood but it is generally agreed that there is invariably a long preliminary period of replication during which the virus spreads and multiplies in many different tissues. In scrapie of sheep, for example, the agent multiplies for many months in the lymphocytic tissues before it appears in the central nervous system and, in Aleutian disease of mink, proliferation of plasma cells over a long period is associated with abnormally high levels of gamma-globulin which produce characteristic glomerular and arterial lesions. Despite the extent of virus multiplication in the affected animal, only a particular cell type undergoes proliferative changes and it has been suggested, therefore, that some defect in the host's defensive mechanism or, indeed, the cumulative reaction of the body's immune system to the persistent infection is responsible for the lesions and the onset of clinical signs of disease.

Slow-virus infections include kuru, Creutzfeldt-Jakob disease and sub-acute sclerosing panencephalitis (SSPE) of man, scrapie of sheep, Aleutian disease and transmissible mink encephalopathy. Chronic infections associated with persistent virus include jaagsiekte, the visna-maedi complex and, possibly, border disease of sheep, equine infectious anaemia, swine fever, African swine fever, bovine virus diarrhoea, lactic dehydrogenase (Riley virus) and lymphocytic choriomeningitis of mice, Marek's disease of poultry and many forms of ribovirus induced tumours. There is also preliminary evidence that a number of commonly occurring human degenerative disorders including multiple sclerosis and rheumatoid arthritis may be the result of slow-virus infection.

Visna-maedi viruses

Definition

Visna and maedi are two clinical and histopathological forms of the same virus infection and are commonly included in the 'slow-virus' group of diseases. Each has an extremely long incubation period, lasting months to several years, followed by a protracted clinical illness which progresses slowly and usually terminates in death.

Visna, which means shrinkage or wasting, is primarily an afebrile demyelinating disease of the central nervous system characterized by indefinite nervous symptoms and an abnormal gait which progresses through paraplegia to complete paralysis and death. Maedi is a highly fatal chronic progressive pneumonia of sheep characterized by dyspnoea (hence the name maedi), and progressive debility.

History and distribution

Both visna and maedi were recognized for the first time in sheep flocks in Iceland in the late 1930s, and both infections are believed to have been introduced into Iceland with a few apparently healthy sheep of the Karakul breed imported from

Germany in 1933 in order to improve the wool industry. The incidence of both diseases varied considerably but when they were at their height, the annual mortality rates in an area containing about 200,000 sheep were about 6–10 per cent for visna and 20–30 per cent for maedi.

As the result of a massive slaughter campaign in the affected areas during the period 1944–52, visna appears to have been completely eradicated from Iceland while the distribution of maedi is now very limited and only isolated outbreaks occur which are quickly brought under control by slaughter.

Several diseases of sheep that are similar clinically and pathologically to maedi have been observed in other countries. These include progressive pneumonia in Montana (U.S.A.), progressive interstitial pneumonia in Germany, la bouhite in France, zwoegerziekte in Holland, Graff-Reinet disease in South Africa, Laikipia lung disease in Kenya and various forms of progressive pneumonias in India, Israel and Peru. The viruses isolated in different countries from visna, maedi, zwoegerziekte and Montana disease appear to be strains of the same virus and it is likely that eventually they will all be classified as a single virus.

Properties of the virus

In negatively stained preparations the visna-maedi virions are approximately spherical bodies measuring between 80 and 120 nm in diameter. Each is surrounded by a clearly defined outer membrane covered with fine, short projections about 8–10 nm in length. The central electron-dense nucleoid contains filamentous structures apparently coiled into a nucleocapsid helix 7–8 nm wide.

Electron microscopy of ultra-thin sections suggests that the mature virions of both visna and maedi viruses are released from the surface of the cytoplasmic membrane of the infected cell as double-walled spherical bodies. The appearance of budding forms and the processes of assembly and release are very similar to those of certain mouse leukaemia and other leukoviruses (oncornaviruses).

Visna virus is readily inactivated at, and below, pH 4.2 and by heating at 50°C for 30 minutes, but survives storage for several months at —70°C. It is sensitive to ether; chloroform, ethanol, metaperiodate and trypsin: and is inactivated by 0.04 per cent formaldehyde or 4 per cent phenol. Maedi virus is similar to visna virus in its sensitivity to physicochemical agents except that it is more sensitive to low pH. Both viruses contain single stranded RNA but their replication is inhibited by 5-bromodeoxyuridine (BUDR), a known inhibitor of DNA synthesis, and by actinomycin D which blocks DNA-dependent RNA synthesis. This does not imply that visna and maedi are DNA viruses

and, since the inhibition is partly overcome by the addition of thymine, this seems to indicate that successful reproduction of visna-maedi virus depends on a DNA-directed RNA synthesis taking place shortly before the formation of the virus. Subsequently it has been shown that visna, maedi, zwoegerziekte and progressive pneumonia (Montana disease) viruses all resemble Rous sarcoma virus and other RNA tumour viruses in that the core of the virion contains an RNA-directed DNA polymerase (reverse transcriptase) that is capable of using the viral RNA as a template for DNA synthesis. In addition they all possess a 60–70 S RNA component. The analogy between visna-maedi virus and the RNA tumour-producing oncornaviruses has been extended by the fact that the morphology and maturation of the viruses are very similar, and that visna virus can also cause transformation of mouse cells in culture. Because the visna-maedi virus complex is now known to possess an antigenically specific RNA-dependent DNA polymerase, it has been suggested that it be included in a genus to be called *Lentivirus* and brought together with oncornaviruses, spumaviruses and other reverse transcriptase containing RNA viruses in the family *Retraviridae*.

Haemagglutination

Contrary to an earlier report, neither haemagglutination nor haemadsorption have been observed with any strain of visna or maedi viruses.

Antigenic properties

Viruses isolated in different countries from sheep with visna, maedi, progressive pneumonia and zwoegerziekte have been characterized in cell cultures and appear to be similar. Cross neutralization tests with sera from experimentally infected sheep indicate that the four viruses are closely related antigenically if not identical. In the visna-maedi complex, antisera against visna virus usually neutralizes maedi virus to a lesser extent than the homologous virus strain, and slight differences have also been observed among strains of each of the two respective viruses.

The role of neutralizing antibody in visna and maedi infections is not well understood. Circulating antibody does not prevent the spread of virus by the blood stream, probably because virus precursors are carried inside blood cells which protect them: and the infected cells are able to release the virus gradually.

Cultivation

The causative agents of visna and maedi have been propagated in cell cultures derived from sheep choroid plexus, kidney and salivary glands, and cause constant and characteristic cytopathic effects leading to cell destruction. The cytopathic effect spreads over the entire monolayer culture converting most of the cells into large stellate forms. In stained preparations, the stellate cells are multinucleated with 2 to at least 20 nuclei often arranged in a circle around the centre of the giant cell. In cell cultures, both viruses have relatively long latent periods, 22 hours for visna and 20 hours for maedi. The cytopathic effect appears within 2–3 weeks but on passage of the virus, the time is shortened to 3–15 days, when large inocula are used. Similar cytopathic effects have been observed in cultures of mouse cerebellum and baby hamster (BHK-21) cells. Other cell systems capable of supporting the growth of visna-maedi virus include primary cultures of bovine, porcine, canine and human choroid plexus cells, as well as cell lines of bovine and porcine origin.

The infection in tissue culture can be considered as 'slow', since the time before the appearance of the cytopathic effect is greatly prolonged when using very small inocula. Moreover, in explants from diseased organs, the infection can persist in the same culture for as long as 4 months since cell growth apparently can, to some extent, keep up with cell death. Despite the relatively rapid type of cytopathic effect in cell cultures, susceptible experimental sheep develop the clinical illness as late as 3–6 years after inoculation, and produce virus throughout all or most of the preclinical period as well as during the clinical phase of the disease.

There is still no clear evidence whereabouts in the host cells the various components of the virions are formed. Staining with acridine-orange indicates that the nucleus is unaffected even in cells showing pronounced cytopathic effects. However, the intensity of red fluorescence in the cytoplasm is enhanced in the infected cells, indicating an increased content of RNA.

In general terms, the cytopathic effect of maedi is similar to that of visna except that it grows more slowly, can be propagated in a wider range of ovine cells but produces fewer large stellate cells. On the other hand visna, but not maedi virus, has been grown in cultures of pig kidney, bovine trachea and cerebellar cells from new-born mice.

The viruses do not grow in embryonated hens' eggs and several attempts to transmit the infections to laboratory animals have failed.

Pathogenicity

Although the viruses of visna and maedi show a close relationship with respect to physical, chemical and biological properties, including serological reactions, and are probably strains of the same virus, they cause two entirely different diseases.

Visna is a slow, demyelinating infection which is, in fact, a subacute encephalitis with a tendency to extend into the white matter around the ventricles. There is a prolonged subclinical meningitis for many months before the onset of clinical signs. The clinical disease is characterized by lip trembling, abnormal head posture, paralysis of the hind legs and other nervous symptoms, which progress slowly to total paraplegia and death within a few weeks to several months. The main pathological changes are those of diffuse encephalomyelitis, lymphocytic and microglial proliferation or infiltration and perivascular cuffing. The primary lesions are followed by a diffuse demyelination of the white matter in the cerebrum, cerebellum, pons, medulla oblongata and spinal cord.

The disease is transmissible to sheep by intracerebral inoculation but produces lesions like maedi when given intranasally. The causative virus is always present in low titres in a variety of tissues including brain, cerebrospinal fluid, lungs, salivary glands, nasal secretions and faeces during the preclinical as well as during the clinical phase of the disease, in spite of high concentrations of neutralizing antibody. Visna-maedi virus appears to have a strong affinity for reticulo-endothelial tissues and it is particularly easy to isolate the virus from spleen and lymph nodes.

Maedi usually occurs in sheep 2 or more years old and is characterized by a chronic interstitial pneumonia. The incubation period of the natural disease is 2–3 years though pathological changes can be detected much earlier. The main symptoms are a gradual loss of condition, dyspnoea and a dry cough. The disease lasts for 3–6 months or longer and almost invariably terminates fatally. At necropsy, the lungs do not collapse when the thorax is opened and are often 2–4 times larger and heavier than normal. They usually have a greyish-yellow to greyish-blue colour and are of spongy consistency. Histological examination shows diffuse perivascular, peribronchiolar and interalveolar infiltration of lymphocytes, monocytes and macrophages, with nodular accumulations of lympoid cells and a degree of thickening of the alveolar septa. The bronchial and mediastinal lymph nodes are frequently hyperplastic and oedematous. In maedi, the intraseptal proliferation usually includes young fibroblasts, whereas in jaagsiekte lungs there is a greater tendency towards 'adenomatosis'.

Immunity

Complement-fixing antibodies are produced 3–4 weeks after infection with visna or maedi viruses, and remain for several years. Neutralizing antibodies appear much later (2–3 months post infection), the titres rise slowly, reach a peak in 2 years and remain high for months or years. The role of neutralizing antibodies in visna-maedi infections is not well understood since circulating antibody does not prevent the spread of virus by the blood stream, and the virus can be isolated both during the pre-clinical and throughout the clinical phase of the disease. In the laboratory, neutralization of the virus is very slow and about 48 hours' incubation at 4°C is required for maximum neutralization. The complement-fixation test is much more sensitive than serum neutralization and is a useful method for the rapid detection of naturally occurring cases of maedi.

Diagnosis
In the final stages of maedi, the clinical signs are similar to jaagsiekte and several other chronic lung diseases of sheep, and a reliable diagnosis can only be made during post-mortem examination. The virus may be isolated from the lungs of affected animals and identified by neutralization tests with specific antisera in cell culture.

In visna, diagnosis is chiefly based on the clinical signs and pathological lesions. It should be noted, however, that mixed cases of both visna and maedi occur frequently in infected flocks.

Control
The most effective means of controlling or eradicating visna and maedi is by slaughtering all sheep in affected flocks and by preventing contact between sheep from different areas.

Scrapie

Synonyms
Cuddie trot: rubbers: la tremblante: maladie tremblante: Zitternkrankheit: Traberkrankheit: Grubberkrankheit: Rida (Iceland).

Definition
An infectious, slowly progressive degenerative disorder of the central nervous system of adult sheep and goats, characterized by an unusually long incubation period (1–5 years), followed by incoordination, paralysis, debility and death. Marked cutaneous irritation is a common sequel of infection but may not be evident in all cases. Inapparent infections are possible.

Scrapie, like mink encephalopathy and kuru of man, is one of the so-called CHINA (*Ch*ronic *i*nfectious *n*europathic *a*gent) or 'slow-virus' diseases.

Hosts affected
Scrapie mostly affects sheep between 2–4 years of age and is seldom seen in young animals less than 18 months old. The disease may occur naturally in goats, whether or not they have been left in contact with sheep, and the incubation period is about the same as in sheep. Apart from sheep and goats, scrapie can be transmitted by various routes to a wide range of host species including, mice, hamsters, rats, gerbils, voles, mink, New World primates (squirrel and spider monkeys) and Old World primates (Cynomolgus monkeys), but rabbits and guinea-pigs are probably resistant.

History and distribution
Scrapie has long been recognised in sheep in the United Kingdom and many severe outbreaks are known to have occurred in England as early as the mid 18th century. The disease is believed to have spread to Scotland in the early years of the 19th century. There is also evidence that the disease existed in Germany prior to 1750, and in France and Spain in 1810. Cases of scrapie have also been reported from Hungary, Finland, Norway and Poland. At the present time, scrapie is still prevalent in many parts of the British Isles but its distribution in Continental Europe is obscure, although it probably occurs in France.

In 1938 scrapie was diagnosed in Canada in a Suffolk ewe imported from Scotland several months before, and from 1943–52 several cases were reported in Cheviot sheep. The first case of scrapie to occur in the U.S.A. was diagnosed in Michigan in 1947 in a sheep that had been imported from the U.K. by way of Canada. In 1952 and subsequently, scrapie was recognized in flocks of purebred sheep in California, Ohio, Illinois, New York and Connecticut. Although the disease is not widespread in the U.S.A., measures have been introduced during the past 20 years to control and eradicate the disease but these have not yet proved successful. In 1955, New Zealand and Australia reported isolated outbreaks in sheep imported from England, but the disease was quickly stamped out by means of a rigorous policy of quarantine and slaughter. There is recent evidence that the infection has been present since the end of the Second World War in hill sheep in the remote regions of Northern India. In Icelandic flocks, a disease called rida, which is a chronic encephalopathy characterized by incoordination of gait but without paralysis, was probably a form of scrapie which is thought to have been imported by sheep from Germany in the mid 1930s. Measures to combat the infection by a massive programme of systematic slaughtering of all sheep in affected areas proved highly successful and Iceland has now been free from rida for many years.

Scrapie has been a continuing problem in Europe for more than two centuries and the early literature shows that a number of devastating outbreaks occurred in Germany and England during the 18th and 19th centuries. Today, the incidence of scrapie in countries where the disease is known to occur varies from flock to flock but is generally low although 10 per cent mortality rates are not uncommon and losses of up to 40 per cent have occasionally been reported in badly affected areas. However, the overall effect on the sheep industry is less serious and nowhere do losses constitute a major economic problem. At present the disease is of rare occurrence in the Southern Hemisphere.

Despite the low incidence of scrapie, it is probably true to say that few areas of biological science have attracted so much attention and so many hypotheses supported by so few experimental data as scrapie has done in recent years: and there is little doubt that the interest in this disease, and similar conditions such as kuru in man, is largely due to the extraordinary nature of their causative agents.

Properties of the scrapie agent

The nature of the causal agent of scrapie has yet to be defined and its properties are so remarkable that many workers are reluctant to accept the 'classic' view that it is a virus.

Compared with the more conventional viruses, the scrapie agent is unusually resistant to heat and will withstand 80°C for half an hour. Although there may be a substantial fall in titre, brain suspensions retain their infectivity even after boiling for 3 hours. The clinical disease can be produced in sheep by the intracerebral inoculation of infected brain tissues previously autoclaved for 30 minutes at 20 lb. per sq. in. Several investigators have confirmed that the scrapie agent also resists exposure to 20 per cent formalin for 18 hours at 37°C and can be stored in 10 per cent formalin at room temperature for up to 28 months. Infected brain material fixed for several weeks in 10 per cent formalin, and then embedded in paraffin, may retain its infectivity on dewaxing 18 months later.

The infectivity titre is reduced (by about 1.5 $\log_{10}$) but not destroyed following treatment with diethyl ether, acetone or chloroform, and is not adversely affected by proteolytic enzymes or other enzymes such as RNAse or DNAse. Acid and alkali have little effect on the activity of the scrapie agent over a pH range of 2.5 to 10.0 but exposure to 5N NaOH results in a dramatic loss of infectivity.

There are many different estimates of the size of the scrapie agent as determined by filtration methods but recent radiation experiments suggest that the agent has a particle size of 7 nm or less, with a molecular weight of $1.5—2.0 \times 10^5$ daltons. Despite intensive efforts, the scrapie agent has not been demonstrated with certainty in tissue homogenates, centrifuged deposits or chromatographic fractions by electron microscopy. Although a report by Canadian workers in 1974 describes small (14 nm) spherical virus-like particles in mouse brain infected with the scrapie agent, but not in normal mouse brain, the significance of this observation in relation to the aetiology of the disease has not been determined.

Although the agent of scrapie undoubtedly increases in quantity by serial animal passage and seems, therefore, to be capable of self-replication, it is not inactivated by exposure to large doses, up to 2.4×10^4 ergs per mm², of ultraviolet light. Thus, the dose of radiation required to inactivate the scrapie agent is far greater than is necessary to destroy even the most resistant organisms by disrupting their genetic material. More recent studies whereby the 'action spectrum' of the scrapie agent can be measured by comparing the relative abilities of ultraviolet light of different wavelengths to de-activate the molecule give results which are almost exactly the reverse of those expected from a nucleic acid or nucleoprotein molecule; instead the 'action spectrum' resembles that of a small protein.

Since the agent has an unusual resistance to formaldehyde, β-propiolactone, ionising radiation and various enzymes which attack nucleic acid, it is unlikely to be composed of nucleic acid and, as it is sensitive to strong solutions of urea, phenol or periodate but insensitive to heat, it is unlikely to be an ordinary protein or carbohydrate. If the recent findings are confirmed and the scrapie agent proves to be some form of self-replicating organism which has no need of DNA or RNA, they will be at variance with the classical Central Dogma of Crick and Watson which stipulates that genetic messages are always coded in the chemical structure of nucleic acid. In other words, information may be transferred from nucleic acid to nucleic acid or from nucleic acid to protein, but transfer from protein to protein or from protein to nucleic acid is impossible.

Thus, the mode of replication of the scrapie agent may well be the first exception to the general rule. Indeed, it has been suggested that the all important factor of scrapie involves an unusual steric rearrangement in the carbohydrate portion of the cell membrane which also contains protein and lipid arranged together with the carbohydrate in a special way. Such a membrane would then have to be able to reproduce by some 'self-copying' process and, if this were possible, scrapie of sheep might be caused by some type of foreign membrane, or part of a membrane, becoming incorporated into the body and being copied or reproduced. There can be no doubt that if these remarkable observations are confirmed it will be difficult to maintain the current view that the causative agent of scrapie should continue to be classified as a virus.

Antigenic properties

Little information is available regarding the antigenicity of scrapie agent, but one of the many remarkable features of the disease is the complete absence of a detectable immunological response to the infection. Thus, no evidence of antibody formation is discernible in cases of natural or experimental disease, nor can differences be shown in the neutralizing capacity of sera obtained from healthy and affected animals. For the same reason it has not been possible to develop serological tests for detecting the agent in infected tissues.

Growth of the agent

Although scrapie was first transmitted experimentally in 1899 by the inoculation of a ewe, it was not until 1936 that it was confirmed that the disease could be produced by the inoculation of healthy sheep with suspensions of brain and spinal cord from affected animals, and that the infection could be transmitted by the intracerebral or subcutaneous routes. Since then, the disease has been transmitted by oral, intracutaneous, intraperitoneal and intramuscular routes, also, The period between inoculation of the agent and the onset of clinical symptoms in sheep varies from up to 2 years or more, but it is generally several months shorter (6–10 months) following intracerebral inoculation, compared with other routes of infection. The goat is a more susceptible experimental animal than the sheep since it is almost 100 per cent susceptible when inoculated with scrapie infected material, and the incubation period is generally shorter (7–30 months) following a single injection. The clinical signs in goats are essentially the same as in sheep, and it is of interest that the appearance of different clinical symptoms in goats inoculated with tissue suspensions from sheep affected with scrapie was the first indication that there might be more than one strain of agent. Indeed, the existence of two distinct strains of scrapie agent, known respectively as 'drowsy' and 'scratching' strains, became more apparent after several serial passages in goats. This was later confirmed and differentiated further in experimentally infected mice (*vide infra*).

An important advance was made in the study of scrapie when it was discovered, in 1961, that laboratory mice inoculated intracerebrally with brain tissues from naturally infected sheep showed almost 100 per cent susceptibility and developed symptoms of the disease with an incubation period of only 4–8 months in later passages. The disease in artificially infected mice is slowly progressive and generally ends in death. Rats and hamsters can also be infected by the intracerebral, intraperitoneal or subcutaneous routes, with an incubation period of 7–8 months or longer. Scrapie infected tissues can also induce encephalopathy in mink.

There is no direct evidence that the scrapie agent replicates in tissue culture and numerous attempts to infect healthy cell lines with the agent have proved unsuccessful. On the other hand, there is good evidence to show that monolayer cultures prepared from brain tissues of sheep affected with scrapie are capable of producing in mice inoculated intracerebrally 15 months previously, a disease with histopathological changes characteristic of early scrapie infection. These cultured cells carrying the scrapie agent have been maintained by repeated subculture through more than 200 passages and the agent appears to multiply in synchrony with, and also as part of, the cell. No specific cytopathic effect has been observed although, in comparison with normal cultures, the carrier cells develop a tendency to proliferate and overlap in the manner of cellular transformation induced by certain oncogenic viruses.

Pathogenicity

Scrapie is essentially a disease of adult sheep and goats, and the duration of the clinical condition extends over weeks, months or even years. In a few instances the clinical manifestations of scrapie run an acute course, often with sudden death after a few days of illness with minimal symptoms. The natural disease is insidious in its onset and almost invariably runs a progressive course which terminates fatally. The incubation period of naturally occurring scrapie is from 1–3 years or longer and the clinical disease is rarely recognised in animals less than 18 months of age.

In the early stages of the illness, the affected sheep usually shows either an apprehensive attitude or hyperexcitability. It tends to carry its head high with erect ears and staring eyes, and runs with a characteristic high-stepping gait. There is no temperature rise. As the disease progresses, locomotor incoordination becomes more severe, particularly of the hind limbs, and in heavily built breeds this ataxia may become pronounced. Fine trembling is often present and cutaneous irritation may accompany the ataxia. A nibbling reflex involving the lips, tongue and jaw is elicited by manual rubbing, scratching or pinching of the skin in the region of the loin or rump or when the animal rubs its body against a firm object. Some animals appear very sleepy and show stupor, whereas others may exhibit intense pruritus and tend to bite the legs, flank and abdomen, or scratch and rub off their wool on fences, gates or other objects. In the terminal stages of the disease ataxia is pronounced and the patient becomes completely immobile and debilitated. Deaths occur most frequently in sheep between 2–5 years of age.

Scrapie has been produced experimentally in sheep and goats by various routes of inoculation. The period between administration of the agent and the development of clinical symptoms is very long, varying from 5 months to several years; but is shorter after intracerebral inoculation than after peripheral injection.

It is now well known that the scrapie agent can be transmitted serially to a number of laboratory animals by the intracerebral, intraperitoneal, subcutaneous or intramuscular routes of inoculation. In mice inoculated subcutaneously, the agent replicates in the tissues and appears in the spleen about one week after inoculation and is present in high titre in the peripheral lymph nodes 4–6 weeks later. At the 3rd week, the titres in the spleen may reach 6.0 $\log_{10}$ ID_{50} units. As the disease develops, the agent spreads slowly to other tissues including the thymus and salivary glands, thence to the lungs, intestines and spinal cord. It finally reaches the brain after about 12–16 weeks. By this time the concentration of agent in the central nervous system is at least 10 fold higher (7.5–8.0 $\log_{10}$ ID_{50}) than that in the spleen, and remains at this level until death supervenes.

The length of the incubation period in experimentally infected mice depends on a number of factors such as the amount of agent injected and the route of inoculation but, especially, on the genotype of mouse selected and on the strain of the agent employed. There is clear evidence that replication of scrapie agent in mice is under the overriding control of a single gene (*sinc*), and that the interaction between the agent and the *sinc* gene is an important factor in the pathogenesis of scrapie and the slow nature of this group of diseases. (The name '*sinc*' is an acronym for '*scrapie inc*ubation). Moreover, the existence of several different strains of scrapie agent was confirmed by measuring the effect of the *sinc* gene on the incubation period of the disease in experimentally infected mice.

It has long been thought that scrapie has certain hereditary features and there are numerous claims that certain breeds of sheep (e.g. Herdwicks and Dalesbreds) are more susceptible than others (e.g. Dorset Downs); also, that scrapie occurs more frequently in purebred than in halfbred animals. Breed susceptibilities to experimental scrapie infection have been investigated by a number of workers but variable results were obtained. However, a marked difference in the incidence of scrapie following subcutaneous inoculation has been demonstrated recently in 2 lines of Cheviot sheep selected from a group of ewes and rams known to be free from the natural disease. In view of these findings and, since it is now evident that a single gene controls recessive resistance to subcutaneous injection of a strain of scrapie agent, it was considered more appropriate to distinguish the 2 Cheviot phenotypes as 'short incubation period' and 'long incubation period' rather than 'susceptible' and 'resistant'. Although genetic variation in the host is either known or suspected to be important in influencing the development of scrapie, the extreme view that it is solely of genetic origin and is caused by a recessive gene, in other words that it is a hereditary disease, is not acceptable to the majority of workers in this field. However, abundant evidence is accumulating which shows that a strong familial pattern exists in scrapie and that the progeny of affected parents usually develop the disease. It seems, also, that where only one parent is affected, the incidence in the progeny matches the ewe's category rather than the ram's.

Pathology

It has long been recognised that the presence of large numbers of vacuolated neurones in almost all parts of the central nervous system is highly characteristic of scrapie, despite the fact that they may also be found singly or in small numbers in the brains of normal sheep. The lesions are found most consistently and are especially prominent in the corpus striatum, diencephalon, brain stem and cerebellar cortex. The cerebral cortex is rarely involved and only minor changes occur in the spinal cord. The typical lesions are mostly bilaterally symmetrical and consist of a progressive degeneration of the neurones and variable spongy rarefaction of the grey matter. Characteristically, the affected neurone shows multilocular vacuolation, the so-called 'bubble cell'', and an eccentrically placed nucleus. Notably, neither inflammation nor overt destruction of myelin occurs and there is no evidence of cellular changes commonly associated with virus encephalitides such as perivascular cuffing or round-cell infiltration.

The presence of spongiform degeneration and pronounced neuronal vacuolation is a common feature of scrapie although these abnormalities are not in themselves pathognomonic of the disease and may be absent in some affected sheep. Indeed, some workers consider that shrinkage and increased basophilia of nerve cells, accompanied by hypertrophy and proliferation of astrocytes, represent the true initial responses to the scrapie agent, and are of greater diagnostic significance.

Scrapie is essentially a disease of the central nervous system and, as such, specific lesions do not occur consistently in other organs of the body. Despite this, however, the agent is widely distributed in the tissues of both naturally and experimentally infected animals.

Ecology

There is disagreement about the mode of spread of the natural disease and some workers have claimed that contagion never, or rarely, occurs on sheep farms. On the other hand, while scrapie has never been regarded as a highly contagious disease there is clear evidence that horizontal transmission can undoubtedly occur under experimental conditions, even when naturally diseased animals are used as donors. Most workers believe that scrapie can be spread indirectly from affected to healthy susceptible sheep as a result of prolonged grazing on contaminated pastures. The agent has also been isolated from placentas of clinically affected ewes and a possible route for contact in the field is by ingestion of this material. Little is known about the route by which the agent enters the body but it is difficult to explain the origin of scrapie in some flocks in any other way than by contact transmission.

Diagnosis

Scrapie is distinguished from other viral infections of the central nervous system by its protracted course and very high mortality rate in clinically affected animals. Unfortunately, the clinical signs are very varied and often may not be sufficiently characteristic for a diagnosis to be made. Indeed, in some sheep the clinical period can be very brief with minimal signs of ataxia or pruritus. Others may run a more acute course with sudden death after only 36–48 hours of clinical illness. In the absence of serological tests and other *in vitro* virological procedures, a confirmatory diagnosis is generally based on histological evidence of neuronal degeneration in the brain stem and on the presence of numerous vacuoles in nerve cells of the medullary region. There is a wide range in the character and severity of the histological lesions in scrapie, and it is well known that some cases of the experimental disease show negligible brain lesions. For this reason it is possible that sheep may die from natural scrapie which goes unrecognised. Thus, a definitive diagnosis largely depends on biological methods for determining the presence of the scrapie agent. It is emphasised that there is no means at present of confirming the presence of scrapie in the living animal.

Control

There are no vaccines available for the prevention of scrapie and in countries where the disease has been recently introduced the only effective means of control is by the slaughter of all affected animals including those known to have been in contact during the previous 3–4 years. In endemic areas, sheep farmers have attempted to protect their flocks by operating a system of rigorous culling of affected maternal lines and close relations of the affected sheep in order to reduce the incidence of scrapie on a particular farm. It is doubtful, however, if these measures have achieved any degree of success.

Transmissible mink encephalopathy

Transmissible mink encephalopathy is a 'slow-virus' infection which occurs sporadically and causes high mortality in adult ranch mink. The incubation period of the naturally occurring disease is between 8 and 18 months or longer, and its clinicopathological features are strikingly similar to those of scrapie in sheep. Affected mink show hyperirritability, compulsive biting, slowly progressive locomotor incoordination, somnolence, terminal prostration and death within 4–7 weeks after the onset of clinical signs. The characteristic histopathological changes in the central nervous system are similar to those of scrapie in sheep except that the principal lesions are mostly distributed in the cerebral cortex, corpus striatum and diencephalon, whereas the more caudal parts of the brain and spinal cord tend not to be affected.

The disease has been transmitted by subcutaneous or intraperitoneal inoculation of mink infected brain tissues to a variety of animals including mink, skunk, racoon, ferret, hamster, goat, sheep and monkey. Mink have also been experimentally infected by intracerebral inoculation of scrapie-infected sheep brain and by feeding of tissues from infected mink carcases. However, the means of natural transmission has not been established.

Although electron microscopy has failed to reveal the aetiological agent of transmissible mink encephalopathy, it is similar to that of scrapie both in size and resistance to heat, formalin, phenol, ether and ultraviolet radiation. Thus, the main differences between the agents of transmissible mink encephalopathy and scrapie lies in their experimental host range. That of transmissible mink encephalopathy causes disease in laboratory primates more readily than scrapie, and while it also induces overt disease in goats and sheep it does not always do so in mice. The agent of transmissible mink encephalopathy is present in many tissues of terminally infected mink and the highest infectivity is in the brain but, like scrapie, it fails to elicit any antibody response in naturally or experimentally infected animals. Vaccines against transmissible mink encephalopathy are not available and treatment is ineffective.

Kuru

One of the disease conditions in man which conforms to the original criteria of slow virus infections is kuru. This is a chronic degenerative disease of the human brain which is similar in many respects to scrapie of sheep.

Kuru was first reported in 1957, as a previously unknown familial degenerative disorder of the central nervous system which accounted for over 50 per cent of all deaths among the South Fore people in a number of adjacent valleys in the mountainous interior of the Eastern Highlands of New Guinea. It also constitutes a serious problem among the North Fore natives and in the villages of adjacent linguistic groups, where intermarriage with Fore peoples is common. The name 'kuru' in Fore dialect means 'to be afraid' or 'to show or tremble with fear or cold'.

In early outbreaks, the disease mostly occurred in women of child-bearing age and children of either sex over five years of age. Adult males were seldom affected but, since 1960, when kuru reached its highest incidence, fewer cases have been reported and these have been equally distributed between men and women.

The disease is of sudden onset and runs a remarkably uniform and progressive course, lasting about 4–24 months. The main symptoms include the inability to maintain balance and difficulty in walking unaided. Many patients show fine, regular tremors resembling shivering and, in some cases, facial incoordination produces involuntary movements of the lips, frequently giving rise to a distorted grin and the appearance of laughter. In the terminal stages of the illness there is marked muscular weakness, inability to feed oneself, and urinary and faecal incontinence.

There are a number of striking similarities between kuru in man and scrapie in sheep, and it is of interest that the ultrastructural changes in these two diseases resemble those found in multiple sclerosis; the most important being localized astroglial proliferation. Almost all patients with kuru or scrapie suffer a continuously progressive illness which usually ends in death in two years or longer. Both diseases have no febrile phase and the main lesions occur only in the central nervous system. There seems little doubt that scrapie and kuru run in families and, in scrapie at least, there is a well recognised familial and breed incidence, whether or not one supports a genetic hypothesis for the disease.

The principal pathological changes in kuru are confined to the central nervous system and are characterized by marked proliferation and hypertrophy of the astrocytes throughout the brain. There is also diffuse neuronal degeneration, which is most severe in the cerebellum, and intracytoplasmic vacuolation in the large neurones.

Little information is available about the properties of the causative agent of kuru, but experimental transmission has been accomplished in chimpanzees

inoculated intracerebrally with a 10 per cent brain suspension from patients with kuru. The incubation period was initially between 18 and 38 months but, after 3 serial passages in chimpanzees, it was reduced to 10–12 months. Although the disease has been transmitted from human patients to rhesus and new world monkeys, there is no evidence that it affects mice and many other species of laboratory animals including poultry. Kuru virus is remarkably stable for many months to several years when stored at —70°C in the form of frozen tissues or brain tissue suspensions. It is also highly thermostable and its infectivity is not appreciably reduced following exposure of the virus to a temperature of 85°C for 30 minutes.

Very little is known about the natural method of spread of kuru. Although most workers believe that it is transmissible horizontally to women and vertically to their children, there is no evidence that outsiders have developed the disease after living in the affected territories. On the other hand, cases have developed over periods of up to several years among natives of the kuru region who have left the area; and in every case it was found that the patient came from families known to have suffered from kuru in the past.

Aleutian disease of mink

Synonyms
Aleutian disease. Viral plasmacytosis of mink.

Definition
Aleutian disease is a slowly progressive debilitating viral infection of mink involving the reticuloendothelial system, and which is characterized by diffuse proliferation of plasma cells, the production of very large amounts of gamma globulin and a persistent viraemia. It appears to be a collagen disease and the lesions are typical of a hypersensitivity or autoimmune phenomenon.

Hosts affected
Mink are the only natural hosts. Ferrets are susceptible to experimental infection and may develop lesions, but rarely succumb to the disease.

History and distribution
Aleutian disease was not recognised until 'blue' mink became fashionable in the 1940s and, as their numbers increased, farmers noted higher mortality rates than in other 'strains' of mink. The first scientific account of this novel disease of mink was published in 1956, and in 1962 three independent groups of workers established that the condition was infectious and probably of viral origin.

Aleutian disease was so named because originally

it was thought to affect only mink with the double recessive colour phase known as Aleutian. This abnormal pigmentation is responsible for the beautiful bluish coats which are highly prized by mink breeders. It is now known that all breeds of mink can contract the disease, although there is a greater hereditary predisposition in the homozygous recessive Aleutian genotype. At present it is one of the most serious infectious diseases of ranch-raised mink throughout the world.

Properties of the virus

The infectious nature of Aleutian disease has been amply confirmed by inoculation of susceptible mink with suspensions of diseased tissues, with cell-free filtrates and with material obtained by ultracentrifugation.

The causative agent is about 25 nm in diameter and is resistant to ether but only partially resistant to formalin (0.3 per cent for 2 weeks) and to heat, remaining infective in tissue suspensions at 80°C for 30 minutes and at 100°C for 3 minutes.

It has been reported that mink inoculated with DNA extracted from diseased spleens develop typical lesions of Aleutian disease, whereas control animals inoculated with enzyme-digested DNA remain healthy.

The agent has not been adapted to other hosts and no tissue culture system is known which supports virus growth.

Pathogenicity

Aleutian disease is a slowly progressive viral infection of mink which invariably terminates fatally after running a course of several months or even years.

Affected animals show progressive loss of weight resulting in severe emaciation, anaemia, uraemia and increased thirst, but no anorexia. There may also be signs of defective haemostasis with bleeding at the mouth and a tendency for haemorrhages to appear in the intestinal tract.

The most pronounced macroscopic lesions are seen in the kidneys which are usually enlarged and congested with petechial haemorrhages scattered over their surfaces in the early stages of the disease but become pale, shrunken and pitted in the later stages of the illness. Other abnormalities include enlargement of the spleen and lymph nodes and yellow-brown mottling of the liver substance.

The main microscopical findings are marked plasmacytosis of the spleen, kidneys, liver, lymph nodes and bone marrow, segmented periarteritis, proliferation of the bile ducts, glomerulitis and degenerative changes of the kidney tubules leading to atrophy and hyaline cast formation.

Serum protein studies show that most affected mink have a systemic proliferation of plasma cells with a marked hypergammaglobulinaemia. The pathological changes such as plasmacytosis, hypergammaglobulinaemia and vascular lesions are suggestive of an autoimmune response. This is supported by the fact that infected mink become positive to the Coombs' test and that the titres obtained parallel the severity of the tissue changes. Infected mink show a progressive increase in the amount of gammaglobulin in the serum which reaches significantly high levels by about 30 days after infection. Although the antibody unites with the virus, it is not able to inactivate the virus nor eliminate it from the host. Moreover, since the virus of Aleutian disease persists in the tissues, chronically infected mink generally develop infectious virus-antibody complexes which circulate in the blood and become deposited in the walls of arterial vessels in kidney glomeruli and other organs and probably give rise to the hyaline degeneration which is characteristic of the disease.

Growth of Aleutian disease virus in experimentally infected mink has a latent period of 6 days, then the virus titres rapidly rise to a peak at the 10th day after infection, when as much as 10^9 ID_{50}/gm of liver can be found. Viral titres subsequently fall to about 10^5 ID_{50}/gm of tissue several months after inoculation. Other genotypes of mink are also susceptible to infection with Aleutian disease virus but overt disease does not occur in experimentally infected ferrets. Natural subclinical infection has been described in ferrets maintained on ranches where Aleutian disease is prevalent in mink.

Ecology

Natural transmission of the agent occurs both horizontally and vertically. Thus, the virus may be transmitted by an affected dam to her kits in utero and also by contact among mink within the same cage. Although virus is shed in the urine, faeces and saliva, contact transmission does not always occur and it has frequently been noticed that only a number of animals in an infected litter develop symptoms of the disease. Moreover, fulminating outbreaks of Aleutian disease are unusual and in most instances losses increase slowly and steadily over the years until, on some ranches, almost all of the mink become affected.

There is a strong genetic predisposition to the disease and mink which are homozygous for the Aleutian gene for coat colour are generally affected with the more rapidly progressive form of the disease, whereas in non-Aleutian breeds the illness runs a more protracted course and may last for several months or years.

Diagnosis

The presence of a progressive, wasting disease and

the characteristic histopathological picture lead to a presumptive diagnosis of Aleutian disease.

A non-specific test called the Iodine Agglutination test (IAT) which detects large amounts of gamma-globulin in the sera, has been widely used to detect mink which should be culled from the breeding stock. The method is as follows: blood obtained by toenail clipping is collected in a capillary tube, allowed to clot and centrifuged. The serum is placed on a glass slide, mixed with a drop of iodine solution and examined for clumping or precipitation of granular material. The method is not very sensitive, however, and mink in the early stages of the disease do not react to the test since it takes between 3–5 weeks for gammaglobulin levels to be sufficiently high to be detectable by the IAT. Thus, false positive and false negative reactions may be obtained and these can result in either the destruction of animals which are not infected with Aleutian disease or the survival of infected animals with false negative reactions thereby perpetuating the infection on the farm. In 1971, however, Canadian workers devised a more sensitive method for detecting infection in naturally and experimentally infected mink. The technique known as counter-electrophoresis (CEP) involves electrophoresis of suspect serum and purified viral antigen in an agar gel and readily demonstrates specific antibody in sera from infected animals in the early stages of the disease. The method has the additional advantage that it also detects antibodies to Aleutian disease in infected mink that are not homozygous for the Aleutian gene and which show only a temporary increase in gammaglobulin levels. The viral antigen employed in the CEP test is prepared by fluorocarbon extraction from the spleen, liver and lymph nodes of experimentally infected mink 10 days after inoculation and prior to the onset of clinical signs of the disease. In the test system, the purified antigen diffuses towards the anode and the antibody towards the cathode, producing a thin line of precipitation if antibody is present. Antibodies against Aleutian disease can also be detected as early as 10 days after infection by means of an indirect immunofluorescence test. Conventional attempts to measure antibody have been unsuccessful and neither complement-fixation nor latex agglutination tests give unequivocal evidence of antinuclear or antigammaglobulin antibodies.

Control

There are no effective methods of prophylaxis and the most satisfactory means of control is based on the early detection of infection by counter-electro-phoresis tests and prompt slaughter of reacting animals from the stock.

Comment

Features of Aleutian disease which are shared by other slow virus infections include the following: slow insidious nature of the disease, inevitable development of clinical illness which terminates fatally after running a prolonged course of several months or years, persistent infection often associated with persistent viraemia, peaceful co-existence of virus and antibody, failure of immunity, genetic predisposition, vertical transmission and familial occurrence.

Viroids

The term 'viroid' has been introduced to denote a new class of subviral elements which are believed to be the smallest known agents of infectious disease. The first was discovered in 1967 during attempts to purify and characterize the causative agent of potato spindle tuber disease, and all viroids isolated sub-sequently have been from species of higher plants.

Viroids consist solely of a short strand of free nucleic acid with a molecular weight of approximately $7—10 \times 10^3$ daltons, which is much smaller than the genome of any known virus. Although the small amount of genetic material that viroids introduce into their hosts is sufficient only to code for 70 to 80 amino acids and, therefore, barely adequate to code for a very small protein, they are able to multiply in host cells and produce disease. The mechanisms by which they replicate are not understood, but it is possible that they are not a single molecular species but rather a population of several RNA molecules of similar length, with different nucleotide sequences, which together may comprise a double-stranded RNA genome of conventional size. This would explain how these agents can contain sufficient genetic information to cause replication in susceptible hosts.

Although the viroids so far identified cause disease of higher plants, it is tempting to speculate that they, or other low molecular weight RNAs, may be associated with a number of animal diseases e.g. scrapie, where viral aetiology has been suspected but where the causal agent has never been identified. Scrapie is the most likely candidate because of its resistance to nucleases and ultraviolet irradiation.

Further reading

ALPER T., CRAMP W.A., HAIG D.A. AND CLARK M.C. (1967) Does the agent of scrapie replicate without nucleic acid? *Nature*, **214**, 764.

ALPER T.D., HAIG D.A. AND CLARKE M.C. (1966) The exceptionally small size of the scrapie agent. *Biochemical and Biophysical Research Communications*, **22**, 278.

BRODY J.A., HENLE W. AND KOPROWSKI H. (1967) Chronic infectious neuropathic agents (CHINA) and other slow virus infections. *Current Topics in Microbiology and Immunology*, **40**, 1.

DICKINSON A.G. (1976) Scrapie in sheep and goats. In *Slow virus diseases of animals and man*. Ed. R.H. Kimberlin, pp. 210–241. Oxford, North-Holland Publishing Company.

DICKINSON A.G., MEIKLE V.M.H. AND FRASER H. (1968) Identification of a gene which controls the incubation period of some strains of scrapie agent in mice. *Journal of Comparative Pathology and Therapeutics*, **78**, 293.

DICKINSON A.G., STAMP J.T. AND RENWICK C.C. (1974) Maternal and lateral transmission of scrapie in sheep. *Journal of Comparative Pathology and Therapeutics*, **84**, 19.

DIENER T.O. (1972) Is the scrapie agent a viroid? *Nature (London)*, **235**, 218.

EKLUND C.M., HADLOW W.J. AND KENNEDY R.C. (1963) Some properties of the scrapie agent and its behaviour in mice. *Proceedings of the Society for Experimental Biology and Medicine*, **112**, 974.

EKLUND C.M., KENNEDY R.C. AND HADLOW W.J. (1967) Pathogenesis of scrapie virus infection in the mouse. *Journal of Infectious Diseases*, **117**, 15.

FIELD E.J. (1969) Slow virus infections of the nervous system. *International Review of Experimental Pathology*, **8**, 129.

FUCCILLO D.A., KURENT J.E. AND SEVER J.L. (1974) Slow virus diseases. *Annual Review of Microbiology*, **28**, 231.

GAJDUSEK D.C. (1967) Slow virus infections of the nervous system. *New England Journal of Medicine*, **276**, 392.

GAJDUSEK D.C. AND ZIGAS V. (1959) Kuru: clinical, pathological and epidemiological study of acute progressive degenerative disease of central nervous system among natives of Eastern Highlands of New Guinea, *American Journal of Medicine*, **26**, 442.

GAJDUSEK D.C., GIBBS C.J. AND ALPERS M. eds. (1965). Slow, latent and temperate virus infections. National Institute Neurol. Dis. Blind, Monograph No. 2. PHS Publication No. 1378, Washington, U.S. Government Print Office.

GORDON D.A., FRANKLIN A.E. AND KARSTAD L. (1967) Viral plasmacytosis (Aleutian disease) of mink resembling human collagen disease. *Canadian Medical Association Journal*, **96**, 1245.

GUDNADOTTIR M. (1974) Visna-Maedi in sheep. *Progress in Medical Virology*, **18**, 336.

HADLOW J. (1959) Scrapie and Kuru. *Lancet*, **2**, 289.

HOTCHIN J. (1967) Immune and autoimmune reactions in the pathogenesis of slow virus disease.

Current Topics in Microbiology and Immunology, **40**, 33.

HOTCHIN J. (1971) A concept of persistent virus infection. In, Viruses affecting man and animals, eds. M. Sanders M. Schaeffer. p. 213. St. Louis: Warren H. Green, Inc.

HUNTER G.D. (1972) Scrapie. A prototype slow infection. *Journal of Infectious Diseases*, **125**, 427.

HUNTER G.D. (1974) Scrapie. *Progress in Medical Virology*, **18**, 289.

KARSTAD L. (1967) Aleutian disease of mink. *Current Topics in Microbiology and Immunology*, **40**, 9.

MARSH R.F. AND HANSON R.P. (1969) Physical and chemical properties of the transmissible mink encephalopathy agent. *Journal of Virology*, **3**, 176.

MARSH R.F., SEMANCIK J.S., MEDAPPA K.C., HANSON R.P. AND RUECKERT R.R. (1974) Scrapie and transmissible mink encephalopathy: search for infectious nucleic acid. *Journal of Virology*, **13**, 993.

PATTISON I. (1965/6) Scrapie. In, Veterinary Annual, ed. W.A. Pool, Seventh edition, p. 138. Bristol: John Wright & Sons Ltd.

PATTISON I.H. AND JONES K.M. (1967) The possible nature of the transmissible agent of scrapie. *Veterinary Record*, **80**, 2.

PORTER D.D. (1971) A quantitative review of the slow virus landscape. *Progress in Medical Virology*, **13**, 339.

PORTER D.D., LARSEN A.E. AND PORTER H.G. (1969) The pathogenesis of Aleutian disease of mink. I. *In vivo* viral replication and the host antibody response to viral antigen. *Journal of Experimental Medicine*, **130**, 575.

SIGURDSSON B. (1954) Rida, a chronic encephalitis of sheep. With general remarks on infections which develop slowly and some of their special characteristics. *British Veterinary Journal*, **110**, 341.

SIGURDSSON B., THORMAR H. AND PALSSON P.A. (1960) Cultivation of visna virus in tissue culture. *Archiv für die gesamte Virusforschung*, **10**, 368.

STAMP J.T. (1967). Scrapie and its wider implications. *British Medical Bulletin*, **23**, 133.

STAMP J.T., BROTHERSTON J.G., ZLOTNIK I., MACKAY J.M.K. AND SMITH W. (1959) Further studies on scrapie. *Journal of Comparative Pathology and Therapeutics*, **69**, 268.

THORMAR H. (1965) A comparison of visna and maedi viruses. I. Physical, chemical and biological properties. *Research in Veterinary Science*, **6**, 117.

THORMAR H., LIN F.H. AND TROWBRIDGE R.S. (1974) Visna and maedi viruses in tissue culture. *Progress in Medical Virology*, **18**, 323.

THORMAR H. AND PALSSON P.A. (1967) Visna and maedi—two slow infections of sheep and their etiological agents. *Perspectives in Virology*, **5**, 291.

WALKER D.L. (1964) The viral carrier state in animal cell cultures. *Progress in Medical Virology*, **6**, 111.

WARD R.L., PORTER D.D. AND STEVENS J.G. (1974) Nature of the scrapie agent: evidence against a viroid. *Journal of Virology*, **14**, 1099.

WILSON D.R., ANDERSON R.D. AND SMITH W. (1950) Studies in scrapie. *Journal of Comparative Pathology and Therapeutics*, **60**, 267.

Index

Page numbers of pricipal references are shown in **bold** print
Page numbers of figures are shown in *italics*.

A

B

D

E

F

G

H

I

M

N

T